PRINCIPLES OF
Inpatient Psychiatry

PRINCIPLES OF
Inpatient Psychiatry

Editors

Fred Ovsiew, MD

Professor of Clinical Psychiatry and Behavioral Sciences
Feinberg School of Medicine
Northwestern University
Fellow and President
American Neuropsychiatric Association
Chicago, Illinois

Richard L. Munich, MD

Clinical Professor of Psychiatry
Weill-Cornell Medical College
Training and Supervising Analyst
Center for Psychoanalytic Training & Research
Columbia University College of Physicians & Surgeons
New York, New York

Wolters Kluwer | Lippincott Williams & Wilkins
Health
Philadelphia · Baltimore · New York · London
Buenos Aires · Hong Kong · Sydney · Tokyo

Acquisitions Editor: Charley Mitchell
Managing Editor: Sirkka Howes
Project Manager: Cindy Oberle
Manufacturing Manager: Kathleen Brown
Marketing Manager: Sharon Zinner
Design Coordinator: Steven Druding
Production Services: Laserwords Private Limited, Chennai, India

Printed in the USA

Library of Congress Cataloging-in-Publication Data

Principles of inpatient psychiatry / editors, Fred Ovsiew, Richard Munich.—1st ed.
   p. ; cm.
  Includes bibliographical references and index.
  ISBN-13: 978-0-7817-7214-3
  ISBN-10: 0-7817-7214-1
  1. Psychiatric hospital care. I. Ovsiew, Fred, 1949- II. Munich, Richard.
  [DNLM: 1. Mental Disorders—diagnosis. 2. Mental Disorders—therapy. 3. Hospitalization. WM 140 P957 2009]
  RC439.P8145 2009
  362.2'1—dc22

            2008035986

Care has been taken to confirm the accuracy of the information presented and to describe generally accepted practices. However, the authors, editors, and publisher are not responsible for errors or omissions or for any consequences from application of the information in this book and make no warranty, expressed or implied, with respect to the currency, completeness, or accuracy of the contents of the publication. Application of the information in a particular situation remains the professional responsibility of the practitioner.

The authors, editors, and publisher have exerted every effort to ensure that drug selection and dosage set forth in this text are in accordance with current recommendations and practice at the time of publication. However, in view of ongoing research, changes in government regulations, and the constant flow of information relating to drug therapy and drug reactions, the reader is urged to check the package insert for each drug for any change in indications and dosage and for added warnings and precautions. This is particularly important when the recommended agent is a new or infrequently employed drug.

Some drugs and medical devices presented in this publication have Food and Drug Administration (FDA) clearance for limited use in restricted research settings. It is the responsibility of health care providers to ascertain the FDA status of each drug or device planned for use in their clinical practice.

To purchase additional copies of this book, call our customer service department at (800) 638-3030 or fax orders to (301) 223-2320. International customers should call (301) 223-2300.

Visit Lippincott Williams & Wilkins on the Internet: at LWW.com. Lippincott Williams & Wilkins customer service representatives are available from 8:30 AM to 6 PM, EST.

                                  10 9 8 7 6 5 4 3 2 1

For LL, G, and A—FO

For Adrienne, Matthew, Edwin, and Andrea—RLM

List of Contributors

George S. Alexopoulos, MD
Professor of Psychiatry
Weill Medical College of Cornell University;
Director, Weill-Cornell Institute
 of Geriatric Psychiatry
New York Presbyterian Hospital
White Plains, New York

James J. Amos, MD
Associate Professor of Psychiatry
University of Iowa;
Psychiatrist
The University of Iowa Hospitals and Clinics
Iowa City, Iowa

Arnold E. Andersen, MD
Professor of Psychiatry
University of Iowa;
Medical Director
Eating Disorder Program
Department of Psychiatry
University of Iowa Hospitals and Clinics
Iowa City, Iowa

C. Alan Anderson, MD
Professor of Neurology, Psychiatry, and Emergency
 Medicine
University of Colorado Denver - School of Medicine
Aurora, Colorado;
Staff Neurologist
Denver Veterans Affairs Medical Center
Denver, Colorado

Arash Ansari, MD
Instructor
Department of Psychiatry
Harvard University;
Attending Psychiatrist
Faulkner Hospital
Boston, Massachusetts

David B. Arciniegas, MD
Associate Professor of Psychiatry and Neurology
University of Colorado Denver - School of Medicine;
Medical Director
Brain Injury Rehabilitation Unit
HealthONE Spalding Rehabilitation Hospital
Aurora, Colorado

Stan D. Arkow, MD
Associate Clinical Professor of Psychiatry
Columbia University College of Physicians
 and Surgeons;
Associate Attending Psychiatrist
Unit Chief of Inpatient Psychiatry
New York Presbyterian Hospital
Columbia-Presbyterian Milstein Pavilion
New York, New York

Anthony W. Bateman, MD, FRCPsych
Consultant Psychiatrist in Psychotherapy
Halliwick Unit, St. Ann's Hospital
Barnet, Enfield, and Haringey Mental Health Trust;
Visiting Professor
University College London
London, England;
Visiting Consultant
The Menninger Clinic
 and the Menninger Department of Psychiatry
 and Behavioral Science
Baylor College of Medicine
Houston, Texas

Mace Beckson, MD
Clinical Professor
Department of Psychiatry and Biobehavioral Science
University of California;
Medical Director
Psychiatric Intensive Care Unit
Department of Psychiatry and Mental Health
VA Greater Los Angeles Healthcare System
Los Angeles, California

W. R. Murray Bennett, MD, FRCPC
Assistant Professor of Psychiatry
University of Washington;
Attending Psychiatrist
Harborview Medical Center
Seattle, Washington

Wayne A. Bowers, PhD
Professor of Psychiatry
University of Iowa;
Director
Eating Disorder Program
Department of Psychiatry
University of Iowa Hospitals and Clinics
Iowa City, Iowa

Peter Burnett, FRANZCP
Clinical Associate Professor
Department of Psychiatry
University of Melbourne;
Medical Director
Orygen Youth Health
Victoria, Australia

Norma V. L. Clarke, MD
Assistant Professor
Menninger Department of Psychiatry
   and Behavioral Sciences
Baylor College of Medicine;
Medical Director
Adolescent Treatment Program
The Menninger Clinic
Houston, Texas

C. Edward Coffey, MD
Kathleen and Earl Ward Chair of Psychiatry
Professor of Psychiatry and Neurology
Wayne State University
Henry Ford Campus;
Vice President
Behavioral Health Services
Henry Ford Health System
Detroit, Michigan

Christine L. Dunn, MA
Research Associate in Psychiatry
Yale University School of Medicine
Yale Program for Recovery & Community Health
Yale-New Haven Psychiatric Hospital
New Haven, Connecticut

Kay Evans, RN, MS, ARNP
Advance Practice Nurse in Psychiatry
University of Iowa;
Eating Disorder Program
Department of Psychiatry
University of Iowa Hospitals and Clinics
Iowa City, Iowa

**Richard Fraser, MBBS, MSc,
MRCPsych, FRANZCP**
Honorary Fellow
University of Melbourne;
Consultant Psychiatrist
Orygen Youth Health
Victoria, Australia

Jeffrey L. Geller, MD, MPH
Professor of Psychiatry;
Director of Public Sector Psychiatry
University of Massachusetts Medical School
Worcester, Massachusetts

Pamela K. Greene, PhD, RN
Adjunct Faculty
Department of Psychiatry
Baylor College of Medicine;
Vice President of Patient Care Services
   and Chief Nursing Office
The Menninger Clinic
Houston, Texas

Sarah Guzofski, MD
Department of Psychiatry
University of Massachusetts Medical School
Worcester, Massachusetts

David A. Kahn, MD
Clinical Professor and Vice Chair for Clinical Affairs
Department of Psychiatry
Columbia University;
Attending Psychiatrist
Columbia University Medical Center
New York Presbyterian Hospital
New York, New York

Balkrishna Kalayam, MD
Associate Professor of Psychiatry
Weill Medical College of Cornell University;
Associate Attending Psychiatrist
New York Presbyterian Hospital
White Plains, New York

Alice Keski-Valkama, MD
Vanha Vaasa Hospital,
Vaasa, Finland

Vicki Kijewski, MD
Clinical Assistant Professor of Medicine
   and Psychiatry
University of Iowa
Iowa City, Iowa

Dimitris N. Kiosses, PhD
Assistant Professor of Psychology
Weill Medical College of Cornell University;
Assistant Attending Psychologist
New York Presbyterian Hospital
White Plains, New York

Sibel A. Klimstra, MD
Associate Professor of Clinical Psychiatry
Weill Medical College of Cornell University
New York, New York;
Associate Vice Chair for Education
Department of Psychiatry
New York-Presbyterian Hopsital-Payne
   Whitney Westchester
White Plains, New York

Walter Knysz, III, MD
Director
Consultation-Liaison Psychiatry;
Assistant Director
Brain Stimulation Center
Department of Psychiatry
Henry Ford Hospital
Detroit, Michigan

Leonard S. Lai, MD
Clinical Instructor
Department of Psychiatry
Harvard Medical School;
Attending Psychiatrist
Faulkner Hospital
Boston, Massachusetts

Vassilios Latoussakis, MD
Research Fellow in Psychiatry
Weill Medical College of Cornell
    University;
Assistant Attending Psychiatrist
New York Presbyterian Hospital
White Plains, New York

Margo Lauterbach, MD
Staff Psychiatrist
Sheppard Pratt Health System
Neuropsychiatry Program
Baltimore, Maryland

David Lovinger, MD
Assistant Professor of Medicine
University of Chicago
Division Chief, Hospital Medicine
NorthShore University HealthSystem
New York

Patrick McGorry, MD
Professor of Psychiatry
University of Melbourne;
Director of Psychiatry
Orygen Youth Health
Melbourne, Australia

Evan D. Murray, MD
Instructor in Neurology
Harvard Medical School
Boston, Massachusetts;
Assistant in Neurology
McLean Hospital
Belmont, Massachusetts

Richard L. Munich, MD
Clinical Professor of Psychiatry
Weill-Cornell Medical College;
Training and Supervising Analyst
Center for Psychoanalytic Training & Research
Columbia University College of Physicians
    & Surgeons
New York, New York

Flynn O'Malley, PhD
Associate Professor
Menninger Department of Psychiatry
    and Behavioral Sciences
Baylor College of Medicine;
Director, Compass Program
Senior Clinical Psychologist
The Menninger Clinic
Houston, Texas

David N. Osser, MD
Associate Professor of Psychiatry
Harvard Medical School
Boston, Massachusetts;
Associate Medical Director
Taunton State Hospital,
Taunton, Massachusetts

Fred Ovsiew, MD
Professor of Clinical Psychiatry
    and Behavioral Sciences
Feinberg School of Medicine
Northwestern University
Fellow and President
American Neuropsychiatric Association
Chicago, Illinois

Kenneth C. Potts, MD
Assistant Professor of Psychiatry
Harvard Medical School;
Associate Chief of Psychiatry
Faulkner Hospital
Boston, Massachusetts

Bruce H. Price, MD
Associate Professor of Neurology
Harvard Medical School
Boston, Massachusetts;
Chief, Department of Neurology
McLean Hospital
Belmont, Massachusetts

Cynthia A. Pristach, MD
Professor of Psychiatry
State University of New York at Buffalo;
Director of Residency Training
Department of Psychiatry
Erie County Medical Center
Buffalo, New York

Richard K. Ries, MD
Professor of Psychiatry
University of Washington;
Director of Outpatient Addictions
Psychiatric and Dual Disorder Services
Harborview Medical Center
Seattle, Washington

L. Mark Russakoff, MD
Director of Psychiatry
Phelps Memorial Hospital Center
Sleepy Hollow, New York

Eila Sailas, MD
National Research Centre for Welfare
   and Health
Helsinki, Finland;
Kellokoski Hospital
Kellokoski, Finland

Paul M. Schoenfeld, MD
Instructor
Department of Psychiatry
Harvard Medical School;
Attending Psychiatrist
Faulkner Hospital
Boston, Massachusetts

William H. Sledge, MD
George D. & Esther S. Gross Professor
   of Psychiatry
Yale University School of Medicine;
Medical Director
Yale-New Haven Psychiatric Hospital
New Haven, Connecticut

Susan Turner, MD
Assistant Clinical Professor of Psychiatry
Columbia University College of Physicians
   and Surgeons;
Assistant Attending Psychiatrist
New York Presbyterian Hospital
Columbia-Presbyterian Milstein Pavilion
New York, New York

Gabor Vari, MD
Chief Resident
Department of Psychiatry
UCLA Semel Institute;
UCLA Neurpsychiatric Hospital
Los Angeles, California

Jason P. Veitengruber, MD
Acting Instructor
Department of Psychiatry
University of Washington;
Assistant Medical Director
Inpatient Psychiatry
Harborview Medical Center
Seattle, Washington

Subhdeep Virk, MD
Assistant Professor of Psychiatry
Ohio State University
Ohio State University Medical Center
Columbus, Ohio

Kristian Wahlbeck, MD, MScD
Department of Psychiatry
University of Helsinki
Helsinki, Finland

Robert Weinstock, MD
Clinical professor
Department of Psychiatry and Biobehavioral Science
University of California
California, Los Angeles

Christine E. Yuodelis-Flores, MD
Clinical Associate Professor of Psychiatry
   and Behavioral Sciences
University of Washington;
Attending Psychiatrist
Harborview Medical Center
Seattle, Washington

Preface

Psychiatry, unlike other medical specialties, originated in hospital practice, namely in the asylums of the early 19th century.[1] In a peculiar reversal over the course of that century, what had been the province of neurology—the outpatient care of patients with "nervous disorders," what we would now likely consider relatively mild forms of mood and anxiety disorders as well as hysteria—became the center of psychiatric practice, and some of what had been the core of hospital psychiatry moved into the domain of neurology and general medicine.[2]

In the last few decades, the distinctive features of hospital care in general medicine have been emphasized, giving rise to a corps of hospitalists who specialize in the inpatient care of the acutely ill. Psychiatry has had its hospitalists for much longer, as for some time psychiatric practice has been split between those more involved in hospital care of the sickest psychiatric patients and those who confine their practice to outpatients. To be frank, psychiatry may have had its hospitalists in part by default, as some psychiatrists who saw only outpatients may have been avoiding the most seriously ill. Yet without doubt the sickest of psychiatric patients are still with us.

It is time, we felt, for the distinctive features of inpatient psychiatric management to come under scrutiny, for hospital psychiatry to take its place beside hospital medicine, surgery, and pediatrics as a self-conscious domain of practice. Further, inpatient psychiatric practice has changed substantially over recent years, and the process of change has not ceased. As length of stay has shortened, many elements once taken for granted as best practice have fallen into disuse: graded privileges, for example, or the routine use of psychotherapeutic interventions. At the same time, our capacity to help patients has advanced because of improvements in both pharmacologic and psychological techniques. It is time as well, we felt, for the principles of best contemporary inpatient practice to come under scrutiny, and for our field to make an effort to preserve what should be preserved from an earlier era of practice. A grasp of contemporary inpatient psychiatry as best practiced, we thought, would be helpful to those just learning about psychiatric illness and management in residency; to those who have occasional inpatient cases and need to know what to hope and work for during the inpatient stay; and to those who (like us) have focused their careers on the inpatient venue. We told our contributors not to review the basics of general psychiatry, and the reader of this volume will not find, for example, discussions of the diagnostic criteria for mania or the epidemiology of schizophrenia. We asked them to discuss what was distinctive and essential in inpatient care. As we worked with them, reviewed their drafts, and read the final product that the reader sees in this volume, we believed we could identify a number of principles of inpatient psychiatry, principles that emerged spontaneously and multicentrically, not because we as editors suggested them but because good clinicians have found common ground.

Let us list some of these principles:

1. A comprehensive database: the inpatient setting offers the opportunity to assemble comprehensive information about and to formulate a comprehensive understanding of patients whose outpatient care may have failed to elucidate the entire clinical picture. Obtaining a detailed history should include requesting medical records from prior care (especially inpatient care) and obtaining reports from collateral informants. A medication history is of particular importance in patients whose presentation suggests treatment-unresponsiveness. The understanding gained from these data may yield ideas for new treatment efforts, both pharmacologic and psychological. The formal diagnosis may change during the admission, but even if it does not the admission may produce an altered understanding of what is central to the patient's care.

---

[1]Ovsiew F, Jobe T. Neuropsychiatry in the history of mental health services. In: Ovsiew F, ed. *Neuropsychiatry and mental health services*. Washington, DC: American Psychiatric Press; 1999:1–21.
[2]Blustein BE. "A hollow square of psychological science": American neurologists and psychiatrists in conflict. In: Scull A, ed. *Madhouses, mad-doctors, and madmen: the social history of psychiatry in the victorian era*. Philadelphia: University of Pennsylvania Press; 1981:241–270.

2. Continuity of care and discharge planning: integrating inpatient care with the outpatient care that preceded it as well as the outpatient care that will follow it is of the highest importance. Failing to do so may mean wasted effort, both in that the inpatient treaters may be attempting interventions already attempted unsuccessfully before admission or failing to utilize those that have proved successful and in that the posthospital treatment may fail to capitalize on the advances achieved during the hospitalization. The hospital stay, for many patients, represents only a small portion of their mental health career. Arrogance on the part of inpatient treaters, acting as if only their own efforts matter, has no place.

3. An integrated team: the inpatient psychiatrist forms part of, and takes a leadership role on, an interdisciplinary team. Certain difficult patients may provoke strains that require explicit attention to the integration of the team, but for all patients attention must be given to the ways the skills and resources of the members of the team can be utilized. Attention to the therapeutic alliance is always of importance, and because patients' relationships to different team members may differ the astute psychiatrist takes advantage of these developing and diverse attachments.

4. Work with families: patients enter the hospital because they are unable to sustain themselves outside the hospital. This simple fact in itself points to the necessity of attending to, working with, and resolving problems in patients' networks of support in their natural environment. Some patients pose problematic behaviors that would tax any family or support network, and no blame should be attached to the presence of problems in the family. But turning away from these problems will not benefit either the patient or the family in the long run.

5. Attention to meaning: the move away from formal psychotherapy over recent years and the impossibility of conducting such treatment in many inpatient cases do not relieve the clinical team of the responsibility to attempt to understand the patient psychologically. Achieving an understanding of the patient pays off in improved specificity and acceptability of interventions in all treatment domains.

6. Medical sophistication: psychiatric patients frequently suffer from general-medical illnesses and frequently have behavioral and social obstacles to obtaining care for these illnesses. These illnesses may contribute to or cause psychiatric symptoms or may result from psychiatric treatments. Inpatient psychiatrists incur responsibility for managing these illnesses (with whatever consultative assistance and whatever degree of urgency are appropriate to the clinical situation). Knowing how to manage these supposedly nonpsychiatric problems is an intrinsic part of inpatient psychiatric practice. Finding ways to integrate psychological, behavioral, psychopharmacological, general-medical, and neuropsychiatric care on the inpatient unit will remain a challenge for the psychiatry of the future.

We have organized the volume in the following way. The first eight chapters, which compose the first section of the book, describe perspectives that are relevant to the care of most or all psychiatric inpatients. In the second section of the book, particular clinical situations or contexts are reviewed with greater specificity. In some chapters, clinical vignettes highlight points of diagnosis or management. Each chapter can stand alone, but frequent cross-references are meant to help the reader pursue matters mentioned in one chapter but discussed in greater detail in another.

Finally, the authors wish to thank Stuart Yudofsky, MD, who recommended that we work together on this book. And both authors gratefully acknowledge the host of mentors, staff members, and patients who have taught us what we know about inpatient psychiatry.

Contents

SECTION I Approaches

SECTION II Clinical Contexts

Approaches

CHAPTER 1

The Ins and Outs of 200 Years of Psychiatric Hospitals in the United States

JEFFREY L. GELLER, SARAH GUZOFSKI, AND MARGO LAUTERBACH

In 1841, Dorothea Dix, then a 39-year-old former school mistress with a history of poor health and groping for a mission, visited the East Cambridge House of Corrections (Massachusetts) on March 28 to find therein a group of women obviously insane.[1] Dix then traveled throughout Massachusetts examining the almshouses and jails, noting specifically the presence and condition of the insane. This resulted in her *Memorial to the Legislature of Massachusetts* in 1843:

> Gentlemen ... I proceed briefly to explain what has conducted me before you unsolicited and unsustained ... I come to present the strong claims of suffering humanity. I come to place before the Legislature of Massachusetts the condition of the miserable, the desolate, the outcast. I come as the advocate of helpless, forgotten, insane, and idiotic men and women; of beings sunk to a condition from which the most unconcerned would start with real horror; of beings wretched in our prisons, and more wretched in our almshouses. And I cannot suppose it needful to employ earnest persuasion, or stubborn argument, in order to arrest and fix attention upon a subject only the more strongly pressing in its claims because it is revolting and disgusting in its details... The condition of human beings, reduced to the extremist states of degradation and misery, cannot be exhibited in softened language, or adorn a polished page.
>   I ... call your attention to the present state of insane persons confined within this Commonwealth, in cages, closets, cellars, stalls, pens! Chained, naked, beaten with rods, and lashed into obedience.[2]

Dix then catalogued specific examples throughout the Commonwealth before indicating,

> This state of things unquestionably retards the recovery of the few who do recover their reason under such circumstances, and may render those permanently insane who under other circumstances might have been restored to their right mind.[2]

Basically, Dix's message provided two reasons to build and/or expand state hospitals: (a) it is the right/moral thing to do and (b) it will return those curable mentally ill to the rolls of taxpayer and remove them from public expense.

Before Dix began her campaign to elicit states' support for the care and treatment of the insane, there had been the establishment of private psychiatric hospitals which met some of the states' needs by having the state purchase hospital beds through various financial arrangements.[3] With some exceptions—Kentucky (1824) and South Carolina (1828)—the earlier states of the United States had private hospitals before they had public ones (see Table 1.1).

States did respond to Dix's plea—by 1845 she had traveled 10,000 miles, visited 18 state penitentiaries, 300 county jails and houses of correction, >500 almshouses, and had assisted in the establishment of 6 hospitals for the insane.[1] But the state hospitals ran into their own financial difficulties as there were too many pauper cases and too few middle class paying patients. State hospitals even advertised to get paying patients including, in some instances, accepting slaves as payment.[4]

TABLE 1.1 OPENING DATES OF FIRST PRIVATE AND FIRST STATE HOSPITAL IN SELECTED STATES

	Facility and Opening Date	
State	**Private**	**Public**
CT	Hartford Retreat (1824)	Connecticut Hospital for the Insane (1868)
MD	Mount Hope Retreat (1840)	Maryland Hospital for the Insane (1798)
MA	McLean Asylum (1818)	Worcester State Lunatic Hospital (1833)
NY	New York Hospital—Bloomingdale (1791/1821)	Utica State Lunatic Asylum (1843)
PA	Pennsylvania Hospital (1752/1841) Friends Asylum (1817)	Pennsylvania State Lunatic Hospital (1851)
RI	Butler Hospital (1847)	Rhode Island State Asylum for the Incurable Insane (1870)
VT	Brattleboro Retreat (1836)	Vermont State Hospital for the Insane (1891)

Noting both prospective patients' needs and the states' struggling finances, Dix modified her approach, moving to the federal government for support. In 1848, Dix presented a *Memorial to the US Congress* requesting 5,000,000 acres (in later versions this was as high as 12,000,000 acres) of federal land, the income from which would be distributed to the states for support of the indigent insane.

Dix made some quite interesting points in her presentation to the legislature about the nature of insanity: the rate of insanity was increasing faster than population growth; many were not well informed about the "great and inadequate relieved distress of the insane;" "statesmen, politicians and merchants" were particularly susceptible to insanity; society was partly to blame because "little care is given in cultivating the moral affections in proportion with the intellectual development of the people;" and insanity, particularly in recently developed cases is curable, but to not treat it is to "condemn them [insane persons] to mental death."[5]

Dix argued that society had obligations to this population. First, she stated, "Humanity requires that every insane person should receive the care appropriate to his condition, in which the integrity of the judgment is destroyed, and the reasoning faculties confused or prostrated." Second, there was an obligation to "secure the public welfare" by protecting citizens from the "frequently manifested dangerous propensities of the insane." Third, public welfare would benefit from the "restoration [of the insane] to usefulness as citizen . . . ."[5]

Dix believed that "under ordinary circumstances, and where there is no organic lesion of the brain, no disease is more manageable or more easily cured than insanity." But to accomplish this, "special appliances" are required and because these are not readily obtainable or sustainable in families, towns, or cities there need to be hospitals.[5]

At the time Dix delivered her address there were, according to her, 20 state hospitals, several incorporated hospitals, and several small private establishments.[5] Contemporary research by one of the authors (JLG) indicates that of psychiatric hospitals actually treating patients, there were 15 state hospitals; 2 county hospitals; 2 municipal hospitals; 6 larger private psychiatric hospitals; and at least 4 other facilities, which were the earliest examples of small psychiatric hospitals, many of which were opened and closed by the same psychiatrist, that is, depended upon him for the treatment of patients.[3,6] These institutions, Dix asserted, could not meet the needs of the insane population of the United States. Dix also noted that the public hospitals were particularly stressed by the number of admissions represented by "uneducated foreigners."[5]

Hospitals were a powerful tool in the fight against insanity: "under well-directed hospital care, *recovery is the rule*—*incurable* permanent insanity the exception." And for those who could not be cured, hospitals would provide a "secure and comfortable" environment. For both classes of the insane, hospitals provided the opportunity for patients "to work under the direction of suitable attendants" such that they "recover from utter helplessness to a considerable degree of activity and capacity for various employments" (an early comment on hospital-initiated rehabilitation and recovery).[5]

Dix lobbied for her bill in Congress through four presidential administrations—Polk (1845 to 1849), Taylor (1849 to 1850), Fillmore (1850 to 1853), and Pierce (1853 to 1857) before it was passed by both houses of Congress. Pierce, however, vetoed the Bill in 1854, indicating:

I cannot but repeat what I have before expressed, that if the several States, many of which have already laid the foundation of munificent establishments of local beneficence, and nearly all of which are proceeding to establish them, shall be led to suppose, as they will be, should this bill become a law, that Congress is to make provision for such objects, the fountains of charity will be dried up at home, and the several States, instead of bestowing their own means on the social wants of their own people, may themselves, through the strong temptation, which appeals to States as to individuals, become humble suppliants for the bounty of the Federal Government, reversing their true relation to this Union.[7]

Interestingly enough, the medical profession favored Pierce's position, not Dix's. An editorial in the *Boston Medical and Surgical Journal*[8] indicated, "asylums are now quite numerous in the States, and gradually increasing, and it seems legitimate to belong to them to provide for the unfortunate lunatics within their own jurisdiction" (p 25). Concern was expressed that if the federal government took responsibility for asylum-based care and treatment, "prodigious efforts would be made to empty local hospitals into the great national reservoir of insanity" (p 25). The *Boston Medical and Surgical Journal* editorialist thought the federal government should be responsible only for "soldiers and sailors who have lost their reason while in the service of their country" (p 26). Perhaps even more surprising, organized psychiatry of the era—the Association of Medical Superintendents of American Institution for the Insane (later to become the American Psychiatric Association)—entirely concurred.[9]

It took a nonpsychiatric physician, but one who had done assessments for the need for psychiatric hospitals and had run a small private facility of his own, Edward Jarvis,[10] to most clearly articulate the 19th century position on the cost of care versus the cost of treatment. Jarvis explained,

A man of twenty years of age, if sane, has an average life of 39.48 years, while if insane he has but an average life of 21.31 years if not restored to health. The average time for restoring to health the insane who apply for treatment upon the early symptoms of disease is twenty-six weeks. At $4 per week, which was the average cost in the three State Lunatic Asylums in Massachusetts for the past year, this amounts to $104, to which is added $30 for each patient, for the cost of rent or interest on the value of the hospital, etc., for six months, making an average cost of $134 for restoration to health. If not restored to health, the family or State must be at an expense of $156 a year for 21.31 years, and must also lose the patient's earnings for the 39.48 years which he would have made if well. The cost of the patient's support is estimated at $2,121, while the loss of his future labor, if he becomes insane at twenty years of age, is estimated at $2,665.37, making a total loss of $4,786.37 if not cured; while, if cured in the average time of twenty-six weeks at a cost of $134, there will be a gain to the family or to the State of $4,652.[10]

Therefore, much of what defines the ensuing social history of the psychiatric hospital through the early years of the 21st century had been laid out by the mid-19th: What role should inpatient treatment play in the care of persons with mental illness? In terms of the public sector, what governmental entity should bear the cost for care and treatment of persons without financial resources who had serious mental illness? If the federal government became more active in this enterprise, would states attempt to cost shift this burden to the federal payor? Should there be separate hospitals for members of the armed forces and for veterans? What was the role of the private sector? What are the public safety functions of psychiatric hospitals—safety to the individual herself/himself and to society at large? Just how dangerous are persons with mental illness, the level and scope of dangerousness determining the magnitude of the number of inpatient psychiatric beds? And how do we balance cost benefit and humanitarian concerns where considering how most effectively we deal with the needs of persons with chronic mental illnesses?

As public psychiatric institutions grew in number and in size, and so too private facilities apparently grew in number (although how many closed in relationship to how many opened is not known) through the second half of the 19th century,[3] the leaders of American psychiatry debated about the clinical methods of inpatient psychiatric treatment. Because all were superintendents of either public or private hospitals, they were quite familiar with the issues. Woodward[11] noted how the insane were benefiting from hospitals' abandonment of punitive treatments and adoption of beneficent ones.

Nichols[12] commented on the decrease in the use of seclusion and restraint. Awl[13] opined that a hospital's reputation was dependent on its cures and discharges, while Ray[14] complained that the distrust of hospitals was due to damning communication by patients to all too "willing ears."

Hospitals, it was noted, needed to be well constructed, for to do otherwise was false economy;[15] were of necessity large, but better if they were small (250 patients in that era);[16] and were overwhelmed by "the rising tide of indiscriminate lunacy pouring through the wards."[17] Contact with family during an episode of illness was a matter of debate: McFarland[18] argued for treatment within the family when possible while Buttolph[19] thought removal to a hospital separated the individual from the persons and place associated with the onset.

The use of biologic treatments in the hospital was also under consideration. Woodward[11] expressed pleasure with the abandonment of the mechanical swing and bloodletting. Nichols[12] remarked that sedation should not be used as a substitute for restraint while Everts warned against what he considered to be the general overuse of medication. Andrews (1893) proclaimed near the end of the century that "remedies are now employed to meet the symptoms of disease in a more rational manner than ever before."

While paying attention to the clinical needs of patients, psychiatric leaders did not disregard issues of costs. Nichols[16] warned how costly treatment is; Earle[20] pointed out that expense did not necessarily correlate with quality; and Ray[14] complained that all too often cost overrode all other considerations in the care and treatment of the insane.

As can be seen, just as with the social questions about psychiatric hospitals, the clinical questions for the ensuing century are pretty much set by the end of the 19th century. How well did the following generations deal with the roles, functions, and financing of psychiatric hospitals laid out by the pioneers of American psychiatric hospitals?

The Development of an Array of Types of Psychiatric Hospitals

The "mental hygiene" movement (1890 to 1950) followed the period of asylum-based care by expanding treatment into alternate psychiatric settings. The integration of psychiatry into general health care began as psychiatric hospitals and clinics focused on the scientific basis of mental illness and on prevention. Mental illness was thought to be a product of faulty environments or genetics, or both. Hence, there was a focus on child guidance clinics and on eugenics. Mental health service expanded to include new disciplines, social workers, and new locations, outpatient clinics.[21]

Despite these efforts, effective treatments for serious mental illness lagged behind, and persons with mental illness continued to suffer as outpatient treatment proved to be no more successful than the care previously received in asylums. This meant that asylums continued to play a key function, but budgetary demands and overcrowding impaired their efficacy. Persons with mental illness and the elderly were being treated ever more aggressively with insulin shock, electroconvulsive therapy, and psychosurgery in attempts to abate the scourge of insanity.[22] Simultaneously, psychoanalysis flourished and psychiatrists began leaving asylums to care for "healthier" patients in private practice.[23]

General hospital psychiatric units date back to Benjamin Franklin and Benjamin Rush who, in 1783, founded the first of such units in the United States at the Pennsylvania Hospital.[24] General hospital psychiatry, however, was largely dormant and did not reemerge until the 1930s. It flourished thereafter due to interweaving forces throughout the medical community. A scientific focus on psychiatry as part of the medical model for illness and the biopsychosocial approach to patients played key roles in this transformation. At its start though, the evolution of psychiatry in the general hospital was driven by the social and economic climate of the era. General hospitals were vulnerable to the rising costs of health care and particularly to unused beds. Moving the treatment of psychiatric patients into general hospitals allowed these hospitals to operate low-cost beds and permitted other medical disciplines to play a larger role in the treatment of those with mental illness. Conversely, psychiatrists could aid medical and surgical specialists as consultants in treating patients with psychosomatic illnesses. That this occurred when individuals with mental illness were beginning to be regarded as patients who had biopsychosocial illnesses warranting multidisciplinary treatment, rather than the "insane" or "lunatics" driven by sin and destined to be locked away in asylums, satisfactorily legitimized the economic argument.[3] Simultaneously, there was a reform in psychiatric and general medical education, placing an emphasis on research and disease prevention, whereby physicians began to focus on the patient and his or her psychology. Theories of psychopathology grew to reflect more dynamic interpretations of illness. These forces, however, did not reach most persons in need of psychiatric treatment. There remained a very significant cohort of undertreated mentally ill, symbolizing society's continued underlying disregard for the psychological influences on diseases.[25]

The first departments of psychiatry in general hospitals were supported by grants from the Rockefeller Foundation, led by Alan Gregg who was the director of the Rockefeller Foundation's Medical Sciences Division. Massachusetts General Hospital (Boston, Massachusetts), Barnes Hospital (St. Louis, Missouri), Duke Hospital (Durham, North Carolina), and Billings Hospital (Chicago, Illinois) were some of the first grant recipients. Funding supported education and fellowships, research, psychoanalytic training, and direct patient care. It appears that Gregg's selective funding for specific research was pivotal in the development of psychosomatic medicine in general hospitals.[25] The Rockefeller Foundation gave approximately $11 million between 1931 and 1941 and created general hospital psychiatry units that to this day continue to make some of the most significant contributions within American academic medicine.[25]

By the early 1940s, approximately 40 inpatient psychiatry units existed in general hospitals in the United States. Post-World War II growth of general hospital psychiatry was fueled by the development of psychiatry units associated with both civilian and military hospitals. By 1952, 205 of the larger US hospitals had psychiatric inpatient units with at least 15 beds.[26]

Psychopathic hospitals were essentially clearinghouses; they would provide temporary treatment for patients with psychiatric illnesses.[27] Psychopathic hospitals received patients with all mental disorders, focusing particularly on patients with acute-onset illnesses. Some of the earliest psychopathic hospitals were the Boston Psychopathic Hospital, Colorado Psychopathic Hospital, Syracuse Psychopathic Hospital, and the Neuropsychiatric Institute at the University of Michigan. Throughout the 1950s more autonomous psychiatric "institutes," such as the institute at Michael Reese Hospital in Chicago, the Langley Porter Clinic in San Francisco, and the Psychiatric Institute at the University of Maryland, were built in direct proximity to general hospitals. These facilities were valuable teaching institutions and research facilities.

An example of a psychopathic hospital is the Boston Psychopathic Hospital, named in 1920, and formerly known as the *Psychopathic Department of Boston State Hospital*, which was founded in 1912. In 1924, the Boston Psychopathic Hospital had 110 beds and a relatively large staff that made up administrative, medical, psychology, laboratory (biochemical and pathology), research, outpatient, social service, occupational therapy, nursing, and clerical departments. The facility supported medical/surgical consultations, and x-ray and dental services. Patients were usually admitted for short periods of time, and disposition planning was based on diagnoses and disease acuity. Many cases came from general hospitals and patients were usually transferred soon after arrival to either state hospitals or discharged to outpatient psychiatric care.[28] Services eventually expanded to include emergency services, child and adolescent units, and patients in the general community. As it became more of a community-based facility, the "Psycho" (as it was called) had its name changed to the Massachusetts Mental Health Center.

The veterans' hospital system was established after World War I when veterans were entitled to health care benefits and compensation. By mid-1919, >3,200 veterans were receiving treatment in US Public Health Service hospitals that were overcrowded, far from patients' homes, and incompatible with rehabilitation and long-term care. Civilian hospitals also cared for veterans, and there was a huge backlog of pending cases. A congressional study estimated there were 204,000 US soldiers who had been "wounded not mortally," and uncounted legions who had tuberculosis and neuropsychiatric conditions.[29] Individual states were unable to create policies to handle this need; hence the federal government became responsible for veterans' health care. Congress, however, was unable to design a national program. Ultimately, the American Legion and the Veterans of Foreign Wars in 1919 served as lobbyists for veterans, supporting, against vocal opposition, the Public Health Service's estimate that >30,000 hospital beds were needed for veterans, predominantly for psychiatry and tuberculosis. On his last day in office in 1921, President Woodrow Wilson signed into law a bill supporting $18.6 million for the establishment of hospitals for veterans.[29]

From 1921 to 1923, under Secretary Andrew Mellon, "consultants on hospitalization" approved the building of >6,000 beds in new veteran's hospitals across the United States.[29] From 1923 to 1945, the Veterans Administration (or VA as of 1930) directed by General Frank T. Hines, saw considerable expansion of hospital beds. Following World War II, new construction led to a revamping of veterans hospitals whereby they were virtually reinvented and rebuilt, and many were affiliated with medical schools; teaching and research became an important focus.[29] Although the VA hospital accounted for only a small percentage of the hospitalized population, trends in care shifted within the VA system toward inpatient care while elsewhere there was a diminution in use of inpatient beds. Between 1955 and 1975, the number of VA inpatient episodes increased by 143%, whereas state and county mental hospitals decreased by 37%.[29]

In contrast to public hospitals, private psychiatric hospitals are generally smaller (50 to 200 beds), more autonomous, with high staff–patient ratios, and offer comprehensive treatment modalities. Historically, private psychiatric hospitals have the potential to adapt to the social and economic changes within their respective communities, and if they cannot meet such demands, they are vulnerable to closure. Financial pressures have always threatened the existence and expansion of private psychiatric facilities.

In 1920, an era in which there was a plethora of psychiatric institutions to care for those with mental illness, most patients were in state hospitals; only 4% were treated in private psychiatric hospitals. Throughout the 1930s private facilities continued to open alongside psychopathic hospitals and general hospital psychiatry units. This expansion slowed down somewhat throughout the 1940s, limited by the high cost of expansion and an inability to afford private treatment. At the same time, the National Mental Health Act (1946) supported research and training in private psychiatric hospitals.

Throughout the 1950s, private psychiatric hospitals, although a small minority of the total number of all psychiatric facilities, admitted 25% to 40% of psychiatric patients annually.[3] However, the public opinion of psychiatry post-World War II was not a favorable one. Crippled by financial strain, a shortage of psychiatrists, and staff dissatisfaction, private facilities fell into bankruptcy throughout the 1950s. Newly developed psychoactive medications offered more effective treatments, and may have fueled, in part, the rebound of the fragile private psychiatric hospitals throughout the 1960s. In 1970, state hospitals represented 91.8% of inpatient beds, general hospitals 5.0%, and private hospitals 3.2% of inpatient beds. By 1998, the total percentage of inpatient beds that belonged to state hospitals had decreased to 42.0% whereas the total percentage of inpatient beds for general hospitals and private hospitals both increased to 35.8% and 22.2%, respectively.

Private psychiatric hospitals continued to increase in number throughout the 1970s and 1980s, and states with the fewest regulations had the most substantial expansions.[3] A concurrent growth in insurance coverage, an increase in the number of mental health providers, and a decrease in social stigma associated with obtaining mental health treatment facilitated the expansion.[30,31] Psychiatric hospitals became potentially lucrative ventures for private corporations. Starting in the 1960s, existing hospitals were being bought by for-profit hospital chains. These investor-owned chains grew in number from 5 psychiatric hospital chains in the late 1960s to 75 in 1984.[3] Four corporations came to dominate this market: Hospital Corporation of America (HCA) in Tennessee; Charter Medical Corporation (CMC) in Georgia; National Medical Enterprises, Inc. (NME), and Community Psychiatric Centers (CPC) in California. Together these corporations owned nearly 10,000 psychiatric beds, controlled 85% of the market, and their profits were in the multimillions.[3]

Although the private chains were in a growth mode, the average length of stay for psychiatric illnesses decreased from 33 days in 1986 to 24 days in 1991, with further decreases over the next decade. Therefore, filling these psychiatric beds became more challenging, and for-profit hospital chains resorted to marketing, advertising, and seeking referrals through community workers including parole officers, police, emergency room staff, self-help groups, and religious workers. These attempts to increase admissions led to alleged fraudulent criminal activity such as paying patients' insurance premiums for them, paying referral sources, and setting referral quotas for hospital employees. Furthermore, reimbursements fueled specific diagnoses and tampering with medical records.[3] Lawsuits and settlements brought by patients, insurers, states, and the federal government led to substantial losses for the for-profit hospital chains. The fine tuning of managed care, the privatization of many public mental health services, and court decisions mandating treatment in the "least restrictive alternative" or "most integrated setting" further altered private psychiatric hospital practice. By the end of the 20th century, private psychiatric hospitals were fewer in number, with fewer beds, and they served a broader range of patients overall.[3]

Attempts at the Movement from Psychiatric Hospitals to Their Alternatives

In 1953, American Psychiatric Association president Kenneth Appel called for a commission to develop a national mental health program, describing the system at that time as consisting of "stopgap" measures that were falling short of the potential to reduce mental illness. This environment, along with the greater context of the civil rights movement, paved the way for the Mental Health Study Act of 1955, in which the legislature called for "an objective, thorough, and nationwide analysis of the human and economic problems of mental illness."[32]

In 1961, the resulting report, *Action for Mental Health*, described a new vision for the treatment of psychiatric illness, one that reflected society's belief that mental illness would be more successfully treated with a focus on community care, active treatment for acute disease, and prevention. State hospitals larger than 1,000 beds would no longer be built, no new patients would be added to hospitals with 1,000 patients, and any existing large hospitals would be converted into facilities specifically for the treatment of chronic mental illness. The new cornerstone of the mental health delivery system would be the Community Mental Health Center (CMHC). In contrast to the traditional mental health system funded by the states, the federal government would assume financial responsibility for the new CMHCs.[32,33]

Funds to build the CMHCs were allocated in 1963 and, in 1965 funds were approved to staff the centers. Under guidelines established by the National Institute for Mental Health, CMHCs were to provide an array of services, including inpatient, partial hospitalization, outpatient, emergency services, consultation, and education.[32] As President John F. Kennedy stated to Congress, there was great hope that the CMHCs would constitute a "bold new approach . . . the reliance on the cold mercy of custodial isolation will be supplanted by the open warmth of community concern and capability" without the need for "prolonged or permanent confinement in huge, unhappy mental hospitals."[32] This new approach was meant to serve two distinct purposes: a renewed effort to prevent mental illness and the creation of an alternative to institution-based treatment for mental disorders.[33]

President Lyndon Johnson's War on Poverty further supported movement of patients out of long-term psychiatric hospitals. In 1965, the Social Security Act created Medicaid and Medicare. The Medicaid program, funded by a combination of federal, state, and local dollars, provides medical care for the poor, including many with mental illness. Medicare, a federally funded program, covers health care for people who are elderly and disabled. These new programs would provide payment for the care of patients transferred from state psychiatric hospitals to nursing homes. States now had a new incentive to shift long-term patients out of the state hospital, where the state paid the entire cost of care, to the nursing home, where the federal government would share the cost.[34–36] Many elderly long-term hospitalized patients were discharged to nursing homes.[37] This was a shift from a long history dating from the mid-19th century of psychiatric hospitals providing custodial care for people affected by diseases that would later be defined as "organic." In this earlier era, when people with epilepsy or tertiary syphilis needed more care than could be provided at home, individuals were not uncommonly admitted to psychiatric hospitals, especially to public facilities.[38]

These social and political changes, more effective medications, and the belief of the psychiatric profession and the general public that psychiatric treatment for people with severe mental illness would be more humane and effective in the community, created the foundation for the large-scale depopulation of state and county psychiatric hospitals, referred to as *deinstitutionalization*. In 1955, there were 558,992 people living in state and county hospitals nationally; by 1976 this number diminished to 193,436.

This non–asylum-based approach was a dramatically different model for treating mental illness, and not all of the consequences of the change were anticipated. For example, the vision of discharged patients living in the community with family was often not attainable. In 1960, 75% of people living in psychiatric hospitals were unmarried, divorced, or widowed, and many did not have connections to people who could care for them.[36] This was a group with few resources at their disposal and maintaining appropriate community housing was challenging. Many of the discharged patients would move from one institution (the state hospital) to another, such as a nursing home or other group living arrangement.[39,40] At the time, there were few state-created residential programs so many patients were discharged to single rooms and boarding houses, often in poor areas of cities. This housing proved to be tenuous and, in the 1970s, many low-income housing options were demolished, limiting the options further. A not insignificant number of former state hospital residents would find themselves homeless[32] or incarcerated.[40,41]

Advocates for the CMHCs had envisioned the centers as a way to revolutionize treatment for persons with chronic mental illness, allowing for discharge from long-term hospitalization into a community where the clinics could provide treatment and care. In reality, between 1968 and 1978, only 3.6% to 6.5% CMHC admissions were state hospital referrals; instead, the CMHCs were reaching a less severely ill, and previously untreated segment of the population, with most patients being seen primarily for outpatient counseling regarding problems of daily living.[32] This trend may have been, in part, a product of the CMHCs mission to prevent mental illness (which may have diminished focus on the treatment of existing mental illness) and the federal-to-local funding mechanism that allowed CMHCs to develop without involving the state mental health authorities.[39] In 1975, legislators responded by refocusing the CMHCs' mandate to treat those with chronic mental illness, including screening patients before state hospital admission and providing follow-up for patients released from state hospitals.[32]

Critiques of deinstitutionalization proliferated. Community treatment was criticized for falling short in providing residential care, case management, rehabilitation services, outpatient treatment, and crisis intervention for the discharged patients. There were deficits in planning and problems in paying for a comprehensive array of community services. Of note, Medicare, Medicaid, and private insurance did not provide reimbursement for many of the support services this group of formerly hospitalized patients required.[42] To get appropriate services, advocates filed class action suits, such as *Brewster v. Dukakis*, in which plaintiffs asserted that patients in the state hospital had the right to treatment outside of the hospital and the state was obligated to develop community services adequate to allow for community discharge.[43,44] Although community tenure could be sustained longer for those patients who have a greater variety of outpatient services[34,45] and while the enhancement of community services made discharge and life in settings outside of the hospital possible for many patients, the state hospital retained an important place in the spectrum of treatment options.[43]

Despite the imperfections of deinstitutionalization, society's values sustained individuals' rights to receive treatment in the community. Some important judicial decisions in the 1960s and 1970s were consistent with these values. The cases of *Lake v. Cameron* (1966) and *Dixon versus Weinberger* (1975) set the legal standard that patients have the right to treatment in the least restrictive setting. This standard of treatment places priority on maintaining a person's autonomy and liberty, and asserts that any limits on personal liberty should be no more than what is necessary for the person's own protection. The treatment community responded by seeking alternatives to inpatient treatment, diverting hospital admissions to other community services, and arranging for discharges to community settings.[46] The case of *Lessard v. Schmidt* (1972) found that to be involuntarily hospitalized for mental illness, a person must pose a danger to self or others; involuntary commitment laws in most states came to reflect this standard.[34] The interpretation of the "least restrictive alternative" as meaning treatment outside of the hospital has been criticized as taking too narrow a view of "restrictiveness." For example, some might argue that for a specific patient, inpatient treatment in her home community with a strong rehabilitation component leading to steady functional improvement may in fact be less restrictive than involuntary depot medication while living in a single room with little contact with service providers.[46,47]

Part of the reality of shifting care from the inpatient setting to the community was learning how to provide adequate care to persons with chronic mental illness outside of the hospital. Some discharged patients fell into a pattern of repeated admissions—rapid stabilizations in the structure of the hospital, followed by relapses upon returning to the community.[41,48] Mental health professionals in Wisconsin, troubled by this pattern, developed Assertive Community Treatment (ACT) as a method to provide this group, who in times past might have been chronically hospitalized, with adequate and appropriate support outside of the hospital.[49,50] Key elements of ACT include assertive, comprehensive, and flexible treatment based on the individual's needs, including support for real-life problems as they arise; building daily living skills; work opportunities; medication; and housing support. Services are provided by a small, closely integrated multidisciplinary team with a typical ratio of one staff person for every ten patients. Treatment contacts are frequent and services are available 24 hours a day, 7 days a week. Typically, Medicaid is the primary funding source, with services billed under rehabilitative or case management categories. However, there are many services provided by ACT that are not reimbursed, requiring programs to seek supplemental funds.[51] Use of ACT has continued to grow and has proved to be a cost-effective means of providing care.[52]

Legal strategies, such as outpatient commitment, have also developed to allow for mandated treatment outside of the hospital for patients at risk for noncompliance and decompensation without treatment. Outpatient commitment generally requires compliance with recommended treatment (such as abstaining from drugs and alcohol and attending appointments), but often does not include provisions for forced medication for people who are competent.[34,53] The criteria for outpatient commitment are in most jurisdictions similar to the standards for inpatient commitment: danger to self or others or inability to care for self. This treatment may be suited to the patient with a history of deteriorations, the likelihood of future deterioration, and the possibility of stabilization if treatment is provided.[53–55] Outpatient commitment is controversial among patients, treatment providers, and the general public, and, to date, insufficient data are available about its impact.[55]

With these legal standards and outpatient services in place, and with social values emphasizing community treatment, it is generally only patients with severe and life-threatening symptoms who currently receive inpatient psychiatric treatment. In recent decades, the inpatient unit has increasingly specialized in the rapid stabilization of acute episodes of psychiatric illness. These are often brief hospitalizations, with the expectation that care even for significantly symptomatic patients will continue in the community. Alternatives to the traditional inpatient unit can be used for diversion or step down. Factors beyond the value placed on community treatment have combined to reinforce this scenario.[56]

Funding for services continues to influence the setting of psychiatric treatment. Medicare and Medicaid payments, which were important in the initial movement of patients from the state hospital to other institutions, are prominent among payers for psychiatric services. This continues to be an incentive to provide care outside of the state hospital system. This funding initially benefited the general hospital psychiatric unit. But, just as in other areas of medicine, attention to the growing costs of health care has resulted in new efforts to "manage" care with attention to cost and efficiency. Decreasing the utilization of *any* inpatient psychiatric care, often seen as the most expensive alternative, receives everbroadening attention.

This tension has resulted in an expansion of the options for psychiatric treatment beyond the traditional dichotomy of inpatient versus outpatient care. A continuum, including partial hospitalization programs, intensive outpatient treatment, and crisis stabilization beds, has developed to provide more flexibility for the more acutely ill person in order to divert them from inpatient treatment.[57–59] Insurers and clinicians attempt to match patients to the most cost-effective level of care from along the continuum.[33,60] For some patients, day hospital and respite care provide suitable and effective alternatives to inpatient hospitalization.[61,62] The more alternatives a community develops, the less that community depends on hospital level care.[43,44]

The influence of managed care continues while the patient is in the hospital. Insurers, both public and private, often require clinical review. Utilization review is a common managed care strategy in which an individual case is reviewed and the insurance company authorizes a limited number of days for treatment; to receive payment for additional treatment, the facility must participate in additional reviews with the insurer. The treatment community has voiced concerns that managed care companies often allow fewer days than the treatment facility requests and many cases require one or more additional reviews in order to be considered for longer treatment, adding to both the administrative burden and cost of providing treatment.[60,63,64]

Managed care has also reached the public sector in an attempt to contain growing expenditures as more patients previously treated in the state hospital are treated with short-term stays in general hospitals.[35] Rather than one longer admission, these patients receive multiple shorter episodes of care, often being admitted to a different treatment site from one hospitalization to the next. In some cases, managed care networks direct admissions to any of a number of hospitals within their network, without necessarily sending patients to units where they have received previous treatment. For the small proportion of patients with frequent admission, this leads to discontinuity of treatment and longer lengths of stay compared to patients admitted to hospitals where they are known.[35,65]

In the mid-1990s, the VA experienced a shift from its traditional focus on inpatient care and dramatically expanded its outpatient services (see Table 1.2); this occurred in the larger context of the reorganization of the Veterans Health Administration into 22 smaller semiautonomous networks.[66] Between 1995 and 2001 the number of occupied annual inpatient psychiatry beds fell by 58% in the VA, the length of stay decreased by 52%, and 27% more veterans were treated in the VA outpatient system.[67]

TABLE 1.2 NUMBERS OF MENTAL HEALTH ORGANIZATIONS, 24-HOUR TREATMENT BEDS, AND FULL-TIME STAFF PSYCHIATRISTS FROM CENTER FOR MENTAL HEALTH SERVICES

	1970	1980	1990	2002
All				
Number of mental health organizations	3,005	3,727	5,284	4,301
Number of 24-h hospital and residential treatment beds	524,878	274,713	272,253	211,199
Number of full-time equivalent psychiatrists	12,938	17,874	18,818	20,233
State and county				
Number of mental health organizations	310	280	273	222
Number of 24-h hospital and residential treatment beds	413,066	156,482	98,789	57,263
Number of full-time equivalent psychiatrists	4,389	3,762	3,849	4,255
Private				
Number of mental health organizations	150	184	462	253
Number of 24-h hospital and residential treatment beds	14,295	17,157	44,871	25,095
Number of full-time equivalent psychiatrists	1,067	1,554	1,582	1,236
Nonfederal general hospital				
Number of mental health organizations	797	923	1,674	1,285
Number of 24-h hospital and residential treatment beds	22,394	29,384	53,479	40,202
Number of full-time equivalent psychiatrists	3,394	6,009	6,500	4,348
VA Medical Center				
Number of mental health organizations	115	136	141	140
Number of 24-h hospital and residential treatment beds	50,688	35,913	21,712	9,672
Number of full-time equivalent psychiatrists	902	2,245	2,103	4,554

VA, Veterans Administration.
(From Foley DW, Manderscheid RW, Atay JE, et al. Center for Mental Health Services. Mental Health, United States, 2002. In: Manderscheid RW, Berry JT, eds. *Highlights of organized mental health services in 2002 and major national and state trends*, DHHS Publication No. [SMA]-06-4195. Rockville: Substance Abuse and Mental Health Services Administration.)

Despite all this, the inpatient unit continues to have a crucial place in psychiatric treatment, although the type of care provided has evolved significantly from its origin. There has been a significant trend toward an increasing volume of acute inpatient admissions (with the number of inpatient admissions quadrupling between 1970 and 1992),[56] and far fewer long-term admissions. Between 1988 and 1994, the number of discharges from general hospitals increased by 35%; over the same time period the number of discharges from public hospitals declined by approximately the same amount.[56] The length of stay in general hospitals decreased from 12.1 to 9.6 days during this same time period.[56] While there are shorter lengths of stay and greater turnover of beds, patients who are admitted have increasingly severe psychiatric and medical illnesses.[68]

Even when enhanced community programs are available, inpatient treatment continues to have an important role in the care of people with chronic mental illness. Many patients do eventually require rehospitalization at some point. In some cases this has been a symptom of inadequate community support and treatment; in other cases, hospitalization for exacerbation of illness is an appropriate component of treatment for a chronic illness.[45] State hospitals continue to provide many important services for patients with exacerbation of chronic illness who are repeatedly at risk for harm to self or others, whose specialized needs cannot be met in the community, and/or who intermittently need backup to the system of community services.[37,48,69]

Because all manner of diversion and alternatives to hospital beds has not eliminated the need for inpatient psychiatric treatment, it is worth examining the changes in which inpatient institutions provide the care. From 1970 to 1998, there was growth in the number of mental health service organizations (from 3,005 to 5,722), followed by a decrease between 1998 and 2002 (Table 1.2).[70] This growth was largely attributable to the growth of general hospitals, residential treatment settings, and

TABLE 1.3 NUMBER OF RESIDENT PATIENTS, NUMBER OF ADMISSIONS TO STATE AND COUNTY PSYCHIATRIC HOSPITALS

Year	Number of Resident Patients	Number of Admissions
1960	535,540	234,791
1970	337,619	384,511
1980	132,164	370,344
1990	92,059	277,813
2000	54,836	158,034
2003	47,247	159,645
2004	52,632	184,301

(From Foley DW, Manderscheid RW, Atay JE, et al. Center for Mental Health Services. Mental Health, United States, 2002. In: Manderscheid RW, Berry JT, eds. *Highlights of organized mental health services in 2002 and major national and state trends*, DHHS Publication No. [SMA]-06-4195. Rockville: Substance Abuse and Mental Health Services Administration.)

other nonhospital mental health organizations such as partial treatment centers. Although the number of organizations has grown, the number of beds decreased from 524,878 in 1970 to 211,199 in 2002. Most of these losses are due to decreases in beds at state psychiatric hospitals, but beds in private and general hospitals have also declined somewhat.[71] There has been a gradual decline in the number of admissions to state psychiatric hospitals since the late 1960s, although in 2003 and 2004, there was an increase in the number of admissions and, for the first time since 1955, an increase in the number of people residing in state hospitals (see Table 1.3).[70]

Many forces combine to shape this pattern. State expenditures on inpatient psychiatric care have decreased, fewer beds are available, and community care and prevention of admissions is emphasized. Fewer facilities provide 24-hour care, and the institutions providing this care have changed over time. More of the 24-hour care is being provided by general hospitals and less by state and county hospitals; in 1955, state hospitals provided 63% of hospital and residential services but in 2002, provided only 13%.[71]

There are important differences between the patient populations served by these institutions. In the 1980s, state, county, and VA hospitals treated more patients with alcohol- and drug-related illness compared to general and private hospitals; this difference dissipated in the 1990s.[37,72] Patients with affective disorders are more likely to be treated at general and private hospitals; county and state hospitals continue to provide a greater share of treatment for patients with schizophrenia.[37,72] Specialized medical-psychiatric units are able to care for people with significant medical comorbidities and some may offer expertise in treating medically or neurologically caused psychiatric symptoms.[68] Uninsured and economically disadvantaged patients are more common in public hospitals.[72] But federal financing for psychiatric care in the general hospital has also grown as more care for this population has shifted from the state hospital to the private and general hospital.[56,73] By 1994, Medicare was the largest payer in private hospitals.[56]

Nor has the workload remained static in these hospitals. In the 1970s, psychiatrists working in public institutions were charged with the care of 45 patients per psychiatrist compared to 8 and 5 patients per psychiatrist in private and general hospitals, respectively. Over time, this disparity has diminished. By the late 1980s, caseloads were 20, 12, and 4.5 per psychiatrist in public, private, and general hospital settings.[35]

There is still much to be learned about which aspects of inpatient care will result in the best outcomes. The link to outpatient services is critical; close coordination with a broad array of outpatient services allows the stabilized patient to continue to recover in the community. Although it may be possible to design improved systems of care and treatment, it remains unclear if there is the will to fund such systems. A significant challenge faced by inpatient psychiatric facilities in the first decade of the 21st century is that reimbursement rates are often less than the cost of care.[73] If this be the case, is it any wonder that persons with severe mental illness fill the roles of the homeless and the incarcerated in the 21st century just as they did in Dorothea Dix's world of the 19th century?

REFERENCES

1. Snyder CM. *The lady and the president. The letters of Dorothea Dix and Millard Fillmore*. Lexington: University Press of Kentucky; 1975.
2. Dix DL. *Memorial to the legislature of Massachusetts*. Boston: Munroe & Francis; 1843.
3. Geller JL. A history of private psychiatric hospitals in the U.S.A.: From start to almost finished. *Psychiatr Q*. 2006;77:1–41.
4. Zwelling SS. *Quest for a cure*. Williamsburg: Colonial Williamsburg Foundation; 1985.
5. Dix DL. Memorial of D.L. Dix, praying a grant of land for the relief and support of the indigent curable and incurable insane in the United States. 33rd Congress, 1st session, Senate Report No. 57, June 27, 1848. Available at: http://www.disabilitymuseum.org/lib/docs/1239cardhtm. Accessed February 27, 2007.
6. Hurd HM, ed. *The institutional care of the insane*. Baltimore: Johns Hopkins Press; 1916.
7. Pierce F. Veto message, May 3, 1954. In: Richardson JD, ed. *A compilation of the messages and papers of the presidents, 1789–1897*, Vol. 5. Washington, DC: Published by the Authority of Congress; 1898:247–256.
8. Accommodations for the insane. *Boston Med Surg J*. 1848;39:25–26.
9. Memorial of D.L. Dix, Praying of congress a grant of land, for the relief and support of the indigent, curable, and incurable insane in the United States. *Am J Insanity*. 1849;5:286–287.
10. Jarvis E. Political economy of health. *Annu Rep Mass State Board Health*. 1874;5:335–338.
11. Woodward SB. Observations on the medical treatment of insanity. *Am J Insanity*. 1850;7:1–34.
12. Nichols CH. Proceedings of the Association of Medical Superintendents for the thirty-first annual meeting. *Am J Insanity*. 1877;34:240–243.
13. Awl W. *Tenth annual report of the direction of the Ohio lunatic asylum, to the forty-seventh general assembly of the state of Ohio, for the year 1848*. Columbus: Medary; 1849.
14. Ray I. The popular feeling towards hospitals for the insane. *Am J Insanity*. 1852;9:36–65.
15. Callender JH. History and work of the Association of Medical Superintendents of American Institutions for the Insane – president's address. *Am J Insanity*. 1883;11:1–33.
16. Nichols CH. Proceedings of the thirty-third annual meeting. *Am J Insanity*. 1879;36:139–223.
17. Godding WW. Aspects and outlook of insanity in America. *Am J Insanity*. 1890;47:1–16.
18. McFarland A. *Eighth biennial reports of the trustees, superintendent and treasurer of the Illinois State Hospital for the Insane at Jacksonville, December 1862*. Chicago: Fulton; 1863.
19. Buttolph HA. *Superintendent's report. In the eighth and ninth annual reports of the managers and officers of the State Asylum for the Insane*. Morristown, 1883, 1884:17–29.
20. Earle P. The curability of insanity: A statistical study. *Am J Insanity*. 1885;41:179–209.
21. Thompson JW. Trends in the development of psychiatric services, 1844–1994. *Hosp Community Psychiatry*. 1994;45:987–992.
22. Valenstein ES. *Great and desperate cures*. New York: HarperCollins; 1987.
23. Grob GN. *Mental illness and American society*. Princeton: Princeton University Press; 1983.
24. Keill SL. Current issues in general hospital psychiatry. Introduction: The evolution of psychiatry in the general hospital. *Gen Hosp Psychiatry*. 1981;3:289–291.
25. Summergrad P, Hackett TP. Alan Gregg and the rise of general hospital psychiatry. *Gen Hosp Psychiatry*. 1987;9:439–445.
26. Greenhill MH. Psychiatric units in general hospitals: 1979. *Hosp Community Psychiatry*. 1979;30:169–182.
27. May JV. The functions of the psychopathic hospital. *Am J Insanity*. 1919;76:21–34.
28. Wood WF. The administrative problems of the Boston psychopathic hospital. *Am J Psychiatry*. 1924;81:297–307.
29. Stevens R. Can the government govern? Lessons from the formation of the veteran's administration. *J Health Polit Policy Law*. 1991;16:281–305.
30. Levenson AI. The growth of investor-owned psychiatric hospitals. *Am J Psychiatry*. 1982;139:902.
31. Dorwart RA, Schlesinger M. Privatization of psychiatric services. *Am J Psychiatry*. 1988;145:543.
32. Talbott JA. *The death of the asylum: a critical study of state hospital management, services, and care*. New York: Grune & Stratton; 1978.
33. Hoge MA, Thakur NM, Jacobs S. Understanding managed behavioral health care. *Psychiatr Clin North Am*. 2000;23:241–253.
34. Durham ML, La Fond JQ. Assessing psychiatric care settings: Hospitalization versus outpatient care. *Int J Technol Assess Health Care*. 1996;12:618–633.
35. Geller JL. A history of the private psychiatric hospital in the USA: From start to almost finished. *Psychiatr Q*. 2006;77:1–41.
36. Grob GN. Public policy and mental illnesses: Jimmy Carter's Presidential Commission on Mental Health. *Milbank Q*. 2005;83:425–456.
37. Thompson JW, Bass RD, Witkin MJ. Fifty years of psychiatric services: 1940–1990. *Hosp Community Psychiatry*. 1982;33:711–717.
38. Ovsiew F, Jobe T. Neuropsychiatry in the history of mental health services. In: Ovsiew F, ed. *Neuropsychiatry and mental health services*.

Washington, DC: American Psychiatric Press; 1999:1–21.

39. Morrissey JP, Goldman HH. Cycles of reform in the care of the chronically mentally ill. *Hosp Community Psychiatry.* 1984;35:785–793.

40. Lamb HR. The new state mental hospital in the community. *Psychiatr Serv.* 1997;48:1307–1310.

41. Lamb HR. When there are almost no state hospital beds left. *Hosp Community Psychiatry.* 1993;44:973–976.

42. Okin RL. State hospitals in the 1980s. *Hosp Community Psychiatry.* 1982;33:717–721.

43. Geller JL, Fisher WH, Wirth-Cauchon JL, et al. Second-generation deinstitutionalization, I: The impact of *Brewster vs. Dukakis* on state hospital case mix. *Am J Psychiatry.* 1990; 147:982–987.

44. Okin RL. *Brewster vs. Dukakis:* Developing community services through use of a consent decree. *Am J Psychiatry.* 1984;141:786–789.

45. Solomon P, Davis J, Gordon B. Discharged state hospital patients' characteristics and use of aftercare: Effect on community tenure. *Am J Psychiatry.* 1984;141:1566–1570.

46. Munetz MR, Geller JL. The least restrictive alternative in the postinstitutional era. *Hosp Community Psychiatry.* 1993;44:967–973.

47. Bachrach LL. Is the least restrictive environment always the best? *Hosp Community Psychiatry.* 1980;31:97–103.

48. Geller JL. In again, out again. A preliminary evaluation of a state hospital's worst recidivists. *Hosp Community Psychiatry.* 1986;37:386–390.

49. Stein LI, Test MA. Alternatives to mental hospital treatment I: Conceptual model, treatment program, and clinical evaluation. *Arch Gen Psychiatry.* 1980;37:392–397.

50. Test MA, Stein LI. Alternatives to mental hospital treatment III: Social cost. *Arch Gen Psychiatry.* 1980;37:409–412.

51. Phillips SD, Burns BJ, Edgar ER, et al. Moving assertive community treatment into standard practice. *Psychiatr Serv.* 2001;52:771–779.

52. Weisbrod BA, Test MA, Stein LI. Alternatives to mental hospital treatment II: Economic benefit-cost analysis. *Arch Gen Psychiatry.* 1980;37:400–405.

53. Schwartz MS, Swanson JW, Kim M, et al. Use of outpatient commitment or related civil court treatment orders in five US communities. *Psychiatr Serv.* 2006;57:343–349.

54. Appelbaum PS. Thinking carefully about outpatient commitment. *Psychiatr Serv.* 2001;52:347–350.

55. Geller JL. The evolution of outpatient commitment in the USA: From conundrum to quagmire. *Int J Law Psychiatry.* 2006;29:234–248.

56. Mechanic D, McAlpine DD, Olfson M. Changing patterns of psychiatric inpatient care in the United States, 1988–1994. *Arch Gen Psychiatry.* 1998;55:785–791.

57. Goldman HH, Thelander S, Westrin C. Organizing mental health services: An evidence-based approach. *J Ment Health Policy Econ.* 2000;3:69–75.

58. Thornicroft G, Tansella M. Components of a modern mental health service: A pragmatic balance of community and hospital care. *Br J Psychiatry.* 2004;185:283–290.

59. Schreter RK. Alternative treatment programs: The psychiatric continuum of care. *Psychiatr Clin North Am.* 2000;23:335–346.

60. Harbin HT. Inpatient services: The managed care view. In: Schreter RK, Sharfstein SS, Schreter CA, eds. *Allies and adversaries: the impact of managed care on mental health services.* Washington, DC: American Psychiatric Press; 1994:11–22.

61. Kluiter H, Geil R, Nienhuis EJ, et al. Predicting feasibility of day treatment for unselected patients referred for inpatient psychiatric treatment: Results of a randomized trial. *Am J Psychiatry.* 1992;149:1199–1205.

62. Sledge WH, Tebes J, Rakfeldt J, et al. Day hospital/crisis respite care versus inpatient care part I: Clinical outcomes. *Am J Psychiatry.* 1996;153:1065–1073.

63. Schlesinger M, Dorwart RA, Epstein SS. Managed care constraints on psychiatrists' hospital practices: Bargaining power and professional autonomy. *Am J Psychiatry.* 1996;153:256–260.

64. Wickizer TM, Lessler D, Travis KM. Controlling psychiatric utilization through managed care. *Am J Psychiatry.* 1996;153:339–345.

65. Geller JL. The effects of public managed care on patterns of intensive use of inpatient psychiatric services. *Psychiatr Serv.* 1998;49:327–333.

66. Desai MM, Rosenheck RA. The interdependence of mental health service systems. *J Ment Health Policy Econ.* 2000;3:61–67.

67. Greenberg GA, Rosenheck RA. Consumer satisfaction with inpatient mental health treatment in the Department of Veterans Affairs. *Adm Policy Ment Health.* 2004;31:465–480.

68. Summergrad P. Medical psychiatry units and the roles of the inpatient psychiatric service in the general hospital. *Gen Hosp Psychiatry.* 1994;16:20–31.

69. Goldman HH, Taube CA, Reiger DA, et al. The multiple functions of the state hospital. *Hosp Community Psychiatry.* 1983;140: 296–300.

70. Atay JE, Crider R, Foley D, et al. Center for Mental Health Services. Mental health, United States, 2002. In: Manderscheid RW, Berry JT, eds. *Admissions and residential patients, state and county mental hospitals,* DHHS Publication No. (SMA)-06-4195. Rockville: Substance Abuse and Mental Health Services Administration.

71. Foley DW, Manderscheid RW, Atay JE, et al. Center for Mental Health Services. Mental Health United States, 2002. In: Manderscheid RW, Berry JT, eds. *Highlights of organized mental health services in 2002 and major national and state trends*, DHHS Publication No. (SMA)-06-4195. Rockville: Substance Abuse and Mental Health Services Administration.

72. Olfson M, Mechanic D. Mental disorders in public, private nonprofit, and proprietary general hospitals. *Am J Psychiatry*. 1996;153: 1613–1619.

73. Geller JL. Excluding institutions for mental diseases from federal reimbursement for services: Strategy or tragedy. *Psychiatr Serv*. 2000;51:1397–1403.

CHAPTER 2

Psychosocial Approaches in Inpatient Psychiatry

RICHARD L. MUNICH AND PAMELA K. GREENE

A dmission to an inpatient psychiatric facility is a major treatment intervention. Its goals include an evaluation of and recovery from disabling symptoms, an assessment and possible modification of precipitating factors, and the promotion of community reintegration and tenure. As described in the first chapter and as will be amply documented throughout this book, the last 60 years have seen radical alterations in the specific goals, structure, and length of stay of this intervention. In the era between 1946 and 1975, admission criteria were expansive, and stays of several months that provided a psychosocial moratorium in a psychotherapeutically oriented and structured milieu were the recognized standard for effective care.[1-4] After the changes in inpatient psychiatry of the last three decades, only a handful of inpatient facilities capable of utilizing such a model of inpatient care continue to exist, some as specialized units within larger psychiatric hospitals.

Advances in treatment, especially psychopharmacologic treatment and more focused psychotherapies, active community interventions, ambiguous results of extended lengths of stay, and powerful economic factors account for contemporary ideology and practice in which less is more and perhaps better, especially with respect to mitigating regressive tendencies and institutional dependency. To complicate matters further, treatment advances utilized in outpatient work in combination with increased financial constraints organized around medical necessity have led to the admission of more complicated and difficult-to-treat patients.

Nevertheless, in many cases the inpatient stay is now 4 to 8 days with rapid assessment, symptom reduction, and environmental manipulation as primary goals. In this time frame, treatment goals must be integrated with discharge planning virtually from the time of admission. In acute care facilities and on psychiatric units in general hospitals, criteria for admission are now more restrictive and include a failure of outpatient treatment, acute and life-threatening symptoms—especially danger to self or others or deteriorating ability to care for oneself—and changes in treatment arrangements that require containment and close monitoring.[5] Diagnostically, these categories generally appear in schizophrenia, schizoaffective and major mood disorders, decompensated borderline personality disorder, substance abuse crisis or withdrawal, severe eating disorders, post-traumatic stress disorder, and situational conditions. Special requirements for extended length of stay are addressed later in this chapter.

Naturally these changes decrease the range and depth of psychosocial approaches available to the hospital psychiatrist. Assessments are perforce somewhat abbreviated and require an intense focus, treatments are barely tested and begun, and precipitants—ideally with family help—identified as clearly as possible. Under these circumstances, the milieu takes on as much a holding and containing as it does a diagnostic and therapeutic function. Staff hierarchy and cohesion and clear delineation of discipline roles take precedence over the less efficient sharing of responsibility and overlap of function. Another constraint, especially for group therapy and milieu functioning, is that the implementation of various approaches is closely related to the degree to which the unit has a diagnostically homogeneous or heterogeneous patient population. It is well known, for example, that the more homogeneous the population, the more coherent and consistent—therefore, the more effective—staff interventions can be. In a heterogeneous patient group, similar cohorts of patients can influence the tenor of a unit in important ways that may be dysfunctional for other cohorts. These shifts are chronicled in many publications, and reflected comprehensively in the review edited in 1992 by Munich and Gabbard,[6] and monographs edited in 1993 by Leibenluft et al.[7] and in 1997 by Sederer and Rothschild.[8] Nevertheless, certain principles prevail whether the patient is in an acute, an intermediate length-of-stay, or residential, or a custodial-care facility.

Much of what follows assumes the ideal access to resources for the inpatient unit. Rarely does the current training situation reference older psychosocial modes of and resources for inpatient practice; therefore, current trainees may remain unexposed to the best of the past. Therefore, the authors elaborate what might be accomplished under the best of circumstances. These resources include adequate time for assessment and implementation, space and facilities, and numbers of trained staff. For example, a carefully calibrated ladder of privileges and responsibilities for the recovering patient to test therapeutic gains will necessarily be modified in a reduced length of stay. Or a group or therapeutic activities program may be constrained by gaps in communication and continuity when the psychiatrists in charge of cases are not part of the unit staff and need to see their patients according to their own busy schedules. Or, even in a closed system or one depending on hospitalists, treatment must be shaped in a more practical and efficient way when the interdisciplinary team simply consists of a psychiatrist and a nursing staff who are responsible for most of the treatment tasks.

Comparing Contemporary Inpatient Settings

Other than the generally accepted notion that a unit functions better and has better outcomes when the staff is of one mind about general principles of treatment delivery, there are no data to justify one method of organizing treatment over the other. Naturally the more extended the length of inpatient stay, the more sophisticated the structures can become, the more focused individual treatments will be, the more opportunities there are for patients to become involved in their treatment (e.g., patient government, unit event planning, creative arts participation, etc.), and the more likely it will be for the treatment milieu to exert its influence. The length of stay also influences the repertoire of specific psychosocial modalities that may be utilized. Therefore, before discussing those modalities, the chapter will briefly compare acute, inpatient specialty and residential treatment settings under the rubrics of admission criteria, average length of stay (ALOS), and treatment focus.

As indicated earlier, admission criteria for acute care settings usually include an emerging crisis in which the patient is a danger to self or others, is unable to care for himself or herself, or where an adjustment in treatment is disruptive enough to require more containment than can be provided in the community. As noted, the ALOS in acute care settings is 4 to 8 days, and the focus of treatment is on symptom reduction, stabilization, and environmental adjustments that facilitate treatment compliance and the initiation or restoration of outpatient treatment.

Admission criteria for inpatient specialty units include unexplained treatment stalemate, recalcitrance, or noncompliance; situations where there have been multiple admissions in a relatively short period of time; diagnostic complexity (multiple diagnoses or various combinations of Axis I and II symptoms); the emergence of new diagnostic information; and dual diagnoses. The length of stay on an inpatient specialty unit varies between 4 and 8 weeks, and the focus is on diagnostic clarity (e.g., how might personality factors be interfering with treatments designed to ameliorate a primary diagnosis), institution of behavioral models to reduce secondary deterioration or gain from illness (e.g., eating disorder, substance abuse, or obsessive compulsive disorder programs), providing a second opinion to faltering outpatient treatment, or helping to start or restart stagnating mental processes that preclude effective treatment. Important goals of an intermediate length of stay are to provide the least restrictive environment and help patients assume more agency for their illness, treatment, and recovery.

Finally, admission criteria for longer-stay, residential treatment include persistent treatment noncompliance, the need for a psychosocial moratorium for a disturbed adolescent who has failed one or two shorter-term admissions, or to provide more time to uncover and understand persistent, complicated, and dysfunctional emotional and behavioral patterns (complicated combinations of diagnoses or Axis I and Axis II psychopathology) for patients who are engaged in treatment on a specialty unit. The ALOS on residential units is 4 to 8 months, and the focus of treatment is on conflict resolution, structural change, and rehabilitation. Wilderness programs with longer lengths of stay may include more explicitly behavioral interventions. Obviously, the potential for behavioral regressions, secondary gain from treatment, and institutional dependency must be carefully monitored in residential programs.

Patients with antisocial personality, most organic syndromes, and previous longer-term hospital treatment are not candidates for inpatient specialty or residential programs. For milieu integrity, staff morale, and utilization review, it is extremely important to differentiate between the severely ill patient who can begin to engage or reengage in a treatment process and one who cannot and, therefore, would benefit from a low-intensity or environment, group home, or custodial facility.

Organization, Structure, and Process

To balance optimum levels of containment, safety, and treatment focus on the one hand and continuity with the referring environment on the other, inpatient units ideally have an organizational structure that provides a coherent and manageable boundary. This boundary is most visibly represented by a Unit Chief or Program Director who has a direct reporting relationship with and accountability to the overall director of the hospital in general or director of the psychiatric service more specifically. In addition and crucially important for effective functioning, the Unit Chief is responsible for the generation of resources for the unit, mobilization of a consensus among the various disciplines involved in providing treatment, and consultation to and evaluation of patients and staff.[9] Invariably, a clinician, usually a psychiatrist (in which case the title may either be Medical or Clinical Director), fills the role. On many units, a psychologist, social worker, or advanced practice nurse fills it. The Program Director usually collaborates in leadership with senior staff including a psychiatrist, nurse manager, social worker, and possibly the director of therapeutic activities.

Whatever the constituency of the unit's senior staff, the Program Director has final responsibility for the unit's structure and performance. This includes the unit's interaction with the admitting office; its overall treatment processes and outcomes; its educational, quality improvement, and safety initiatives; and its relationship with regulatory and accrediting bodies, medical records, and utilization review. Psychiatrists are also responsible to their hospital's Medical Board. The overall hospital administration or medical school Department of Psychiatry conjointly manages many of these elements. Further details of these structures and their interactions are discussed in detail in chapters by Russakoff (see Chapter 6), Pristach (see Chapter 7), and Weinstock (see Chapter 8).

The Interdisciplinary Team

Turning inward, the bulk of the unit's therapeutic work is managed by interdisciplinary teams, the number depending on the unit's census. The interdisciplinary team represents the treatment arm(s) of the unit's senior staff and reports directly to it. The authors prefer the contemporary term *interdisciplinary* to the traditional *multidisciplinary* team designation because it more accurately reflects the interrelated aspect of the various roles and the importance of the collaborative nature of the treatment task. Furthermore, it is basic to the psychosocial approach that there are limitations in the capacity of any one observer or discipline fully to identify and appreciate the many factors involved in a patient's clinical state and hospital course. This limitation is especially true for those patients with multiaxial diagnoses and complex psychosocial situations, who potentially benefit from the different perspectives derived from the unique role and task of each team member. The importance and centrality of collaborative relationships between various team members cannot be overemphasized, and therefore the following descriptions of the roles perforce involve dyads. Congruent with effective treatment and the requirements of most regulatory bodies, the patient is an essential member of the team. This important membership arrangement ideally begins the process of restoring the patient's sense of agency by demystifying the decision making about care and enhancing involvement throughout the hospital stay.

There are many tasks to be accomplished by the interdisciplinary team, most of which, as mentioned, are accomplished in various dyadic configurations. To begin with, the psychiatrist team leader is responsible for working with the patient on the initial diagnostic assessment as well as the overall organization and coordination of the treatment. The psychiatrist is the key figure in determining what other medical or psychiatric resources are required for the assessment. Because the psychiatrist is responsible for many patients, each patient may be assigned a primary clinician with whom the psychosocial and family assessments are completed.

The primary clinician, often a psychologist, social worker, or advanced practice nurse, has a smaller case load and serves as the patient's ombudsperson, meeting daily and linking him or her with individual, group, and family treatments; maintaining contact with the family and referring clinician during the evaluation and treatment; and implementing a discharge plan. On an acute care unit, the primary clinician may also take the role of the individual psychotherapist. Ideally, the primary clinician is present with the psychiatrist during the initial intake. Because of the primary clinician's role in the treatment and familiarity with potential resources to support the treatment, the psychiatrist and primary clinician collaborate in constructing the interdisciplinary treatment plan as well as actively participating in ongoing utilization review.[10]

In an increasingly cost-conscious hospital environment, the primary clinician may be seen as an unnecessary luxury, the main work accomplished by the psychiatrist and the nurse. On teaching units, the role of primary clinician may be filled by residents or even medical students with close supervision and codocumentation by the psychiatrist.

Naturally the psychiatrist and patient's primary nurse are responsible for the ordering and administration of, feedback about, and compliance with somatic therapies. Because of their continuous presence on the unit, nursing staff also has primary responsibility for the milieu as a whole. One reason the primary nurse is so important in this role is that he or she has the most reliable data about the patient's level of functioning with respect to activities of daily living, social and relational skills and deficits; eating and sleeping patterns; and participation in therapeutic activities such as creative arts, occupational therapy and rehabilitation modalities, and spiritual life. The other reason is that the stability and coherence of the milieu has a major impact on individual patients, and it most clearly provides the unit's essential stabilizing and containing functions. The patient's primary nurse or his or her delegate (perhaps a mental health worker) may have regular one-to-one meetings with the patient. On many units, substance abuse counselors, chaplains, and therapeutic activities personnel collaborate with and report through nursing staff, but there is much variability and no standard of practice in this arrangement.

Under the aegis of the psychiatrist and the primary clinician and following the initial assessments of the patient and family, all members of the interdisciplinary team collaborate on constructing the interdisciplinary treatment plan. Ideally signed by the patient, this written document serves as a road map to the treatment, outlining major problems and goals with time frames, and parsing out the various psychosocial modalities and psychopharmacologic treatments that will ensue. Usually the plan is in place within the first 24 hours so that all staff have a sense of who the patient is and where the treatment is meant to go. More than likely, the patient will be more or less restricted within the unit boundaries for at least the first 24 hours to ensure safety, to observe for anything important that might have been missed on admission, and to allow time for the patient to acclimate to his or her new surroundings. For ideal communication with different shifts, the treatment plan is updated regularly and no less than weekly, a process that usually takes place in the context of treatment team meetings after consultation with the patient.

Following the initial period of restriction to the unit, many units have a carefully graded ladder of increasing freedom and responsibility through which patients progress as they recover. The patient's status on the ladder and the initiation of more autonomous activities and therapeutic passes are the responsibility of the primary nurse and the primary clinician. A number of graduated level systems have been developed. The most useful is one that is relatively simple to understand and can be implemented with consistency. Ideally, most patients will see the level system as having value. The idea is for each patient to have as much autonomy or freedom as his or her behavior would indicate to be prudent. The number of different levels and the criteria for each level, needs to be well known by staff and patients and used consistently. That is, each patient who is on a certain level in a given system knows what to expect and expects the same freedom as every other patient on that same level.

The number of different levels in a level system will vary, in part based on the patient population, the geographic setting, and the ALOS. If a patient is admitted in crisis, he or she is initially likely to need a high degree of supervision for safety. As the crisis begins to resolve and staff have an opportunity to become familiar and establish trust with the patient, it may be feasible to allow a patient to join a small group of patients and leave the unit with staff accompaniment, or even go off the unit independent of staff for predetermined lengths of time with specified purposes and destinations. A hospital that is freestanding, contained with an actual structure around the perimeter, an ALOS of 5 to 7 days, and not part of a general hospital will have more options than an inpatient unit with a shorter ALOS. A facility that has a campus-like feel will have more possibilities than a structure that has no outdoor space for leisure time.

As mentioned, the primary nurse and primary clinicians provide the most input about increases in level and are empowered to reduce levels on the ladder. Medical-legal constraints require that increases must go through the psychiatrist team leader, although actual criteria for movement on the ladder are usually more behavioral than medical-psychiatric. For example, the best indicator for an increase in status is how things have gone on the current status; or the best indicator for a therapeutic pass was how the last one or how the last meeting went with the person(s) with whom the patient is to go out. In collaboration with the patient, the primary nurse and the primary clinician are in the best position to assess these factors. The observational and interpersonal roles filled and data obtained by all members of the nursing staff, especially mental health technicians or aides, in the above-mentioned matters cannot be overemphasized.

It is the responsibility of interdisciplinary team members to identify and resolve strain within the team and between the team and the unit, to maintain the flow of information from the patient's various treatment modalities back to the team, to ensure the patient's involvement in treatment and connection to the therapeutic values of the unit, to provide regular updates and modifications of the initial assessment and interdisciplinary treatment plan, and to arrange for a seamless transition to the next level of care. This includes detailed communication with the providers at the next level of care and as complete and timely a discharge summary as possible.

The responsibilities and tasks enumerated earlier are achieved in several ways. On an acute or psychiatric intensive care unit, the team might meet and round with the patient every day or even twice a day. These rounds share information, assess progress, adjust short-term and long-term goals, and distribute treatment responsibilities. As the patient shows improvement and becomes less acutely ill, the rounding schedule usually becomes more flexible. In the spirit of collaboration and to the extent that it is not overly stimulating or disruptive, team meetings may include the patient. Although it is often useful for staff to disagree, negotiate, and resolve issues in the presence of the patient, even the most highly functional teams need at least one meeting a week without their patients present. Many treatment teams schedule a separate case conference to discuss a difficult patient in more depth, and often this can be a unit-based event. Consistent documentation of the patient's progress and the team's observations and work is vitally important. Notes indicating the process and decisions of the team meetings must be signed by each member attending and include his or her role.

Treatment team meetings are different from the unit's weekly staff meeting. The weekly staff meeting is important for the discussion of general matters such as the unit's relation to the overall hospital, introduction of and farewell to staff members and trainees, scheduling of unit events, coordinating changes in coverage, and communication between disciplines. The staff meeting is also important for more complex matters and may be held on an impromptu basis to discuss emergent situations or dysfunctional events, for staff support and morale, the management of collective disturbances, working out more difficult disagreements about treatment issues, or even interdisciplinary matters unrelated to but possibly effecting specific patient care.

Specific Psychosocial Modalities

INITIAL ASSESSMENT

In the following chapters that deal with specific conditions, therapies specific to the disorder are discussed; therefore, this section of the chapter addresses more general considerations. With each patient, however, the initial assessment takes on special significance: First, because the situation is already tense and confusing for the patient and family members and also because this may be the patient's first encounter with a mental health caretaker or hospital psychiatrist. The importance of an accurate diagnosis and unfamiliarity of the setting and time pressures only increase the importance of these first encounters, but there are generally agreed-upon goals and techniques of the initial interview and clear standards about elements that must be assessed. The interviewer must create an atmosphere of relative ease, balancing between the need to provide conditions for as much disclosure as possible with enough structure so that the patient feels safe. There are no hard-and-fast rules about this, but the interviewer might want to invite a patient's significant other into the interview, or for ease of patient egress, or for interviewer safety leave the door to the interview room ajar. The traditionally accepted format is ideal for coming to a categorical or Diagnostic and Statistical Manual of Mental Disorders, Fourth Edition (DSM-IV) diagnosis and includes a more or less systematic collection of the identifying data, chief complaint, history of the present illness, past psychiatric and medical history, family history, and mental status examination. Specific assessment for suicidality and substance abuse are mandatory for initial assessment and treatment planning. Even in the traditional format, an unspoken goal of the initial interview is to make subsequent interviews and assessments possible.

Following on this idea, MacKinnon et al.[11] indicate another way of thinking about the initial data, one that might provide a more dimensional and narrative view of the patient. They divide the important information into three categories: content and process, introspective and inspective data, and affect and thought. Content relates to the factual information that is gathered, and process relates to the way or manner in which the patient relates to the interviewer, including functional and dysfunctional defensive operations. Introspective data are the information the patient provides verbally about his or her mental state and experiences, whereas inspective data involve nonverbal communications. These data also importantly include those limiting factors the patient brings to the situation. Affect, of course, involves the patient's feelings in general and about the current situation specifically. Thought refers to the quality and quantity of thought, especially its content and degree of organization (pp. 7–9). Thinking about the initial interview(s) in the less formal way of these very experienced authors, especially when the interviewer's point of view is also noted and included, may foster a more robust treatment alliance that will facilitate patient participation, acceptance of treatment, and ultimately greater compliance.

In the case of an admission precipitated by the emergence of difficult-to-manage material or transference/countertransference stalemate or other dysfunctional aspect of an outpatient treatment, it is particularly important to have the input of the outpatient treater before proceeding too far. As Adler[12] points out, these data include the history of the treatment, the therapists' formulation, and hypotheses about transference and countertransference issues. Because of the complicated boundary between the inpatient and outpatient setting as well as feelings on both sides, the role of referring clinicians is often minimized or ignored. Therefore, a valuable source of information is lost; and if the patient is referred back, whatever might have transpired in the treatment to precipitate the admission may well be repeated.

It is crucial that there is as much participation as possible by the social worker assigned to the family and the nurse assigned to the patient in the initial assessment. In addition to hearing the story firsthand, they collect vital family and somatic information that will be central to the treatment plan. Not only does this enhance the quality of the data collected but it also provides the fabric for interdisciplinary collaboration around the case. As soon as the acute situation begins to stabilize, ancillary assessments including substance dependence and abuse, and also, in the case of a longer stay, rehabilitation readiness and spiritual needs can play a role. As mentioned earlier, the written treatment plan is entered into the chart and follows as closely as possible the initial assessments and appears following the assessments and precedes the progress notes.

On the basis of the unit's philosophy, ALOS and resources, and the patient's clinical status, a repertoire of psychosocial interventions above and beyond what has been described as basic to the milieu will be available to the patient. Naturally, these treatments are geared to achieving the goals outlined in the treatment plan and may include combinations drawn from the following sections. The reader will find references to these throughout the rest of the volume related to specific syndromes.

INDIVIDUAL PSYCHOTHERAPY

Perhaps the most reasonable outcome for individual work on the inpatient unit is an increasingly clear picture of the patient's psychopathological situation, a determination of what kind of treatment might be most helpful, and finally the patient's capacity and motivation to pursue individual work. During very short stays and with payers' insistence on medical necessity, even these goals may be too ambitious, and whatever exploration that ensues needs to be tempered with much supportive work. It is also often the case that what was expected to be a short stay of a few days more or less suddenly turns into something more complicated and extended. In these cases, it is extremely valuable to have had an individual, such as the primary clinician as mentioned earlier, assigned to the patient for more one-to-one exploration of the complicating factors and support during the treatment complication or impasse that has developed.

Several recent studies have identified those patients who are most likely to benefit from a psychotherapeutic intervention. These patients include those who are open to a psychosocial causal attribution of illness and a psychotherapeutic approach,[13] patients with a moderate as compared with a high level of anxiety,[14] patients who have higher levels of global functioning from the beginning of treatment,[15] patients with whom there appeared to be an initial alliance,[16] and female patients who acknowledged a perception of interpersonal problems and had a low estimation of their capabilities.[17] Specific attachment patterns do not seem relevant for individual psychotherapy, but a secure attachment may predict a better outcome for group psychotherapy.[18] Because special techniques have been developed for many of the clinical situations covered in this book, the reader is referred to the specific chapter for particular approaches in individual treatments.

Obviously, the psychological signs and symptoms leading to the present admission assume priority in the individual psychotherapy. As Bennett[19] points out, the precipitants most often represent a failure of the individual to adapt to a stressful situation. The stressors might include the loss of a significant relationship or job, the loss of hope, or a major problem in the outpatient treatment; but what usually leads the person into the crisis is a failure of his or her adaptive defenses or absence of important interpersonal support. In focal psychotherapy, while more medical-psychiatric means are addressing the underlying illness, the first step might be to assist the patient in identifying and restoring those usually effective defenses that have failed. Notably, in one patient group studied, turning against the self was the most frequent and ineffective defense mechanism used.[20]

Insofar as psychotherapy is an element of the treatment plan, the assigned psychotherapist usually has more responsibility for collecting relevant psychiatric data and bringing together the biologic and psychosocial data about the patient. Unlike outpatient treatment and in the case of a therapist-administrative split on longer-term units, the individual therapist must coordinate the work with the interdisciplinary team and milieu while making every effort to maintain confidentiality. Naturally, confidentiality does not extend to self-destructive or treatment- and milieu-destructive behaviors, but other personal matters may be kept between patient and therapist. After the initial assessment, the therapist necessarily takes a more active and interactive stance, saving exploratory and expressive techniques for later so as to protect vulnerability and minimize emotional distress. Because of regressive tendencies, cognitive-behavioral (see also Chapter 10) and mentalization-based techniques (see also Chapter 14) are often more useful at this point to learn more about how the patient was thinking. In fact, a growing body of evidence suggests that cognitive techniques are superior to dynamically oriented treatments for patients with psychotic disorders.[21]

Although usually provided in groups on inpatient units, a growing utilization of and evidence for the effectiveness of dialectical behavior therapy (DBT) on an individual, group, and inpatient basis is reported.[22,23] DBT is especially useful in the treatment of suicidal, parasuicidal, or dangerous dissociative episodes and other dysfunctional behaviors that may be associated with the need for admission. Basically a cognitive and behavioral technique and utilizing target lists (as in a treatment plan), it combines sequenced and focused interventions with a validating environment. During the inpatient stay, the goal is to focus on the current episode, leaving more chronic patterns for longer inpatient and outpatient treatments. Treatment proceeds in three phases—commitment, restoring control, and getting out—and is reinforced in individual, group, and milieu contexts. The result is an increase in distress-tolerance, emotion-regulation, mindfulness, and self-management skills.

No matter what sort of individual therapy is provided, the degree of support, exploration, reinforcement, interpretation, and confrontation utilized by the individual psychotherapist will be determined by many of the factors suggested earlier. Valuable here-and-now information derived from the enactments of basic interpersonal relationship patterns and interactions between the patient, the team, and the milieu enrich the psychotherapy, preventing it from turning into an unhelpful refuge.[24,25] By providing a consistent figure, a regular and private space, and an agreed-upon session length and time, not only does an inpatient psychotherapy provide an opportunity for the patient to unburden himself or herself, understand much of the mystery of what is happening, and receive much-needed support but it also illuminates for the therapist much more about the impact of the patient's relatedness in the world. Naturally, problems that arise between therapist and patient are often reflective of the kinds of difficulties the patient encounters in life in general and provide even more information to support treatment efforts. Although this is extremely valuable information for the patient's treatment, it puts additional pressure on the shoulders of the individual psychotherapist. Such issues have been amply described in works about psychodynamically informed hospital treatment from Main[1] and Burnham[26] to Gabbard[27] and Munich and Allen.[28]

When patients have the psychological and material resources to benefit from a longer (several weeks to a few months) hospital stay, the individual psychotherapy usually takes on a more important role in the treatment plan. In most treatment centers that provide such treatment and depending on how disturbed the patient is, the psychotherapy function is carried out by someone different from the person or interdisciplinary team responsible for the clinical-administrative aspects of the patient's care. In this way, the individual psychotherapist is able to get a better picture of the patient's patterns of manifest and more subtle adaptive and maladaptive behaviors and ways of thinking, illuminate any tendency to provoke conflicts (splitting) between significant figures, and identify important transference and countertransference trends. This capacity is true whether or not psychodynamic, mentalization-based, dialectical, or cognitive-behavioral techniques are being employed in the psychotherapy. Because inpatients are very often more fragile than outpatients, staff members as well as psychotherapists must perform auxiliary ego functions such as reality testing, assistance with impulse control, anticipation of consequences (judgment), and sharpening of thinking and boundaries. In addition, the therapist must maintain contact with the team around such issues as attendance and general themes, and especially when the patient, another patient, or a staff member may be in some danger. Therefore, because of the holding nature of the inpatient milieu, the availability of and more frequent contact with the psychotherapist, inpatient psychotherapy is inherently less confidential and more supportive.[29]

GROUP THERAPY

Group therapies of various sorts are likely the most widely utilized mode of providing psychosocial treatment on the inpatient unit. Since their inception, there have been many forms of group interventions ranging from traditional process and exploratory techniques to more structured and educative models through problem-solving and social-skills groups, to those organized around a specific technique for specific illnesses (body-image disturbance, substance abuse). Insofar as one of the main reasons for hospital treatment relates to the deterioration or loss of an important relationship and its support, the inpatient group that focuses on interpersonal relations becomes a key therapeutic instrument.

General principles for group work on the inpatient unit as outlined by Yalom,[30] Kibel,[31] and Kemker and Kibel[32] include ensuring that the group is fully authorized and integrated into the unit structure with regular scheduling, leadership, and time and space boundaries. Insofar as possible, patients should not miss or be called from the group for other appointments. Because of the rapid turnover of patients, their heterogeneity of psychopathology, and varying levels of motivation and intactness, groups may be organized according to the interdisciplinary team responsible for their treatment or according to level of severity of illness. This kind of grouping facilitates the group process that ideally focuses on the here-and-now interpersonal factors relevant to the admission, minimizes conflict, and attempts to create a safe, supportive, and constructive atmosphere. Leadership should help the group form agendas and otherwise be active and directive to facilitate the emergence of relevant issues, especially interpersonal concerns. Generally speaking about units with a shorter length of stay, the authors cited earlier indicate the importance of not trying to "fix" problems, reducing a focus on the past, and minimizing critical feedback and confrontation.

The goals of inpatient group therapy on the contemporary inpatient unit have mainly to do with giving patients the idea that expressing their issues will be helpful, that doing so will promote therapeutic processes and engagement. Furthermore, participation in group therapy will decrease both the isolation that has come about from the stigma of his or her illness and the anxiety associated with a hospital stay that includes witnessing conflicts and disturbed behaviors in the milieu. Recent studies have demonstrated the effectiveness of inpatient group therapy, especially in patients who exhibited symptoms of mood disorder,[33] in utilizing cognitive therapy techniques for patients with active symptoms of schizophrenia,[34,35] in patients having vocational strains and conflicts,[36] in helping survivors of incest improve coping strategies,[37] and in catalyzing continuity of treatment after discharge.[38]

Naturally, a more extended length of stay and stable group membership create the potential for more ambitious goals and expansive exploratory techniques, consistent with those sought in outpatient treatment. These include a less directive approach by the therapist, more focus on group process and dynamics, and therefore more tolerance for interpersonal conflict and confrontation. Inpatient group therapy on the intermediate and longer length-of-stay unit will have a greater relationship to processes on the overall milieu than on the shorter-term unit and therefore can become a valuable learning tool for the individual's relationship to his or her social environment.

PSYCHOEDUCATION

The last decade has seen a great increase in psychoeducational techniques employed on inpatient units, usually practiced in a group format. On the basis of success with family groups[39] and patient satisfaction data indicating that patients have a great interest in learning more about their illness and obtaining techniques for coping, these groups are focused on such matters as details of etiology and symptoms of various illness configurations, affect regulation and management, mindfulness, relationship building, the many issues related to medication utilization and compliance, trauma, and social skills training. The groups are enhanced by an active and interactive stance of the leader(s), didactic elements and problem-solving exercises, role playing, and homework assignments. These techniques support the reestablishment of patient agency by reducing stigma, modifying guilt and blame, and expecting participation that involves patients more actively in their treatment. Other than in the realm of psychoeducational work with families, there is far less published evidence for the effectiveness of these techniques on the inpatient service than there is for group therapy.[40,41]

The first extensions of psychoeducation beyond its use with families were for patients with trauma and personality disorders and then with a wide range of problems and disorders.[42] It was demonstrated that psychoeducational programs were an important way to strengthen the relationship between patient and clinician, that information about the illness was effectively transmitted in this manner, and that patient's motivation for seeking future treatment was enhanced.[43,44] In units with a longer length of stay, psychoeducational techniques may be used extensively to provide more in-depth information about relationships, illness configurations, and coping skills. As with group psychotherapy in these units, the work is facilitated by having homogeneous patient groupings.

Allen[45] outlined a set of general principles guiding psychoeducational work for patients with serious mental disorders who had sustained trauma in important relationships. These include organizing the educational content into a simple, conceptual framework; involving the patients in the educational process; helping patients learn to communicate their difficulties with others; fostering a group climate conducive to self-disclosure, exploration, and learning; addressing resistance before encouraging change; keeping constructive coping in views; and, while acknowledging the severity of the problems and the difficulty overcoming them, also fostering hope (pp. 353–354).

FAMILY AND MARITAL INTERVENTIONS

In the contemporary era, the question is not whether to involve the patient's family in hospital treatment; rather, the issue is the timing and intensity of that involvement, which ideally takes place from the earliest contacts, even before the actual admission. Because it is often the case that patients come to the hospital from a family context and will very likely return there, effective treatment must involve the significant other or family members. The question of timing and intensity is represented in the differentiation between and developing processes in alliance and assessment, support and psychoeducation, and discharge planning and continuing care and possible therapy. In the ideal circumstance, the family moves from being a member of the treatment team during the assessment to a full participation in the treatment in the ongoing hospital and outpatient phases. In the case of readmissions, especially with an aware and motivated family, the focus can shift from assessment to psychoeducation and therapy much more quickly. Many inpatient units also run psychoeducational groups for their patients and families.

Earlier in this chapter, it was noted that the patient's primary clinician has responsibility for the interface between the interdisciplinary team and the family. This important relationship affects the quality of the alliance with the family, the evaluation of their connection with the patient and their own needs and dynamics, and thus what tasks need to be accomplished to help everyone through this phase of the illness. Glick and Clarkin[46] identified six goals for the family work: (a) accepting the reality of the illness and understanding the current episode, (b) identifying current episodic stressors,

(c) identifying potential future stressors with and outside the family, (d) elucidating stressful family interactions, (e) planning strategies for managing or minimizing future stressors, and (f) accepting the need for continued treatment (pp. 342–344).

Techniques to achieve these goals require collaboration, facilitation of openness, establishment of trust, consultation, and psychoeducation. It is worth noting here that the terms *family systems* and *dynamics* are minimized, especially during the acute phase and most likely during the course of shorter hospital stays. In a longer-term environment, especially with a family which has been through previous acute stays and psychoeducational approaches, a more formal family therapy process may be instituted in which the exploration of dynamics and long-standing underlying conflicts may take place with the hope of resolution and change.

Important assumptions underlying family work include an appreciation of the psychosocial factors in psychopathology, the central role of the family in recovery from virtually every diagnostic entity, the burden of illness a family regularly sustains, and the importance of the family's traditional ways of coping. In this last regard, an important factor supported by considerable evidence is the role of expressed emotion in many families with a psychiatrically ill member.[47] Although the overt expression of emotion in a closed system does not cause illness, it can make adaptation to it much more difficult. Furthermore, the modulation of that same emotion has been shown to enhance positive outcomes. Finally, it has been shown that the appropriately engaged family plays a significant role in helping the patient understand and maintain medication and treatment compliance over the course of illness.[48,49]

REHABILITATION AND CREATIVE ARTS THERAPIES

The last decade has witnessed the emergence of a considerable evidence base for the utilization of rehabilitative techniques to help patients normalize their functioning and acquire knowledge about disease management in such diverse areas as personal goals and roles, quality of life issues, medication maintenance, functional living skills, management of symptoms, improved cognitive skills, and the utilization of the full range of supportive social services.[50,51] Rehabilitation services depend on a collaborative approach, systematic assessment, staged educational exercises and experiences, and the involvement of family members when possible. Although the range of techniques is not easy to establish and follow through on an acute care unit, certain ways to assess rehabilitation readiness can be utilized given the availability of published instruments or appropriately trained staff. Some techniques have been developed for use on short-term units.[52]

As might be inferred from the information provided in the previous text, a major contribution of rehabilitation techniques is in helping patients with discharge readiness, especially for those with serious mental illness and longer lengths of inpatient stays. Community reentry programs led to slightly higher attendance at first appointments after discharge,[53] enhanced physical well-being of the patients and reintegration into the community, and facilitated community placement.[54]

Rehabilitation psychiatry, sometimes under the purview of the occupational therapist, is competing for inpatient budget resources with traditional creative arts therapies such as music, art, and drama therapies. The last decade has seen a distinct diminishment in utilization of the latter modalities except in longer-term specialty hospitals.

NONSPECIFIC OBSERVING AND THINKING ABOUT PATIENT BEHAVIORS

It is a premise of a psychosocial approach that symptoms and behaviors have complex determinants and meanings. Furthermore, patients are often communicating on different levels and in different ways at the same time. Although interpretations of such behaviors are usually in the province of the therapist to whom the behavior is presented or in the context of a specific treatment relationship, this may not be the case and therefore thoughtfulness should usually precede any interpretation or action. For example, a patient who is recovering from a psychotic episode is stating that he wants to leave the hospital but is regularly not far from sight of the nursing station where he has nothing to say when approached. Is he communicating that his needs are not being recognized or that he does not feel part of decision making in his treatment, or is he simply testing boundaries or expressing some ambivalence about the nature of his request?

Or does the young woman with a borderline personality disorder and a history of probable traumatic sexual abuse who is complaining about the attention of a male nursing aide have a legitimate point to make or is she signaling her readiness to begin talking about and exploring the details of her history? And if the latter is true, is there an adequate therapeutic and containing context for her to do so during this stay, or would it be better for her to wait to explore this material until after discharge? And is the older, widowed patient with a severe depression who seems suddenly better, brighter, and more interactive on the way to recovery or is he now quietly committed to carrying out the suicide plan for which he was admitted? And while most staff know not to argue the point with a delusional patient, what approach should they take when alone with the patient or off the unit before automatically looking for help, returning to the unit, or pressing for more antipsychotic medication? These and other questions may well fall between the individual or group therapist and other staff members in the milieu but require thoughtful and measured responses in the service of good treatment.

In this regard and also by way of introducing the next section on the treatment milieu, it is important to note here the important but often underestimated interaction between the individual patient and the milieu in which his or her thoughts, feelings, and behaviors take place. There has been much written to describe, explicate, and analyze this complicated interaction such that no matter how ill the patient or extreme the specific behavior, an adequate psychosocial approach to patient care cannot consider that behavior without also considering and appreciating its context. In other words, not only does the treatment milieu described in subsequent text provide holding and containment but also when disrupted play a role in the exacerbation or facilitation of suicidal and aggressive behaviors as well as such events as collective disturbances and elopements.

Beginning with the documentation of the influence on social system processes that value systems can have on inpatient treatment,[55] to the relation of collective disturbances occurring when there is disorganization with the staff hierarchy,[3] to dysfunctional group processes mobilizing primitive object relations that lead to regressive behaviors among group members,[56] to the effect that special patients have on a vulnerable staff,[57,58] to the effect of the disruption of a unit's boundaries on group and intergroup processes,[59] to the contribution of intergroup and intragroup tensions to dysfunctional behaviors,[60] there is compelling evidence for the interaction between the ward milieu and individual patient behaviors. Some of the symptoms of a disrupted milieu that leaders need to be alert to include demoralization, excessive and sustained countertransference reactions, severe intrastaff conflict, the unavailability of staff (due to excessive turnover or illness), acting out of conflicts, failure of group task accomplishment, and collective disturbances.[61]

The Treatment Milieu

Just as the contemporary standard of care supports the presence of the patient on the interdisciplinary team, the discussion of complicated unit events often benefits from the involvement of the patient community as well as the staff. For at least 60 years, effective inpatient units have actively cultivated a treatment milieu that is therapeutic as well as containing. By tradition and because of their 24-hour presence, the milieu is generally considered the domain of nursing. The underlying premise of the milieu is that all aspects of the environment in an inpatient setting can contribute to patient care. This includes the interpersonal and social aspects as well as the organizational rules and the actual physical elements of the environment. Its goals include providing a holding environment, diagnostic field, community surrogate, and treatment potential. In the ideal situation, both staff and patients are the beneficiaries of these arrangements.

On an acute unit, creating and managing the environment in a way that maintains a therapeutic atmosphere has become increasingly challenging. The challenge is to maintain continuity in the therapeutic elements of the milieu with the rapid turnover of patients and with patients who are typically admitted in the midst of crisis. Patients may be suicidal or have repeated episodes of deliberate self-harm behaviors including cutting and burning. Patients may be confused, sexually disinhibited, or prone to elopement.[62] On a longer-term and more stable milieu, the inevitable emergence of complex patient and staff dynamics provide the challenge. Nevertheless, it is still feasible to manage the environment actively and provide a setting where social interactions, therapeutic activities, role modeling by staff, and the physical setting can discourage pathology, support adaptive behaviors and attitudes, and foster experiences that benefit patients.

A number of treatment models have been used to guide the development of therapeutic milieus. Rehabilitation models focus on the development or restoration of skills that permit an individual to return to more independent living outside the hospital setting. The focus of object relations models is to help patients reestablish their own internal world. Crisis intervention models take a problem-solving approach, with a short-term focus. Behavior rather than inner psychic states is the focus of behavior models of milieu care. There are a number of other models, but as previously noted there is no clear evidence that one model is superior to another. What appears to matter most is having a treatment model that the interdisciplinary team agrees upon, understands, and can use to develop, implement, and maintain the environment.[63]

Whatever treatment model is used, the five functions of the milieu formulated by Gunderson[64] over 30 years ago continue to be useful in the conceptualization of a treatment environment. These overlapping functions or techniques are containment, support, structure, involvement, and validation.

CONTAINMENT

Containment has to do with the provision of a structure that fosters physical and emotional safety, a holding environment where patients feel nurtured. Staff who can "connect" with patients and convey a sense of warmth, availability, and caring promote an environment where patients feel accepted. Staff intervene with patients in the management of intense, overwhelming emotional urges, preventing impulses from being acted out behaviorally. Patients need to know the environment will be an auxiliary ego of sorts and provide what they, themselves, may temporarily not be able to manage.[63]

The physical environment cannot be overlooked and has been recognized since the time of Florence Nightingale. Nightingale espoused the need for proper ventilation and cleanliness. Seemingly simple elements can have a substantial impact. One of these elements has to do with the type and arrangement of the furniture. Furniture is often selected with durability and safety in mind. Comfort and esthetic qualities also need to be taken into account. It is disconcerting to walk into an inpatient community space and find straight-backed chairs lining the walls. Careful consideration should be given to what will welcome patients and enhance social interaction among patients and between patients and staff. Too much space can inhibit conversation and promote isolation, whereas overcrowding can contribute to anxiety and irritability. Easily rearranged furniture allows for reconfiguring to facilitate a range of activities. An open nursing station influences the patient's perception of nurses' availability.

Torre[65] addressed the use of color in healing environments. Color can affect an entire setting and change the essence of the space. Blue and green are examples of colors that promote relaxation, whereas orange and yellow activate or energize the space. Lighter hues can make a room seem more spacious. The environment can be further enhanced and made more soothing with the addition of art, plants, or an aquarium. Even in brief hospitalizations, patients may find it comforting to have personal items such as a special pillow or family photo.

SUPPORT

Support is a function of the therapeutic milieu that contributes to patients' sense of security. Experiences that allow patients the opportunity to gain a sense of competence and confidence are important. Providing verbal reassurance and reinforcement that is genuine and realistic are beneficial to patients.

Staff members are instrumental in helping those patients who need assistance with activities of daily living. The staff needs to be prepared to assist with the basics of bathing and dressing in some treatment settings. There is a delicate balance to be achieved. The patient needs assistance, yet part of the assistance is helping in a manner that promotes the patient's autonomy, agency, and readaptation as much as possible. It can be labor intensive and time consuming to *assist with* rather than *doing for* the patient. The value and potential gains for the patient may be difficult to see but must not be sacrificed for perceived efficiency.

STRUCTURE

Structure, the third function of the milieu identified by Gunderson, refers to the framework that is provided. The framework contributes to a sense of security and can help the patient think before acting. Functional components for orientation need to be readily available. Clocks that are easy to read and set to the correct time and daily newspapers are considered advisable. A warm welcome upon arrival to the unit can instill an initial sense of security. It is also an opportunity to provide an orientation that can convey the basic framework of the milieu.[66] Most individuals respond better when they know what is expected and when. Schedules or routines that are accurately and clearly stated along with the rules, for example, no smoking inside, are very helpful. The orienting information needs to be presented in a way that is not overwhelming and may need to be reviewed several times. Having a printed handout that highlights the information is valuable. Staff identification is part of providing clear structure. Who are these staff members and what are their roles? At the very least, all staff members need to introduce themselves and wear name badges that are easy to read. Privilege systems or graduated levels of responsibility are yet another aspect of the structure within the milieu. Ideally, it is woven into the overall treatment for each patient in a way that is motivating and not used to punish a patient.

The overall amount of structure is an issue that has to be deliberately managed and evaluated periodically by the interdisciplinary team. A structure that is too rigid can become antitherapeutic and prevent growth opportunities. Too little structure, structure that is not clear, or inconsistencies can contribute to confusion and unsafe conditions for staff and patients. In the process of day-to-day management of the milieu, it is not unusual for nursing staff to make temporary changes in the structure. A common change applies to the privilege level of an individual patient. When an individual regresses, it may be necessary to increase the level of supervision or decrease the amount of freedom that had been allowed. When this occurs, it is important for the team to support the change, a change that should be consistent with what is needed to optimize the treatment conditions for a patient, including the patient's personal safety. These adjustments in structure generally should not be made as a unilateral decision, nor should the decisions be made in anger with intent to punish. There can be a fine line between providing natural consequences and punishing when a privilege is withheld based on a patient's behaviors within the milieu. It is important for staff to be comfortable setting limits, and staff need to know that the team will support their decisions. This is an issue that typically surfaces regularly in the overall management of the dynamics that emerge with the ever-changing treatment environment.

INVOLVEMENT

The processes that encourage patients to interact and engage within the milieu are termed *involvement*. Involvement as a function of the milieu allows the patient opportunities to practice new skills and ways of modifying maladaptive interpersonal patterns. Even with brief hospital stays, patients can work on improving social skills when the milieu emphasizes collaboration, cooperation, and involvement.

Before hospitalization, it is not unusual for patients to have experienced a sense of isolation, which may continue into the hospital setting. Staff, in the context of the milieu, should make an effort to create opportunities for interpersonal interactions that are nonthreatening and feasible for individuals who have limited internal resources. Patients cite the opportunity for interpersonal interaction with peers as the most valuable aspect of inpatient psychiatric care.[67]

VALIDATION

The fifth function of the milieu Gunderson identified is validation. Validation, the affirmation of individuals, can be an antidote for hopelessness and helplessness.[63] It is achieved through one-to-one interactions between staff and patients. These private talks may not be formal psychotherapy but they can be therapeutic nonetheless. Validation may also be experienced by the patient through formal and informal group interactions. A key feature is that the patient is able to express concerns and describe troubling symptoms without fear of being criticized or experiencing punitive responses.

STAFF CONSIDERATION AND THE MILIEU

The five functions of the milieu are not automatic. Containment, support, and structure can be achieved only through careful design and ongoing collaborative efforts of the staff. Time constraints in short-term hospitalizations may reduce the degree to which substantive involvement and validation can occur. Therefore, nurses are strongly encouraged to remain mindful of every aspect of the environment, knowing that virtually its every aspect could be therapeutic, and patients have limited time in the treatment setting. There must be keen sensitivity to barriers interfering with therapeutic interactions. For example, simultaneous use of a computer to chart while talking with a patient during an assessment interview could easily interfere with the initiation of rapport. Because of the close proximity of the work done by the nursing staff within the patients' community space, there are nearly constant opportunities for nursing staff to role model interactions. The need for self-awareness cannot be overstated and is an essential element to building the therapeutic milieu.

Ensuring that the team recognizes and resolves conflict is particularly critical to the health of the milieu. When a milieu begins to feel as though it is unraveling, struggling to function in a way that is therapeutic, it can be instructive for the team to take a step back and examine the team dynamics. A patient or group of patients may be taking on the distress or dysfunctional behaviors of the team, as was the case in the following scenario.

Case Vignette

Persistent gossip, conflict, and discord between the nursing staff on different shifts had escalated to the point that they were palpable. The nurse manager called a meeting with all nursing staff to address the concerns. Initially staff members were defensive and no one was willing to engage in the exploration of the dynamics or accept responsibility.

With the skillful intervention by the nurse manager, some initial resolution began to take place with plans for follow-up meetings. Behavioral expectations were stated and plans were made to continue the process of resolving the conflicts and reestablish appropriate working relationships.

Later in the day, during a community meeting, patients complained bitterly about one another, about the lack of trust within the patient group, and problems with gossip. The community meeting was almost a caricature of the staff meeting.

The nurse manager was able to seize this opportunity to teach staff about the power of the parallel process.

The circumstances within the patient community served as an unusually clear example of the parallel process. Typically the problems are first recognized in the patient community as illustrated as far back as the reports of Stanton and Schwartz on "collective disturbances" in 1954[3] and in the classic article "The Coffee-Pot Affair: An Episode in the Life of a Therapeutic Community."[68] Whether the terminology used is parallel process, transference/countertransference, or projective identification, the concept must be acknowledged and addressed openly and on an ongoing basis.

SAFETY

Safety is always a primary consideration in inpatient psychiatric-mental health care settings. Staff members who feel their safety is threatened cannot be effective, and patients will struggle with engagement in treatment when there is a question of safety. Therefore, this volume specifically addresses safety both in this chapter on general psychosocial approaches and in Chapter 12 on the assessment, management, and prevention of agitation and aggression.

The milieu is especially vulnerable when there has been a change in venue or leadership, an influx of new staff that has not yet been integrated into the team, or an unusually large number of new patients who have not been incorporated into the milieu.

It may not be possible to manage the rate at which patients are admitted, but attending to staff retention and managing turnover rates is paramount to the success of an interdisciplinary team and to the stability of the treatment milieu. The potentially dysfunctional impact of using "float" staff or staff from agencies should not be underestimated. This extends to the support staff such as those in housekeeping. What initially may seem to be saved fiscally by contracting services may in fact be lost in the long run with the ongoing failure of continuity and stability.

Even when the milieu is functioning well, it is feasible for a patient's behavior to escalate to the point of being out of control. Behaviors can erupt suddenly with great intensity.[69] If the milieu is cohesive and the team is intact, it is quite possible to respond rapidly by de-escalating the situation, judiciously using the quiet room and constant observation, and therefore decompressing an incident of extreme escalation with minimal disruption. Although such episodes may lead to the use of seclusion and restraint, it is important to note that it is now a principle of regulatory and accrediting bodies that the use of seclusion or restraint is ideally the last resort.

The concept of preventing violence and therefore the use of seclusion and restraint is multifaceted and includes, but is not limited to, specific assessment criteria that help identify risk for violence, well-designed and meaningful treatment, use of safety plans, and quiet rooms.[70] One recommended approach, the Public Health Prevention Model (PHPM), begins with the identification of factors contributing to an individual's difficulty maintaining behavioral control. The identification process is initiated during the admission process and a plan is developed with the individual patient ideally resulting in preventing, minimizing, or mitigating problem behaviors. The patient and possibly family provide input to the plan based on past experiences. Primary prevention is achieved through interventions designed to anticipate and head off the development of situations that put an individual in a situation of risk.[70]

A quiet room is a room or area within the milieu where a patient elects to spend time to reduce stimulation and prevent behavior escalation. The use of this room or special space allows the patient to regain a calmer composure, beginning with the patient choosing to use the space, in other words, being in as much control as reasonably possible. The use of the quiet space can be preplanned with the patient so that he or she can identify triggers or patterns for which the quiet room would be helpful. The patient is not locked or otherwise forcefully detained in a quiet room. Interventions are individualized to support de-escalation. There is a wide gamut of interventions that a patient may find helpful ranging from the use of soothing music, having a comfort object such as a blanket or photo, talking with a staff member, or journaling among others.

The language that the staff uses is powerful as it can fuel or prevent problems. Because how we speak about something or someone reflects how we value and treat that something or someone,[71] person-first language in the treatment setting is strongly encouraged. Person-first language centers on each patient as a unique individual and eliminates dehumanizing labeling and judgmental comments such as "that borderline" or "they are just manipulating." In person-first language there is sensitivity to the aggression in terms such as *take downs*. Speaking of an individual, rather than a diagnostic category could clearly impact the dynamics in an interaction. A particularly difficult rhetorical usage is one that begins with a staff member saying to a patient, "you need to ... " This construction can easily be construed as provocative by the agitated or aggressive patient and confusing by the patient in a psychotic state. Usually, the staff member is conveying a need of his or her own rather than one of the patient.

Another specific example of attitude or mindset has to do with the approach to physical containment when a patient is violent. With one intervention program, the term for a number of staff coming together to intervene is *show of force*. Typically, the idea is to have enough staff present that the patient sees he or she is definitely outnumbered and acquiesces to the direction and expectations of the staff. If this does not occur in a very brief time span, there is a "take down." The patient is physically held and escorted with force or possibly put on the floor, and then carried by staff to a seclusion area.

By contrast, "show of support" results in a number of staff coming together, but the idea is to support the de-escalation. The staff may actually stay close, but not necessarily visible, to the patient, so as not to convey intimidation or threat to the patient. The qualitative experience as well as outcome for the patient and staff tends to be quite different from the "show of force" intervention style.

Seclusion and Restraint

As physical injury and psychological damage can be inflicted on patients as well as staff, with ensuing liability risk, there is inherent danger in each use of seclusion or restraint. As a result of changing practices and research findings, there is now an intense focus on reducing the use of seclusion and restraints in clinical settings.[70] At times conflict is unavoidable, and perhaps even necessary, in the treatment process. The secondary level of prevention in the PHPM involves early recognition of problematic thoughts, feelings, and behaviors followed by interventions to minimize and resolve these before behaviors escalate. When, because of extreme behavioral dyscontrol, seclusion, or restraint is unavoidable, tertiary prevention would be appropriate. Tertiary prevention would call for postseclusion and postrestraint interventions designed to mitigate the impact of the seclusion/restraint episode by analyzing the event, taking corrective action, and preventing a reoccurrence.[70]

In this regard, the need for staff education and training is supported by research findings that reveal staff–patient interactions are closely linked with conflicts that arise. Huckshorn[70] reported that researchers found violence is associated with environmental triggers, including an atmosphere of staff "taking control," focusing on "managing" patients, failure to individualize treatment, idiosyncratic and arbitrary rule enforcement, and patient boredom.

A number of available programs focus on the use of therapeutic communication and other de-escalating skills to promote improved staff interaction with patients, with the hope of lowering the incidence of seclusion and restraint. To reduce the danger of physical injury and emotional trauma for patients and staff and improve patient outcomes, having staff trained in one standardized approach within a facility is imperative. No matter which program is selected, the common element in all reputable programs will be a shared understanding among staff as to how to physically approach and contain a violent patient when other interventions have failed to de-escalate the behaviors. To ensure safety of patients and staff, regular practice of acquired strategies and techniques is important. The use of de-escalation techniques, quiet rooms, constant observation, and seclusion and restraint are discussed in further detail in Chapter 12 on the assessment, management, and prevention of agitation and aggression.

Debriefing

As mentioned with the PHPM, debriefing is an important element in different stages; immediately following a seclusion or restraint event, the debriefing is led by a senior staff member who was not directly involved in the event. The intent is to ensure the well-being of everyone involved and to review the event with a focus on reducing future use of seclusion or restraints. The initial debriefing also addresses the documentation and aims to stabilize the milieu. It is useful to have a template or guide for the process. A second debriefing should be conducted. The use of behavior chain analysis or an approach similar to that used in a root cause analysis can be helpful to systematically examine what occurred. The aim is to identify anything that could be improved to avoid a similar event forwarding the future. Both debriefing times have a prevention/education focus, not blame for staff or the patients involved.

SUICIDAL BEHAVIOR AND ITS MANAGEMENT

Suicidality is a common precipitant to hospitalization. Although it is difficult to acknowledge, staff as well as patients know hospitalization will not necessarily ensure the preservation of life. The underlying expectation is that when people are admitted to hospitals their safety will be maintained. Because a suicidal patient presents complex emotional and legal challenges that can elicit strong reactions in even the most experienced staff, clinicians typically do not relish the opportunity to work with an individual contemplating suicide. Consequently, mental health professionals have recognized the need for more empiric evidence to guide clinical practice. The Suicide Resource Prevention Center in collaboration with the American Association of Suicidology have identified core competencies, based on research evidence and clinical expertise, to be used by mental health professionals to guide practice in the assessment and management of suicide risk.

Managing one's own reactions to the suicidal patient is the first and perhaps the most important of the competencies.[72] Persistent self-reflection and clinical supervision are vital to the mental health professional's ability to manage reactions and countertransference. Managing one's own reactions is fundamental to the overall process of establishing a therapeutic alliance with a patient who is suicidal. It is within the context of the therapeutic alliance that patients can confide the extent of their suicidal thoughts and plans and warning signs can be identified.

Suicide warning signs are the earliest detectable signs that indicate an elevated risk for suicide in the near term (minutes, hours, or days). Warning signs are subjectively expressed or behaviorally implied, or both.[73] Specifically, an individual who has made a very recent suicide threat or is searching for a means is said to be exhibiting warning signs. Additional warning signs supported by evidence include the following:

- Hopelessness
- Rage, anger, seeking revenge
- Acting reckless, engaging in risky activity, seemingly without thinking
- Feeling trapped, seeing no way out
- Increasing alcohol or other drug use
- Withdrawal from family, friends, or society
- Anxiety, agitation, inability to sleep, or sleeping excessively
- Dramatic mood changes
- No reason for living, no sense of purpose

Warning signs become the target for interventions when there is a high risk for suicide in the near term.

The use of warning signs in assessment and management of suicide risk is a shift from the traditional attention to risk factors. There is a plethora of statistically significant risk factors identified in the literature. Risks are an integration of biological, psychological, social, and cultural factors that are correlated with increased risk that one day an individual will die by suicide.[72] Risk factors are not predictors of suicide. That being said, identifying the risk factors for any given patient is still an absolute necessity in the provision of care. Because suicidal behavior cannot be reliably predicted, an assessment of risk should be made and documented for every patient.[74] At a minimum, this assessment of risk needs to include questions about suicidal thoughts, plans, intent, and actions along with past history of suicidality. The assessment should encompass known risk and protective factors. On the basis of clinical observations as well as the individual patient's responses, the clinician is expected to understand what contributes to escalating suicide risk and make an educated judgment as to the degree of acute risk for suicidal behavior and specifically document that judgment. Clinical interventions based on reducing or resolving modifiable risk factors and strengthening protective factors are essential. The reduction of risk factors or enhancing protective factors can result in a different trajectory for an individual who is or has been at risk for suicide. Effective treatment for the sources of the underlying psychological pain is also imperative.

During hospitalization, it is important for staff to be attentive to risk factors, warning signs, psychological stressors, and the mental status of every individual patient in an ongoing assessment process. The use of standardized scales or tools can be helpful in the assessment process. Objective data that can be collected at intervals can be beneficial in the ongoing assessment process. Assessment tools are often best when combined with the interactive interview as it could be misleading to reduce the overall suicide risk to a number on a scale.

During interactions aimed at assessing suicidality, it is important for the clinician to maintain a matter-of-fact demeanor and be fully present to the patient. This increases the likelihood that the patient will be able to sense the ability of the clinician to tolerate whatever he or she has to reveal. When there is an initial denial of suicide, particularly during an initial interview, it is important to find a way to ask the question again. The case example illustrates the benefit of asking a second time.

Case Vignette

During the admission of a young woman, the psychiatrist asked the patient about suicidal ideation to which the patient responded, "Occasionally I have thought of killing myself, but I do not think I would ever do it (suicide). It would hurt my parents too much." The psychiatrist then commented "I understand that you would not want your parents to be hurt. I wonder though, when you have had thoughts of suicide, do you ever think about how you would kill yourself?" To this, the young woman replied, "Oh, yes, I actually have the plans to build a guillotine in my garage."

It is easy to see, from the patient's first response to the second, ideas about the patient's risk for suicide change. Factors that may influence the patient's willingness to be candid include the ability of the clinician to be direct in the communication. Asking a follow-up question helps convey to the patient that there is a genuine interest and that the clinician can tolerate hearing the answer.

Suicidal individuals often struggle with ambivalence about living and dying. There may be ambivalence about whether to trust the clinician enough to disclose their suicidality. Suicidal individuals may have difficulty articulating their suicidal ideation if it is the first time they have verbalized their ideation. Adequate time must be allowed for patients to formulate their responses to questions, and the clinician has to be comfortable with silence during this time of formulation.

Clinicians need to consider whether the patient has reason to minimize or exaggerate risk.[72] For instance, if a patient has previously been at high risk for imminent suicide and hospitalized, he or she may have been placed on one-to-one supervision, always in the visual field of a staff member who remains within arm's length. This can be experienced by the patient as intolerably intrusive. The patient understandably would want to avoid being placed in that situation again. Or a patient may be motivated to exaggerate suicidality, dreading a pending discharge because of fears about being discharged from the security of the hospital environment.

A collaborative approach to assessment and management of suicide risk is widely recommended.[75,76] Insofar as the patient is viewed as a partner, an active participant with the treatment team, the clinical staff has to manage the delicate balance of taking appropriate responsibility rather than taking total control. One intervention is the use of a written crisis response plan or safety plan, developed collaboratively with the patient and members of the team. These plans reduce the reliance on so-called and basically ineffective "no-suicide contracts" and provide the patient with tangible ideas for what can be done when suicidal urges are present. The crisis response plan is a living, evolving document that can be modified during the course of treatment and at the time of discharge to be used to help the patient cope as he or she transitions from the hospital, a known high-risk time for reoccurrence of suicidal urges.[73,77]

Reconciling the difference and potential conflict between the clinician's goal to prevent suicide and the patient's goal to eliminate psychological pain is essential to the success of interventions with suicidal patients.[72] A strong focus on supporting the patient in reducing the emotional pain needs to be incorporated into the plan of care. This extends to the need for staff to hold hope for the patient, particularly when the patient is not able to find hope.

Providing a safe holding environment is fundamental to the well-being of a suicidal patient. This can include using varying levels of precautions, anticipating obvious means to suicide available in the physical environment, and making necessary modifications in the environment. Staff may need to remove select objects, and increase the frequency of documented watchfulness or observation of patient behaviors, strongly consider restricting the patient to the unit, while allowing the patient as much control and input into the process as possible. Meal trays may need to be delivered to the unit for the patient rather than allowing him or her to leave the unit. The trays often have plastic utensils rather than regular silverware.

There are times when a patient will need to be placed on "one-to-one" with staff. The staff member literally stays within arm's reach of the patient and keeps the patient in view at all times. The one-to-one level of supervision is intended to be more than a physical intervention. The staff member providing this supervision will interact with the patient and encourage the patient to be involved in appropriate activities. The interdisciplinary team needs to develop clear intervention strategies during the time of this heightened level of supervision. For example, the team will have to determine which, if any, on-unit groups or activities the patient should attend with the one-to-one staff at their side. Finally, when a patient is placed on one-to-one, confidentiality, milieu implications, and other expectations regarding treatment need to be considered and clearly understood by all staff. All ongoing assessments need to be documented along with the risk-benefit rationales for decisions.[74]

Each year, there are hundreds of completed suicides which occur in hospital settings. When a suicide occurs in the hospital setting, it is a traumatic event for staff and patients. There is sudden and understandable concern by patients for their own safety and fears related to loss of control.[63] Patients will need support for appropriate containment and mourning. There will be a potential for the contagion affect that will need to be managed as well.

Simultaneously, staff needs support for it can be devastating, even career ending for clinicians if appropriate supervision and support are not available. The staff must resume meaningful work and receive care for themselves at the same time. Reactions will vary; there can be everything from minimizing to physiological manifestations or symptoms of posttraumatic stress. It is important to provide a forum for staff to express and share feelings and reactions in a safe, nonjudgmental atmosphere. Not everyone will be ready to use this forum at the same time; therefore, consideration has to be given to how long and how often this forum is made available. Employee assistance programs may be indicated for select individuals.

Conducting a root cause analysis, with the intent to learn, not blame, can be critical for the future of the staff and for any given treatment program. The overall impact of a suicide on an individual staff member or the treatment team as a whole should not be underestimated. The benefits of the information gathered from these so-called psychological postmortems can be illuminating, far reaching, and long lasting.[78]

COMMUNITY/PATIENT–STAFF MEETINGS—REGULATING THE ENVIRONMENT

Since the time of Maxwell Jones,[79] the weekly or biweekly patient–staff or community meeting of all patients and staff (on duty) has long been the traditional centerpiece of the therapeutic milieu. Although the goals of such a meeting vary greatly with the unit's specialty designation and patient's ALOS, it is the social system's quintessential observatory of ongoing group and organizational processes, general unit morale, the level of strain within and among various staff and patient groups, and the capacity of recovering patients to manage and regulate their reintegration into something resembling the complexity of a community. It is also an opportunity for staff members to evaluate their capacity to be a genuine part of the inpatient world.

Beyond those larger benefits, the meeting manages several practical matters that include the introduction and farewell to patients and staff; the announcements of various unit functions and events; schedule changes; and the description, discussion, and possible resolution of specific unit problems including patient and staff complaints. The meeting offers unique opportunities to educate patients about the impact of sociocultural factors on their illness as well as to demonstrate the dysfunctional and defensive aspects of scapegoating processes. It is important that these meetings have consistent leadership and an available agenda (often coconstructed with a patient representative) as it is rarely useful, especially with an acutely ill and rapidly changing population, to have the meeting proceed in an unstructured way. Less structured meetings are often useful in accomplishing the more general goals listed earlier on longer length-of-stay units.[80,81]

General Comments

It is clear from the earlier discussion that the treatment milieu can serve diagnostic, management, and therapeutic ends as well as holding and containing ones. By observing a patient's response to and interaction with a relatively small and well-managed milieu, the staff has opportunities beyond individual interactions with clinicians to learn about a version of the patient in the world. Often patients are more "themselves" in the milieu than in individual or small-group and scheduled therapeutic sessions. Leadership and followership proclivities, styles of interpersonal relating, and adaptive capacities emerge that reveal otherwise hidden skills and deficits. By witnessing and participating in individual and community crises, individuals can learn ways to manage symptoms and regulate affect. In the present authors' experience, many patients feel they gain as much from the way a milieu is managed and daily interactions with floor staff and fellow patients as they do from more formal interventions.

The Discharge Phase

Continuity of care is crucial to ensure treatment compliance, to maintain recovery and adaptation, and to facilitate community reintegration and tenure. Although most patients are desirous of leaving the hospital, discharge is invariably a tense time when new or originally presenting symptoms and resistances emerge or reemerge. Leaving the inpatient haven brings up issues of separation and loss, heightens anxiety about how much has actually been accomplished, raises the specter of stigma and acceptance by the outside world, and may even lead to new symptoms or those that precipitated the admission in the first place. These anxieties are usually more relevant the longer the hospital stay. Furthermore, the vicissitudes of reimbursement pressure the treatment staff from the moment acute symptoms wane. Therefore, as soon as possible after the initial assessment is completed and active treatment commences, discharge planning assumes an important priority in the treatment.

Ideally, the admission process itself has included a thorough accounting of relevant benefits and finances, and clinicians are aware of the patient's social supports and aftercare options. As part of the initial assessment, issues and problems with the patient's prior outpatient arrangements—from individual treatment to placement—are part of the history of the present illness. This and admission data make it possible for the team to begin exploring possibilities with the patient and family in the context of treatment. In many cases, following safety and containment, an inpatient stay is the best context for launching an outpatient treatment. Just as the interdisciplinary team needed a strong connection with the referring clinician and agency, that same connection must be established with the clinician and agency to which the patient will be referred. This connection is always needed; but it is especially important when the inpatient team has questions about the value of the prior outpatient treatment. In this case, every effort must be made, often with the help of or consultation with the Unit Chief, to resolve matters in the best interest of the patient.

The timing and process of discharge are also important. The patient will benefit from as thorough a knowledge of the discharge plan as possible; and in the best of reimbursement circumstances he or she will have made at least one if not more visits to the outpatient situation as well as home before the actual discharge date (see especially Chapter 13). For those patients who have been admitted in the midst of suicidal or violent ideation or episodes, a thorough predischarge assessment of those factors must be done and documented. It is useful for the patient to have a written summary of discharge plans that includes the name and dosage of all medicines, as well as the names and telephone numbers of and times of first appointments with the clinicians and agencies to which he or she is referred.

Depending on the clinical situation, a discharge just before the weekend might leave the patient with too much unstructured time before first outpatient appointments, whereas a discharge too early in the week might leave the patient in a too-empty house. Many programs prefer to discharge in the early part of the week so as to maximize continuity of care and diminish the loss of structure. Remembering how intense the introduction to the unit might have been, inpatient staff, particularly members of the patient's team, are encouraged to provide a formal and individualized opportunity for the patient to bring up final concerns and say good-byes. (Refer to Chp. 12, esp. pp 247–248).

Continuing Care and Alternatives to Hospitalization

As will be clear from virtually every chapter that follows, an inpatient admission is only one stage in an ideal continuum of care for the vast majority of patients who are recovering. Depending on how much support is required to sustain community tenure and reintegration, this continuum can range from a return to individual therapy with the patient's referring clinician to effective step-down options that include family involvement in that treatment, partial or day hospitalization, intensive outpatient services that include some group work,[82] or assertive community treatment[83] and case management.[84] These venues share a philosophy of providing treatment in much less restrictive environments and reinforcing individual agency by emphasizing rehabilitation and adaptation to real-world situations.

The effectiveness of day-hospital programs has been demonstrated for patients with schizophrenic,[85] personality,[86,87] eating,[88] and substance abuse disorders.[89] Detoxification from substances and electroconvulsive therapy, at one time considered only to be done on an inpatient basis, are now being undertaken on an outpatient basis in selected situations.

Decisions about alternatives to hospital care are covered in many of the chapters that follow and depend on many factors. These factors include the need for safety and containment, the degree of regression or decompensation, past response to treatment, available alternatives, and familial and financial resources. From a common sense point of view and in the authors' experience, the more seamless the transition from inpatient to outpatient care, the better the outcome for the patient.

Challenges in the Role of Hospital Clinician

In the last two decades, fewer and fewer clinicians of any mental health discipline are interested in pursuing or sustaining a career doing inpatient work. Reductions in length of stay coupled with the admission of more difficult-to-treat patients heighten the pressure on all staff members and provide scant respite from a burdensome workload. Although advances in the development of the role of nonpsychiatric hospitalists and in step-down programs alleviate some of this strain, the pace of care remains intense and relentless. Beyond ensuring safety and providing immediate symptom relief for patients, further gratifications from the work are hard to come by. If one adds the burdens of stringent documentation, negotiations with third-party payers, and enhanced regulatory requirements to the mix, the promise of gaining greater knowledge while providing care for the mentally ill person, once major attractions to the field of inpatient psychiatry, seems easier to fulfill in a variety of outpatient settings.

In addition, psychiatrists are now more drawn to careers in neuroscience, neuropsychiatry, or outpatient psychopharmacologic practice. There are very limited roles in the contemporary inpatient setting for psychologists, and intensive psychotherapy, projective testing, and neuropsychologic testing are done mainly on an outpatient basis. Psychologists are attracted by the dramatic advances in cognitive sciences. As noted earlier, there is often no time on the inpatient service for social workers to do family and couples work beyond early intervention and assessment. The effects of the national nursing shortage are pervasive in virtually all hospital units, making the competition for resources between directors of nursing and services more onerous. Creative arts therapies are all but extinct in the inpatient world. Therefore, mental health workers, traditionally the least trained personnel on the front line in the provision of inpatient care, have become critical factors in maintaining quality of care.

So what kind of attractions does contemporary inpatient work offer? Certainly, the motivated clinician should like a challenge, working with patients who are suffering maximally. These patients include those who have a lot at stake, for whom other interventions have failed, whose thinking appears beyond repair, who have no hope for living, whose key relationships are in jeopardy or at an end, or who are otherwise living utterly isolated lives. The clinician contemplating inpatient work should have a high tolerance for this suffering and be reasonably content with partial results. He or she needs to be people-oriented, drawn to working on an interdisciplinary team of changing composition and in which there is likely to be an intense mixture of collaboration and conflict, cooperation, and competition, and taking both leadership and followership roles.

The hospital clinician will perforce be part of a larger institutional context that provides certain security and benefits while placing less value on stimulation and autonomous functioning. The latter value may be enhanced somewhat by the special challenges and rewards of an academic setting or the opportunity to do teaching. Part of this larger context is a closer relationship to other fields of medicine as well as an identification with the particular intensity and drama of hospital life itself. Much like an emergency room clinician, the contemporary inpatient clinician needs an action orientation, and comfort with crisis, chaos, and aggression. The constant replication of family dynamics in the work with patients and in staff-to-staff interactions may be exciting or represent yet another strain in the work. It is possible that successful hospital clinicians have a unique mixture of narcissism and masochism; that is, their self-esteem is supported by being "on" while sustaining work in the midst of difficult experiences and painful situations. The gratifications that ensue from the above-mentioned attractions are in marked distinction from those obtained in outpatient work.

There are other satisfactions in the work. Although it is true that recovery is usually partial, the observed changes can be dramatic and the restoration of hope in an otherwise complicated and despairing situation remarkable. The gratitude of many patients and their families is a meaningful counter to the endless challenges provided by emergency admissions, hospitals, medicolegals, and regulatory constraints and the vicissitudes of staff life. Hospital clinicians become comfortable with seeing beyond the presenting issues and become excited about identifying otherwise missing factors that can make a fundamental difference in a patient's ongoing treatment. These can be seen in something as basic as finding a more effective medicine to getting in touch with a personality factor that interferes with recovery from a depression to seeing how the misuse of a substance is masking a developing thought disorder. Providing a useful second opinion to equally burdened outpatient agencies and clinicians or successfully tweaking a faltering treatment plan are among the achievements that make the work worthwhile; the accomplishments can be seen in discovering an issue in treatment noncompliance or noting how the inclusion of another family member reinforces the progress and continuation of the treatment.

Some of the above-mentioned strains and satisfactions of inpatient work are both mitigated and enhanced in specialty or longer length-of-stay units. Data supporting longer stays are sparse and are complicated by the fact that the usual patient admitted there is very often complicated with multiple diagnoses as well as noncompliant with and otherwise resistant to treatment. Nevertheless, hospital clinicians working in such settings have the satisfaction of participating in more in-depth treatment alliances, the development of a broader view of patients and their history and circumstances, and the possibility of making a more substantial difference in treatment outcome.

Because of the intensity of the work and necessary commitment to unit life, hospital clinicians must always be on guard not to become alienated from the outpatient context. This alienation might take the form of diminished respect for and contact with the referring clinician or agency. This issue may need to be monitored by the chief of service or other hospital official or group such as the departments of quality assurance and marketing. Naturally these groups can be experienced as anathema to the hard-working clinician, but they exist for the overall benefit of the hospital. Equally important, the nature of the work can lead to individual strain, the loss of a feeling of worth and hopefulness, and role-related burnout. Warning signs may include an increase in previously latent symptoms, patient complaints, unexplained tardiness or absences, heightened conflict and contentiousness, and questionable judgments. In this regard, staff members who struggle with substance abuse or paranoid or antisocial traits are vulnerable to have these tendencies exacerbated, are particularly difficult for a unit's functioning, and usually require immediate attention. Unit Chiefs, Program Directors, and Discipline Heads must be especially alert to these issues while also needing some sort of backup of their own. Time off, referral for personal counseling, and continuing medical education are important hedges, but nothing is more supportive in this regard than a sensitive and involved leadership who are not reticent about intervening and demonstrating concern.

In conclusion, the authors' experience and belief are that the inpatient unit, a treatment locus under siege, can be a source of great personal satisfaction. The rewards of ongoing professional collaboration include constant stimulation and in the appropriately managed setting, an opportunity for personal growth. From an intellectual point of view, there is no greater laboratory for an ongoing view into the complex relationship between individual identity and dynamics and the vicissitudes of social reality. Because of the complicated challenges and rewards in the role of the hospital clinician, it is part of the task of those in leadership positions to look continually for ways to improve the psychosocial situation in which their staff work and their patients receive treatment, thereby providing the conditions in which staff members can maximize their professional gratifications.

REFERENCES

1. Main TF. The hospital as a therapeutic institution. *Bull Menninger Clin.* 1946;10:66–70.
2. Jones M, Baker A, Freeman T, et al. *The therapeutic community: a new treatment method is psychiatry.* New York: Basic Books; 1953.
3. Stanton AH, Schwartz MS. *The mental hospital.* New York: Basic Books; 1954.
4. Edelson M. *Sociotherapy and psychotherapy in the treatment of schizophrenia.* Chicago: University of Chicago Press; 1970.
5. Sederer L. Brief Hospitalization. In: Tasman A, Riba M, eds. *Review psychiatry,* Chapter 26, Vol. 11. Washington, DC: American Psychiatric Press; 1992:518–534.
6. Munich RL, Gabbard GO. Hospital psychiatry. In: Tasman AT, Reba MD, eds. *Review of psychiatry,* Vol.11. Washington DC: American Psychiatric Press; 1992:501–604.
7. Leibenluft E, Tasman A, Green SA. *Less time to do more: psychotherapy on the short term inpatient unit.* Washington: American Psychiatric Press; 1993.
8. Sederer LI, Rothschild AJ. *Acute care psychiatry: diagnosis and treatment.* Baltimore: Williams & Wilkins; 1997.
9. Munich RL. The role of the unit chief: An integrated perspective. *Psychiatry.* 1986;49:325–336.
10. Haslam-Hopwood GTG. The role of the primary clinician in the multidisciplinary team. *Bull Menninger Clin.* 2003;67:5–17.
11. MacKinnon RA, Michels R, Buckley PJ. *The psychiatric interview in clinical practice,* 2nd ed. Washington: American Psychiatric Press; 2006.
12. Adler G. Individual Psychodynamic Psychotherapy. In: Leibenluft E, Tasman A, Green S, eds. *Less time to do more,* Chapter 3. Washington, DC: American Psychiatric Press; 1993:39–58.
13. Schneider W, Klauer T. Symptom level, treatment motivation, and the effects of inpatient psychotherapy. *Psychother. Res.* 2001;11(2):153–167.
14. Thunnissen M, Remans Y, Trijsburg W. Premature termination of short-term inpatient psychotherapy: client's perspectives on causes and effects. *Int J Ther Support Organ.* 2006;27(2):265–273.
15. Hauff E, Varvin S, Laake P, et al. Inpatient psychotherapy compared with usual care for patients who have schizophrenic psychoses. *Psychiatr Serv.* 2002;53(4):471–473.
16. Svensson B, Hansson L. Therapeutic alliance in cognitive therapy for schizophrenic and other long-term mentally ill patients: development and relationship to outcome in an inpatient treatment programme. *Acta Psychiatr Scand.* 1999;99(4):281–287.
17. Loffler-Staska H, Voracek M, Leithner K, et al. Predicting psychotherapy utilization for patients with borderline personality disorder. *Psychother Res.* 2003;13(2):255–264.
18. Strauss B, Kirchmann H, Eckert J, et al. Attachment characteristics and treatment outcome following inpatient psychotherapy: Results of a multisite study. *Psychother Res.* 2006;16(5):573–586.
19. Bennett M. Focal psychotherapy. In: Sederer LI, Rothschild AJ, eds. *Acute psychiatry,* Chapter 17. Baltimore: Williams & Williams; 1997:355–374.
20. Geiser F, Shultz-Werner A, Imbierowicz K, et al. Impact of the turning-against-self defense mechanism on the process and outcome of inpatient psychotherapy. *Psychother Res.* 2003;13(3):355–370.
21. Fenton W. Individual and family therapies. In: Gabbard G, ed. *Treatments of psychiatric disorders.* Washington: American Psychiatric Association Press; 2007:345–360.
22. Swenson C, Sanderson C, Dulit R, et al. The application of dialectical behavioral therapy for patients with borderline personality disorder on inpatient units. *Psychiatr Q.* 2001;72(4):307–324.
23. Swenson C, Witterholt C, Bohus M. Dialectical behavior therapy on inpatient units. In: Dimeff L, Kerner K, eds. *Dialectical behavior therapy in clinical practice.* New York: Guilford Press; 2007:69–110.
24. Stasch M, Cierpka M, Hillenbrand E, et al. Assessing reenactment in inpatient psychodynamic therapy. *Psychother Res* 2002;12(3):355–368.
25. Skogstad W. Internal and external reality in inpatient psychotherapy: Working with severely disturbed patients at the Cassel Hospital. *Psychoanal Psychother.* 2003;17(2):97–118.
26. Burnham D. The coffee-pot affair: An episode in the life of a therapeutic community. *Hosp Community Psychiatry.* 1972;23(2):33–38.
27. Gabbard G. Splitting in hospital treatment. *Am J Psychiatry.* 1989;146(4):441–461.
28. Munich RL, Allen J. Psychiatric and sociotherapeutic perspectives on the difficult-to-treat patient. *Psychiatry.* 2003;66(4):346–357.
29. Gabbard G. Treatments in dynamic psychiatry III: dynamically informed hospital treatment. *Psychodynamic psychiatry in clinical practice*; American Psychiatric Press; 1990:125–146.
30. Yalom ID. The specialized therapy group. *The theory and practice of group psychotherapy.* New York: Basic Books; 1985:456–485.
31. Kibel H. Group psychotherapy. In: *Less time to do more: psychotherapy on the short term inpatient unit.* Washington: American Psychiatric Press; 1993:89–109.

32. Kempker S, Kibel H. Group Psychotherapy. In: Sederer LI, Rothschild AJ, eds. *Acute care psychiatry: diagnosis and treatment.* Baltimore: Williams & Wilkins; 1997:375–390.

33. Kosters M, Burlingame G, Nachtigall C, et al. A meta-analytic review of the effectiveness of inpatient group psychotherapy. *Group Dyn.* 2006;10(2):146–163.

34. Bechdolf A, Kohn D, Knost B, et al. A randomized comparison of group cognitive-behavioral therapy and group psychoeducation in acute patients with schizophrenia: Outcome at 24 months. *Acta Psychiatr Scand.* 2005;112(3):173–179.

35. Hayes S, Hope D, Terryberry-Spohr L, et al. Discriminating between cognitive and supportive group therapies for chronic mental illness. *J Nerv Ment Dis.* 2006;194(8):603–609.

36. Beutal M, Knickenberg R, Krug B, et al. Psychodynamic focal group treatment for psychosomatic inpatients – with an emphasis on work-related conflicts. *Int J Group Psychother.* 2006;56(3):285–305.

37. DiVitto S. Empowerment through self-regulation: Group approach for survivors of incest. *J Am Psychiatr Nurses Assoc.* 1998;4(3):77–86.

38. Farkas-Cameron M. Inpatient group therapy in a managed health care environment: Application to clinical nursing practice. *J Am Psychiatr Nurses Assoc.* 1998;4(5):145–152.

39. Simon C. Psychoeducation: a contemporary approach. In: Watkins TR, Callicutt JW, eds. *Mental health policy and practice today.* London: Sage Publications Inc; 1997:129–145.

40. Anderson CM, Hogarty GE, Reiss DJ. Family treatment of adult schizophrenia patients: A psycho-educational approach. *Schizophr Bull.* 1980;6(3):490–505.

41. Potter M, Williams R, Costanzo R. Using nursing theory and a structured psychoeducational curriculum with inpatient groups. *J Am Nurses Assoc.* 2004;10(3):122–128.

42. Siegmann R, Long G. Psychoeducational group therapy changes the face of managed care. *J Pract Psychiatry Behav Health.* 1995;29–36.

43. D'Silva K, Duggan C. Service innovations: Development of a psychoeducational programme for patients with personality disorder. *Psychiatr Bull R Coll Psychiatr.* 2002;26(7):268–271.

44. Pratt S, Rosenberg S, Mueser K, et al. Evaluation of a PTSD Psychoeducational program for psychiatric inpatients. *J Ment Health.* 2005;14(2):121–127.

45. Allen J. Psychoeducational approaches. *Traumatic relationships and serious mental disorders.* West Sussex: John Wiley and Sons; 2001:347–372.

46. Glick ID, Clarkin JF. Family support and intervention. In: Sederer LI, Rothschild AJ, eds. *Acute care psychiatry: diagnosis and treatment.* Baltimore: Williams & Wilkins; 1997:337–354.

47. Micklowitz DJ, Goldstein MJ, Nuechterlein KH, et al. Family factors and the course of bipolar affective disorder. *Arch Gen Psychiatry.* 1988;45(3):225–231.

48. Schooler N, Keith S, Severe J, et al. Relapse and rehospitalization during maintenance treatment of schizophrenia. *Arch Gen Psychiatry.* 1997;54:453–463.

49. Pitschel-Walz G, Leucht S, Bauml J, et al. The effect of family interventions on relapse and rehospitalization in schizophrenia – a meta-analysis. *Schizophr Bull.* 2001;27(1):73–92.

50. Munich RL, Lang E. The boundaries of psychiatric rehabilitation. *Hosp Community Psychiatry.* 1993;44:661–665.

51. Kopelowicz A, Wallace CJ, Lieberman RP. Psychiatric rehabilitation. In: Gabbard G, ed. *Treatments of psychiatric disorders.* Washington: American Psychiatric Publishing; 2007:361–379.

52. Kopelowicz A, Lieberman R, Zarate R. Recent advances in social skills training for schizophrenia. *Schizophr Bull.* 2006;32(Suppl 1): S12–S23.

53. Wirshing D, Pierre J, William C, et al. Letters to the editors: Community re-entry program training module for schizophrenic inpatients improves treatment outcomes. *Schizophr Res.* 2006;18(1–3):338–339.

54. Smith R. Implementing psychosocial rehabilitation with long-term patients in a public psychiatric hospital. *Psychiatr Serv.* 1998;49(5):593–595.

55. Caudill W, Redlich FC, Gilmore HR, et al. Social structure and interaction processes on a psychiatric ward. *Am J Orthopsychiatry.* 1952;22:314–334.

56. Kernberg O. Regression in groups. *Internal world and external reality.* New York: Jason Aronson; 1980:211–234.

57. Gabbard GO. The treatment of the "special" patient in a psychoanalytic hospital. *Int Rev Psychoanal.* 1986;13:333–347.

58. Main TF. The ailment. *Br J Med Psychol.* 1957;30:129–145.

59. Edelson M. *Sociotherapy and psychotherapy.* Chicago: University of Chicago Press; 1970.

60. Smith T, Munich RL. Analysis of a series of violent episodes on an in-patient unit. *Int J Ther Commun.* 1991;12(4):217–232.

61. Smith TE, Munich RL. Suicide, violence, and elopement: prediction, understanding, and management. In: Tasman E, Riba MB, eds. *Review of psychiatry,* Vol. 11. Washington, DC: American Psychiatric Press; 1992:535–554.

62. Bowers L, Brennan G, Flood C, et al. Preliminary outcomes of a trial to reduce conflict and containment on acute psychiatric wards: city nurses. *J Psychiatr Ment Health Nurs.* 2006;13:165–172.

63. Soth NB. *Informed treatment: milieu management in psychiatric hospitals and residential treatment center.* Summit: Scarecrow Press; 1997.

64. Gunderson JG. Defining the therapeutic processes in psychiatric milieus. *Psychiatry.* 1978;41(4):327–335.

65. Torre MA. Creating a healing environment. *Perspect Psychiatr Care.* 2006;42(4):262–264.

66. Kneisl CR, Wilson SH, Trigoboff E. *Contemporary psychiatric-mental health nursing.* New Jersey: Pearson Education, Inc.; 2004.

67. Thomas SP, Shattell M, Martin T. What's therapeutic about the therapeutic milieu? *Arch Psychiatr Nurs.* 2002;16(3):99–107.

68. Bradshaw WH. The coffee-pot affair: An episode in the life of a therapeutic community. *Hosp Community Psychiatry.* 1972;23(2):33–38.

69. Johnson ME, Delaney KR. Keeping the unit safe: The anatomy of escalation. *J Am Psychiatr Nurses Assoc.* 2007;13(1):42–52.

70. National Association of State Mental Health Program Directors. *The restraint and seclusion: a risk management guide page.* Available at: http://www.nasmhpd.org/general_files/publications/ntac_pubs/R-S%20RISK%20MGMT%2010-10-06.pdf. Accessed December 17, 2007.

71. Snow, Kathie. *Disability is Natural. The People First Language page.* Available at: http://ftp.disabilityisnatural.com/documents/PFL8.pdf. Accessed January 15 2008.

72. Suicide Prevention Resource Center in collaboration with the American Association of Suicidology. *Assessing and managing suicide risk: core competencies for mental health professionals,* 2006.

73. Rudd MD, Berman AL, Joiner TE, et al. Warning signs for suicide: Theory, research, and clinical applications. *Suicide Life Threat Behav.* 2006;36(3):255–261.

74. Berman AL. Risk management with suicidal patient. *J Clin Psychol.* 2006;62(2):171–184.77.

75. Jobes DA. *Managing suicidal risk: a collaborative approach.* New York: Guilford Press; 2006.

76. Shea SC. *The practical art of suicidal assessment: a guide for mental health professionals and substance abuse counselors.* West Sussex: John Wiley and Sons; 2002.

77. Lewis LM. No-harm contracts: A review of what we know. *Suicide Life Threat Behav.* 2007;37(1):50–57.

78. Munich RL. Suicide on an inpatient unit: A sociotherapeutic view. *Int J Ther Commun.* 1983;4(3):196–211.

79. Jones M, Baker A, Freeman T, et al. *The therapeutic community: a new treatment method in psychiatry.* New York: Basic Books; 1953.

80. Swenson CR, Munich RL. Types of large-group meetings in the therapeutic community: With special emphasis on the long-term unit. *Psychiatry.* 1989;52:437–445.

81. Russakoff LM, Oldham JM. The structure and technique of community meetings: The short-term unit. *Psychiatry.* 1982;45:38–44.

82. McKay J, Cacciola J, McClellan A. An initial evaluation of the psychosocial dimensions of the American Society of Addiction Medicine Criteria for inpatient versus intensive outpatient substance abuse. *J Stud Alcohol.* 1997;58:239–252.

83. Olfson M. Assertive community treatment: An evaluation of the experimental evidence. *Hosp Community Psychiatry.* 1990;41:634–641.

84. Sledge W, Astrachan B, Thompson K, et al. Case management in psychiatry: An analysis of tasks. *Am J Psychiatry.* 1995;152:1259–1263.

85. Hoge MA, Davidson L, Hill WL, et al. The promise of partial hospitalization: A reassessment. *Hosp Community Psychiatry.* 1992;43(4):345–354.

86. Piper W, Rosie J, Azim H, et al. A randomized trial of psychiatric day treatment for patients with affective and personality disorders. *Hosp Community Psychiatry.* 1993;44:757–763.

87. Karterud S, Pedersen G, Bjordal E, et al. Day treatment of patients with personality disorders: Experiences from a Norwegian treatment research network. *J Personal Disord.* 2003;17: 2436–2462.

88. Zipfel S, Reas D, Thornton C, et al. Day hospitalization programs for eating disorders: A systematic review of the literature. *Int J Eat Disord.* 2002;31:105–117.

89. Alterman A, O'Brien C, McClellan A. Effectiveness and costs of inpatient versus day hospital rehabilitation. *J Nerv Ment Dis.* 1994;182:157–163.

Pharmacologic Approach to the Psychiatric Inpatient

ARASH ANSARI, DAVID N. OSSER, LEONARD S. LAI, PAUL M. SCHOENFELD,
AND KENNETH C. POTTS

Characteristics of Inpatient Treatment

The role of inpatient psychiatric treatment has evolved in recent decades. Psychopharmacologic advances have enabled more successful treatment of major mental illnesses. The movement to deinstitutionalize psychiatric patients and shift care to community-based agencies and the economic realities of the health care marketplace have had major impact to reduce the length of stay. Nevertheless, a recent study by the U.S. Health and Human Services Agency for Healthcare Research and Quality[1] found that in 2004, 1.9 million out of 32 million admissions (6%) to US community hospitals were primarily for a mental health or substance abuse diagnosis, while an additional 5.7 million admissions (18%) also involved depression, bipolar disorder, schizophrenia, or other mental health diagnoses or substance abuse–related disorders as a secondary diagnosis. The top five diagnoses reported were mood disorders, substance abuse–related disorders, delirium/dementia, anxiety disorders, and schizophrenia. The average length of stay for a patient with a primary mental health or substance abuse diagnosis was 8 days compared to 5 days for nonmental health–related diagnoses.

Because of time limitations, the goals of inpatient psychiatry have shifted from striving to achieve full remission to symptom alleviation through the judicious use of psychotropic medication so that the stay can be brief. Patients may therefore be discharged as long as they are evaluated to be unlikely to harm themselves or others, even though only some of the most distressing symptoms have improved, for example, agitation, anxiety, or insomnia. Medication treatment plans focus on these symptoms with the understanding that the full effect and benefit may not occur for several weeks. Psychosocial treatments such as intensive short-term individual psychotherapy, group therapy, and milieu interventions that apply the principles of psychodynamic, cognitive, behavioral, and dialectic behavioral techniques are vital in helping patients reduce problematic thoughts, behavior, feelings, and other responses to their stressors and symptoms in the inpatient setting. As no patient exists in a vacuum, outreach to families, significant others, and social supports to address possible acute psychosocial precipitants will contribute to helping reduce the likelihood of a relapse or a recurrence. Consultations with outpatient providers can be of critical importance. The inpatient stay can often provide an opportunity to clarify how the community treatment network can be made more efficient and responsive to the patient's needs.

Factors Influencing Pharmacotherapy on an Inpatient Unit

Publicly and privately funded inpatient psychiatric treatment is usually authorized for patients who present a danger to themselves or to others or who have demonstrated that they are unable to care for themselves. Inpatient treatment is monitored closely by mental health review agencies hired to ensure that this most expensive level of psychiatric care is used effectively and minimally in order to contain costs. Inpatient treatment teams must be vigilant about the time limitations imposed on each admission. This is made more difficult by the fact that the safety concerns that open the door to an inpatient admission generally are often found to be complicated by a myriad of additional reasons for which the patient has come to the attention of health care providers. Thorough assessment and formulation of why the patient is in a crisis must be done quickly and with a careful evaluation of which symptoms and contributing factors are the most important to address. These factors can range from noncompliance with treatment because of poor insight to limited treatment access and to destabilizing forces such as homelessness and family or relationship conflicts. Patients have comorbid medical illnesses or substance abuse–related factors that confound and prevent successful outpatient interventions. Therefore, the challenge for the inpatient multidisciplinary treatment team is to be able to evaluate and stabilize the sickest patients in the psychiatric care continuum in the shortest time possible.

In some cases, keeping the inpatient stay brief may be therapeutic, especially in the more character-disordered where the inpatient treatment milieu may encourage regressive behaviors.

Goal of Inpatient Treatment as Related to Pharmacotherapy

The task of the psychiatrist is to alleviate some of the presenting symptoms. This may mean the commencement of a new medicine or the resumption or adjustment of a medication regimen that has been effective in the past. The choices made have to enable prompt and effective symptom relief while the patient is in the hospital and to be feasible for the outpatient treatment team to continue in the community. Some medicines will be effective in the short run, for example, benzodiazepines for anxiety, whereas other medicines such as antidepressants are initiated with the expectation that in time a more definitive effect will occur. In other situations, it may be preferable to withhold initiation of pharmacologic treatment, such as when the presenting picture is complicated by significant substance abuse that obscures determination of whether Axis I pathology is primary or secondary. The opportunity to observe the initial response to medication will also allow evaluation of side effects, such as excess sedation or akathisia, which may preclude the use of that particular drug.

Close observations by the treatment team facilitate psychopharmacology decisions dependent on symptoms rather than syndromal diagnoses. For example, medicine may be given to target anxiety symptoms while it is determined if the symptoms are part of a mood disorder or an independent anxiety disorder.

It is important to explain to the patient and his or her family that the short length of stay allowed does not commonly result in full remission. They need to understand that the goal is to reduce troubling symptoms and to enable the patient to feel safer, be in better behavioral control, and to be able to function better with or without the assistance of others in the community. Often the suicidal or homicidal ideation that prompted the admission will resolve soon after admission because of the containment and structure of the supportive inpatient milieu. The focus will then quickly shift to the crucial question of whether the patient still requires inpatient level of care.

Selecting Treatment

Selecting initial psychopharmacologic treatment for a newly admitted patient can be a complicated process and is based on multiple considerations and variables. Often the prescribing physician must weigh many of these variables simultaneously and rapidly given the complicated psychiatric, medical, and psychosocial presentations of most hospitalized patients. Ten factors that influence choice of initial agent will be reviewed.

SYMPTOM CONTROL—THE AGITATED PATIENT AND THE USE OF P.R.N. MEDICATION

The inpatient psychiatrist is faced with the challenge of making a provisional diagnosis and an initial treatment plan for the patient. Sometimes this diagnosis is based on very limited or even contradictory clinical and historical data. The clinician must be aware that new information may come to light, and the diagnoses may need to be modified. Recalling the guiding principles of "safety first" and "do no harm" is frequently helpful.

It is important to identify and treat the most serious symptoms regardless of diagnosis—these include violence, aggression, assault, self-harm, suicide, disorganizing psychosis, agitation, and risk of dying from inanition or other complications of poor oral intake and immobility (e.g., deep venous thrombosis [DVT], aspiration pneumonia, and skin breakdown). A symptom-based approach to psychopharmacologic treatment in an inpatient setting is therefore often necessary. This section will focus on the treatment of the agitated patient and the use of p.r.n. medication.

The Agitated Patient

A patient may become agitated at any time during the admission. Upon entry to the hospital, factors include the effects of being confined, the change in environment, and the loss of autonomy. A patient may become agitated later in the admission, such as if too rapidly allowed out of a contained situation or denied privileges. Nicotine-dependent patients can become extremely agitated if not permitted to smoke when they want. Interestingly, a recent study found that when units become smoke-free, incidents of agitation and restraint are markedly reduced.[2]

The violent, aggressive, or out-of-control patient can be very difficult to manage. The risk of assault or of self-harm must be assessed and reassessed. Prevention is the best approach, of course, with active treatment of any patient who may be at risk.

Certainly, the intensive use of the structure of the inpatient milieu can be instrumental in minimizing the need for medication. The containment of quiet rooms and destimulation can reduce potentially stressful situations for the patient, allowing time for a treatment plan to help an agitated patient.

However, there are situations where all the best efforts fail. Safety of the patient or staff is at risk, and sometimes urgent medication is necessary. When a rapid response is required, parenteral medication is indicated (although in less acute situations oral medication should be considered). A combination of an intramuscular typical antipsychotic and a benzodiazepine has been shown to be more effective than either one used alone.[3] This combination can avoid the need for an adjunctive dose of an anticholinergic; extrapyramidal symptoms (EPS) are infrequent. The advantages are avoiding both additional injections and anticholinergic toxicity. A common combination includes haloperidol 2 to 5 mg along with lorazepam 1 to 2 mg intramuscularly (in the same syringe) given every 30 to 60 minutes, up to three doses. Haloperidol is often considered first-line because of its relative safety profile, the lack of an established ceiling dose, and years of clinical experience. Other typical antipsychotics are less often used in this situation and have become less available. Intramuscular chlorpromazine is not recommended because of its high risk of hypotension. Intramuscular droperidol should not be used in the emergency treatment of agitation because of the increased risk of QTc prolongation with this agent.

The role of intramuscular atypical antipsychotics (i.e., ziprasidone, olanzapine, aripiprazole) is less clear. The upper limit of dosing and risks of drug interactions (e.g., QTc prolongation issues) may preclude ongoing use in an agitated patient. Although these drugs are heavily promoted by their manufacturers and many clinicians use them, the evidence base is unsatisfactory. All have been compared with haloperidol alone, without lorazepam or concomitant anticholinergic agents.[4–6] This gave the atypicals an unfair advantage.

One alternative to consider is monotherapy with parenteral lorazepam. This can be a valuable option when exposure to a typical antipsychotic is undesirable. A usual dose may be 1 to 3 mg intramuscularly hourly up to three doses. Some clinicians may be hesitant to use benzodiazepines with a substance-using patient. However, its efficacy in treating agitation in an emergency may well outweigh these concerns. Some clinicians are also concerned about the risk of "disinhibition" or a paradoxical reaction. There are no clear risk factors for this, and it appears to be rare. The risk of respiratory depression with repeated doses of benzodiazepines should be taken into account, especially if the patient has other sedating drugs on board, or has pulmonary insufficiency. As with all medication, an elderly agitated patient may require significant dose reduction and greater intervals between dosing.

Use of p.r.n. Medication

The use of so-called p.r.n. medication (*pro re nata*—"as the thing is born") is common in inpatient psychiatry to treat a variety of symptoms, including agitation (see preceding text), anxiety, breakthrough psychotic symptoms, and insomnia. Judicious use of p.r.n. medication can be very helpful in evaluating the need to change the standing medication plan. For example, the psychotic patient who is not "held" by his standing medication and needs "extra" doses may need a reevaluation of the standing medication dose.

However, there are also potential pitfalls. There is the risk of forming an association, on the part of the patient, between an undesirable behavior and taking an extra pill, thereby reinforcing drug-seeking behavior and externalization of responsibility. On many units, the culture is to actively encourage patients, if in distress, to ask for a p.r.n. medication. The astute clinician then helps the patient identify the precipitating factor and solve the problem, thereby fostering more of a sense of self-control on the part of the patient.

The milieu effect of p.r.n. medication is important to consider. Asking for extra medicine may be a patient's way of communicating the need for more contact, especially in a busy inpatient unit. The patient may then feel heard, attended to, and held, even if medicine is not offered. The interaction allows for more patient–staff contact. In addition, nursing staff often feel safer if p.r.n. medication is "on the books" for a challenging patient. The placebo effect of p.r.n. medication must not be overlooked.

The choice of a p.r.n. agent should take into account the relevant symptom and the current medication list. Attention should be paid to the total daily dose (standing plus p.r.n. available) so as to avoid exceeding maximum recommended doses. When treating psychosis or mania, p.r.n. medication should ideally be the same as the standing medication, so as to avoid the risks of polypharmacy, including the risks of adverse (e.g., cardiac) effects. Adjunctive use of benzodiazepines can be very helpful in psychotic patients.[3]

In patients with anxiety, short-acting or intermediate acting benzodiazepines are often used. Although not approved by the U.S. Food and Drug Administration (FDA), many clinicians use low-dose antipsychotics in these patients, especially if substance abuse is an issue. Low-dose antipsychotics may be particularly helpful in patients with anxiety or agitation associated with personality disorders[7,8] (see subsequent text). Trazodone is a cost-effective alternative that needs further study. Prazosin can be useful as a p.r.n. during the day for patients with post-traumatic stress disorder (PTSD) as well as at night for sleep.[9,10]

Insomnia is probably the single symptom for which p.r.n. medication is most frequently requested. Insomnia may be due to the environment, a side effect of medication, a complication of a general medical condition (such as restless legs syndrome [RLS] or obstructive sleep apnea), a consequence of excessive intake of caffeine or nicotine, a symptom of withdrawal, and so on. Although sleep hygiene should be addressed, often medication is required. Choices include antihistamines, benzodiazepines, trazodone, low-dose sedating tricyclic antidepressants, prazosin, and newer hypnotics.

Psychotropic medicines, both p.r.n. and standing, also play a crucial role in the treatment of patients with borderline personality disorder (BPD). Often patients with BPD are admitted to inpatient units when they are emotionally overwhelmed, regressed, and in poor behavioral control. Heightened emotional lability, irritability, anger, impulsivity, transient psychosis, and agitation can all be present. Frequently p.r.n. medicines are used to decrease the intensity of these symptoms, and, if helpful, may be continued as standing treatment. When the patient with BPD exhibits dangerous agitation that places the patient or others directly at risk of harm, then, as is the case in the schizophrenic or manic patient, intramuscular or oral antipsychotics are likely to be needed. Overall total doses needed are usually less than those employed in manic or psychotically agitated patients. Even when immediate dangerousness is not an issue, antipsychotics can be used to decrease patient hostility and transient psychosis.[11] Although there is no reason to believe that any one antipsychotic is more effective than any other, in acute situations many clinicians prefer to use an antipsychotic that can have immediate and observable effect (e.g., perphenazine, haloperidol, or risperidone). Quetiapine is also frequently used for p.r.n. treatment of anxiety in patients with BPD. Disinhibition from benzodiazepines (which as previously noted is of limited concern when treating violent behavior in general) is of particular concern in patients with BPD and may lead to further behavioral dyscontrol;[12] benzodiazepines, therefore, should not be used to treat anxiety in these patients. Once acuity has decreased and transient psychotic phenomena have subsided, continuing an antipsychotic as a standing medication may help reduce impulsivity and aggression, and improve overall functioning.[13] Again, total doses needed are usually lower than those needed for the ongoing treatment of a primary psychotic disorder.[14,15] Quetiapine and aripiprazole may also be helpful for ongoing mood and anxiety symptoms in these patients.[8,16] Serotonergic antidepressants and mood stabilizers may help primarily with affective lability and anger.[11,13] One controlled study of 30 patients suggested that omega-3 fatty acids may reduce depression and aggression in patients with moderate BPD.[17] On the other extreme with respect to toxicity, clozapine has been reported in several uncontrolled studies to be helpful in reducing morbidity in some treatment refractory patients.[18,19]

PATIENT'S PSYCHOPHARMACOLOGIC HISTORY

An advantage the inpatient psychiatrist has is extended time to obtain a history of the psychopharmacologic treatment the patient has received. It is time well spent. The psychiatrist should have several interviews with the patient over a few days to ascertain as much detail as possible about what the patient remembers about his medication history. Information about dose, efficacy, side effects, duration of treatment, and use of different medication combinations is necessary to formulate an approach and apply relevant treatment algorithms. The level of functional recovery with previous treatment interventions is critical to assess. An understanding of the factors that contribute to compliance or noncompliance is essential for establishing the ongoing medication treatment alliance. Repeating treatment trials that have failed in the past is to be avoided if possible. It is important to obtain a comprehensive list of all prescribed and over-the-counter medicines used by the patient for general medical ailments to evaluate for possible drug interactions.

Careful medication reconciliation on admission is required. The physician must accurately determine what the patient was taking immediately before admission. For each identified item, there should be clear documentation of the plan to continue, change, or stop the medication. This practice promotes the accurate administration of medication.

Because the patient may be an unreliable informant, collateral information from outpatient clinicians and family members should be actively sought as soon as possible. They often have critical insights and observations about how effective different psychopharmacologic interventions have been.

When medical records are available to supplement the data collected from patients and significant others, history gathering is easier. Fortunately, more and more health care organizations are switching to electronic information systems that enable all clinicians to have fast, convenient, and accurate access to psychiatric and general medical histories at the touch of a keyboard. However, when the patient is treated in multiple unrelated health care systems, it can still be extremely difficult to obtain accurate, sequenced historical information in a timely manner for a short inpatient stay. Error-prone educated guesswork can often not be avoided especially in the early days of an admission.

PREEXISTING GENERAL MEDICAL CONDITIONS

There are certain common general medical concerns that influence the selection of pharmacologic agents. Very early in the decision-making process, many physicians first glance at the patient's past medical history to clarify the "medical milieu" in which they will be prescribing. Rapid access to laboratory data as well as other testing (e.g., electrocardiogram [ECG]), and review of general medical history especially in an electronic medical record, when available, are extremely helpful.

Cardiac

Many psychotropics can affect cardiac conduction, with the potential to delay conduction enough to lead to fatal arrhythmias. There is an association between sudden death and the use of antipsychotics[20] and tricyclic antidepressants at high doses[21] (but not selective serotonin reuptake inhibitors [SSRIs]), although causality has not been completely established, and there may be multiple etiologies. The cardiovascular effects of psychotropics should therefore be taken into account before beginning treatment.

Prolonged QT interval (reported as QTc when corrected for heart rate) is believed to be associated with *torsades de pointes*, a potentially fatal ventricular arrhythmia. The QT interval includes both the QRS interval as well as the ST segment. Whereas QRS (depolarization phase) lengthening is primarily associated with the use of tricyclic antidepressants (or low-potency typical antipsychotics with tricyclic structure) and their effect on sodium channels, atypical antipsychotics may potentially prolong the ST segment (repolarization phase) through their effect on potassium channels.[22] Although there is some question whether QT prolongation is a reliable indicator for the risk of *torsades de pointes*,[23] measuring this interval is the simplest way to estimate this risk.

Antipsychotics are not equal in their potential to affect the QT interval. Thioridazine, mesoridazine, pimozide, and droperidol[24] have shown significant potential to prolong QT and should generally be avoided. Among the newer antipsychotics, ziprasidone is considered to have the greatest potential to lengthen QT.[22] Some postmarketing studies such as the Clinical Antipsychotic Trials of Intervention Effectiveness (CATIE) have not confirmed this.[25,26] Premarketing data with aripiprazole indicate little risk.[27] Clozapine may contribute to QT prolongation primarily in patients with other risk factors.[28] The other cardiac risks of clozapine, that is risk of developing myocarditis or cardiomyopathy, are etiologically independent of its effect on cardiac conduction.

Tricyclic antidepressants, especially at high doses (particularly in the setting of overdose), have long been known for their potential to interfere with cardiac conduction and have traditionally been used with caution in patients with cardiac disease. Lithium may worsen sick sinus syndrome, produce blockade of the sinoatrial node, and also prolong QT.[29] SSRIs do not appear to significantly prolong QT, although there has been concern regarding their potential to induce bradycardia.[30-32]

Patients at higher cardiac risk should be identified before starting treatment with antipsychotics, tricyclic antidepressants, and lithium. Caution should be used in the care of the elderly, those with preexisting cardiac disease or preexisting QT prolongation, bradycardia, hypokalemia, or hypomagnesemia, and in those taking concomitant medication with proarrhythmic potential. A baseline ECG should be obtained in these patients; if the QTc is >440 to 450 msec, the patient should be monitored more carefully, and a QTc >500 msec should greatly increase concern for arrhythmias. Ziprasidone is contraindicated if the QTc is >500 msec. Magnesium and potassium abnormalities should be corrected early on. In high-risk patients, medicines with lower potential for cardiac toxicity should be used, and an effort should be made to use the lowest effective dose. Additionally, the clinician should be aware of medication interactions that may increase the serum level of the selected agent (see section on Medication Interactions). The clinician should also consider obtaining repeat ECGs on any patient who is being treated with two or more psychotropics with high risks of QT prolongation as the doses of these medications are titrated.

Blood Pressure

Many commonly used psychotropics have α-adrenergic blocking effects and can therefore lower blood pressure. Some of the observed cases of sudden death in patients taking antipsychotics or tricyclic antidepressants may be primarily due to severe hypotension rather than to cardiac arrhythmias. Vital signs, commonly checked on admission and daily thereafter, can identify those with preexisting hypotension. Patients at risk for orthostatic hypotension include the elderly, those with cardiac disease, and those taking other medicines that can lower blood pressure. Medicines whose propensity to lower blood pressure mandates caution are clozapine, chlorpromazine, risperidone, quetiapine, tricyclic antidepressants, and trazodone. Clozapine, which carries the highest risk of causing orthostasis, requires a very gradual and careful titration (i.e., starting at 12.5 mg once or twice a day with increases starting with 25 mg increments daily). In the patient who has been noncompliant it should not be restarted at prior doses if treatment has been interrupted for 2 or more days. Chlorpromazine administered intramuscularly or at sudden high oral doses carries a similar risk. Although tolerance to this side effect usually develops, care should be exercised when starting these medicines (or restarting them at previously prescribed high doses in patients who may have been recently nonadherent to their regimen). Increased fluid intake should be encouraged as tolerated and orthostatic blood pressure should be monitored in symptomatic patients until the appropriate dose is reached.

In regard to the risk of increasing blood pressure, there has been concern regarding the use of serotonin and norepinephrine reuptake inhibitors (SNRIs) in patients at risk for hypertension. Venlafaxine used at high doses can increase blood pressure.[33,34] This effect may be less pronounced with duloxetine and may not be clinically significant.[35,36] Patients with stable, effectively treated hypertension have not been found to show an increase in blood pressure from venlafaxine.[37]

Hepatic

There are two considerations regarding choice of psychiatric drug in a patient with compromised hepatic function. The first is the issue of hepatotoxicity with certain medicines, and the second is the use of hepatically metabolized agents in patients with preexisting liver disease. Baseline liver function tests should be measured, and if high, should influence care when using certain psychotropics.

Valproate, olanzapine, and quetiapine can cause hepatotoxicity. Although in the vast majority of cases any elevation in transaminases is mild and transient, these medicines should be used cautiously. The presence of clinically active liver disease or cirrhosis would suggest use of other agents (e.g., lithium rather than valproate for mania). If, during early inpatient treatment, transaminase levels increase to more than three times the upper end of the normal range, discontinuing or decreasing the dose of the offending agent should be considered. Patients with previous exposure to hepatitis B or C virus who are not acutely ill can still be treated with these medicines, although transaminases should be carefully monitored.[38,39] Given the concern that one would be exposing these patients with potentially worsening liver disease to yet another toxic insult, alternative nonhepatotoxic agents (e.g., lithium) should be considered when appropriate. Valproate may also rarely cause hyperammonemic encephalopathy without causing transaminase elevation,[40] although this is controversial.[41]

In the case of a patient admitted with preexisting liver disease, medicines which are primarily hepatically metabolized should be started at lower doses and increased slowly and agents with shorter half-lives should be used preferentially.

Renal

Measurement of kidney function, that is serum creatinine, is routinely done upon admission to an inpatient unit. Lithium, topiramate, and gabapentin are cleared by the kidneys, and any decrease in renal function warrants dose reduction of these medicines.

A common scenario is the admission to the inpatient unit of a patient whose lithium has been discontinued as an outpatient, because of concerns regarding worsening renal function (as can occur in up to 20% of patients on long-term lithium treatment).[42] Often the patient had been previously well maintained for many years on lithium. Once lithium is discontinued, however, the patient may decompensate and require multiple alternative medication trials and multiple hospitalizations for recurrent manic or depressive episodes. In these patients, the overall risks of morbidity and mortality may be less with rechallenge with lithium than if lithium treatment is withheld. After a clear risk and benefit assessment, and in close consultation with a nephrologist, it may be clinically appropriate for these patients to resume taking lithium. Close monitoring from then on, while avoiding further episodes of lithium toxicity, and administration of lithium once a day at bedtime, may decrease the risk of worsening renal effects.[43]

Metabolic Syndrome

Metabolic syndrome is characterized by dyslipidemia, hyperglycemia, and weight gain and is a major risk associated with some second-generation antipsychotics.

Hyperglycemia/Diabetes

The prevalence of diabetes is higher in patients with schizophrenia (in part because of unhealthy lifestyles) independent of treatment with antipsychotics.[44] Clozapine and olanzapine have clearly been implicated in increased risk of onset of hyperglycemia and diabetes, and in the exacerbation of preexisting diabetes, even leading to diabetic ketoacidosis. The propensity of quetiapine to cause hyperglycemia is numerically greater than that of other second-generation antipsychotics but less than that of the two agents mentioned earlier.[25] The data regarding risperidone are mixed.[45] One putative mechanism is that some of these agents rapidly induce insulin resistance, with or without causing weight gain.

Measuring fasting plasma glucose and inquiring about a patient's personal and family history of hyperglycemia and/or diabetes can help identify those at risk for developing diabetes, and determining hemoglobin A_{1c} can provide a measure of recent glycemic control. In patients at high risk of developing diabetes, aripiprazole or ziprasidone should be considered.[46] If fasting glucose is elevated, a glucose tolerance test has excellent predictive value regarding who is going to develop overt diabetes.[47]

Weight Gain

The risk of significant weight gain, particularly in the first few months of treatment, should be considered when prescribing atypical antipsychotics. A 2- to 3-kg weight gain early in the course of treatment (i.e., within the first 3 weeks) often predicts the risk of substantial weight gain over the long term.[48] However, different antipsychotics are not equal in their propensity to cause obesity. Clozapine and olanzapine are generally considered to be more likely to cause weight gain than quetiapine and risperidone, and in turn aripiprazole and ziprasidone are the least likely to contribute to weight gain.[49] Measuring baseline body mass index (BMI) and waist circumference are recommended by recent guidelines.[46] A patient's admission weight must be measured to establish a pretreatment baseline.

Hyperlipidemia

Antipsychotics that have the highest propensity to cause weight gain also carry the highest risk of worsening lipid profile. Risperidone may be more neutral in this regard, and ziprasidone may actually improve lipid profile.[25] Triglycerides are the lipids most affected by the use of atypical antipsychotics.[50] A fasting lipid profile can identify those patients already at higher cardiac risk and again serve as a pretreatment baseline. Pharmacotherapy of hyperlipidemia may be necessary. Also education on diet and lifestyle changes necessary to manage these side effects is essential, although compliance with these changes over time can be more unsatisfactory than compliance with the antipsychotic treatment itself.[51]

Leukopenia, Thrombocytopenia

Although many psychotropics (e.g., antipsychotics) can cause leukopenia, clozapine and carbamazepine are the primary medicines that need to be avoided in leukopenic patients. Of the antidepressants, mirtazapine may be associated with leukopenia, although causality has not been established and this has been rarely observed in clinical practice.[52] Gabapentin can also infrequently have a mild leukopenic effect.[27] Lithium, on the other hand, has been suggested for treatment of leukopenia and may be beneficial in this regard;[53] the mechanisms for increased white blood count may include demarginalization of neutrophils as well as possible release of colony-stimulating factors.[54–56]

The use of mood stabilizers such as carbamazepine, oxcarbazepine,[57] and valproate[58,59] is problematic in patients with preexisting thrombocytopenia because of their potential for lowering platelet count. Even when platelet count is normal, valproate may cause platelet dysfunction and prolong bleeding time.[60,61] Therefore, patients taking valproate should be assessed for bleeding risk before any invasive surgical procedures.

Hyponatremia

The syndrome of inappropriate antidiuretic hormone secretion (SIADH), resulting in hyponatremia, has been documented in patients, especially the elderly, who have been taking antidepressants. In addition to SSRIs, mirtazapine, duloxetine, and bupropion have all been implicated.[62–64] Among mood stabilizers, carbamazepine and oxcarbazepine can both cause hyponatremia,[65] although the mechanism is not secondary to SIADH and is not well understood.[66]

Neurologic Disease

Seizures

Patients with seizure disorders provide challenges in the choice of medication. Antidepressants and antipsychotics are thought to lower seizure threshold and this effect is generally dose dependent.[67] The most likely to do so are clozapine, chlorpromazine, olanzapine, quetiapine, tricyclic antidepressants, and bupropion (contraindicated in patients with seizure disorders). The risk with monoamine oxidase inhibitors (MAOIs) and SSRIs and other new antidepressants are considered to be low.[68] This is controversial, however. Depression itself appears to increase seizure risk and a review of FDA clinical trial data for antidepressants has shown a possible anticonvulsant effect of newer antidepressants at therapeutic doses[69] (although in overdoses antidepressants are still considered to increase seizure risk). Among antipsychotics, haloperidol and risperidone are less likely to affect seizure threshold.[70] All psychotropics should be used cautiously in patients with seizure disorders or when patients are seizure-prone (e.g., during alcohol or benzodiazepine withdrawal).

Stroke

Antipsychotics increase the incidence of stroke in patients with dementia.[71–73] First- and second-generation antipsychotics likely pose equal risk.[74] Possible etiologies for stroke may be related to cardiovascular effects or changes secondary to excessive sedation. In patients with dementia and significant behavioral dyscontrol or assaultiveness, SSRIs,[75] trazodone, or mood stabilizers should be considered.[76] However given their more rapid onset of action, antipsychotics should not be withheld if there is imminent risk of harm secondary to behavioral dyscontrol. The clinician should be aware that the use of both typical and atypical antipsychotics may be associated with an increased risk of death in patients with dementia.[71]

Extrapyramidal Symptoms

Patients with a prior history of dystonic reactions or substance abuse, and young, male patients are at higher risk for developing acute dystonias. Dystonias are primarily caused by typical antipsychotics but can occur with any antipsychotic with higher D_2 receptor occupancy (e.g., risperidone). Olanzapine, especially in high doses, can also cause EPS, although at lower rates than typical antipsychotics, possibly because of its own anticholinergic effects.[45] Quetiapine and clozapine are least likely to cause dystonias and parkinsonism.

Clozapine should also be considered in a patient presenting with tardive dyskinesia (TD), although all antipsychotics may mask, and therefore appear to improve, symptoms with treatment. Clinicians should attempt to avoid using typical antipsychotics in patients with preexisting abnormal movements. If abnormal movements again develop during treatment, clinicians should be aware that withdrawing the offending agent (especially if done too rapidly) could unmask and thereby worsen symptoms of TD. Patients at higher risk for TD are the elderly, women, those with prolonged treatment or past treatment with high doses of neuroleptics, those who developed significant parkinsonian side effects initially, and those with a history of affective disorders.

In contrast to other EPS, akathisia rates are generally similar among atypical antipsychotics, although there are lower overall rates with atypicals when compared with typical antipsychotics (10% to 20% vs. 20% to 50%, respectively).[45] Identifying akathisia as the cause of agitation, restlessness, or even worsening psychosis or suicidality is crucial because treatment would include decreasing rather than increasing antipsychotic dose.

Restless Legs Syndrome

RLS has been reported with the use of antidepressants such as SSRIs,[77] venlafaxine,[78] and mirtazapine[79] (as well as with several antipsychotics). Preliminary case reports suggest that bupropion, through modulation of dopaminergic effect, may be a better alternative antidepressant in patients with either preexisting or antidepressant-induced RLS.[80]

Women of Childbearing Age

Careful attention should be given to the choice of medication in young women. The general areas of concern are (a) the possibility of unplanned pregnancy while taking psychotropics and subsequent potential harm to the fetus (discussion of the care of the pregnant patient can be found in Chapter 14) and (b) the hormonal effects of medications on nonpregnant women.

Valproate may play a role in the development of polycystic ovary syndrome in women of reproductive age,[81] thereby affecting fertility (although there is a lack of clarity regarding rates given a higher-than-baseline occurrence of polycystic ovaries in bipolar patients not taking valproate).[82] In general, the use of mood stabilizers in young women can be very problematic given the possibility of interfering with fertility (e.g., valproate), interacting to decrease effectiveness of oral contraceptives (e.g., carbamazepine), and then increasing the chances of congenital malformations (e.g., valproate, carbamazepine, and to a lesser extent lithium) should pregnancy ensue. Considering alternatives to treatment with mood stabilizers and providing patient education are particularly important when treating women of childbearing age.

Another endocrine risk in women is the propensity of many antipsychotics to increase prolactin. Of the newer antipsychotics risperidone is the most problematic. Olanzapine, which is generally unlikely to increase prolactin, may do so at higher than usual doses (e.g., 30 mg per day).[83]

MEDICATION INTERACTIONS

The potential for interactions among psychotropics, or interactions between psychotropics and other classes of medication, often influences the inpatient clinician's choice of therapeutic agent. Although occasionally the likelihood of interactions clearly precludes the use of certain agents, more commonly the concern about interactions necessitates caution when introducing a new medicine. A complete list of interactions is beyond the scope of this chapter. The inpatient psychiatrist is well advised to consult the several available databases (web-based [e.g., www.genemedrx.com],[84] print,[85] etc.) when using multiple medicines. Nevertheless, there are commonly encountered types of interactions, both pharmacokinetic and pharmacodynamic, that should be kept in mind when choosing treatment for the hospitalized psychiatric patient. Patients at particularly high risk for dangerous medication interactions include those with impaired drug metabolism (including the elderly and those with organ insufficiencies) and those with chronic conditions (e.g., chronic psychiatric conditions, human immunodeficiency virus [HIV], cardiac patients) who require long-term complex pharmacotherapy.

Antidepressants

SSRIs are well known for their ability to interact with other medicines by affecting the hepatic cytochrome P-450 system. A primary concern is the potential for an SSRI to inhibit the enzymatic activity of specific P-450 isoenzymes, thereby increasing the serum levels of other hepatically metabolized medications (i.e., substrates), such as tricyclic antidepressants, antipsychotics, and warfarin.[86] Potentially harmful dose-dependent side effects (e.g., effects on cardiac conduction secondary to increased plasma concentrations of tricyclic antidepressants and antipsychotics, or increased bleeding secondary to increased warfarin levels) could develop. Not all SSRIs are equal in their potential for dangerous interactions. Fluoxetine, paroxetine, and fluvoxamine are more likely to inhibit hepatic enzymes; fluoxetine's inhibition of CYP2C9 and CYP2D6, paroxetine's inhibition of CYP2D6, and fluvoxamine's inhibition of CYP1A2, CYP2C9, CYP2C19, and CYP3A4 are of particular concern. Additionally, these three SSRIs exhibit nonlinear dose–concentration kinetics and small changes in dose may result in greater than expected enzyme inhibition and serum concentrations of substrates. These SSRIs should be used with caution when combined with other medication.[87]

Among SSRIs, citalopram and escitalopram have the least potential to affect serum levels of other medicines through enzymatic inhibition and should be selected preferentially in patients taking multiple medicines (however, citalopram can markedly increase clozapine levels through a mechanism that has not yet been elucidated).[88,89] Sertraline also generally causes less enzymatic inhibition than fluoxetine, paroxetine, and fluvoxamine. Other non-SSRI antidepressants that also should be favorably considered in the setting of medication combinations are venlafaxine and mirtazapine, both of which have a very low risk of medication interactions. However, although citalopram, venlafaxine, and mirtazapine are not likely to clinically affect the activity of hepatic enzymes, they themselves are substrates of these enzymes and their plasma concentrations can increase if used in combination with other enzyme-inhibiting SSRIs, thereby increasing the chances of unexpected or unwanted serotonergic effects.

Other antidepressants can also inhibit cytochrome P-450 enzymes. Duloxetine and bupropion can both moderately inhibit CYP2D6. Nefazodone is a potent CYP3A4 inhibitor and this can affect the metabolism of many common substrates such as macrolide antibiotics, statins, calcium channel blockers, and many HIV protease inhibitors, as well as many antipsychotics including ziprasidone (see subsequent text).[87,90]

The concomitant use of MAOIs and serotonergic antidepressants is contraindicated because of the potential to cause serotonin syndrome. A washout period of 2 weeks (5 weeks after discontinuation of fluoxetine) should be allowed before starting an MAOI. Two weeks should be allowed before switching from MAOIs to other antidepressants.[91] SSRIs also should not be used with linezolid, an antibiotic used for the treatment of infections caused by gram-positive bacteria, because of this drug's weak MAOI properties.[92]

Antipsychotics

Although newer antipsychotics do have weak cytochrome enzyme-inhibiting activity (and first-generation antipsychotics, such as phenothiazines, are stronger enzyme inhibitors), they are themselves substrates of P-450 enzymes and as such can be affected by enzyme-inducing and enzyme-inhibiting agents. As noted earlier, certain SSRIs, as well as other medicines (such as valproate and the frequently used antibiotic ciprofloxacin), can inhibit the metabolism of many old and new antipsychotics, thereby increasing their plasma concentrations. Specifically, clozapine and olanzapine are substrates for CYP1A2; haloperidol, risperidone, clozapine, and olanzapine are substrates for CYP2D6; and haloperidol, clozapine, risperidone, quetiapine, and ziprasidone are substrates for CYP3A4.[90] When metabolism of these antipsychotics is inhibited, there is a higher potential for side effects such as EPS or cardiac toxicity.

Using two or more antipsychotics or combining antipsychotics with other medicines that prolong the QT interval could be problematic and would require close monitoring. The addition of ziprasidone, which some studies find to have a higher propensity to cause QT prolongation, to other QT-prolonging drugs such as pentamidine, or class Ia (e.g., procainamide, quinidine) or class III (e.g., amiodarone) antiarrhythmics, should be avoided.[24]

Clozapine should not be combined with other medicines, such as carbamazepine, which can cause leukopenia. The combination of clozapine and benzodiazepines may rarely cause fatal respiratory suppression and therefore should generally be used cautiously.[93]

Clozapine and olanzapine are metabolized by CYP1A2, and cigarette smoking can decrease their levels through induction of this isoenzyme. Consequently, a newly admitted inpatient who is restricted from smoking may experience an increased plasma clozapine concentration and therefore should be monitored for increased risk of adverse effects.[90] Enzyme induction by cigarette smoke is primarily a function of polycyclic aromatic hydrocarbons found in tobacco smoke rather than of nicotine—the use of nicotine replacement therapy would not therefore cause similar induction.[94] Although paroxetine and fluoxetine can increase clozapine levels through enzyme inhibition, the use of fluvoxamine is of particular concern. Fluvoxamine can increase clozapine concentrations 5- to 10-fold through CYP1A2 inhibition[87,90] and this combination should usually be avoided or used very cautiously. Interestingly, however, the addition of fluvoxamine has been used as a strategy to boost low clozapine levels and possibly minimize adverse effects of the metabolite norclozapine, including weight gain.[95]

Mood Stabilizers

Carbamazepine is an inducer of many hepatic enzymes (CYP1A2, CYP2C9, CYP2C19, CYP3A4) and as such can lower the concentration of other medicines including many tricyclic antidepressants, antipsychotics, benzodiazepines, and other mood stabilizers, including lamotrigine, as well as nonpsychotropic medications such as warfarin.[90] In the manic patient who requires rapid behavioral control, and who may be receiving carbamazepine in addition to an antipsychotic and/or a benzodiazepine, the clinician should be aware that these adjunctive or other medicines may not be providing full clinical effect because of decreased plasma levels. This effect seriously limits the utility of carbamazepine in these situations. (In this regard the clinician should also be aware that in addition to carbamazepine, the antiepileptic drugs phenobarbital, phenytoin, and primidone also have similarly strong enzyme-inducing properties.)[96]

Along with carbamazepine, oxcarbazepine, high-dose topiramate,[97] and possibly lamotrigine may also stimulate the metabolism of oral contraceptives, and if used would require patients to undertake additional precautions to avoid pregnancy and/or a change to a stronger contraceptive dose.[98] In women relying on oral contraceptives, alternative treatments should be considered. Valproate and gabapentin are less likely to affect oral contraceptive levels.[96]

Valproate can inhibit the glucuronidation of lamotrigine, and this combination requires very slow titration of lamotrigine to decrease the risk of dangerous rash.[96,99] Sertraline, possibly also through inhibition of glucuronidation, may also significantly increase lamotrigine levels.[100] Valproate can also increase the plasma levels of substrates of CYP2C9 and CYP2C19 such as phenobarbital, phenytoin, many tricyclic antidepressants, and warfarin. Valproate is also highly protein bound and competition in protein binding with warfarin can cause a significant increase in the free fraction of warfarin and the prothrombin time.[27,101]

Lithium and gabapentin are renally excreted and are not likely to interact with other mood stabilizers.[102] Lithium levels, however, can increase with concomitant use of nonsteroidal antiin-flammatory drugs (NSAIDs), thiazide diuretics, angiotensin-converting enzyme (ACE) inhibitors, metronidazole, and tetracyclines.[103]

SPEED OF RESPONSE

In the acute inpatient setting, speed of pharmacotherapy response is critical. Unfortunately, there has been little study focused on speed as the primary outcome measure. Clinicians have been forced to rely on their clinical experience or that of trusted colleagues and form their own opinion. The present authors will survey the applicable or possibly applicable literature on strategies for maximizing speed of response to treatment of schizophrenia, mania, and depression.

Antipsychotics in Schizophrenia and Schizoaffective Disorder

Osser and Sigadel in 2001[3] published a comprehensive review of antipsychotic response speed in schizophrenia. This review concluded that risperidone may work faster than other antipsychotics, and that olanzapine worked fastest when started at relatively higher doses (e.g., 15 mg daily) compared with lower doses (e.g., 5 or 10 mg daily). Risperidone was the only second-generation antipsychotic that appeared to work faster than the control first-generation antipsychotic. However, that difference was not statistically significant, and it was of questionable clinical significance because the data on which it was based were not primary outcome data in the studies from which it was derived. Notably, quetiapine and ziprasidone numerically trailed the control first-generation antipsychotic in the first week or two of treatment. However, the authors of these studies did not note this in their discussions, although the implications for antipsychotic therapy in the acute inpatient setting might be important. This could be because the studies were not designed to focus on the outcome at 1 or 2 weeks.

Recent studies have suggested that rapid, as opposed to conventional, dosing of quetiapine speeds response in acute schizophrenia during the first week of treatment.[104] The starting dose of rapid treatment was 200 mg on the first day, followed by 400 mg on the second day, 600 mg on the third day, and 800 mg on day 4. However, the conventional dosing was to begin with 50 mg on day 1, 100 mg on day 2, 200 on day 3, 300 on day 4, and 400 mg on day 5. This is slower than most clinicians would go, but the side effects of dizziness, restlessness, and excess sedation on the faster titration were significant.

The possibility of early onset of therapeutic response to risperidone versus conventional antipsy-chotics was confirmed in a more recent review.[105] In this *post hoc* analysis of four studies involving 757 patients, a significantly greater proportion of patients at weeks 1 or 2 achieved a 20% reduc-tion in Positive and Negative Syndrome Scale (PANSS) total scores with risperidone, compared with perphenazine (mean dose 28 mg daily) or haloperidol 10 to 20 mg daily. This may be clinically important because a meta-analysis has shown that failure to achieve a 25% reduction of symptoms on an antipsychotic in the first 2 weeks predicts poor outcome at 4 weeks (positive predictive value of 63%).[106]

The large National Institute of Mental Health (NIMH)-sponsored CATIE study could have been an opportunity to collect prospective data on early response, but the investigators did not design the study to shed light on this. The first evaluation point was 1 month after starting randomized antipsychotic therapy.

The short-term comparative effectiveness of antipsychotics was tested in another recent randomized trial that was not supported by pharmaceutical companies.[107] Three hundred and twenty seven acute schizophrenia and schizoaffective patients who were newly admitted to a public sector hospital were randomized in a 3-week open-label study to haloperidol (mean maximum dose 16 mg), aripiprazole (22 mg), olanzapine (19 mg), quetiapine (650 mg), risperidone (5.2 mg), or ziprasidone (150 mg). Effectiveness was defined, controversially, as whether the patient was well enough for discharge. By this criterion, haloperidol (89%), olanzapine (92%), and risperidone (88%) were significantly more effective than aripiprazole (64%), quetiapine (63%), and ziprasidone (64%) over the 3-week period of the study.

Secondary outcome measures involving various rating scales did not show significant differences. This "pragmatic" outcome measure of dischargeability could have been subject to a variety of biases, but the study is interesting in that it supports the suggestion that not all antipsychotics are equal in rapidity of response and finds olanzapine, the conventional antipsychotic, and (again) risperidone to work faster.

When antipsychotics do work, they work fairly quickly. Leucht et al. pooled data from seven randomized trials of one antipsychotic (amisulpride, not available in the United States) and found that more reduction of positive and total symptoms occurred in the first 2 weeks than in the second 2 weeks ($p < 0.0001$).[108] By the end of 4 weeks, 68% of the improvement that will be found at 1 year was already achieved.

Speed of Response in Mania

Rapid response is highly desirable in the management of the acutely manic patient, especially when there is extreme hyperactivity or serious medical illness that may be exacerbated by the manic state. For this reason, many clinicians combine mood stabilizers and antipsychotics early, for example, in the first week of admission. Some evidence supports this, but the relevant studies did not compare untreated patients assigned to either cotherapy or monotherapy. Rather, the patients studied had already been treated with mood stabilizers and had failed on them (or received inadequate doses) after which they had an antipsychotic or placebo added.[109] Often, newly admitted patients will have been tried on monotherapy with a mood stabilizer or antipsychotic in the community before needing admission; therefore, it is certainly reasonable for them to get early combination treatment once hospitalized.

Regarding the choice of which antipsychotic to add, typical or atypical, naturalistic data seem to favor the atypicals at least with respect to extrapyramidal side effects,[110] but head-to-head comparisons (e.g., olanzapine vs. haloperidol) have found no efficacy differences in mania.[111]

If monotherapy is to be initiated in a first-onset or untreated, newly admitted patient, it is difficult to discern what choice would work most rapidly. There is no clear evidence to favor a mood stabilizer or an antipsychotic as monotherapy. However, oral-loaded divalproex seems to work faster than standard-titration methods.[112] With rapid oral loading, the patient is given (in one method) 30 mg/kg/day on days 1 and 2, followed by 20 mg/kg/day on subsequent days. In a pooled analysis of three studies involving 348 patients, this approach worked faster than lithium (300 mg three times daily for 2 days followed by titration to levels 0.4 to 1.5 mEq per L), and it worked equally rapidly to olanzapine 10 mg for 2 days followed by increase to a maximum of 20 mg daily.[112]

All five atypical antipsychotics have been approved by the FDA for the treatment of acute mania based on placebo-controlled studies. However, it must be kept in mind that the ethical requirements of placebo-controlled studies mandated that the sicker patients were not included.[113] Therefore, the effectiveness of monotherapy with atypicals in real-world patients is unclear.

Although there have been claims that the evidence suggests some atypicals work faster than others in mania, this seems to be an artifact of design variations in the registration trials.[114] Risperidone and ziprasidone patients were first rated at 1 and 2 days, aripiprazole at 4 days, and olanzapine at 7 days in these trials. Doses used were risperidone 1 mg every 6 to 8 hours, with maximum 6 to 10 mg daily; aripiprazole 30 mg daily (although a recent study used 15 mg and it worked well[115]); ziprasidone 40 mg twice daily with food, increased to 60 to 80 mg twice daily on the second day; olanzapine 15 mg daily to start and then adjusted to 5 to 20 mg daily. As is the case in schizophrenia treatment, quetiapine may work most rapidly in mania with an oral-loading schedule of 200 mg on day 1 with daily increases of 200 mg until 800 mg is reached by day 4, given in two divided doses.[116]

Patients who have new-onset bipolar mania who do not need urgent behavioral control are best treated with monotherapy with lithium. Although slower in treating the acute episode, no other treatment has performed as well in preventing recurrences of mania and depression and in reducing risk of suicidal behavior.[117] Observational data indicate that monotherapy with lithium, if initiated, is more likely to be sustained as a monotherapy, compared with anticonvulsants and antipsychotics which lead more often to polytherapy.[118]

Speed of Response in Depression

There has been a long-standing interest in finding ways to increase the response rate to antidepressants because of the clinical impression that they require many weeks to work. However, is this impression based on fact? According to a meta-analysis of 47 double-blind, placebo-controlled trials that evaluated the progression of improvement weekly or biweekly, >60% of the improvement that was going to occur on medication occurred in the first 2 weeks.[119] Also, the biggest differences between drug and placebo were seen during this initial period, suggesting that this initial improvement was a true antidepressant effect. This analysis also failed to support another long-standing impression, that rapid early response is a predictor of placebo response.

Are there any differences in the speed of response of different individual antidepressants? In a recent meta-analysis of all antidepressant controlled trials by the U.S. Agency for Healthcare Research and Quality,[120] one antidepressant had sufficient evidence to deserve mention as possibly having a faster onset of action. Mirtazapine, in seven studies, all sponsored by the manufacturer, consistently had faster effect in comparison with four different SSRIs. The effect size was moderate; the number needed to treat to yield one additional responder after 1 to 2 weeks of treatment was 7. Also, one antidepressant seemed to work consistently slower than at least four other antidepressants—fluoxetine. This is presumed to be due to the long half-life of fluoxetine and its metabolite norfluoxetine, which results in a long period (which can be months) until development of steady-state levels when the patient is started on the lowest effective dose of 20 mg daily.[121]

Augmentation strategies to speed response have been the subject of interest for decades. Prospects that have had periods of popularity include combining SSRIs and tricyclic antidepressants and adding pindolol to SSRIs (which seems to speed response in Europe but not in the United States).[122] More recently, studies in which atypical antipsychotics are added to SSRIs have been financed by the atypical antipsychotic drug companies.[123] This costly approach can augment a partial response to an SSRI, but there have been no studies evaluating whether initial cotherapy would speed response.

There is a possibility that antidepressants will be developed that have a much more rapid onset, even within hours, based on recent studies with intravenous infusions of the N-methyl-D-aspartate receptor agonist ketamine.[124] More research is needed to find a way of sustaining the benefits and dealing with toxicity, but the findings are of great interest.

Suicidal depressed patients present a particular challenge. There is an urgent need to see rapid improvement in suicidal thinking. With effective treatment, most patients will become less suicidal, but for a few, suicidal ideation and activity may increase, or occur *de novo*, in the early weeks of treatment. This has been observed since the beginning of the antidepressant era. It was thought to be due to a progression of response to antidepressants. Patients might initially show improvement in psychomotor retardation, with a lag in improvement in mood, leading to increased risk of suicidal actions. Possibly, this might be the mechanism with antidepressants like tricyclics with their primarily noradrenergically mediated pharmacodynamics. Other causes of increased suicidality have been proposed with the SSRIs and other second-generation antidepressants, including an activation or akathisia-like effect associated with dysphoria. All antidepressants could cause the emergence of a mixed state in a latent bipolar patient. The FDA has recently, though controversially, determined that the risk for antidepressant-emergent suicidality is higher in children, adolescents, and young adults, and required package insert alerts to watch for this adverse effect.[125] In any case, it is reasonable to monitor all patients closely when they are started on antidepressants.

MATCHING SIDE EFFECT PROFILES TO PRESENTING SYMPTOMS

A simple, yet common, consideration when choosing among treatment options concerns the issue of attempting to match the immediate effects (or side effects) of medication to patients' presenting symptoms. For example, while waiting for the effect of an antidepressant on the primary depressive disorder, the patient may have prominent neurovegetative symptoms that cause much distress. Choosing an antidepressant that could ameliorate, or at least not worsen, these symptoms may decrease the need to use multiple drugs and increase the likelihood of continued treatment adherence.

Sleep Changes

When choosing an antidepressant, mirtazapine or nefazodone given at bedtime may be more helpful than other serotonergic antidepressants for a patient with insomnia. On the other hand, patients prescribed paroxetine may subjectively feel more tired but are just as likely to have continued insomnia.[126] Bupropion or fluoxetine given during the day may be better suited for a depressed patient with somnolence. Among antipsychotics, quetiapine and olanzapine would probably help more with sleep, whereas aripiprazole or ziprasidone might be better suited for the already somnolent or anergic psychotic patient.

Appetite Changes

If the depressed patient is cachectic, mirtazapine can increase appetite and oral intake earlier than the time required for the antidepressant effect to occur. In contrast, bupropion, nefazodone, or venlafaxine would be good choices for an overweight patient. In a bipolar patient, lithium and valproate can be helpful if weight loss is a presenting symptom. Among antipsychotics, olanzapine and quetiapine could be chosen if weight gain would actually be desirable. However, the risks would include increased triglycerides, hyperglycemia, and insulin resistance. For the already overweight psychotic patient, aripiprazole or ziprasidone may be more appropriate.

POLYPHARMACY

Polypharmacy—or more appropriately "polytherapy"—may be defined as the concomitant use of two or more agents within the same class (e.g., two antipsychotics). The addition of medication from other classes, possibly for amelioration of side effects or improved control of symptoms (e.g., an antipsychotic plus a mood stabilizer for acute mania), is not always considered to be polytherapy. However, these combinations may still constitute "relative" polytherapy if the use of an available alternative single agent would have worked equally well.

Most practice guidelines and evidence-based algorithms recommend the use of sequential trials of monotherapy for treatment of acute episodes of psychiatric illness and may suggest polytherapy only as a last resort. There continues to be a dearth of controlled trials studying the use of polytherapy in hospitalized patients. Still, if one considers the use of combination psychotropics across different classes of medication, then clearly the use of polytherapy is the norm rather than the exception in the hospitalized patient.[127] However, the concomitant use of multiple drugs within the same class (e.g., two or more antipsychotics) is also highly prevalent—40% to 50% for antipsychotics in schizophrenic and schizoaffective patients[128,129]—and this use has increased over time.[130] Probable reasons for both types of increase likely include the availability of a greater number of pharmacotherapeutic agents and the presumed increase in safety of many of the newer available agents. Furthermore, psychiatric units provide treatment for patients with (a) severe mental illness, (b) histories of multiple past hospitalizations and medication trials, (c) treatment resistance, and/or (d) dangerous behavioral problems, indicating the likelihood of an even greater perceived need for polytherapy for symptom control. The pressure from managed care for more rapid control of symptoms during briefer inpatient stays has also contributed to the use of polytherapy in this population. Understandably, in the absence of evidence, factors such as personal preference, historical patterns of practice, and pressures from milieu and nursing staff to treat patients more aggressively[131] have further contributed to the continued prevalence of polytherapy in inpatient clinical practice.

Although it is frequently unclear if there is any added benefit from the use of multiple medicines, the downsides and risks of polytherapy are clear. These include the risks of increased (a) medication-related adverse effects,[132] (b) dangerous drug–drug interactions, (c) medication errors, (d) mortality rates,[133] (e) medication nonadherence after discharge, and (f) cost.[134] Inpatient polytherapy has also been associated with longer hospital stays, although this may be because the most ill patients may be the most likely to be treated with multiple medicines.[132] It is reasonable then that generally polytherapy should be avoided when possible. To this end the use of treatment algorithms, periodic reviews of inpatient practice, and raising awareness regarding the risks of polytherapy can decrease its use in the inpatient setting.[135] However, there are certain circumstances in which, after a clear review of risks and benefits, polytherapy may be appropriate in hospitalized patients.

Cross-Titration

Clinicians commonly use cross-titration when adding a new medicine while discontinuing a previously ineffective one. The first agent is not discontinued abruptly in an effort to decrease the risks of withdrawal or discontinuation-related phenomena or worsening due to loss of an occult partial response. In the case of antipsychotics, for example, a 3-week taper can significantly reduce crossover exacerbations.[136] Frequently, however, as the patient improves with the addition of the second drug, the clinician is tempted to believe that the combination therapy (rather than the second drug alone) is responsible for this improvement and hence both medicines are continued. However, if one assumes that the response to the first drug was unsatisfactory despite an appropriate trial (i.e., dosing was appropriate and duration of treatment was adequate), it is not likely that it would have new-found effectiveness at a subsequently lower dose. In most cases it is recommended that the cross-titration continue until a clear switch is made to the second drug.[137] Completing the cross-titration switch need not occur in the hospital and may continue on an outpatient basis after the patient is well enough to be discharged. In these circumstances, clear communication with outpatient providers is necessary to convey the inpatient team's treatment plan in order to decrease the chance of continued polytherapy.

The Agitated Manic and/or Psychotic Patient

In manic patients, mood stabilizers may not be immediately effective in the treatment of mania and a 1- to 2-week time period or longer may be needed to achieve significant therapeutic effect. Preliminary studies comparing olanzapine, risperidone, or quetiapine in combination with lithium or valproate versus the use of either mood stabilizer alone suggest that the combination treatments may be more effective—although the addition of an antipsychotic increased the rate of adverse effects.[138–142] It is not clear, however, whether polytherapy results in earlier response. Also, as noted earlier, in these studies patients had a second agent added because they were not satisfactorily responding to monotherapy; the studies did not evaluate whether it is more desirable to commence treatment with the two agents simultaneously.

In schizophrenic patients there can be variable response time with the use of different antipsychotics.[3] In both the agitated manic patient and the agitated psychotic patient, there can be a real need early on for adjunctive medications such as benzodiazepines. Clinical experience suggests that adjunctive first-generation antipsychotics may acutely decrease the risk of harm secondary to behavioral dyscontrol. They may also be needed for severe insomnia. The rationale for adding typical antipsychotics should not be to hasten overall recovery—a prospect for which there is no good evidence—but in the hope of decreasing dangerous behavior in the short term. Clinicians should take into account the risks of medication interactions and the increase in risk of antipsychotic-related adverse effects and carefully balance these against the potential benefits when considering adding neuroleptics. Once the patient's behavior improves and remains stable, adjunctive drugs such as benzodiazepines and typical antipsychotics can be withdrawn. If the patient has required high doses of these agents, it is recommended that they be tapered and not abruptly discontinued, and again, clear communication with the outpatient psychiatrist is essential to ensure that the taper continues following discharge.

In the nonagitated psychotic patient there is less justification for adjunctive polytherapy. If there is no response to the first antipsychotic drug within the first week, increasing to more optimal dosing or switching to a new antipsychotic (to clozapine if appropriate) should be considered.[3] The temptation to use polytherapy within the first week (or to change to another antipsychotic prematurely) occurs if there is little response in terms of targeted psychotic symptoms. With partial response, deciding on the next step is complicated by the possibilities that (a) the patient may respond better given enough time and that (b) the observed improvement may be due to placebo effect or to other therapeutic effects of hospitalization.[3] The clinician should ensure that optimum dosing is being used and despite the uncertainty the best course of action may be to allow for gradual response. If after 2 to 3 weeks of optimal dosing—by which time most of the improvement that one is likely to see will have occurred[143]—there is still insufficient response, the antipsychotic agent should be changed. (This would constitute a briefer trial and more rapid switch than recommended by algorithms based on outpatient treatment.[144]) Again if appropriate the change should be to clozapine. A lengthy taper of the first agent is usually not needed under these circumstances.

The Depressed Patient

In depressed patients, unless multiple monotherapies have failed, the use of combination antidepressant therapy is usually not needed and a relatively rapid taper can precede the use of a new antidepressant. The concomitant use of two SSRIs should be avoided due to the risk of serotonergic side effects. If a combination of antidepressants is considered, then agents with different mechanisms of action should be used,[145] although dose increase to the optimal or maximal dose of the first agent should be tried before adding a second antidepressant. In addition, clinicians should not underestimate the effectiveness of psychotherapy when combined with antidepressant therapy and its ability to reduce the need for antidepressant polytherapy.[146–148]

Adding an antidepressant to an acutely psychotic schizophrenic patient's antipsychotic regimen is generally not helpful and may cause symptom exacerbations or drug interactions. Mood symptoms generally improve as the patient responds to the prescribed antipsychotic.[149]

In the patient with bipolar depression, lithium[150] or quetiapine[151] and possibly lamotrigine[152] may be used as monotherapies, although there are three unpublished negative or failed studies with lamotrigine monotherapy.[103] However, if these agents cannot be used, then antidepressants may need to be considered, despite disappointing data on the efficacy of antidepressants over the long term.[153] In these cases, it may be prudent to treat the patient with another mood stabilizer (and to reach therapeutic serum levels if applicable) before carefully introducing an antidepressant, thereby reducing the risk of inducing mania.

TREATMENT RESISTANCE

Patients who are admitted to acute psychiatric units have frequently had a number of medication trials with unsatisfactory results, leading to their need for admission. Therefore, treatment resistance is a typical challenge encountered in this setting. There are also more severe levels of treatment resistance. Exhaustive trials may have already occurred in recidivistic patients, and it will be difficult to determine what to do next. Or the patient may have had more than one significant trial during the present admission, without success, and the length of stay to that point may require that the patient be transferred to a tertiary-care facility.

Although detailed algorithms for the approach to treatment-resistant problems would require going beyond the scope of this chapter, a list of sometimes overlooked or avoided options that are especially worthy of consideration will be offered. As a general principle, making one medication change at a time, and giving it adequate time to be dosed properly, produces better and faster results than "treatment as usual" that lacks this organized and consistent approach.[154]

Schizophrenia and Schizoaffective Disorder

In the treatment of schizophrenia and schizoaffective disorder, one must first rule out the perhaps most frequent cause of poor response—noncompliance (e.g., cheeking, self-induced vomiting, purging). The most evidence-supported pharmacotherapy option after there have been a minimum of two adequate monotherapy trials of antipsychotics is clozapine.[155,156] The two trials should include one first-generation antipsychotic and either risperidone or olanzapine. The resistance to using clozapine comes from fear of side effects and concern about the amount of time it takes to start a reasonable trial. Also, a very common conceptual obstacle on the part of the physician is the assumption that a previously noncompliant patient would not be willing or able to adhere to the monitoring regime (i.e., blood draws) that would be needed with clozapine treatment. This concern is usually misplaced, however, given that if the patient responds well to clozapine, outpatient compliance could be much better than expected. The physician has to be prepared to make an appropriately positive and convincing description of the potential benefits versus the risks of this option during the consent process. This is the true "art" of medicine—the ability to persuade the patient (and the managed care reviewer) to agree to an effective, highly evidence-based, but arduous treatment course. The improvisational throwing together of unproven combinations of multiple classes of disparate psychotropic agents is closer to alchemy than to art. (Clozapine is also an important option for treatment-resistant cases of bipolar disorder and BPD.)[18,19]

If clozapine cannot be used, many patients have never had an adequate trial of a reasonably well-tolerated first-generation antipsychotic such as perphenazine, and may benefit substantially even if the more esteemed second-generation drugs have been ineffective. Fully a quarter of well-defined treatment-resistant patients with schizophrenia had a substantial response (>30% improvement in PANSS score) with perphenazine in a controlled study at a dose of approximately 40 mg daily.[157]

Surprisingly, aripiprazole at a dose of 30 mg did equally well in this trial, although there were somewhat more dropouts due to side effects.

Finally, in thinking about treatment resistance in the pharmacotherapy of schizophrenia, it is useful to recall the original observations of Dr. Heinz Lehmann from the 1950s regarding the phases of response to chlorpromazine.[158] He observed three phases, as follows:

1. Medicated cooperation. The patient is no longer assaultive or uncooperative but does not interact socially and still has persistent delusions, hallucinations, or formal thought disorder. This phase is usually achieved within the first week of treatment.
2. Socialization. The patient is able to interact reasonably well but still has persistent psychotic symptoms on questioning. It may take 4 to 6 weeks to achieve this phase.
3. Elimination of thought disorder. The patient is in substantial remission, with refinement of social and occupational capacities. It may take several months to reach this phase, if it occurs at all.

If the patient's improvement seems to have plateaued at level (1) or (2), further medication trials including clozapine are indicated. One may then have the opportunity to observe the patient progressing further on this continuum of response.

Mania

In the treatment of mania, lithium may be the most overlooked option in the United States currently.[159] Marketing influences may have led American physicians to routinely overlook the significant benefits of lithium over the long term, particularly for suicidal patients and others with resistant depression, and underestimate the risks of alternative agents (e.g., the greater weight gain and teratogenicity associated with valproate).

Depression

Inpatients with psychotic depression are often not given the most evidence-supported pharmaco-therapy,[160] which is to use full doses of antipsychotics and antidepressants in combination.

In the approach to pharmacotherapy-resistant nonpsychotic depression, it is important to delineate and intervene to ameliorate stress-related and personality style-mediated contributions to the depressed state.[161] Beyond that, Sequenced Treatment Alternatives to Relieve Depression (STAR*D) has suggested that thyroid hormone augmentation of an SSRI, and the quadruple-action combination of venlafaxine and mirtazapine may deserve more consideration than previously thought.[162,163] ECT, with its high remission rates,[164] deserves consideration as an alternative to either of these options.[165] Unfortunately, the likelihood of use of ECT is strongly dependent on its availability in the hospital to which the patient is admitted.

PHARMACOGENETICS

Pharmacogenetics, the study of genetically determined drug response, can guide treatment selection by helping to predict how an individual patient would respond to specific agents. A brief discussion of promising developments can shed light on the ways in which better understanding of genetically determined factors can affect clinical treatment. Pharmacogenetic understanding holds significant potential to decrease morbidity by decreasing the risk of adverse drug effects and decreasing overall treatment time—time that would otherwise be spent trying ineffective treatments. At a minimum, it is important to obtain the family history of drug response in patients admitted to the psychiatric unit. It may also be of value to think about how psychopharmacologic choices may be influenced by ethnic and population-based considerations.[166]

A primary area has been the improved understanding of genetic polymorphisms in CYP450 enzymes, especially the CYP2D6 and CYP2C19 variants, and their impact on the pharmacokinetics of drug response and tolerance.[167] Laboratory testing for 19 genes is now available[168] but not yet part of mainstream clinical practice, in part because it is not covered by any insurance programs. Individual genotypes can be identified based on the function of the enzymatic phenotype (e.g., poor, intermediate, extensive, or ultrarapid metabolizers). For example, "ultrarapid" metabolizers may carry three or more active CYP2D6 alleles, whereas "poor metabolizers" may lack enzymatic activity. Poor metabolizers may therefore be at higher risk of adverse effects if treated with medicines that are substrates of this isoenzyme, whereas ultrarapid metabolizers may not show clinical response. Ultrarapid metabolism, for example, may be one reason for treatment refractoriness to antipsychotics, many of which are metabolized by CYP2D6. What is additionally important is that relevant genotypes are represented differently in different populations. For example, approximately 30% of patients from North Africa and the Middle East may be ultrarapid metabolizers of CYP2D6 substrates;[167] up to 50% of Asians may have a partially deficient form of the CYP2D6 allele.[169] A web-based computer program is available that combines genetic and drug interaction information to predict troublesome drug interactions (www.genemedrx.com).

Pharmacodynamic implications of genetically determined response could also have direct influence on choice of treatment. A major area of study is that of the genetic variants of the serotonin transporter gene (*SLC6A4*). The "short" form of the serotonin transporter gene promoter has a polymorphism that has been associated with decreased response to SSRIs, whereas the presence of the long allele is associated with positive drug response.[170] Also interestingly the short allele variant may be associated with increased risk of antidepressant-induced mania.[171] This correlation of long versus short forms of the alleles with treatment response, however, may apply only to SSRIs and not to antidepressants with other mechanisms of action (e.g., mirtazapine).[172]

For antipsychotics, polymorphisms in receptor genes have been associated with both effectiveness and with the risk of adverse effects. Examples particularly relevant to inpatient psychiatry are studies showing the possibility of an association between variations in D2-receptor genes and the speed of response to antipsychotics[173] and effects of variations in D$_3$-receptor genes on the development of TD.[170] There also could be important economic ramifications—the potential to predict those who can benefit from more affordable first-generation antipsychotics without being genetically predisposed to TD would significantly influence treatment decisions.[174]

In regard to mood stabilizers, the study of lithium responders and genetic inheritance of bipolar disorder may eventually guide treatment. Positive response to lithium may be associated with bipolar disorder that is more genetically based.[175] A known clear family history of bipolar disorder therefore may argue for the selection of lithium for these patients.

MANAGED CARE AND FINANCIAL CONSIDERATIONS

Although physicians would like to feel that they have the autonomy, right, and responsibility to prescribe whatever they think is best, the reality is that health care resources are limited and it is impossible to avoid oversight by managed care. Questions will be raised about the high costs of certain medicines. At the same time, the primary interest of managed care review teams is to keep the length of stay as short as possible and their criteria mainly focus on safety issues and ensuring that "active treatment" is occurring. Often this means to them that there have to be frequent medication changes. They see this as concrete evidence of active interventions, whereas the other no less important and effective inpatient interventions such as intensive individual or group psychotherapy are less appreciated in justifying ongoing inpatient stay. There is often scant acknowledgment that most psychotropic medicines have latency periods before their onset of action and often it is the therapeutic milieu that is responsible for the rapid initial improvement in the patient's distress.

Nevertheless, difficult as it is, psychiatrists should avoid the temptation, fanned by the impatience of managed care reviewers, to increase doses too rapidly or to add additional medicines before current ones have had a reasonable chance to take effect. Evidence-supported approaches should influence treatment decisions and not the usually unseen managed care criteria for allowing additional days of inpatient care that usually have little scientific basis.

Drug formularies inform physicians of the availability of more economical choices when selecting medication. The hope and expectation is that these lists are guided not only by economic concerns but also by the realities of clinical practice. Requests by physicians for exceptions based on these realities should follow from thoughtful, cost-effective, stepwise sequences of choices that can be justified to the cost managers in terms that they will understand.

With a significant proportion of the population in the United States lacking health benefits, the psychiatrist may have to opt for alternative medication to accommodate a patient's ability to pay for it.

Sometimes, this may expose the patient to the risk of more side effects compared with a newer drug. For example, the atypical antipsychotics have fewer motor side effects but they are not currently available in a generic formulation and therefore none may be affordable without health benefits. Even if the health plan allows the use of newer medicines, they may still be unaffordable because of the high copayments or limited allowable yearly coverage. Psychiatrists in many parts of the world confront this problem routinely. As the costs of health care continue to escalate and fewer financial resources are available for patient care, physicians can expect to be required to factor economics more and more into their clinical decisions.

Improving Outcome after Discharge

Up to 50% of discharged psychiatric inpatients may be readmitted within 1 year of discharge.[176] Many factors can help prevent readmission but the two most important ones are compliance with treatment appointments and medication. Studies have shown that up to half of discharged patients with schizophrenia or related disorders miss their first follow-up appointment after their hospital release.[177] Boyer et al.[178] reported that aftercare appointment compliance can be enhanced by three clinical "bridging strategies." These are (a) communication between inpatient and outpatient providers about discharge plans, (b) starting outpatient programs before discharge, and (c) family involvement during the hospitalization.

Disease-management programs promoted by managed care companies for medical diagnoses are beginning to be developed for psychiatric illnesses. Kopelowicz et al.[179] demonstrated that patients and their families who received skills training had better outcomes in the first 9 months in regard to relapse, functioning, and rehospitalization. Psychoeducation of patients, especially when their families are involved, has produced reduction of relapse and readmission rates of up to 50%. Inpatient teams should therefore take advantage of the ability to involve family members in meetings during the hospital stay.

Finally, compliance is negatively associated with the complexity of a medication regimen. The inpatient psychiatrist has the opportunity to examine closely whether polytherapy regimens that require multiple daily doses of various therapeutic agents are really necessary. Simplification of a patient's pharmacotherapeutic regimen can significantly contribute to continued improvement and stability after discharge from the inpatient setting.

Summary

The pharmacologic approach to the psychiatric inpatient is influenced by multiple considerations. Treatment needs to be provided for the most severely psychiatrically ill patients within a short period of time and it needs to be safe and effective and also to increase the likelihood that patients remain well after discharge.

1. The provision of safe treatment means that any dangerous or assaultive behavior has to be treated urgently, often before a definitive diagnosis is reached. Typical antipsychotics and benzodiazepines remain the mainstay for rapid parenteral treatment.
2. In decreasing patient distress, p.r.n. medication does play a role in decreasing patient distress, although the request for such medication by patients and staff may suggest a need to consider psychological methods of managing this distress.
3. Efforts should be made to clarify patients' past pharmacotherapeutic treatments. Collateral information is often necessary. Data regarding past medication trials, both successful and otherwise, as well as information regarding reasons for past medication nonadherence, can be invaluable.
4. In all patients, but particularly in those with concomitant medical illness, the choice of agent should be guided by an effort to decrease overall medical risk and to avoid worsening the patient's medical comorbidities. The effect of psychiatric medication on all major systems, including cardiovascular, neurologic, hematologic, hepatic, renal, metabolic, and reproductive should be considered, and adequate steps should be taken to identify high-risk patients and monitor them when appropriate.
5. Antipsychotics, antidepressants, and mood stabilizers carry the risk of dangerous medication interactions. In the patient being treated with multiple medicines, psychiatric or otherwise, an effort should be made to decrease the risk of these interactions.

6. Although some agents may bring about response quicker than others (e.g., risperidone for psychosis, mirtazapine for depression), dose and speed of titration also likely affect speed of response for antipsychotics (e.g., olanzapine and quetiapine) and for mood stabilizers (e.g., valproate).

7. Psychiatric medicines should be used that would preferentially improve, rather than worsen, patients' associated neurovegetative symptoms, such as sleep and appetite changes, by matching side effect profiles to these symptoms.

8. Polytherapy should be minimized when there is a lack of evidence for its effectiveness and risk of increased overall side effects. However, in certain contexts (e.g., during cross titrations, or while treating agitated manic or psychotic patients) polytherapy may be temporarily necessary.

9. Treatment resistance constitutes a significant problem in the inpatient population. Clozapine use should not be avoided when there is clear treatment resistance to multiple other antipsychotics. In patients with bipolar disorder, lithium should not be overlooked. In refractory depressed patients, ECT and evidence-supported antidepressant combinations (e.g., venlafaxine and mirtazapine) should be considered.

10. Pharmacogenetic factors may explain lack of response to, or lack of tolerability of, certain medications in specific patients. Laboratory testing for genetic polymorphisms will increasingly aid in the identification of patients who would be likely to respond to certain therapies earlier during inpatient treatment.

11. Efforts should be made to resist managed care reviewers who push for aggressive psychopharmacologic interventions when psychotherapy is more appropriately indicated. On the other hand, outpatient insurance formularies, and patients' lack of ability to afford expensive prescribed medications after discharge cannot be ignored when deciding the inpatient choice of treatment.

12. The inpatient psychiatrist should keep in mind that for any pharmacotherapeutic regimen to be successful it should be tied to psychosocial interventions. Individual and group psychotherapy, family involvement in patient treatment, communication with outpatient systems of care, and strategies to increase likelihood of treatment adherence are all critical for a successful outcome. Comprehensive treatment of the whole patient is necessary for the ongoing provision of safe and effective treatment.

REFERENCES

1. Agency for Health Care Research and Quality. *Care of adults with mental health and substance abuse disorder in U.S. community hospitals: Health and Human Services Agency for Health Care Research and Quality,* 2004.

2. Woodward SA, Zeiss RA, Wheeler R, et al. Smoking Cessation and Decreased Behavioral Restraints in Inpatient Psychiatry. *American Psychiatric Association Annual Meeting,* New Research Poster NR 579. San Diego, 2007.

3. Osser DN, Sigadel R. Short-term inpatient pharmacotherapy of schizophrenia. *Harv Rev Psychiatry.* 2001;9(3):89–104.

4. Brook S, Walden J, Benattia I, et al. Ziprasidone and haloperidol in the treatment of acute exacerbation of schizophrenia and schizoaffective disorder: Comparison of intramuscular and oral formulations in a 6-week, randomized, blinded-assessment study. *Psychopharmacology (Berl).* 2005;178(4):514–523.

5. Breier A, Meehan K, Birkett M, et al. A double-blind, placebo-controlled dose-response comparison of intramuscular olanzapine and haloperidol in the treatment of acute agitation in schizophrenia. *Arch Gen Psychiatry.* 2002;59(5):441–448.

6. Tran-Johnson TK, Sack DA, Marcus RN, et al. Efficacy and safety of intramuscular aripiprazole in patients with acute agitation: A randomized, double-blind, placebo-controlled trial. *J Clin Psychiatry.* 2007;68(1):111–119.

7. Raj YP. Psychopharmacology of borderline personality disorder. *Curr Psychiatry Rep.* 2004;6(3):225–231.

8. Villeneuve E, Lemelin S. Open-label study of atypical neuroleptic quetiapine for treatment of borderline personality disorder: Impulsivity as main target. *J Clin Psychiatry.* 2005;66(10):1298–1303.

9. Taylor FB, Lowe K, Thompson C, et al. Daytime prazosin reduces psychological distress to trauma specific cues in civilian trauma posttraumatic stress disorder. *Biol Psychiatry.* 2006;59(7):577–581.

10. Raskind MA, Peskind ER, Hoff DJ, et al. A parallel group placebo controlled study of prazosin for trauma nightmares and

sleep disturbance in combat veterans with post-traumatic stress disorder. *Biol Psychiatry.* 2007;61(8):928–934.

11. Binks CA, Fenton M, McCarthy L, Lee T, et al. Pharmacological interventions for people with borderline personality disorder. *Cochrane Database Syst Rev.* 2006(1):CD005653.

12. Cowdry RW, Gardner DL. Pharmacotherapy of borderline personality disorder. Alprazolam, carbamazepine, trifluoperazine, and tranylcypromine. *Arch Gen Psychiatry.* 1988;45(2):111–119.

13. Nose M, Cipriani A, Biancosino B, et al. Efficacy of pharmacotherapy against core traits of borderline personality disorder: Meta-analysis of randomized controlled trials. *Int Clin Psychopharmacol.* 2006;21(6):345–353.

14. Bellino S, Paradiso E, Bogetto F. Efficacy and tolerability of quetiapine in the treatment of borderline personality disorder: A pilot study. *J Clin Psychiatry.* 2006;67(7):1042–1046.

15. Soler J, Pascual JC, Campins J, et al. Double-blind, placebo-controlled study of dialectical behavior therapy plus olanzapine for borderline personality disorder. *Am J Psychiatry.* 2005; 162(6):1221–1224.

16. Nickel MK, Loew TH, Gil FP. Aripiprazole in treatment of borderline patients, part II: An 18-month follow-up. *Psychopharmacology (Berl).* 2007;191(4):1023–1026.

17. Zanarini MC, Frankenburg FR. Omega-3 fatty acid treatment of women with borderline personality disorder: A double-blind, placebo-controlled pilot study. *Am J Psychiatry.* 2003;160(1):167–169.

18. Chengappa KN, Ebeling T, Kang JS, et al. Clozapine reduces severe self-mutilation and aggression in psychotic patients with borderline personality disorder. *J Clin Psychiatry.* 1999;60(7):477–484.

19. Benedetti F, Sforzini L, Colombo C, et al. Low-dose clozapine in acute and continuation treatment of severe borderline personality disorder. *J Clin Psychiatry.* 1998;59(3):103–107.

20. Straus SM, Bleumink GS, Dieleman JP, et al. Antipsychotics and the risk of sudden cardiac death. *Arch Intern Med.* 2004;164(12):1293–1297.

21. Ray WA, Meredith S, Thapa PB, et al. Cyclic antidepressants and the risk of sudden cardiac death. *Clin Pharmacol Ther.* 2004;75(3):234–241.

22. Glassman AH, Bigger JT Jr. Antipsychotic drugs: Prolonged QTc interval, torsade de pointes, and sudden death. *Am J Psychiatry.* 2001;158(11):1774–1782.

23. Shah RR. Drug-induced QT dispersion: Does it predict the risk of torsade de pointes? *J Electrocardiol.* 2005;38(1):10–18.

24. Fayek M, Kingsbury SJ, Zada J, et al. Cardiac effects of antipsychotic medications. *Psychiatr Serv.* 2001;52(5):607–609.

25. Lieberman JA, Stroup TS, McEvoy JP, et al. Effectiveness of antipsychotic drugs in patients with chronic schizophrenia. *N Engl J Med.* 2005; 353(12):1209–1223.

26. Breier A, Berg PH, Thakore JH, et al. Olanzapine versus ziprasidone: Results of a 28-week double-blind study in patients with schizophrenia. *Am J Psychiatry.* 2005;162(10):1879–1887.

27. *Physician's desk reference.* Montvale: Thomson PDR; 2007.

28. Merrill DB, Dec GW, Goff DC. Adverse cardiac effects associated with clozapine. *J Clin Psychopharmacol.* 2005;25(1):32–41.

29. Mamiya K, Sadanaga T, Sekita A, et al. Lithium concentration correlates with QTc in patients with psychosis. *J Electrocardiol.* 2005;38(2):148–151.

30. Brucculeri M, Kaplan J, Lande L. Reversal of citalopram-induced junctional bradycardia with intravenous sodium bicarbonate. *Pharmacotherapy.* 2005;25(1):119–122.

31. Isbister GK, Prior FH, Foy A. Citalopram-induced bradycardia and presyncope. *Ann Pharmacother.* 2001;35(12):1552–1555.

32. Pae CU, Kim JJ, Lee CU, et al. Provoked bradycardia after paroxetine administration. *Gen Hosp Psychiatry.* 2003;25(2):142–144.

33. Mbaya P, Alam F, Ashim S, et al. Cardiovascular effects of high dose venlafaxine XL in patients with major depressive disorder. *Hum Psychopharmacol.* 2007;22(3):129–133.

34. Johnson EM, Whyte E, Mulsant BH, et al. Cardiovascular changes associated with venlafaxine in the treatment of late-life depression. *Am J Geriatr Psychiatry.* 2006;14(9):796–802.

35. Raskin J, Goldstein DJ, Mallinckrodt CH, et al. Duloxetine in the long-term treatment of major depressive disorder. *J Clin Psychiatry.* 2003;64(10):1237–1244.

36. Wohlreich MM, Mallinckrodt CH, Prakash A, et al. Duloxetine for the treatment of major depressive disorder: Safety and tolerability associated with dose escalation. *Depress Anxiety.* 2007;24(1):41–52.

37. Feighner JP. Cardiovascular safety in depressed patients: Focus on venlafaxine. *J Clin Psychiatry.* 1995;56(12):574–579.

38. Felker BL, Sloan KL, Dominitz JA, et al. The safety of valproic acid use for patients with hepatitis C infection. *Am J Psychiatry.* 2003;160(1):174–178.

39. Lott RS, Helmboldt KM, Madaras-Kelly KJ. Retrospective evaluation of the effect of valproate therapy on transaminase elevations in patients with hepatitis C. *Pharmacotherapy.* 2001; 21(11):1345–1351.

40. Mallet L, Babin S, Morais JA. Valproic acid-induced hyperammonemia and thrombocytopenia in an elderly woman. *Ann Pharmacother*. 2004;38(10):1643–1647.

41. Carr RB, Shrewsbury K. Hyperammonemia due to valproic acid in the psychiatric setting. *Am J Psychiatry*. 2007;164(7):1020–1027.

42. Lepkifker E, Sverdlik A, Iancu I, et al. Renal insufficiency in long-term lithium treatment. *J Clin Psychiatry*. 2004;65(6):850–856.

43. Gitlin M. Lithium and the kidney: An updated review. *Drug Saf*. 1999;20(3):231–243.

44. Dixon L, Weiden P, Delahanty J, et al. Prevalence and correlates of diabetes in national schizophrenia samples. *Schizophr Bull*. 2000;26(4):903–912.

45. Shirzadi AA, Ghaemi SN. Side effects of atypical antipsychotics: Extrapyramidal symptoms and the metabolic syndrome. *Harv Rev Psychiatry*. 2006;14(3):152–164.

46. Clark NG. Consensus development conference on antipsychotic drugs and obesity and diabetes. *Diabetes Care*. 2004;27(2):596–601.

47. van Winkel R, De Hert M, Van Eyck D, et al. Screening for diabetes and other metabolic abnormalities in patients with schizophrenia and schizoaffective disorder: Evaluation of incidence and screening methods. *J Clin Psychiatry*. 2006;67(10):1493–1500.

48. Lipkovich I, Citrome L, Perlis R, et al. Early predictors of substantial weight gain in bipolar patients treated with olanzapine. *J Clin Psychopharmacol*. 2006;26(3):316–320.

49. Gentile S. Long-term treatment with atypical antipsychotics and the risk of weight gain: A literature analysis. *Drug Saf*. 2006;29(4):303–319.

50. Osser DN, Najarian DM, Dufresne RL. Olanzapine increases weight and serum triglyceride levels. *J Clin Psychiatry*. 1999;60(11):767–770.

51. Piette JD, Heisler M, Ganoczy D, et al. Differential medication adherence among patients with schizophrenia and comorbid diabetes and hypertension. *Psychiatr Serv*. 2007;58(2):207–212.

52. Anghelescu I, Klawe C, Dahmen N. Venlafaxine in a patient with idiopathic leukopenia and mirtazapine-induced severe neutropenia. *J Clin Psychiatry*. 2002;63(9):838.

53. Sedky K, Lippmann S. Psychotropic medications and leukopenia. *Curr Drug Targets*. 2006;7(9):1191–1194.

54. Hager ED, Dziambor H, Hohmann D, et al. Effects of lithium on thrombopoiesis in patients with low platelet cell counts following chemotherapy or radiotherapy. *Biol Trace Elem Res*. 2001;83(2):139–148.

55. Hager ED, Dziambor H, Winkler P, et al. Effects of lithium carbonate on hematopoietic cells in patients with persistent neutropenia following chemotherapy or radiotherapy. *J Trace Elem Med Biol*. 2002;16(2):91–97.

56. Gallicchio VS, Messino MJ, Hulette BC, et al. Lithium and hematopoiesis: Effective experimental use of lithium as an agent to improve bone marrow transplantation. *J Med*. 1992;23(3–4):195–216.

57. Mahmud J, Mathews M, Verma S, et al. Oxcarbazepine-induced thrombocytopenia. *Psychosomatics*. 2006;47(1):73–74.

58. Conley EL, Coley KC, Pollock BG, et al. Prevalence and risk of thrombocytopenia with valproic acid: Experience at a psychiatric teaching hospital. *Pharmacotherapy*. 2001;21(11):1325–1330.

59. Trannel TJ, Ahmed I, Goebert D. Occurrence of thrombocytopenia in psychiatric patients taking valproate. *Am J Psychiatry*. 2001;158(1):128–130.

60. Gerstner T, Teich M, Bell N, et al. Valproate-associated coagulopathies are frequent and variable in children. *Epilepsia*. 2006;47(7):1136–1143.

61. De Berardis D, Campanella D, Matera V, et al. Thrombocytopenia during valproic acid treatment in young patients with new-onset bipolar disorder. *J Clin Psychopharmacol*. 2003;23(5):451–458.

62. Kruger S, Lindstaedt M. Duloxetine and hyponatremia: A report of 5 cases. *J Clin Psychopharmacol*. 2007;27(1):101–104.

63. Ladino M, Guardiola VD, Paniagua M. Mirtazapine-induced hyponatremia in an elderly hospice patient. *J Palliat Med*. 2006;9(2):258–260.

64. Bagley SC, Yaeger D. Hyponatremia associated with bupropion, a case verified by rechallenge. *J Clin Psychopharmacol*. 2005;25(1):98–99.

65. Dong X, Leppik IE, White J, et al. Hyponatremia from oxcarbazepine and carbamazepine. *Neurology*. 2005;65(12):1976–1978.

66. Sachdeo RC, Wasserstein A, Mesenbrink PJ, et al. Effects of oxcarbazepine on sodium concentration and water handling. *Ann Neurol*. 2002;51(5):613–620.

67. Alldredge BK. Seizure risk associated with psychotropic drugs: Clinical and pharmacokinetic considerations. *Neurology*. 1999;53(5 Suppl 2):S68–S75.

68. Montgomery SA. Antidepressants and seizures: Emphasis on newer agents and clinical implications. *Int J Clin Pract*. 2005;59(12):1435–1440.

69. Alper K, Schwartz KA, Kolts RL, et al. Seizure incidence in psychopharmacological clinical trials: An analysis of Food and Drug Administration (FDA) summary basis of approval reports. *Biol Psychiatry*. 2007;62(4):345–354.

70. Pisani F, Oteri G, Costa C, et al. Effects of psychotropic drugs on seizure threshold. *Drug Saf*. 2002;25(2):91–110.

71. Schneider LS, Dagerman KS, Insel P. Risk of death with atypical antipsychotic drug treatment for dementia: Meta-analysis of randomized placebo-controlled trials. *JAMA.* 2005;294(15):1934–1943.

72. Schneider LS, Dagerman K, Insel PS. Efficacy and adverse effects of atypical antipsychotics for dementia: Meta-analysis of randomized, placebo-controlled trials. *Am J Geriatr Psychiatry.* 2006;14(3):191–210.

73. Herrmann N, Lanctot KL. Do atypical antipsychotics cause stroke? *CNS drugs.* 2005;19(2): 91–103.

74. Gill SS, Rochon PA, Herrmann N, et al. Atypical antipsychotic drugs and risk of ischaemic stroke: Population based retrospective cohort study. *Br Med J.* 2005;330(7489):445.

75. Pollock BG, Mulsant BH, Rosen J, et al. Comparison of citalopram, perphenazine, and placebo for the acute treatment of psychosis and behavioral disturbances in hospitalized, demented patients. *Am J Psychiatry.* 2002;159(3):460–465.

76. Salzman C. Treatment of the agitation of late-life psychosis and Alzheimer's disease. *Eur Psychiatry.* 2001;16(Suppl 1):25s–28s.

77. Yang C, White DP, Winkelman JW. Antidepressants and periodic leg movements of sleep. *Biol Psychiatry.* 2005;58(6):510–514.

78. Salin-Pascual RJ, Galicia-Polo L, Drucker-Colin R. Sleep changes after 4 consecutive days of venlafaxine administration in normal volunteers. *J Clin Psychiatry.* 1997;58(8):348–350.

79. Agargun MY, Kara H, Ozbek H, et al. Restless legs syndrome induced by mirtazapine. *J Clin Psychiatry.* 2002;63(12):1179.

80. Kim SW, Shin IS, Kim JM, et al. Bupropion may improve restless legs syndrome: A report of three cases. *Clin Neuropharmacol.* 2005;28(6): 298–301.

81. Bilo L, Meo R. Epilepsy and polycystic ovary syndrome: Where is the link? *Neurol Sci.* 2006; 27(4):221–230.

82. Klipstein KG, Goldberg JF. Screening for bipolar disorder in women with polycystic ovary syndrome: A pilot study. *J Affect Disord.* 2006;91(2–3):205–209.

83. Wilson DR. High dose olanzapine and prolactin levels. *Presented at the 51st American Psychiatric Association Institute on Psychiatric Services.* New Orleans, 1999.

84. www.genemedrx.com.

85. Ciraulo DA, ed. *Drug interactions in psychiatry,* 3rd ed. Philadelphia: Lippincott Williams & Wilkins; 2006.

86. Sayal KS, Duncan-McConnell DA, McConnell HW, et al. Psychotropic interactions with warfarin. *Acta Psychiatr Scand.* 2000;102(4): 250–255.

87. Ereshefsky L, Jhee S, Grothe D. Antidepressant drug-drug interaction profile update. *Drugs R D.* 2005;6(6):323–336.

88. Borba CP, Henderson DC. Citalopram and clozapine: Potential drug interaction. *J Clin Psychiatry.* 2000;61(4):301–302.

89. Novartis. Product Information: Drug Warning and New Information, Clozaril(R), clozapine. 2005.

90. Spina E, Scordo MG, D'Arrigo C. Metabolic drug interactions with new psychotropic agents. *Fundam Clin Pharmacol.* 2003;17(5): 517–538.

91. Boyer EW, Shannon M. The serotonin syndrome. *N Engl J Med.* 2005;352(11):1112–1120.

92. Huang V, Gortney JS. Risk of serotonin syndrome with concomitant administration of linezolid and serotonin agonists. *Pharmacotherapy.* 2006;26(12):1784–1793.

93. Grohmann R, Ruther E, Sassim N, et al. Adverse effects of clozapine. *Psychopharmacology (Berl).* 1989;99(Suppl):S101–S104.

94. Kroon LA. Drug interactions with smoking. *Am J Health Syst Pharm.* 2007;64(18):1917–1921.

95. Lu ML, Lane HY, Lin SK, et al. Adjunctive fluvoxamine inhibits clozapine-related weight gain and metabolic disturbances. *J Clin Psychiatry.* 2004;65(6):766–771.

96. Perucca E. Clinically relevant drug interactions with antiepileptic drugs. *Br J Clin Pharmacol.* 2006;61(3):246–255.

97. Bialer M, Doose DR, Murthy B, et al. Pharmacokinetic interactions of topiramate. *Clin Pharmacokinet.* 2004;43(12):763–780.

98. Crawford P. Interactions between antiepileptic drugs and hormonal contraception. *CNS Drugs.* 2002;16(4):263–272.

99. Yuen AW, Land G, Weatherley BC, et al. Sodium valproate acutely inhibits lamotrigine metabolism. *Br J Clin Pharmacol.* 1992;33(5):511–513.

100. Kaufman KR, Gerner R. Lamotrigine toxicity secondary to sertraline. *Seizure.* 1998;7(2): 163–165.

101. Guthrie SK, Stoysich AM, Bader G, et al. Hypothesized interaction between valproic acid and warfarin. *J Clin Psychopharmacol.* 1995; 15(2):138–139.

102. Spina E, Perucca E. Clinical significance of pharmacokinetic interactions between antiepileptic and psychotropic drugs. *Epilepsia.* 2002;43(Suppl 2):37–44.

103. Janicak PG, Davis JM, Preskorn SH, et al. *Principles and practice of psychopharmacotherapy,* 4th ed. Lippincott Williams & Wilkins; 2006.

104. Pae CU, Kim JJ, Lee CU, et al. Rapid versus conventional initiation of quetiapine in the treatment of schizophrenia: A randomized, parallel-group trial. *J Clin Psychiatry.* 2007; 68(3):399–405.

105. Glick ID, Shkedy Z, Schreiner A. Differential early onset of therapeutic response with

risperidone versus conventional antipsychotics in patients with chronic schizophrenia. *Int Clin Psychopharmacol.* 2006;21(5):261–266.

106. Leucht S, Busch R, Kissling W, et al. Early prediction of antipsychotic nonresponse among patients with schizophrenia. *J Clin Psychiatry.* 2007;68(3):352–360.

107. McCue RE, Waheed R, Urcuyo L, et al. Comparative effectiveness of second-generation antipsychotics and haloperidol in acute schizophrenia. *Br J Psychiatry.* 2006;189:433–440.

108. Leucht S, Busch R, Hamann J, et al. Early-onset hypothesis of antipsychotic drug action: A hypothesis tested, confirmed, and extended. *Biol Psychiatry.* 2005;57(12):1543–1549.

109. Smith LA, Cornelius V, Warnock A, et al. Acute bipolar mania: A systematic review and meta-analysis of co-therapy versus monotherapy. *Acta Psychiatr Scand.* 2007;115:12–20.

110. Letmaier M, Schreinzer D, Reinfried L, et al. Typical neuroleptics versus atypical antipsychotics in the treatment of acute mania in a natural setting. *Int J Neuropsychopharmacol.* 2006;9(5):529–537.

111. Rendell JM, Gijsman HJ, Keck P, et al. Olanzapine alone or in combination for acute mania. *Cochrane Database Syst Rev.* 2003;CD004040.

112. Hirschfeld RMA, Baker JD, Wozniak P, et al. The safety and early efficacy of oral-loaded divalproex versus standard-titration divalproex, lithium, olanzapine, and placebo in the treatment of acute mania associated with bipolar disorder. *J Clin Psychiatry.* 2003;64(7):841–846.

113. Licht RW, Gouliaev G, Vestergaard P, et al. Generalisability of results from randomized drug trials: A trial on antimanic treatment. *Br J Psychiatry.* 1997;170:264–267.

114. Goodwin FK, Jamison KR. *Manic-depressive illness: bipolar disorders and recurrent depression,* 2nd ed. New York: Oxford University Press; 2007.

115. Keck PE, Sanchez R, Torbenys A, et al. Aripiprazole monotherapy in the treatment of acute bipolar I mania: A Randomized Placebo and Lithium Controlled Study. *American Psychiatric Association Annual Meeting,* New Research Poster NR 304. San Diego, 2007.

116. Hatim A, Habil H, Jesjeet SG, et al. Safety and efficacy of rapid dose administration of quetiapine in bipolar mania. *Hum Psychopharmacol.* 2006;21(5):313–318.

117. Baldessarini RJ, Tondo L, Hennen J, et al. Is lithium still worth using? An update of selected recent research. *Harv Rev Psychiatry.* 2002;10(2):59–75.

118. Baldessarini RJ, Leahy L, Arcona S, et al. Patterns of psychotropic drug prescription for U.S. patients with diagnoses of bipolar disorders. *Psychiatr Serv.* 2007;58(1):85–91.

119. Posternak MA, Zimmerman M. Is there a delay in the antidepressant effect? A meta-analysis. *J Clin Psychiatry.* 2005;66(2):148–158.

120. Gartlehner G, Hansen RA, Thieda P, et al. *Comparative effectiveness of second-generation antidepressants in the pharmacologic treatment of adult depression: comparative effectiveness review No. 7.* Rockville: Agency for Healthcare Research and Quality; 2007.

121. Janicak PG, Davis JM, Preskorn SH. *Principles and practice of psychopharmacotherapy,* 4th ed. New York: Lippincott Williams & Wilkins; 2006:228.

122. Ballesteros J, Callado LF. Review: Combining pindolol with an SSRI improves early outcomes in people with depression. *J Affect Disord.* 2004;79:137–147.

123. Berman RM, Marcus RN, Swanink R, et al. The efficacy and safety of aripiprazole as adjunctive therapy in major depressive disorder: A multicenter, randomized, double-blind, placebo-controlled study. *J Clin Psychiatry.* 2007;68(6):843–853.

124. Zarate CA Jr, Singh JB, Carlson PJ, et al. A randomized trial of an N-methyl-D-aspartate antagonist in treatment-resistant major depression. *Arch Gen Psychiatry.* 2006;63(8):856–964.

125. Leon AC. The revised warning for antidepressants and suicidality: Unveiling the black box of statistical analyses. *Am J Psychiatry.* 2007;164(12):1786–1788.

126. Preskorn S. *Outpatient management of depression,* 2nd ed. Caldo: Professional Communications, Inc; 1999.

127. Rittmannsberger H, Meise U, Schauflinger K, et al. Polypharmacy in psychiatric treatment. Patterns of psychotropic drug use in Austrian psychiatric clinics. *Eur Psychiatry.* 1999;14(1):33–40.

128. Jaffe AB, Levine J. Antipsychotic medication coprescribing in a large state hospital system. *Pharmacoepidemiol Drug Saf.* 2003;12(1):41–48.

129. Procyshyn RM, Thompson B. Patterns of antipsychotic utilization in a tertiary care psychiatric institution. *Pharmacopsychiatry.* 2004;37(1):12–17.

130. Botts S, Hines H, Littrell R. Antipsychotic polypharmacy in the ambulatory care setting, 1993-2000. *Psychiatr Serv.* 2003;54(8):1086.

131. Ito H, Koyama A, Higuchi T. Polypharmacy and excessive dosing: Psychiatrists' perceptions of antipsychotic drug prescription. *Br J Psychiatry.* 2005;187:243–247.

132. Centorrino F, Goren JL, Hennen J, et al. Multiple versus single antipsychotic agents for hospitalized psychiatric patients: Case-control study of risks versus benefits. *Am J Psychiatry.* 2004;161(4):700–706.

133. Waddington JL, Youssef HA, Kinsella A. Mortality in schizophrenia. Antipsychotic polypharmacy and absence of adjunctive anticholinergics over the course of a 10-year prospective study. *Br J Psychiatry*. 1998;173:325–329.

134. Stahl SM, Grady MM. High-cost use of second-generation antipsychotics under California's Medicaid program. *Psychiatr Serv*. 2006;57(1):127–129.

135. Patrick V, Schleifer SJ, Nurenberg JR, et al. Best practices: An initiative to curtail the use of antipsychotic polypharmacy in a state psychiatric hospital. *Psychiatr Serv*. 2006;57(1):21–23.

136. Viguera AC, Baldessarini RJ, Hegarty JD, et al. Clinical risk following abrupt and gradual withdrawal of maintenance neuroleptic treatment. *Arch Gen Psychiatry*. 1997;54(1):49–55.

137. Stahl SM. Antipsychotic polypharmacy: Evidence based or eminence based?. *Acta Psychiatr Scand*. 2002;106(5):321–322.

138. Tohen M, Chengappa KN, Suppes T, et al. Efficacy of olanzapine in combination with valproate or lithium in the treatment of mania in patients partially nonresponsive to valproate or lithium monotherapy. *Arch Gen Psychiatry*. 2002;59(1):62–69.

139. Sachs GS, Grossman F, Ghaemi SN, et al. Combination of a mood stabilizer with risperidone or haloperidol for treatment of acute mania: A double-blind, placebo-controlled comparison of efficacy and safety. *Am J Psychiatry*. 2002;159(7):1146–1154.

140. Yatham LN, Grossman F, Augustyns I, et al. Mood stabilisers plus risperidone or placebo in the treatment of acute mania. International, double-blind, randomised controlled trial. *Br J Psychiatry*. 2003;182:141–147.

141. Sachs G, Chengappa KN, Suppes T, et al. Quetiapine with lithium or divalproex for the treatment of bipolar mania: A randomized, double-blind, placebo-controlled study. *Bipolar Disord*. 2004;6(3):213–223.

142. Yatham LN, Paulsson B, Mullen J, et al. Quetiapine versus placebo in combination with lithium or divalproex for the treatment of bipolar mania. *J Clin Psychopharmacol*. 2004;24(6):599–606.

143. Leucht S, Busch R, Hamann J, et al. Early-onset hypothesis of antipsychotic drug action: A hypothesis tested, confirmed and extended. *Biol Psychiatry*. 2005;57(12):1543–1549.

144. Miller AL, Chiles JA, Chiles JK, et al. The Texas Medication Algorithm Project (TMAP) schizophrenia algorithms. *J Clin Psychiatry*. 1999;60(10):649–657.

145. Dodd S, Horgan D, Malhi GS, et al. To combine or not to combine? A literature review of antidepressant combination therapy. *J Affect Disord*. 2005;89(1–3):1–11.

146. Simon J, Pilling S, Burbeck R, et al. Treatment options in moderate and severe depression: Decision analysis supporting a clinical guideline. *Br J Psychiatry*. 2006;189:494–501.

147. Keller MB, McCullough JP, Klein DN, et al. A comparison of nefazodone, the cognitive behavioral-analysis system of psychotherapy, and their combination for the treatment of chronic depression. *N Engl J Med*. 2000;342(20):1462–1470.

148. Schramm E, van Calker D, Dykierek P, et al. An intensive treatment program of interpersonal psychotherapy plus pharmacotherapy for depressed inpatients: Acute and long-term results. *Am J Psychiatry*. 2007;164(5):768–777.

149. Levinson DF, Umapathy C, Musthaq M. Treatment of schizoaffective disorder and schizophrenia with mood symptoms. *Am J Psychiatry*. 1999;156(8):1138–1148.

150. Goodnick PJ. Bipolar depression: A review of randomised clinical trials. *Expert Opin Pharmacother*. 2007;8(1):13–21.

151. Keating GM, Robinson DM. Quetiapine: A review of its use in the treatment of bipolar depression. *Drugs*. 2007;67(7):1077–1095.

152. Goldsmith DR, Wagstaff AJ, Ibbotson T, et al. Lamotrigine: A review of its use in bipolar disorder. *Drugs*. 2003;63(19):2029–2050.

153. Leverich G, Altshuler L, Suppes T, et al. Risk of switch in mood polarity to hypomania or mania in patients with bipolar depression during acute and continuation trials of venlafaxine, sertraline, and bupropion as adjuncts to mood stabilizers. *Am J Psychiatry*. 2006;163(2):232–239.

154. Adli M, Bauer M, Rush AJ. Algorithms and collaborative-care systems for depression: Are they effective and why? A systematic review. *Biol Psychiatry*. 2006;59:1029–1038.

155. Kane JM, Honigfeld G, Singer J, et al. Clozapine for the treatment-resistant schizophrenic: A double-blind comparison with chlorpromazine. *Arch Gen Psychiatry*. 1988;45(9):789–796.

156. McEvoy JP, Lieberman JA, Stroup TS, et al. Effectiveness of clozapine versus olanzapine, quetiapine, and risperidone in patients with chronic schizophrenia who did not respond to prior atypical antipsychotic treatment. *Am J Psychiatry*. 2006;163(4):600–610.

157. Kane JM, Meltzer HY, Carson WH, et al. Aripiprazole for treatment-resistant schizophrenia: Results of a multicenter, randomized, double-blind, comparison study versus perphenazine. *J Clin Psychiatry*. 2007;68(2):213–223.

158. Lehmann H. On acute schizophrenia patients. In: Lehmann H, Ban T, eds. *The butyrophenones in psychiatry*. Montreal, Canada: Quebec Psychopharmacological Research Association; 1964.

159. Baldessarini RJ, Leahy L, Arcona S, et al. Patterns of psychotropic drug prescription for U.S. patients with diagnoses of bipolar disorders. *Psychiatr Serv.* 2007;58(1):85–91.

160. Andreescu C, Mulsant MH, Peasley-Miklus C, et al. Persisting low use of antipsychotics in the treatment of major depressive disorder with psychotic features. *J Clin Psychiatry.* 2007;68(2):194–200.

161. Parker G, Manicavasagar V. *Modelling and managing the depressive disorders: a clinical guide.* New York: Cambridge University Press; 2005.

162. McGrath PJ, Stewart JW, Fava M, et al. Tranylcypromine versus venlafaxine plus mirtazapine following three failed antidepressant medication trials for depression: A STAR*D report. *Am J Psychiatry.* 2006;163:1531–1541.

163. Nierenberg AA, Fava M, Trivedi MH, et al. A comparison of lithium and T3 augmentation following two failed medication treatments for depression: A STAR*D report. *Am J Psychiatry.* 2006;163(9):1519–1530.

164. Husain MM, Rush AJ, Fink M, et al. Speed of response and remission in major depressive disorder with acute electroconvulsive therapy (ECT): A Consortium for Research in ECT (CORE) report. *J Clin Psychiatry.* 2004;65(4):485–491.

165. McCall WV. What does STAR*D tell us about ECT? *J ECT.* 2007;23(1):1–2.

166. Ruiz PE. *Review of psychiatry, Ethnicity and psychopharmacology*, Vol. 19. American Psychiatric Publishing, Inc; 2000.

167. de Leon J, Armstrong SC, Cozza KL. Clinical guidelines for psychiatrists for the use of pharmacogenetic testing for CYP450 2D6 and CYP450 2C19. *Psychosomatics.* 2006;47(1):75–85.

168. De Leon J. Amplichip CYP450 test: Personalized medicine has arrived in psychiatry. *Expert Rev Mol Diagn.* 2006;6(3):277–286.

169. Bertilsson L. Geographical/interracial differences in polymorphic drug oxidation. Current state of knowledge of cytochromes P450 (CYP) 2D6 and 2C19. *Clin Pharmacokinet.* 1995; 29(3):192–209.

170. Malhotra AK, Murphy GM Jr, Kennedy JL. Pharmacogenetics of psychotropic drug response. *Am J Psychiatry.* 2004;161(5):780–796.

171. Mundo E, Walker M, Cate T, et al. The role of serotonin transporter protein gene in antidepressant-induced mania in bipolar disorder: Preliminary findings. *Arch Gen Psychiatry.* 2001;58(6):539–544.

172. Murphy GM Jr, Hollander SB, Rodrigues HE, et al. Effects of the serotonin transporter gene promoter polymorphism on mirtazapine and paroxetine efficacy and adverse events in geriatric major depression. *Arch Gen Psychiatry.* 2004;61(11):1163–1169.

173. Lencz T, Robinson DG, Xu K, et al. DRD2 promoter region variation as a predictor of sustained response to antipsychotic medication in first-episode schizophrenia patients. *Am J Psychiatry.* 2006;163(3):529–531.

174. Ozdemir V, Aklillu E, Mee S, et al. Pharmacogenetics for off-patent antipsychotics: Reframing the risk for tardive dyskinesia and access to essential medicines. *Expert Opin Pharmacother.* 2006;7(2):119–133.

175. Alda M. Pharmacogenetics of lithium response in bipolar disorder. *J Psychiatry Neurosci.* 1999;24(2):154–158.

176. Bridge JA, Barbe RP. Reducing hospital readmission in depression and schizophrenia: Current evidence. *Curr Opin Psychiatry.* 2004;17(6):505–511.

177. Klinkenberg WD, Calsyn RJ. Predictors of receipt of aftercare and recidivism among persons with severe mental illness: A review. *Psychiatr Serv.* 1996;47(5):487–496.

178. Boyer CA, McAlpine DD, Pottick KJ, et al. Identifying risk factors and key strategies in linkage to outpatient psychiatric care. *Am J Psychiatry.* 2000;157(10):1592–1598.

179. Kopelowicz A, Zarate R, Gonzalez SV, et al. Disease management in Latinos with schizophrenia: A family-assisted, skills training approach. *Schizophr Bull.* 2003;29(2):211–227.

CHAPTER 4

General Medical Evaluation and Management of the Psychiatric Inpatient

FRED OVSIEW AND DAVID LOVINGER

P sychiatrists' skill in providing general medical care has been in question since the foundation of the profession. In 1894, the prominent American neurologist Silas Weir Mitchell was invited to speak to the American Medico-Psychological Association, the precursor to the American Psychiatric Association. He took note of the geographic isolation of psychiatric practice in the asylums away from the rest of medical practice, and then he said:

> When we ask for your asylum notes of cases, or by some accident have occasion to look over your case books, we are too often surprised at the amazing lack of complete physical study of the insane, at the failure to see obvious lesions, at the want of thorough day by day study of the secretions in the newer cases, of blood-counts, temperatures, reflexes, the eye-ground, color-fields, all the minute examination with which we are so unrestingly busy.[1]

In this chapter, we address general medical evaluation and management of the psychiatric inpatient. The chapter does not aim at comprehensive coverage; a psychiatric patient could have any disease. The goal is to help the psychiatrist gain a deeper scientific and clinical understanding of a set of general medical problems that arise commonly in psychiatric inpatients, so that assessment and intervention occur more thoughtfully, less by rote, and with greater understanding and expertise, whether the psychiatrist seeks consultation or not. The integration of general health care with mental health care raises important policy issues, which are not addressed in this clinically oriented chapter.[2]

Separate chapters in this volume describe problems in the inpatient psychiatric care of patients with known, active, serious general medical or neurologic comorbidity. We do not duplicate that material. Chapter 5 offers recommendations for a neuropsychiatric approach to differential diagnosis of common psychiatric syndromes presenting for inpatient care. In this chapter, we document the common concurrence of general medical illness in psychiatric inpatients, describe the tools useful for identifying concurrent general medical conditions in psychiatric inpatients and the interpretation of common abnormalities in screening laboratory tests, suggest strategies for clinical and laboratory evaluation when common conditions are suspected, and offer management recommendations for some common general medical problems that arise as the consequence of psychiatric illness or its treatment.

Prevalence of General Medical Illness in the Psychiatric Population

Knowledge of the domain we discuss is not incidental to inpatient psychiatric practice but a core component of it in most, perhaps all, psychiatric inpatient settings, because concurrent general medical illness is so common and so important. Psychiatric inpatients suffer from an excess of general medical illness, compared with the general population, and these disorders are associated with increased mortality. Further, the illnesses are often undiagnosed or unknown to the inpatient treaters. A brief review of the data supporting these assertions is in order.

Many investigations have demonstrated that concurrent general medical disorders are present in excess of the population prevalence in patients with serious mental illness.[3–5] In a large sample of Medicaid patients, those with a psychotic disorder were significantly more likely than those without a psychotic disorder to have each of the eight conditions studied: diabetes, hypertension, heart disease, asthma, gastrointestinal disorders, skin infections, malignancies, and acute respiratory disorders. Heart disease showed the largest differential, with an odds ratio (OR) of 4.24 for the comparison of all psychotic patients with the general population and 3.19 when only non–substance abusers were considered.[6] Risk for heart disease may be especially elevated in younger people with serious mental illness.[7] In a different sample of chronically mentally ill outpatients on Medicaid, 75% had at least one chronic health problem and 50% had at least two chronic health problems.[8] Chronic lung disease was the most common condition; nearly a third of the sample had medium to high severity of chronic pulmonary disease. In a study of privately insured patients, disorders in almost every organ system were significantly more common in patients with schizophrenia than in comparison patients, including neurologic disorders (OR up to 9.76), hepatitis C (OR 7.54), hypothyroidism (OR 2.62), diabetes with complications (OR 2.11), and chronic obstructive lung disease and asthma (OR 1.88 and 1.80, respectively).[9]

Patients with schizophrenia have a life expectancy approximately 15 years shorter than the general population, almost a 20% reduction.[10] A longitudinal study of a schizophrenia cohort found an elevated risk of death (all-cause standardized mortality ratio [SMR]) of approximately threefold, comprising a twofold increase in risk of death for natural causes.[11] In a different population, the relative risk of mortality, in comparison with the general population, was 2.59, a significant elevation, even after the marked elevation in risk of death from suicide (relative risk of 9.9) was excluded.[12] In yet another sample, comprising patients from a public psychiatric hospital of whom 43% had a schizophrenia spectrum diagnosis, SMRs for chronic pulmonary disease and heart disease were 5.5 and 3.8, respectively.[13]

Mood disorder similarly is associated with increased mortality from cardiac disease.[14] A long-term follow-up of patients hospitalized for mood disorders showed a significantly elevated SMR of 1.41 for causes of death other than suicide and in particular a significantly elevated SMR of 1.63 for "all vascular diseases."[15] In a study of patients with type 2 diabetes, the presence of depression conferred roughly a twofold increase in mortality risk, which remained significant even after adjustment for potential behavioral mechanisms of increased risk.[16] Similarly, the risk of myocardial infarction was approximately tripled in those who had been hospitalized for depression (and quintupled in those admitted for psychotic depression), and the elevated risk remained significant when conventional risk factors for myocardial infarction were controlled for.[17]

Despite such evidence that depression itself, independent of typical risk factors, may elevate risk of adverse health outcomes, clearly "lifestyle" factors such as smoking, diet, and physical inactivity explain a substantial portion of the excess morbidity and mortality found in patients with major psychiatric disorders.[18] Obesity is a factor of particular importance. Compelling data suggest that obesity is highly prevalent in the seriously mentally ill and that its elevated rate is in part independent of medication-related weight gain.[13,19,20]

The toxicity of psychiatric medicines may explain a portion of the elevated mortality rate. Weight gain due to psychotropic drugs is of substantial health importance and an important determinant of quality of life and probably of compliance with medication.[21] Fontaine et al. offered a crude estimate of the mortality due to clozapine-induced weight gain; they calculated that it roughly offset the demonstrable suicide-prevention benefit of clozapine.[22] This estimate of elevated cardiovascular risk left out of account the additional diabetogenic effect of antipsychotic medicines, which is partly independent of weight gain and due to insulin resistance, and their adverse effects on lipid profile.[23]

The combination of central obesity, hypertension, insulin resistance with glucose intolerance, hypertriglyceridemia, high low-density lipoprotein (LDL) cholesterol, and low high-density lipoprotein (HDL) cholesterol—the metabolic syndrome—is a major cardiovascular risk factor and is now recognized to be a common consequence of psychiatric medicines. By most estimates, the metabolic syndrome is present in more than one third of severely mentally ill patients, a figure substantially greater than the population prevalence.[24–26] Nonalcoholic fatty liver disease has more recently been recognized as an aspect of the metabolic syndrome and a potential complication of psychotropic drugs.[27]

Seriously mentally ill patients suffer as well from social and financial obstacles to obtaining medical care. A longitudinal study of patients with schizophrenia offered poignant vignettes of deaths recorded as "avoidable": patients, carers, and sometimes physicians failed to identify medical illness or to pursue its treatment in an ordinary way.[11]

Case Vignettes

A middle-aged man died of pulmonary edema shortly after leaving an emergency room; he had failed to wait to be seen. Two female nursing home residents died of pneumonia, which had been untreated despite medical evaluation. A homeless woman who had refused general medical and psychiatric care died of diabetic ketoacidosis.

Indeed, some evidence suggests that medical care of inadequate quality is responsible for a substantial portion of the elevated risk of death. Druss et al. found a 19% increase in 1-year mortality after myocardial infarction for patients with mental disorders, but the differential disappeared with statistical control for indicators of quality of care.[28] Such findings emphasize the widely recognized principle that psychiatrists often serve as the gatekeepers (and advocates) for general medical care for their seriously ill patients.

The data in this section justify a high level of attention to concurrent general medical illness in psychiatric inpatients. That such illness is often unknown to the inpatient staff at the time of admission underlines the importance of a thorough clinical approach. Seriously mentally ill patients do not give adequate medical histories,[29] and medical records may be hard to obtain in a timely manner. The patients' mental disorders may have led to inadequate preadmission general medical evaluation, with inadequate history taking and physical and cognitive examination probably the major contributors to missed diagnoses.[30–32]

Of additional and urgent concern is that general medical disorders, recognized or unrecognized, may be contributing to or causing the psychiatric symptoms that lead to admission. A review of studies from various psychiatric settings found that more than one fourth of patients had general medical illnesses producing psychiatric symptoms and that more than half of such illnesses were previously undiagnosed.[33] In a large study in the California public mental health system, Koran et al. found that more than a third of the patients had important general medical disease and of those the system was unaware of more than half (although the patient was aware of the illness in approximately half the missed cases). Approximately 6% of patients were thought to have diseases producing their mental symptoms, and most of these diseases had been recognized by the mental health system.[34] In a more recent study confined to inpatients, Koran et al. reviewed a group of 289 patients in a public-sector inpatient unit.[35] Of these patients, 84 (29%) had "active and important physical disorders." In 3 patients the authors judged that a previously unrecognized disorder was causing or contributing to mental symptoms; in 14 patients, previously recognized disorders were causing or exacerbating the psychiatric symptoms. Therefore for 17/289 (5.9%) patients, a general medical condition was ultimately thought to be directly relevant in the pathogenesis of psychiatric symptoms.

The methods, both of detecting general medical illness and of judging its relationship to psychiatric symptoms, vary substantially among studies, and a secular change in the rate of such causation or of its being missed on initial evaluation is a possibility. Whether the number is relatively small or impressively large, inpatient psychiatrists do not want to miss somatic disease causing psychiatric symptoms in their inpatients.

In a naturalistic study that did not attempt to attribute causation, Lyketsos et al. observed that active concurrent general medical disorders were present in a substantial minority of patients admitted to a tertiary-care psychiatric unit, and they found that their presence was associated with poorer outcomes in regard to psychiatric symptoms and functional status and with increased length of stay.[36] They concluded that attention to concurrent general medical disorders was not only good practice in itself but that it might well improve the psychiatric outcome of an inpatient stay.

General medical illness coincident with psychiatric illness, in part related to behavioral factors and causing substantial impairment and mortality; morbidity and mortality consequent to psychiatric treatment; and general medical illness producing the symptoms leading to psychiatric admission or leading to more difficult and less effective psychiatric hospitalizations: these are conceptually distinct categories, but they call univocally for a high level of general medical skill and attention on the part of the inpatient psychiatrist. Moreover, the data reviewed suggest that trying to exclude patients with active general medical illness from admission to psychiatric inpatient units, by insisting on "medical clearance," substantially mistakes the needs of the seriously psychiatrically ill. A population of patients in need of psychiatric inpatient care will perforce require general medical care, and it seems wiser for inpatient psychiatrists and facilities to prepare for this than to try to ignore and exclude it.

Medical History Taking in Psychiatric Inpatients

Taking a general medical history should be a routine part of the psychiatric diagnostic interview, but textbooks of diagnostic interviewing pay little attention to this feature of the diagnostic process. For example, a chapter on diagnostic interviewing in a major text indicates that the data collected in a psychiatric interview should include "all medical disorders past and present and their treatments and childhood disorders that involve the central nervous system" (p 794)—a formidable task! However, the remainder of the lengthy chapter offers almost no instruction on how to perform this task.[37]

In the authors' opinion, inpatient psychiatrists should not routinely defer taking the general medical history to a consultant. First, the psychiatrist, not the consultant, should be the expert on interviewing psychotic or otherwise severely mentally ill patients. Second, the psychiatrist, not the consultant, should be the expert on what general medical conditions might affect, or even cause, the psychiatric symptoms at hand. Third, the psychiatrist, who often elsewhere in the hospital preaches the virtue of integrating psychological with somatic medicine, should practice this virtue on the psychiatric unit. Fourth, the psychiatrist, if he or she is to manage the patient properly during the hospitalization and after discharge, needs to be closely familiar with the patient's general medical status. For example, drug interactions may need to be considered. Reading a consultant's note is just not the same as taking the history oneself. Fifth, as general medical illness and its treatment may be important psychosocial stressors, the psychiatrist needs to hear directly about their nature, chronology, and impact. Sixth, the psychiatrist can take a step toward a therapeutic alliance with certain recalcitrant patients by marking himself or herself as a physician by asking physicianly questions (and performing a physical examination, as discussed in subsequent text). All this, of course, is not to argue against consultation when appropriate, merely to underscore the importance of a personally taken history as delineated here.

The extent of the general medical history obtained by the psychiatrist naturally depends on the clinical situation. In many instances, a brief survey of the patient's health status with an appropriate review of systems is sufficient. In other instances, details of the patient's severe or chronic illnesses need to be explored. Whenever possible, medical records should be reviewed to supplement, confirm, and correct the admission interview.

A few simple inquiries can accomplish a great deal. "Have you had any problems with your heart (lungs, liver, kidneys, joints, skin, thyroid gland, blood pressure, sugar [diabetes], cancer)?"—together with appropriate follow-up questions—can elicit much of the needed information.

Case Vignette

A psychiatric resident, having taken the psychiatric history from a new patient with depression, was eagerly observing his attending's administration of the Hamilton Depression Rating Scale. As he sat back in his chair doing so, thus relieved of the still-new task of formulating questions for the patient and listening "with the third ear" to the answers, he noticed for the first time that the patient had a thyroidectomy scar on her neck. When the supervisor finished, the resident inquired about the scar and learned that the patient had recently stopped taking her thyroid replacement pills.

Along with this "past medical history," the psychiatric admission interview should include a review of systems. The psychiatrist should be comfortable inquiring about constitutional symptoms (fever, weight loss, malaise, fatigue), endocrine symptoms (heat or cold sensitivity, constipation or diarrhea, alopecia or change in texture of the hair, change in menses), rheumatic disease symptoms (joint swelling or pain, rash, oral ulcers, dry eyes or mouth, past miscarriages), cardiopulmonary symptoms (shortness of breath, chest pain and its characteristics, irregular heartbeat, cough), and so on. Again, the extent of inquiry should be guided by the clinical situation and a grasp of the "pretest" likelihood of disease based on the epidemiologic data reviewed earlier. Atypical features of the psychiatric presentation—such as late age of onset, unexpected cognitive problems, or the absence of a prodrome or family history—should lead to a greater emphasis on potential discovery of systemic illness explanatory of the psychiatric symptoms.

Taking the history of past cerebral disease is discussed in Chapter 5.

THE PSYCHIATRIC PHYSICAL EXAMINATION

"Good psychiatry begins with a responsible Doctor undressing the patient and carrying out a proper physical examination."
   — Pediatrician and psychoanalyst (but not psychiatrist) Donald Winnicott (quoted by Issroff[38])

Whether psychiatrists should perform physical examinations—and, if they should, whether they actually do—has been repeatedly addressed in the psychiatric literature over the past several decades.[39] Some clinicians have argued that the physical contact between psychiatrist and patient is unwise and that in any event psychiatrists lack the necessary skills to perform an adequate examination. The latter point is quite possibly correct, although the evidence as to the skills of internists is not reassuring either.[40] However, skills in physical diagnosis will not be improved by their neglect; rather, such skills should be taught to trainees and practiced, as other diagnostic skills are practiced, through one's career.[41]

That physical examination by psychiatrists has adverse emotional consequences has often been taken for granted, although powerful voices have been raised to the contrary, as the epigraph to this section illustrates. At the height of psychoanalytic dominance in American psychiatry, the psychiatrist and psychoanalyst Karl Menninger wrote:

The physical examination of the psychiatric patient is not only a diagnostic procedure, but may constitute one of the most important steps in the therapy. Sometimes it is indeed the very keystone of the therapeutic relationship. It serves to identify the physician in his professional capacity, and to establish, by means of a now familiar and conventional procedure, a confidence in the examiner as a doctor. ... The "laying on of hands" has a deep and powerful significance to the patient. ... Personally I doubt if it causes as many difficulties as does its omission or its delegation to others. It may be that we psychoanalysts rationalize the fact that some of us do not like to do physical examinations, or do not feel competent to do them properly, and discard or delegate a valuable medical prerogative.[42] (pp. 48–49.)

Of course, this is not to deny potential complications of the psychiatrist's performing a physical examination (as Menninger sensitively described in parts of the passage not quoted). Proper facilities must be available, not always the case on a psychiatric inpatient unit. In most instances, in part because of the potential ambiguity of "laying on of hands," especially for an acutely disturbed psychiatric patient, the physician should be accompanied by a "chaperone," for example a unit nurse or, on a teaching unit, one or more trainees. The chaperone should as a rule be of the opposite gender to the psychiatrist. In certain instances (perhaps the hospital care of a patient in intensive psychotherapy with the psychiatrist), physical examination may be unwise. At times, the physical examination allows the patient and doctor to discuss matters that were ignored, missed, or minimized during the preceding interview, for example, the patient's feelings about a disfiguring injury or the origins of scars from self-cutting. By performing an examination, the physician can bring these facts into the conversation. At other times, a patient's misinterpretation of the procedure is clear during the examination and should be addressed explicitly by the examiner.

What has perhaps been lacking is the construction of a physical diagnostic approach to psychiatric patients that emphasizes the domains of concern and the likely findings. What is required is a psychiatric physical examination, just as other specialists have taken the physical diagnosis toolbox and chosen instruments from it as being of special use in the patient populations of interest to them. Fortunately, not only are there excellent texts of physical diagnosis,[43,44] which pay attention to the sensitivity and specificity of traditional maneuvers, but also some psychiatric authors have begun the process of constructing a psychiatric physical examination.[45–48] A fuller discussion of the psychiatric physical examination is offered elsewhere.[49–51] Here we briefly highlight findings that the inpatient psychiatrist should be closely familiar with. Somewhat artificially, for the purposes of exposition the neurologic examination is discussed in a different chapter, along with other aspects of the neuropsychiatric evaluation.

General Appearance

Height and weight should always be measured on hospital admission, and the body mass index can be calculated from these figures (e.g., using an online calculator such as the one found at http://nhlbisupport.com/bmi/bminojs.htm). Short stature or unusual height, both assessed in relation to the patient's biological family, raise questions of developmental disorders (fetal alcohol syndrome, mitochondrial disorders, Down syndrome, homocysteinuria, Marfan syndrome, etc.). Weight loss should not be attributed to behavioral factors (such as depression) without further consideration of systemic illness, such as a neoplasm. Weight gain may be due to psychiatric medicines but also to an endocrinopathy. Along with weight and height, admission assessment should include measurement of waist circumference. Waist circumference is an element of the metabolic syndrome and marks the contribution to cardiovascular risk of a central distribution of fat accumulation.[52]

Vital Signs

Abnormalities of pulse, blood pressure, respiratory rate, and temperature should never be discounted as consequences of the patient's psychiatric state. To be sure, at times an anxious or depressed patient has mild tachycardia. Catatonic patients, even while immobile, may show tachycardia as a manifestation of overarousal. Nevertheless, abnormal vital signs always require attention.

   Elevated heart rate may represent sinus tachycardia or a ventricular or supraventricular arrhythmia. (Tradition to the contrary notwithstanding, normal heart rate is 50 to 90.[53]) An electrocardiogram should be obtained to differentiate among these possibilities. Sinus tachycardia may derive from various pathophysiologies (see Table 4.1). Of these, volume depletion and pulmonary embolus (both possible consequences of immobility in psychiatrically ill patients) deserve mention as common, dangerous, and potentially lacking other immediate red flags. In any patient on an antipsychotic (or other dopamine-blocking drug), tachycardia not susceptible to an alternative immediate explanation should raise consideration of neuroleptic malignant syndrome. Although tachycardia alone does not meet the syndromal criteria, not infrequently in the earliest (and most easily reversible) stages only a partial syndrome is present. Similarly, tachycardia can be a feature of the serotonin syndrome.

TABLE 4.1 SOME CAUSES OF SINUS TACHYCARDIA

Pain
Infection
Noninfectious systemic inflammation
Hypovolemia
Hypoxia
Pulmonary embolism
Acute coronary ischemia
Heart failure
Dysautonomia (e.g., neuroleptic malignant syndrome, fatal familial insomnia)
Stimulants and other drugs
Anemia
Pheochromocytoma
Hyperthyroidism

Case Vignette

A late adolescent with schizophrenia was hospitalized for osteosarcoma. On the oncology service, he was treated with haloperidol and risperidone concurrently. On transfer to a psychiatry floor, he was consistently tachycardic but had no other abnormal physical findings (except the absence of a leg). Nonetheless, creatine kinase (CK) was measured and was elevated. Laboratory data did not reveal evidence of infection. In the absence of other explanations for either tachycardia or elevated CK, the antipsychotic drugs were stopped, and the tachycardia immediately ceased; CK elevation resolved over the next few days.

Tachypnea may derive from chronic pulmonary disease, very common in the chronically mentally ill,[8] or a more acute process, such as pulmonary embolus. Some clinicians have argued for measurement of oxygen saturation by pulse oximetry as a routine vital sign. Yawning occurs with sedation but also in opiate withdrawal and as a consequence of serotonergic and dopaminergic drugs.[54] Sighing, on the other hand, appears to be nonorganic. Irregular respiration, which may be attributed to anxiety, occurs more frequently than realized as a manifestation of tardive dyskinesia.

Blood pressure should be measured with the patient supine or sitting (with the arm at the level of the heart) using a cuff with a bladder that covers at least 80% of the arm's circumference. The patient should be at rest for at least 5 minutes before the measurement is made; many expert physical examiners measure the blood pressure late or last in the examination. Measuring orthostatic pulse and blood pressure on admission may detect dehydration and provides a baseline should the patient have an adverse reaction to medication. To obtain orthostatic vital signs the clinician should perform first supine and then standing measurements with the latter taken 1 minute after the patient assumes the upright posture.

Elevated body temperature requires immediate attention. Infectious or inflammatory disease, adverse drug reactions, neoplasms, and other conditions can produce fever, which is defined as a temperature higher than the 99th percentile of the normal range. Because body temperature varies during the course of the day by approximately $0.5°C$ ($0.9°F$), different values apply in the morning and the evening, with the upper limit of normal in the evening being $37.7°C$ ($99.9°F$); tympanic membrane temperature is commonly lower than oral temperature by $0.4°C$ ($0.7°F$). Despite these complications, ordinarily a temperature simply $>38°C$ ($100.4°F$) is taken as a fever requiring evaluation. Any patient on antipsychotic agents should be considered suspect for neuroleptic malignant syndrome unless an immediately compelling alternative explanation for fever is identified, and serotonin syndrome must be considered in appropriate circumstances.

Head, Eyes, Ears, Nose, and Throat

Minor physical anomalies relevant to neurodevelopmental disorders, including psychosis, cluster in this region. A V-shaped palate, "cuspidal ear" (with a sharp angulation of the external ear), and reduced head circumference can be identified at the bedside.[55,56] Cleft lip and palate are associated with frontal lobe disorder both anatomically and neuropsychologically.[57] Dentition should be noted as a potential domain of ill health in the chronically mentally ill.[58,59] Uveitis, oral ulcers, and sicca symptoms (dry eyes, dry mouth) are associated with autoimmune disease.[60] Details of assessing visual and auditory acuity are discussed in Chapter 5.

Neck

Neck stiffness should be sought in a delirious patient. Thyroid enlargement or signs of previous thyroid surgery (as in the case mentioned in an earlier vignette) should be assessed.

Heart and Vessels

Observation of the jugular venous pressure is crucial in assessment of volume overload and congestive heart failure, although estimation of right-sided pressures is difficult for those without much practice. Pedal edema may signify volume overload, hypoalbuminemia, or an adverse drug reaction. Distal pulses should be palpated.

The stethoscope, sometimes forgotten, and its use have long been the hallmark of the physician.[39] Auscultation of the carotids for bruits is simple and apparently relevant to cerebrovascular disease but an unfortunately poor index of low flow. Auscultation of the heart can reveal the S_3 of heart failure, the S_4 of left ventricular stiffness, the pericardial knock or rub of pericardial disease, and the well-known array of murmurs. The latter are relevant to stroke, infectious endocarditis, and numerous other conditions. One of the authors well recalls, as a resident, finding the murmur of a ventricular septal defect in a young schizophrenic man; in distant retrospect, the diagnosis of psychosis related to the velocardiofacial syndrome (22q11.12 deletion), then unknown, can only be conjectured.

Lungs

As discussed earlier, chronic pulmonary disease is highly prevalent in the chronically mentally ill. Auscultation for breath sounds may help identify patients with emphysema (wheezing, prolonged expiratory phase) as well as those with other acute and chronic lung disorders.

Abdomen

Signs of liver disease, such as ascites and liver enlargement or tenderness, should be sought especially in patients with alcohol abuse.

Central Nervous System

The neurological examination is discussed in detail in Chapter 5.

Laboratory Evaluation of Psychiatric Inpatients

Laboratory tests are widely used for screening purposes upon psychiatric admission. "Screening" in this context refers to obtaining laboratory data when specific indications for the test do not emerge from the history or physical examination. Therefore, obtaining a chest x-ray on every patient admitted to a psychiatric unit would be "screening;" obtaining a chest x-ray on a patient who has a cough and fever would not. Screening may aid in the detection of unrecognized disease, especially when history taking and physical examination are hampered by the patient's psychiatric illness; may make both patient and physician more confident of the absence of disease; and may provide baseline data should developments require further assessment of laboratory parameters (e.g., if treatments may alter laboratory findings). Often studies of the utility of screening tests take into account only the first of these purposes.

No consensus exists on an appropriate panel of screening laboratory tests for psychiatric inpatients.[61,62] However, the available data suggest that an extensive battery of tests is not cost effective and moreover may be clinically misleading. The false-positive rate of even a relatively specific laboratory test is high if the pretest probability of a positive result (i.e., the prevalence of the true-positive result in the population) is very low. Therefore, scattershot testing is likely to produce false-positive results that lead to further testing and to a satisfying feeling of being careful and thorough on the doctor's part, a feeling that does not correspond to any benefit for the patient. A competent history and physical examination, by allowing an estimate of the pretest probability of disease, make the laboratory tests more informative. Furthermore, as already discussed, evidence suggests that history taking and examination are the best techniques for uncovering general medical illness in psychiatric inpatients.[30,31]

A further limitation on the practice of ordering extensive batteries of tests is imposed by the common readmission of chronically mentally ill patients. Whatever the value of a screening laboratory panel, surely its value is far less when the patient is readmitted the following month. Review of available data should take the place of rote test ordering.

Therefore, the authors recommend that only a limited panel of tests be undertaken beyond those arising from findings in the history and examination. In certain populations, notably the elderly, substance abusers, and those with severe psychiatric or social obstacles to obtaining good medical care, a more extensive laboratory screening approach may be appropriate. The authors tentatively recommend a screening battery including a complete blood count, a chemistry panel (including fasting glucose, electrolytes, renal function tests, CK, liver enzymes, and albumin), thyrotropin and free thyroxine (see subsequent text), cobalamin (vitamin B_{12}, see subsequent text), a serum pregnancy test in women of reproductive potential, and urine toxicology. A screening role for the sedimentation rate, chest x-ray, and electrocardiogram is not supported by available data, although certainly these and other tests may be indicated by the history and physical examination. Routine urinalysis is often suggested in the literature, but evidence for its utility as a screening test is lacking. Certain other screening tests are indicated under specific circumstances, as discussed in more detail in subsequent text. These include tests for syphilis, measurement of lipids (for which there are consensus guidelines), and assays for human immunodeficiency virus (HIV), hepatitis C, and tuberculosis (TB) infection in patients with risk factors.

A more detailed discussion of the interpretation and use of findings in commonly ordered laboratory tests follows.

THYROID DISEASE

The thyroid gland secretes thyroid hormone in the form of thyroxine (T_4) and some triiodothyronine (T_3). Much of circulating T_4 is protein bound, and the unbound (free) portion can be measured as the free thyroxine index (FTI) or directly (fT_4). T_4 is converted in peripheral tissues to the metabolically active form of the hormone, T_3, and a biologically inactive form, reverse T_3 (rT_3). T_4 and to a lesser extent T_3, by feedback at the level of the pituitary, influence the level of the pituitary hormone thyrotropin (thyroid-stimulating hormone [TSH]), which regulates secretion of T_4. Thyroid disease is often due to an autoimmune process, associated with antibodies to thyroid peroxidase (antiTPO) and thyroglobulin (antiTg). Overt primary hypothyroidism is marked by elevated serum TSH with decreased fT_4 and T_3; hyperthyroidism due to thyroid disease is indicated by suppression of serum TSH, usually to undetectable levels, with elevated T_4 or, at times, an increase of T_3 only (T_3 thyrotoxicosis). Central thyroid disease, although uncommon, produces a different pattern of abnormalities in thyroidal laboratory tests (discussed briefly in subsequent text).

A common pattern of thyroid test results in newly admitted psychiatric patients is normal TSH with mild elevation of T_4 in a patient without evidence of thyroid disease by history or examination.[63,64] This state, known as *euthyroid hyperthyroxinemia*, represents a stress response in the hypothalamic-pituitary-thyroid axis and requires no treatment. Measurement of thyroid tests in a few weeks' time is likely to demonstrate resolution of the anomalous pattern.

Patients with acute systemic illness, including alcoholism, often show a pattern of thyroid tests called the *nonthyroidal illness* (or *euthyroid sick*) syndrome.[63] In mild cases, T_3 is low, and rT_3 is raised. With more severe illness, T_4 is also low, but TSH usually remains normal. Whether this state represents genuine hypothyroidism has been controversial,[65] but few, if any, experts would recommend its "correction" in patients on psychiatric units.

Anomalous patterns of thyroid tests can result from the effect of psychotropic drugs. Lithium produces hypothyroidism by interfering with production of thyroid hormone at several steps, notably release from the thyroid gland. This consequence of lithium therapy is strongly associated with the presence of antithyroid antibodies.[66] Carbamazepine and oxcarbazepine produce reductions in T_4 and FTI without corresponding increases in TSH and with no clinical evidence of hypothyroidism.[67] Furthermore, assays of fT_4 by direct methods give normal results.[68] Valproate, lamotrigine, and topiramate do not produce this effect. Opiates increase the concentration of thyroid-binding globulin and therefore the total T_4 but do not change thyroid function as measured by fT_4 and TSH. Reports conflict as to production of subtle hyperthyroidism by stimulants such as amphetamine and cocaine (and subtle hypothyroidism by their withdrawal).[69,70]

In hypothyroidism, TSH rises above normal even before free T_4 and T_3 fall below normal, a state called *subclinical hypothyroidism*. The name derives from the absence of systemic symptoms responsive to thyroid hormone. Therefore, patients with normal T_4 and mildly elevated TSH who complain of feeling tired all the time or being unable to lose weight generally do not respond to treatment with levothyroxine (L-T$_4$).[71,72] Under these circumstances, antithyroid antibodies should be assayed, because their presence predicts progression to overt hypothyroidism. Usual endocrinologic practice would be to reassess patients with mild elevations of TSH (<10) and normal T$_4$ at intervals. Larger TSH increases, markedly high autoantibody titers, or the presence of a goiter would mandate earlier treatment.

However, the proper threshold for treatment with L-T$_4$ in "subclinical" hypothyroidism may differ in patients with depression. Even if fT$_4$ is normal, an elevation of TSH may increase risk for depression or for failure to respond to pharmacotherapy for depression.[73–75] In contrast to somatic symptoms, mood and cognitive symptoms in patients with mild TSH elevations may respond to L-T$_4$.[71] The authors' practice is to give L-T$_4$ to depressed patients with normal T$_4$ but elevated TSH.

In the patient without evidence of thyroid disease by history or examination, guidelines for screening for increased or decreased thyroid function recommend measurement of TSH alone.[76] However, this approach risks missing hypothyroidism due to pituitary disease (central or secondary hypothyroidism), in which the TSH may be in the lower portion of the normal range but the fT$_4$ low. Secondary hypothyroidism may be more common than once thought, and its symptoms may be subtle.[77,78] Because obtaining a detailed and reliable history may be impossible in a severely ill psychiatric inpatient, measuring fT$_4$ as well as TSH for screening purposes may be reasonable, especially given the evidence that pretreatment fT$_4$ may correlate with response to treatment.[74,75]

An occasional indication for assaying antithyroid antibodies is suspicion of the encephalopathy associated with autoimmune thyroid disease (Hashimoto encephalopathy).[79] These patients typically present with subacutely evolving cognitive impairment, myoclonus, and seizures, so that Creutzfeld-Jakob disease may be in the clinician's differential diagnosis. Psychotic symptoms are not infrequent. Patients may have a history of thyroid disease but are characteristically euthyroid at the time of presentation. However, antithyroid antibodies are present, although probably not directly involved in the pathogenesis of the syndrome.

ADRENAL DISEASE

Patients with adrenal insufficiency generally have nonspecific complaints of lassitude and fatigue, myalgias, gastrointestinal symptoms, weight loss, sexual dysfunction, postural hypotension, hyperpigmentation, hyponatremia (in the large majority of cases), and hyperkalemia (somewhat less frequently). These patients commonly have mood symptoms and apathy, and occasionally they have psychosis or delirium.[80] The risk of mood disorder and the other psychiatric symptoms may not be due entirely to cortisol deficiency itself.[81,82] The commonest cause of adrenal insufficiency is autoimmune adrenalitis (which can be identified by assaying antibodies against 21-hydroxylase) and therefore tends to coexist with other autoimmune diseases, especially autoimmune thyroid disease but also gonadal failure and type 1 diabetes mellitus.

Patients with cortisol excess have hypertension, glucose intolerance, abdominal striae, hirsutism, acne, facial plethora, and truncal obesity with characteristic fat deposition in cervical, supraclavicular, and temporal areas. The combination of hypertension, diabetes, and obesity is so common that searching for Cushing syndrome as its cause should be reserved for patients with some of the more specific features of the syndrome. Many patients with cortisol excess are depressed.[83] Several idiopathic psychiatric states, notably depression, are associated with elevated levels of cortisol. This adds to the challenge of identifying a primary endocrinopathy as the cause of associated psychopathology. However, although cortisol excess may be demonstrated biochemically in depressed patients, these patients rarely have the physical signs of Cushing syndrome.

The cortex of the adrenal gland secretes cortisol; secretion is regulated by adrenocorticotrophic hormone (ACTH), released by the pituitary. As with thyroid hormone, cortisol exists in the blood in both a bound and an unbound form, but current techniques are inadequately reliable to measure serum free cortisol. Testing for deficiency or excess of cortisol is more complicated than testing thyroid function because of the pulsatile nature of secretion and its circadian variation. An early morning cortisol level >18 μg per dL excludes adrenal insufficiency.[81] A low morning serum cortisol (<5 μg per dL) level has very high specificity for adrenal insufficiency but is only approximately 36% sensitive. For adequate assessment, measuring baseline ACTH and serum cortisol both before and after adrenal stimulation with synthetic ACTH is generally required. Healthy subjects should be able to attain a peak stimulated cortisol >21 μg per dL. Even normal results do not completely exclude adrenal insufficiency, because the identification of secondary adrenal insufficiency (due to pituitary or hypothalamic disease) requires further complex stimulation tests.[81]

Testing for cortisol excess usually begins with measuring 24-hour urinary free cortisol. A markedly elevated result (greater than three times the upper limit of normal) implies Cushing syndrome. Equivocal levels (one to three times the upper limit of normal) may be seen in patients with depression and alcoholism as well as other states that mimic Cushing syndrome. An alternative approach is to measure late evening (11 PM or midnight) serum or salivary cortisol. In Cushing syndrome, but not in depression, the diurnal variation of cortisol secretion is blunted, so an appropriately low late-evening cortisol level (<5 μg per dL) makes Cushing syndrome unlikely, and an elevated midnight serum cortisol level (>7.5 μg per dL) sensitively identifies Cushing syndrome.[84] This approach, in contrast to attempting to collect a 24-hour urine sample in an acutely ill psychiatric patient, may be a suitable in-hospital diagnostic method.

B$_{12}$ AND FOLATE DEFICIENCY

Deficiency of vitamin B$_{12}$ (cobalamin) characteristically produces a megaloblastic anemia, with reduced hemoglobin and hematocrit and elevated mean corpuscular volume. However, the central nervous system manifestations of cobalamin deficiency—the syndrome of subacute combined degeneration, with peripheral neuropathy, myelopathy, cognitive impairment, and psychiatric symptoms—frequently occur without anemia, and psychiatric or cognitive symptoms can occur without physical signs.[85] Moreover, tissue deficiency of cobalamin may be present when serum cobalamin measurements are in the low-normal range. Some 5% to 10% of patients with serum cobalamin between 200 and 300 prove to have tissue cobalamin deficiency.[86,87] Because untreated cobalamin deficiency can produce permanent nervous system damage, whereas in the early stages the process is correctable, clinicians should have a low threshold for searching for cobalamin deficiency.

Therefore, a low *or low-normal* (below 300) serum B$_{12}$ result should prompt further investigation. In particular, serum homocysteine and methylmalonic acid (MMA) better indicate tissue cobalamin deficiency because cobalamin is a cofactor for the enzymatic steps that metabolize homocysteine and MMA, which thereby build up in the absence of cobalamin. Elevated MMA is the more specific indicator of cobalamin deficiency, as homocysteine elevations can result from folate deficiency as well. However, the MMA level may be equivocal, and longitudinal follow-up may be required.[88] Furthermore, MMA reduction may be insufficiently sensitive to identify all potentially cobalamin-responsive states. One confounding factor is renal insufficiency; MMA increases with reduction in renal function, so elevated MMA is less specific for cobalamin deficiency in this setting.[89]

If both MMA and homocysteine are normal, deficiency of cobalamin is excluded with a high degree of confidence.[90] If MMA is elevated, the patient may have pernicious anemia (PA), which results from destruction of the gastric parietal cells that secrete intrinsic factor (IF) necessary for the efficient transport of ingested cobalamin. Therefore at this point in the workup, antibodies to IF and parietal cells should be assayed, although these tests sometimes give false-negative results, especially in white patients.[91] If antibodies are not present, other causes of low cobalamin must be considered. Beyond confirming or refuting the diagnosis of PA in the cobalamin-deficient patient, the clinician should consider exploring whether nervous system damage has occurred by assaying the integrity of white-matter pathways using magnetic resonance (MR) imaging, evoked potentials, and nerve conduction studies.

The neuropsychiatric syndrome due to folate deficiency is similar to that of cobalamin deficiency, although peripheral neuropathy is less common and mood disorder more common.[85] As with cobalamin deficiency, anemia and macrocytosis may not be present in the patient presenting neurologically or psychiatrically. Measuring serum folate is an adequate screen for folate deficiency unless the patient has already begun to eat a hospital diet; in such cases red blood cell folate is the more accurate measure. In the equivocal case, serum homocysteine should be assayed. The evidence of prominent psychiatric symptoms in folate deficiency is matched by preliminary evidence for improved response to psychopharmacologic treatment in patients concurrently supplemented with folic acid.[92]

BONE HEALTH

Seriously mentally ill patients appear to be at elevated risk of low bone mineral density (BMD) and consequent fracture.[93,94] The risk may arise from disease-related factors, such as elevated cortisol in mood disorder; or from medication-related factors, such as hyperprolactinemia due to antipsychotic drugs, reduced osteoblast activity due to serotonin reuptake inhibitors, or reduced serum vitamin D and increased bone turnover due to certain antiepileptic drugs.[95–99] No consensus recommendations for screening for reduced BMD (osteopenia or osteoporosis) and management of bone health in psychiatric patients have been proposed. In epileptic patients, expert guidelines suggest screening with measurements of calcium, phosphorus, alkaline phosphatase, and a scan of BMD and giving supplemental daily calcium and vitamin D.[97] Although psychiatric patients do not share with epileptic patients the risk factor of trauma during convulsions, the elevated risk of fracture in epileptic patients is not entirely attributable to this factor; seriously mentally ill and epileptic patients may share the risks of reduced exposure to sunlight, reduced physical activity, and exposure to bone-toxic medication. Although further research is needed to specify appropriate practices, the inpatient psychiatrist should consider BMD scanning and prophylaxis with calcium and vitamin D for patients treated with antipsychotic agents that increase prolactin, with antiepileptic drugs including divalproex, or with serotonin reuptake inhibitors.

SYPHILIS

Neurosyphilis is a classic cause of psychiatric disturbance; 100 years ago, as many as 20% of patients in psychiatric hospitals were there because of the ravages of general paresis of the insane.[100] Even now, syphilis is a cause that must not be missed of cognitive decline and psychiatric symptoms. Neurosyphilis still commonly presents with the classic physical signs: pupillary abnormalities, present in approximately half the cases, or absent tendon jerks. Evaluation of the patient with a relevant history or signs should include laboratory testing for neurosyphilis. However, consensus guidelines for laboratory screening (i.e., in those without such a history or findings) in newly presenting dementia recommend syphilis tests only for those patients who have lived in areas of high prevalence of the disease, roughly a broad band across the southern United States and the major metropolitan areas elsewhere in this country.[101]

An important determinant of the testing strategy for syphilis is that the reagin test (rapid plasma reagin [RPR], Venereal Disease Research Laboratory [VDRL]) often reverts to normal either spontaneously or because of intercurrent antibiotic treatment insufficient to treat neurosyphilis. Therefore, reagin tests have a sensitivity of only approximately 70% for neurosyphilis, inadequate for screening purposes.[102] When the purpose of testing is to rule out neurosyphilis (as against, e.g., making a diagnosis of a rash that may betray primary or secondary syphilis), a specific treponemal test (such as the Fluorescent Treponemal Antibody Absorption Assay [FTA-ABS]), which turns positive early in the disease and remains positive forever, must be obtained. If it is positive, a quantitative RPR should be obtained. Also, if test results for syphilis are positive, strong consideration must be given to testing for other diseases potentially transmitted by the same route, notably HIV. Considerations regarding cerebrospinal fluid (CSF) examination in patients with positive serologic test results for syphilis are discussed in Chapter 5 on neuropsychiatric issues.

SLEEP APNEA

The importance of identifying sleep apnea relates not only to its long-term adverse effects on cardiopulmonary health but also to its consequences for mood and cognition.[103] It should be considered one of the reversible contributors to dementia[104] and to depression as well.[105] Just as bed partners often provide the clinician with the grounds for suspecting the disorder, so night nurses can observe snoring and breathing disturbances in sleeping hospitalized patients; some instruction for inpatient staff on the disorders and technique of observation may be necessary. An interesting observation by a trainee appears to hold up as a diagnostic pointer: a patient with sleep apnea may snore while asleep, but that patient does not snore when catatonic despite immobility and unresponsiveness superficially similar to the sleeping state. When sleep apnea is suspected, polysomnography should be performed to confirm the diagnosis and determine the treatment regimen. The capacity to provide continuous positive airway pressure treatment during sleep should be available on psychiatric units.

MUSCLE ENZYMES

Elevated CK can occur in psychiatric patients for multiple reasons: overactivity, intramuscular injections, seizures, crush injury (e.g., due to unconsciousness after a suicide attempt), cocaine or alcohol abuse, the effects of psychiatric medicines, and acute psychosis itself. Although elevation of CK is well known as a feature of neuroleptic malignant syndrome, it occurs at times as a consequence of the use of atypical antipsychotics even in the absence of neuroleptic malignant syndrome or indeed of any clinical correlate.[106] Further, its utility as a marker of neuroleptic malignant syndrome is sometimes overestimated, because CK may be elevated in febrile patients on psychotropic agents even when infection is the cause of the fever.[107] In the authors' view, given these complexities, routine measurement of CK on hospital admission is useful as a baseline datum. Markedly elevated CK indicates a risk of myoglobinuric renal injury and requires intravenous (IV) fluid therapy.

INFECTIOUS DISEASES

Infection with HIV and the consequent acquired immunodeficiency syndrome (AIDS) are not uncommon among the mentally ill, with a prevalence many times the population prevalence.[108] Risk factors for infection include injection-drug abuse and high-risk sexual activity, including unprotected sex. Some psychiatric patients may engage in high-risk sexual activity because of impulsivity due to psychosis or mania, others because of vulnerability to sexual exploitation. The threshold for screening psychiatric patients on admission to the hospital should be low. Initial testing is usually with an enzyme immunoassay method; positive results are checked using a Western blot method before being reported as positive. The sensitivity of the test is extremely high, well over 99%, for infection of more than 3 months' duration. Patients testing positive should have HIV viral load and CD4 lymphocyte counts determined. All such patients should be seen by specialists in AIDS; infectious disease specialists and internists with a special expertise in AIDS deliver better care than nonspecialized primary care physicians.[109]

The presence of HIV infection creates several complications for inpatient psychiatric management. First, HIV infection can produce psychiatric symptoms. Second, interactions between psychiatric drugs and antiretroviral agents must be taken into account. In lieu of detailed consideration of this issue, and given the rapid changes in recommended HIV regimens, the authors urge clinicians to consult databases of drug interactions whenever treatment of a patient on antiretrovirals is contemplated. Two further pharmacologic concerns are that antiretrovirals may cause psychiatric symptoms and psychiatric medicines may affect HIV replication. Thoughtful collaboration is important in the management of these complex patients. Third, discharge planning must specifically address the importance of compliance not only with psychiatric treatment but also with antiretroviral therapy. In some venues, the AIDS crisis has led to the provision of public services for management of HIV-infected patients, which may serve well the chronically mentally ill.

Hepatitis C virus (HCV) infection—the most common blood-borne infection—can cause hepatic cirrhosis and hepatocellular carcinoma. Its prevalence is elevated in psychiatric inpatient populations, even apart from the substantial elevation related to substance abuse. Rates of infection in psychiatric populations up to 11 times the population prevalence have been reported, often without abnormal liver enzymes.[110] Consensus guidelines recommend screening in high-risk populations,[111] and psychiatric inpatients, on present evidence, especially those who abuse substances, should therefore be considered candidates for screening. One reason to ascertain HCV status is that the combination of hepatitis C and alcohol abuse increases the risk of liver damage.

Appropriate clinical suspicion of TB is required for initiating a diagnostic evaluation, and infectious disease consultation should be sought for patients who are suspects. Symptoms typically begin insidiously and nonspecifically and include fatigue, cough, weight loss, and fever. Active disease usually, though not always, represents a reactivation of a previous infection. Patients at elevated risk for TB include those with HIV or who are otherwise immunosuppressed (>15 mg prednisone per day, organ transplant recipients, etc.), those with recent close contact with a patient with active TB, nursing-home residents, drug users, patients of low socioeconomic status, diabetic patients, and patients immigrated from countries with a high prevalence of TB (the developing world). Patients in whom active TB is suspected require isolation until active disease can be ruled out. Since very few if any psychiatric units have negative-pressure rooms, these standards entail that if TB is so much as under consideration patients must be admitted to or transferred to a general medical unit with a negative-pressure room. Because TB should be suspected in any patient at high risk (as specified earlier) with a cough or fever, and because exposure puts other patients and staff at risk, patients in whom the consideration might arise should be evaluated, at least with chest x-ray, before admission to a psychiatric unit. Tuberculin skin testing, with the purified protein derivative (PPD), should be performed, though a positive test indicates only a history of infection and cannot by itself be used to diagnose active TB. To do that, a chest x-ray must be performed and three daily-sputum samples collected and examined for acid-fast bacilli. A negative chest x-ray does not exclude TB in patients with AIDS.

Management of Common General Medical Problems on the Inpatient Psychiatric Unit

IMMOBILITY

Decreased physical activity is a common finding among hospitalized patients, regardless of the reason for hospitalization. Among psychiatric patients, reduced activity features in states of severe depression and catatonia. Such patients may also have reduced oral intake, an issue discussed in subsequent text. Immobility has many sequelae, including venous thromboembolism (VTE) and pressure ulcers, both of which are serious and potentially life-threatening conditions. Deconditioning, another consequence of immobility, holds particular significance for the elderly. Fortunately, a number of interventions are available to physicians and other caregivers in the hospital setting.

Prophylaxis against VTE has been studied in a variety of settings, although primarily in medical and surgical patients.[112] Prolonged immobility is a recognized risk factor, and when other risk factors (age, obesity, and other comorbidities) are also present pharmacologic or mechanical prophylaxis is warranted. Psychiatrists must give consideration to the degree of immobility because depressed patients with moderate psychomotor slowing present a different risk for VTE from catatonic patients for whom death from VTE is a well-documented complication.[113] One reasonable approach is to use Pendleton schema of major and minor risk factors for VTE (see Table 4.2) and to consider immobility a minor risk factor.[114] The presence of any other risk factor, major or minor, would warrant the institution of VTE prophylaxis.

An additional consideration is that antipsychotic drugs appear to produce an elevated risk for VTE.[115,116] Although the data are not fully consistent and controlled-trial data regarding interventions are lacking, it appears reasonable to take into account this risk factor, like that of oral contraceptives or estrogen, in deciding whether to prescribe pharmacologic VTE prophylaxis. In cases where the threshold for using heparin is judged not to be reached, adequate hydration should still be ensured and patients mobilized as best possible as steps to reduce the risk of VTE.

Appropriate pharmacologic regimens include enoxaparin (low molecular weight heparin, Lovenox) 40 mg, subcutaneously every day, or unfractionated heparin 5,000 units, subcutaneously every 8 hours. The use of low molecular weight heparin, although more expensive, carries a lower risk of heparin-induced thrombocytopenia, a serious complication of prophylaxis. A platelet count should be performed every other day for the first 2 weeks of therapy for patients on any form of heparin. Complete blood counts do not need to be followed regularly unless there are signs of bleeding. Patients with mild renal insufficiency (glomerular filtration rate 30 to 59 mL per minute) require adjustment of enoxaparin dose. For patients with a contraindication to anticoagulant prophylaxis, such as a bleeding diathesis, the authors recommend the use of mechanical prophylaxis with graduated compression stockings and intermittent pneumatic compression devices.

Pressure ulcers are another common consequence of immobility, with incidence rates as high as 8% of all hospitalized patients.[117] The elderly and bed-bound patients have even higher rates of ulcer development. The development of pressure ulcers is the result of a combination of external factors, such as prolonged pressure, friction, and moisture, and host factors, such as patients who are elderly, have diabetes or other vascular diseases, or have poor nutrition.[118] Prevention of pressure

TABLE 4.2 RISK FACTORS FOR VENOUS THROMBOEMBOLISM (VTE)

Major risks (any one warrants prophylaxis)
- Acute respiratory failure
- Heart failure as admission diagnosis
- Age older than 70
- Malignancy (active)
- Acute stroke or myocardial infarction
- Major surgery in last 30 days
- Critical illness
- History of VTE
- Known thrombophilia
- Central venous catheter

Minor risks (any two warrant prophylaxis)
- Obesity (>120 kg)
- Infectious disease as admitting diagnosis
- Estrogen/oral contraceptive
- Chronic heart failure
- Age 40–70
- Nephrotic syndrome
- Acute inflammatory bowel disease or rheumatic disease as admit diagnosis
- Chronic lung disease
- Varicose veins
- Family history of VTE

ulcers is a cornerstone of hospital care and a standard part of nursing assessment. The Braden scale, typically performed by a floor nurse, evaluates patients in six subscales using scores ranging from 1 to 3 or 4: sensory perception, moisture, activity, mobility, nutrition, and friction and shear. The maximal total score is 23; a score of 18 or less indicates high risk. By identifying patients at high risk and instituting a comprehensive prevention plan, such as turning patients every 2 hours, providing pressure-reducing surfaces and mattresses, and addressing nutrition, mobility and incontinence, the incidence of pressure ulcers can be reduced.

NUTRITIONAL SUPPORT AND CHOICE OF DIETS

Dietary choice and nutritional support are complex topics worthy of advanced study, and special problems in patients with eating disorders are covered in Chapter 19. Presented here are some basic guidelines for choosing a diet for hospitalized patients. For patients without swallowing difficulties and who lack concurrent general medical conditions such as hypertension, congestive heart failure, or renal disease, a regular diet is an appropriate first choice. Patients with hypertension need a low-salt diet; patients with renal disease need a diet low in both sodium and potassium. Patients with hyperlipidemia and coronary artery disease should receive a low-fat diet. For patients with diabetes, it is customary to specify an American Diabetes Association (ADA) diet and a particular number of kilocalories (kcal), with 1,800 or 2,000 kcal being the most common. Another name for a diabetic diet is consistent carbohydrate, to reflect the need that diabetic patients have for a controlled amount of carbohydrates when dosing insulin. These diets can be combined, so that a diabetic patient with hyperlipidemia and hypertension can receive a 2,000 kcal, low-fat, low-salt ADA diet.

For patients who are not able to eat a standard meal, supplemental fluids must be provided and supplemental feeding may be necessary as well. Typically, if the duration of inadequate oral feeding will be a week or less and the patient is not obviously malnourished, supplemental feeding is not needed. Consultation with a nutritionist can help to sort out who does and who does not need supplemental feeding and what type of feeding is appropriate for those who do.

Patients who do not eat need supplemental fluid within the first 24 hours of beginning to fast and can receive maintenance fluid, which is equal to their daily needs and accounts for losses through urine, stool, and sweat. The standard method for calculating the maintenance fluid rate is 40 mL per hour for the first 10 kg of patient body weight, plus 20 mL per hour for the second 10 kg of patient body weight, plus 1 mL per hour for every subsequent 1 kg of patient body weight. This formula simplifies to a maintenance fluid rate (in milliliters per hour) equal to weight (in kilograms) plus 40. A typical maintenance fluid solution is 0.45 (half-normal) saline, with or without 20 mEq of potassium in each liter. Patients receiving IV fluid as their sole fluid and nutritional intake should have their urine output monitored ($\geq$0.5 mL/kg/hour) and should have a basic metabolic panel checked daily to evaluate for the development of electrolyte abnormalities, metabolic acidosis, or renal failure.

DEHYDRATION

Poor oral intake and dehydration are another common set of consequences of conditions that can accompany or lead to hospitalization of any type. Although the body is very good at regulating fluid balance, there are obligate losses of both fluids and electrolytes in urine, stool, and sweat. Nausea, vomiting, and diarrhea are common precipitants of dehydration or, more properly, hypovolemia. In the psychiatric population, hypovolemia may result from the problems that can lead to psychiatric hospitalization, including substance abuse, confusional states, catatonia, and depression.

The signs, symptoms, and evaluation strategies of hypovolemia are likely to be similar no matter what the cause. Elements in the history that suggest the possibility of volume depletion include the above-mentioned nausea, vomiting, and diarrhea as well as chronic diuretic use, muscle weakness (due to hypokalemia or hyperkalemia), and thirst, which is a natural response to volume depletion as well as to hypernatremia. In more severe cases, lethargy, confusion, seizures, and coma may result from hyponatremia or hypernatremia. Clinical findings include tachycardia, postural (orthostatic) or even frank hypotension, and decreased urine output. Common laboratory findings are concentrated urine (elevated specific gravity), low urine sodium (<10 mEq per L), elevated blood urea nitrogen (BUN)/creatinine ratio (>20), and elevation of the serum creatinine over baseline. Other abnormalities, such as hyponatremia or hypernatremia, should result in a prompt medical evaluation, for the consequences of these conditions can be quite severe. Shock is the final common pathway for hypovolemia of all causes and is a medical emergency best treated in a critical care setting.

Treatment of mild to moderate hypovolemia (without hypotension or acute renal failure) can be begun with IV fluids. A liter of 0.9 (normal) saline is a good initial choice in most situations, particularly for patients who are orthostatic. Lactated Ringers, or LR, is another reasonable choice in patients without significant renal failure or liver disease. This has somewhat less sodium and has small amounts of potassium and of lactate, which is converted to bicarbonate by the liver. There is no standard method for determining the rate of IV replacement in hypovolemic patients, but 50 to 100 mL per hour over the maintenance rate is a safe and reasonable place to begin. This translates to 200 to 250 mL per hour. For treatment of psychiatric patients not on a medical floor, the authors suggest a limit to volume repletion of 1 to 2 L. If concern remains for hypovolemia, evaluation by an internist is advised.

CONSTIPATION

Constipation is common in hospitalized patients and may result from factors such as poor diet and reduced physical activity. Although symptom relief is usually achieved with a combination of dietary changes and medication, clinicians should be alert to other possible causes of constipation and evaluate patients properly. Common medical causes of constipation include hypothyroidism, medicines such as antipsychotics, antidepressants, and calcium channel blockers, and autonomic neuropathy from diabetes mellitus (although diarrhea can also be a consequence).

Asking patients to increase dietary fiber and fluid intake is an approach that most clearly mirrors normal physiology and has the benefit of being highly effective. This may be as simple as increasing the number of servings of fruits, vegetables, and whole grains. Metamucil or Citrucel are over-the-counter fiber supplements that work by retaining water, bulking and softening the stool, and promoting more frequent bowel movements. Abdominal bloating and gas are common side effects. Stool softeners such as docusate sodium (Colace) are essentially mild detergents and work by making stool softer and more slippery. Although they can be useful for prophylaxis, stool softeners are generally less effective than other agents once constipation has developed. More effective is the wide variety of osmotic agents. Lactulose and sorbitol are sugars that are not absorbed and serve the purpose of drawing water into the stool. Polyethylene glycol is a synthetic osmotic laxative that works in the same manner. All osmotic laxatives are very effective. Stimulant laxatives, such as bisacodyl or senna, work primarily by stimulating gut motility. Although effective, stimulant laxatives should not be used chronically unless the patient does not respond to other measures.

FALLS: RISKS AND PREVENTION

Falls are more common in hospitalized patients than is realized, the potential for serious injury is high.[119] Fall rates for hospitalized patients vary from just under 2 to approximately 18 falls per 1,000 patient days, which amounts to between 2% and 17% of patients, depending on the population.[120] One fourth of those falls result in injury.[121] Although elderly patients are at particular risk, all hospitalized patient are at risk, especially those with orthostatic hypotension, visual impairment, impairment of gait or balance, medication use, limitations in basic or instrumental activities of daily living, and cognitive impairment, are at risk.[122] In addition, hospitalization-specific causes, such as delirium, Foley catheters, nasogastric tubes, and IV lines, increase the risk of a fall. Fortunately, fall prevention programs can reduce fall rates by 20% to 30%. Successful programs typically take a multidisciplinary approach to fall prevention and address patient factors such as weakness or confusion, and medical factors such as medication, bedrails, and catheters. From a physician standpoint, a less formal approach could involve avoiding the improper use of medicines that can alter the sensorium, such as anticholinergics, or induce postural hypotension, such as antihypertensives, particularly α-adrenergic receptor antagonists. In addition, the judicious use of supervision can play a role. Restraints are contraindicated; although they are often justified as fall prevention, their use can precipitate falls, serious injury, and even death.

OBESITY AND METABOLIC CONDITIONS

Obesity is increasingly common in hospitalized patients as it is in the population as a whole. The particularly high prevalence of obesity in the mentally ill was cited earlier. Although the contribution of obesity to mortality is the subject of debate and excess mortality may not be associated with obesity *per se*,[123,124] nonetheless obesity is associated with other conditions such as diabetes, hypertension, hyperlipidemia, and inactivity that do make substantial contributions to morbidity and mortality. The metabolic syndrome too, comprising type 2 diabetes, dyslipidemia, hypertension, and obesity, is highly and excessively prevalent in the chronically mentally ill. Consensus guidelines for management of psychotic patients, and in particular patients treated with atypical antipsychotic drugs, emphasize screening for and monitoring of abnormalities of body mass index, glucose, and lipids.[125,126] For the most part, available guidelines focus on long-term outpatient management of the seriously mentally ill; adaptation of the guidelines to inpatient care is thus far a matter of judgment. However, for many patients, the only reliable occasion for testing and treatment planning is the inpatient stay, and in our judgment a liberal testing strategy is appropriate. For example, while guidelines suggest testing lipids at 1 year after initiation of an antipsychotic, performing the test upon hospital admission 9 months on may well be reasonable.

As discussed earlier, measurement of height and weight and calculation of the body mass index should be routine aspects of hospital admission. If present, obesity should be identified as a problem—sometimes the patient's most life-threatening problem—and a treatment plan devised. This plan could include selection of the least toxic psychotropic drugs, pharmacologic strategies to minimize weight gain or produce weight loss, health education, behavioral therapy oriented to weight loss, and consideration of bariatric surgery.[126–129] Development of educational groups on the psychiatric unit related to diet and exercise would be a useful addition to many treatment programs.

Screening for diabetes mellitus, specifically type 2, is beneficial because of the commonly long asymptomatic period, effective treatments, and substantial benefit of early diagnosis and treatment. In addition, in the prediabetes state of impaired fasting glucose or impaired glucose tolerance, lifestyle modification can prevent or delay the onset of overt diabetes. There is some debate about who should be screened for diabetes, but all patients on antipsychotic medication are considered high risk and therefore appropriate candidates for screening. Among other patients, a strict evidence-based approach would limit screening to patients with hypertension or hyperlipidemia,[130] although many experts would expand screening to include patients who are older than 45, overweight, have a family history of diabetes mellitus in a first-degree relative, are physically inactive, belong to a high-risk ethnic or racial group (African American, Hispanic, Native American, Asian American, and Pacific Islanders), have a history of gestational diabetes mellitus, have polycystic ovary syndrome, or have a history of vascular disease.[131]

The screening process itself is straightforward and does not require an oral glucose tolerance test. A patient with a fasting plasma glucose of 126 mg per dL or higher on two separate occasions has diabetes mellitus. A patient with a fasting plasma glucose level of 100 to 125 mg per dL on two separate occasions has impaired fasting glucose. Additionally, a nonfasting (random) glucose level of 200 mg per dL or greater, in a patient with the typical symptoms of diabetes (polyuria, polydipsia, and unexplained weight loss) meets the criteria for diabetes.[132] Patients with a new diagnosis of diabetes should have a glycosylated hemoglobin (hemoglobin A_{1c}) checked, be screened for dyslipidemias, and be referred to a primary care physician or medical consultant.

Dyslipidemia is a heterogeneous grouping of disorders of cholesterol metabolism and includes elevations in the LDL cholesterol and triglycerides as well as lowered levels of HDL cholesterol. What makes these disorders significant is their relation to atherosclerosis in the coronary beds and elsewhere throughout the body. Dyslipidemia is often asymptomatic until substantial end-organ damage is present. Given that there are highly effective treatments, this makes screening beneficial for reasons similar to those elaborated for diabetes. Both the National Cholesterol Education Program (NCEP) and the U.S. Preventive Services Task Force guidelines relate to screening for dyslipidemia, although they take different approaches. The authors focus on the NCEP recommendations here.[133]

The NCEP recommends screening all adults aged 20 years or more with a fasting lipid panel every 5 years. A fasting lipid panel consists of a measured total cholesterol, HDL cholesterol, and triglycerides. From these values LDL cholesterol can usually be estimated. Considered together with demographic variables related to cardiovascular risk, knowledge of risk factors makes possible an estimate of a patient's 10-year risk of coronary heart disease (CHD). The standard (Framingham) risk factors are cigarette smoking, hypertension ($\geq$140/90 mm Hg or on treatment), low levels of HDL cholesterol (<40 mg per dL), age (45 years or older in women, 55 years or older in men), and the presence of premature CHD in a first-degree relative (younger than 55 years in male relatives, younger than 65 years in female relatives). Patients with established CHD or CHD equivalents (diabetes mellitus, symptomatic carotid artery disease, peripheral arterial disease, or an abdominal aortic aneurysm) are at the highest risk and warrant the most aggressive treatment. In general, patients with 0 to 1 CHD risk factors should have an LDL value of <160 mg per dL, patients with 2 or more CHD risk factors should have an LDL or <130 mg per dL, and patients with established CHD or a CHD equivalent should have an LDL of <100 mg per dL or even lower in certain cases. Drug therapy with HMG-Co-reductase inhibitors (statins) is commonly instituted to achieve these results. The details of this therapy are beyond the scope of this discussion; patients with dyslipidemias should have medical consultation or referral.

Hypertension is another common metabolic condition the aggressive management of which can have substantial health benefits. The seventh Joint National Committee Report on the Prevention, Detection, Evaluation, and Treatment of High Blood Pressure (JNC VII)[134] divides blood pressure into three broad groups: normal, which is a reading that is <120/80 mm Hg; prehypertension, which is 120 to 139/80 to 90 mm Hg; and hypertension, which is 140/90 mm Hg or higher. Hypertension is then subdivided into stage 1 hypertension, which is 140 to 159/90 to 99 mm Hg, and stage 2 hypertension which is 160/100 mm Hg or greater. The patient's blood pressure category is determined by the higher of the systolic and diastolic pressures. Patients with diabetes or chronic kidney disease have the more stringent goal of a blood pressure <130/80 mm Hg. The recommended initial treatment is typically a thiazide diuretic for patients with stage 1 hypertension and a two-drug regimen including a thiazide for stage 2. If there are other diagnoses such as chronic kidney disease or CHD, other medicines may be indicated or even first line, such as angiotensin-converting enzyme (ACE) inhibitors, angiotensin receptor blockers, or β-blockers.

Typically, patients with stage 1 hypertension (<160/100 mm Hg) will follow up with an outpatient physician 4 to 6 weeks after the initiation of therapy, but in the hospitalized patient, one need not wait so long. Diuretics take several days to a week to have full effect, and most other long-acting medication (once daily) takes 1 to 3 days to have a full effect. Patients with stage 2 hypertension or anyone with signs or symptoms of end-organ damage (chest pain, renal insufficiency, headaches, etc.) should be seen by a consultant as soon as is feasible. Short-acting calcium channel blockers should generally be avoided without expert guidance, as they have been associated, in certain circumstances, with increased mortality.[135]

IMMUNIZATION

A hospitalization is an opportunity, often missed, to vaccinate patients at risk for common infections. Although vaccination rates for children are quite good, and those of older adults (older than 65 years) are steadily improving, those of young and middle-aged adults are typically poor. In general, a patient's need for vaccination depends on age, gender, and health status. Some medical conditions, such as diabetes or chronic kidney disease, increase the need for recommended immunizations, whereas others, particularly immunosuppression, make certain vaccinations, such as those with live organisms, contraindicated. General recommendations for adults, focusing on influenza, pneumococcal, and hepatitis vaccinations, will be discussed. More and continually updated information is available from the Centers for Disease Control at http://www.cdc.gov/vaccines/.

Influenza is a serious viral illness, characterized by a high fever, myalgias, and upper respiratory symptoms, which occurs in annual outbreaks worldwide in the winter months. One hallmark of influenza virus is that the high rate of mutation in the envelope glycoproteins helps the virus evade the immune system of its host. As a result, immunity is not long lasting; the vaccine needs to be redesigned annually. High mortality rates during influenza epidemics have been attributed to a lack of antibody protection due to unexpected major changes in the virus. Current vaccination strategy is primarily focused on individuals at highest risk for complications. Although influenza is often a self-limited viral illness, in the elderly or chronically ill complications, such as bacterial pneumonia, are more frequent. Current recommendations are to vaccinate everyone aged 50 and older, as well as residents of nursing homes or chronic care facilities of any age. In addition, adults with chronic pulmonary disease (including asthma), cardiovascular disease (but not hypertension), renal or hepatic disease, diabetes mellitus, immunosuppression, or HIV should also be immunized. Adults with neurologic disorders that can impair handling of secretions (neuromuscular weakness, cognitive dysfunction, and seizure disorders) and women who will be pregnant during the influenza season should also be vaccinated. Obviously, these guidelines include a large proportion of chronically mentally ill patients.

Invasive pneumococcal disease, in particular pneumococcal pneumonia, is clinically serious and potentially fatal. Widespread use of a pneumococcal vaccine in children has led to a substantial reduction in the burden of disease in both children and adults,[136] and vaccine use in adults has resulted in a reduction in serious disease as well.[137] Current recommendations are for a one-time vaccination of all adults older than 65 years and a repeat vaccination for those adults if they were younger than 65 at the time of the last vaccination and the prior vaccination was ≥5 years earlier. Adults aged 19 to 64 should be vaccinated only if they have chronic pulmonary disease (excluding asthma), chronic cardiovascular disease, diabetes mellitus, chronic liver disease, chronic alcoholism, chronic kidney disease, functional or anatomic asplenia, immunosuppressive conditions, cochlear implants, or CSF leaks. Again, these criteria will identify a substantial proportion of the chronically mentally ill.

There are two types of hepatitis for which it is possible and useful to vaccinate. Hepatitis A is an acute illness characterized by nausea, vomiting, jaundice, and right upper quadrant pain and is transmitted by the fecal–oral route. Symptoms typically last 4 to 6 weeks. Although the infection is typically self-limited, fulminant liver failure occasionally occurs, typically in patients with preexisting liver disease, such as hepatitis C. There is no carrier state and no chronic hepatitis. Vaccination is administered with a course of two injections separated by 6 months and is recommended for patients with liver disease (such as cirrhosis or hepatitis C), IV drug users, men who have sex with men, and patients who receive clotting factor concentrates. Hepatitis B has a similar clinical picture to hepatitis A, although the course is usually more prolonged. Hepatitis B is transmitted sexually or percutaneously (through injection-drug use) and may also be transmitted perinatally. Fulminant liver failure may occur, and unlike hepatitis A there can be a carrier state and associated chronic hepatitis, which is a risk factor for cirrhosis and hepatocellular carcinoma. Vaccination is administered as a three-injection course, at 0, 1, and 6 months, and is recommended for the same groups as for hepatitis A, and additionally patients on hemodialysis, with HIV, or who are not in monogamous relationships.

INFECTION CONTROL

Infection control policies vary somewhat among institutions, but there are certain common themes in all health care environments. All policies are dependent on the adherence of health care practitioners. One of the most effective practices and the hallmark of universal precautions is routine hand washing, either with plain or antimicrobial soap, before and after every patient contact. Unfortunately, nonadherence to good health practices is not limited to patients.[138] Alcohol or chlorhexidine-based gels are similarly effective, and ease of application may improve adherence of clinicians. This simple practice remains a powerful tool in reducing nosocomial infections and should be observed with all patients when there is physical contact, however brief.[139,140]

Various isolation precautions are employed in specific situations where there is an established or suspected infection or a high risk of infection. Contact isolation is used for patients with enteric infections, particularly *Clostridium difficile*, and infections or colonization with multidrug resistant organisms (methicillin-resistant *Staphylococcus aureus* and vancomycin-resistant *Enterococci*). With *C. difficile*, a documented infection is not required; the suspicion of this virulent pathogen is enough to require contact isolation pending laboratory confirmation. Precautions are limited to gloves and gowns for clinicians or visitors and confinement to a private room for the patient. Droplet precautions, primarily for influenza (although other infections, such as pertussis and some viral infections, require these precautions), simply require a surgical mask to be worn. As in the case of *C. difficile*, the clinical suspicion of an infection is enough to require isolation to be instituted. Droplet precautions should not be confused with airborne precautions, required for patients with TB and varicella, which entail a respirator for clinicians and a negative-pressure room for patients.

Summary and Conclusions

General medical disorders are common in psychiatric inpatients and cause excess mortality. Moreover they may cause psychiatric symptoms and may be caused by psychiatric treatments. Relying on a misbegotten concept of "medical clearance" leads inpatient psychiatrists to pay less attention to concurrent general medical illness than the evidence reviewed here mandates.

To be sure, psychiatric units should not take on cases they are not prepared to manage, and excluding patients with unstable cardiac rhythms or acute hypoxemia is more than sensible. However, the patients not excluded as unstable are still likely to have a substantial burden of systemic illness and may require interventions that can be safely performed on a properly prepared psychiatric unit. Further, expanding the boundaries of safe management on the psychiatric unit may allow better care of patients who are acutely psychiatrically ill. For example, an acutely suicidal patient who is mildly dehydrated may be better served by admission to a (relatively) "suicide-proof" unit where IV fluids can be administered than by admission to a general medical floor where psychiatric issues are largely unaddressed while fluids are administered.

The inpatient psychiatrist should have access to expert consultation from general internists, internal medicine subspecialists, and other medical specialists. But it remains the psychiatrist's responsibility to integrate complications and interventions in other domains into the formulation of the patient's psychiatric status and the advice from other physicians into the plan of care. To make informed use of consultants, the inpatient psychiatrist must be knowledgeable about aspects of general medical illness and skilled in elements of general medical management. All in all, in the authors' view, the principle on the inpatient unit is: doctor first, then psychiatrist.

REFERENCES

1. Mitchell SW. Address before the 50th annual meeting of the American Medico-Psychological Association, held in Philadelphia, May 16th, 1894. *J Nerv Ment Dis.* 1894;21:413–437.
2. Horvitz-Lennon M, Kilbourne AM, Pincus HA. From silos to bridges: Meeting the general health care needs of adults with severe mental illnesses. *Health Aff.* 2006;25(3):659–669.
3. Yates BL, Koran LM. Epidemiology and recognition of neuropsychiatric disorders in mental health settings. In: Ovsiew F, ed. *Neuropsychiatry and mental health services.* Washington, DC: American Psychiatric Press; 1999:23–46.

4. Mitchell AJ, Malone D. Physical health and schizophrenia. *Curr Opin Psychiatry.* 2006;19(4):432–437.

5. McIntyre RS, Soczynska JK, Beyer JL, et al. Medical comorbidity in bipolar disorder: Reprioritizing unmet needs. *Curr Opin Psychiatry.* 2007;20(4):406–416.

6. Dickey B, Normand S-LT, Weiss RD, et al. Medical morbidity, mental illness, and substance use disorders. *Psychiatr Serv.* 2002;53(7): 861–867.

7. Osborn DPJ, Levy G, Nazareth I, et al. Relative risk of cardiovascular and cancer mortality in people with severe mental illness from the United Kingdom's General Practice Research Database. *Arch Gen Psychiatry.* 2007;64(2):242–249.

8. Jones DR, Macias C, Barreira PJ, et al. Prevalence, severity, and co-occurrence of chronic physical health problems of persons with serious mental illness. *Psychiatr Serv.* 2004;55(11):1250–1257.

9. Carney CP, Jones L, Woolson RF. Medical comorbidity in women and men with schizophrenia: A population-based controlled study. *J Gen Intern Med.* 2006;21(11):1133–1137.

10. Hennekens CH, Hennekens AR, Hollar D, et al. Schizophrenia and increased risks of cardiovascular disease. *Am Heart J.* 2005;150(6):1115–1121.

11. Brown S, Barraclough B, Inskip H. Causes of the excess mortality of schizophrenia. *Br J Psychiatry.* 2000;177(3):212–217.

12. Heila H, Haukka J, Suvisaari J, et al. Mortality among patients with schizophrenia and reduced psychiatric hospital care. *Psychol Med.* 2005;35(5):725–732.

13. Miller BJ, Paschall CB III, Svendsen DP. Mortality and medical comorbidity among patients with serious mental illness. *Psychiatr Serv.* 2006;57(10):1482–1487.

14. Rugulies R. Depression as a predictor for coronary heart disease: A review and meta-analysis. *Am J Prev Med.* 2002;23(1):51–61.

15. Angst F, Stassen HH, Clayton PJ, et al. Mortality of patients with mood disorders: Follow-up over 34-38 years. *J Affect Disord.* 2002;68(2-3):167–181.

16. Katon WJ, Rutter C, Simon G, et al. The association of comorbid depression with mortality in patients with type 2 diabetes. *Diabetes Care.* 2005;28(11):2668–2672.

17. Janszky I, Ahlbom A, Hallqvist J, et al. Hospitalization for depression is associated with an increased risk for myocardial infarction not explained by lifestyle, lipids, coagulation, and inflammation: The SHEEP Study. *Biol Psychiatry.* 2007;62(1): 25–32.

18. Brown S, Birtwistle J, Roe L, et al. The unhealthy lifestyle of people with schizophrenia. *Psychol Med.* 1999;29(3):697–701.

19. Thakore JH, Spelman L. Obesity and psychotic disorders. In: McElroy SL, Allison DB, Bray GA, eds. *Obesity and mental disorders.* New York: Taylor & Francis Ltd; 2006:21–40.

20. McElroy SL, Kotwal R, Nelson EB, et al. Obesity and mood disorders. In: McElroy SL, Allison DB, Bray GA, eds. *Obesity and mental disorders.* New York: Taylor & Francis Ltd; 2006: 41–92.

21. Allison DB, Mackell JA, McDonnell DD. The impact of weight gain on quality of life among persons with schizophrenia. *Psychiatr Serv.* 2003;54(4):565–567.

22. Fontaine KR, Heo M, Harrigan EP, et al. Estimating the consequences of anti-psychotic induced weight gain on health and mortality rate. *Psychiatry Res.* 2001;101(3):277–288.

23. Newcomer JW. Second-generation (atypical) antipsychotics and metabolic effects. *CNS Drugs.* 2005;19(Suppl 1):1–93.

24. Saari KM, Lindeman SM, Viilo KM, et al. A 4-fold risk of metabolic syndrome in patients with schizophrenia: The Northern Finland 1966 Birth Cohort Study. *J Clin Psychiatry.* 2005;66(5):559–563.

25. Mackin P, Bishop D, Watkinson H, et al. Metabolic disease and cardiovascular risk in people treated with antipsychotics in the community. *Br J Psychiatry.* 2007;191: 23–29.

26. Correll CU, Frederickson AM, Kane JM, et al. Metabolic syndrome and the risk of coronary heart disease in 367 patients treated with second-generation antipsychotic drugs. *J Clin Psychiatry.* 2006;67(4):575–583.

27. Delgado J-S. Evolving trends in nonalcoholic fatty liver disease. *Eur J Intern Med.* 2008;19(2): 75–82.

28. Druss BG, Bradford WD, Rosenheck RA, et al. Quality of medical care and excess mortality in older patients with mental disorders. *Arch Gen Psychiatry.* 2001;58(6):565–572.

29. Kilbourne AM, McCarthy JF, Welsh D, et al. Recognition of co-occurring medical conditions among patients with serious mental illness. *J Nerv Ment Dis.* 2006;194(8):598–602.

30. Olshaker JS, Browne B, Jerrard DA, et al. Medical clearance and screening of psychiatric patients in the emergency department. *Acad Emerg Med.* 1997;4(2):124–128.

31. Tintinalli JE, Peacock FW, Wright MA. Emergency medical evaluation of psychiatric patients. *Ann Emerg Med.* 1994;23(4):859–862.

32. Reeves RR, Pendarvis EJ, Kimble R. Unrecognized medical emergencies admitted to psychiatric units. *Am J Emerg Med.* 2000;18(4): 390–393.

33. Koranyi EK, Potoczny WM. Physical illness-es underlying psychiatric symptoms. *Psychother Psychosom*. 1992;58(3-4):155–160.

34. Koran LM, Sox HC Jr, Marton KI, et al. Medical evaluation of psychiatric patients. I. Results in a state mental health system. *Arch Gen Psychiatry*. 1989;46(8):733–740.

35. Koran LM, Sheline Y, Imai K, et al. Medical disorders among patients admitted to a public-sector psychiatric inpatient unit. *Psychiatr Serv*. 2002;53(12):1623–1625.

36. Lyketsos CG, Dunn G, Kaminsky MJ, et al. Medical comorbidity in psychiatric inpatients: Relation to clinical outcomes and hospital length of stay. *Psychosomatics*. 2002;43(1):24–30.

37. Othmer E, Othmer SC, Othmer JP. Psychiatric interview, history, and mental status examination. In: Sadock BJ, Sadock VA, eds. *Comprehensive textbook of psychiatry*, 8th ed. Philadelphia: Lippincott Williams & Wilkins; 2005:794–826.

38. Issroff J. Winnicott and Bowlby: personal reminiscences. In: Issroff J, ed. *Winnicott and Bowlby: personal and professional perspectives*. London: H. Karnac Books Ltd; 2005:13–69.

39. McIntyre JS, Romano J. Is there a stethoscope in the house (and is it used)? *Arch Gen Psychiatry*. 1977;34(10):1147–1151.

40. Vukanovic-Criley JM, Criley S, Warde CM, et al. Competency in cardiac examination skills in medical students, trainees, physicians, and faculty: A multicenter study. *Arch Intern Med*. 2006;166(6):610–616.

41. Norton J. The importance of the physical examination in a psychiatry residency program. *Acad Psychiatry*. 2001;25(4):236–237.

42. Menninger KA, Mayman M, Pruyser PW. *A manual for psychiatric case study*, 2nd ed. New York: Grune & Stratton; 1962.

43. McGee SR. *Evidence-based physical diagnosis*, 2nd ed. Philadelphia: WB Saunders; 2007.

44. Sapira JD. *The art and science of bedside diagnosis*. Baltimore: Urban & Schwarzenberg; 1990.

45. Summers WK, Munoz RA, Read MR. The psychiatric physical examination – part I: Methodology. *J Clin Psychiatry*. 1981;42(3):95–98.

46. Summers WK, Munoz RA, Read MR, et al. The psychiatric physical examination – part II: Findings in 75 unselected psychiatric patients. *J Clin Psychiatry*. 1981;42(3):99–102.

47. Garden G. Physical examination in psychiatric practice. *Adv Psychiatr Treat*. 2005;11(2):142–149.

48. Sanders RD, Keshavan MS. Physical and neurologic examinations in neuropsychiatry. *Semin Clin Neuropsychiatry*. 2002;7(1):18–29.

49. Ovsiew F. Neuropsychiatric physical diagnosis in context. In: Yudofsky SC, Kim HF, eds. *Neuropsychiatric assessment*. Arlington: American Psychiatric Publishing; 2004:1–38.

50. Ovsiew F. Neuropsychiatric approach to the patient. In: Sadock BJ, Sadock VA, eds. *Comprehensive textbook of psychiatry*. Philadelphia: Lippincott Williams & Wilkins; 2005:323–349.

51. Ovsiew F. Bedside neuropsychiatry: eliciting the clinical phenomena of neuropsychiatric illness. In: Yudofsky SC, Hales RE, eds. *American psychiatric publishing textbook of neuropsychiatry and behavioral neurosciences*. Washington, DC: American Psychiatric Publishing; 2007:137–187.

52. Hu FB. Obesity and mortality: Watch your waist, not just your weight. *Arch Intern Med*. 2007; 167(9):875–876.

53. Spodick DH, Raju P, Bishop RL, et al. Operational definition of normal sinus heart rate. *Am J Cardiol*. 1992;69(14):1245–1246.

54. Sommet A, Desplas M, Lapeyre-Mestre M, et al. Drug-induced yawning: A review of the French pharmacovigilance database. *Drug Saf*. 2007;30(4):327–331.

55. Lloyd T, Dazzan P, Dean K, et al. Minor physical anomalies in patients with first-episode psychosis: Their frequency and diagnostic specificity. *Psychol Med*. 2008;38(1):71–77.

56. Yoshitsugu K, Yamada K, Toyota T, et al. A novel scale including strabismus and 'cuspidal ear' for distinguishing schizophrenia patients from controls using minor physical anomalies. *Psychiatry Res*. 2006;145(2-3):249–258.

57. Boes AD, Murko V, Wood JL, et al. Social function in boys with cleft lip and palate: Relationship to ventral frontal cortex morphology. *Behav Brain Res*. 2007;181(2):224–231.

58. Friedlander AH, Marder SR. The psychopathology, medical management and dental implications of schizophrenia. *J Am Dent Assoc*. 2002;133(5):603–610.

59. McCreadie RG, Stevens H, Henderson J, et al. The dental health of people with schizophrenia. *Acta Psychiatr Scand*. 2004;110(4):306–310.

60. Ovsiew F, Utset T. Neuropsychiatry of the rheumatic diseases. In: Yudofsky SC, Hales RE, eds. *American psychiatric publishing textbook of neuropsychiatry and clinical neurosciences*, 4th ed. Washington, DC: American Psychiatric Publishing; 2002:813–850.

61. Anfinson TJ, Kathol RG. Screening laboratory evaluation in psychiatric patients: A review. *Gen Hosp Psychiatry*. 1992;14(4):248–257.

62. Kim HF, Yudofsky SC. Neuropsychiatric laboratory testing. In: Yudofsky SC, Kim HF, eds. *Neuropsychiatric assessment*. Washington, DC: American Psychiatric Publishing; 2004:105–153.

63. Langton JE, Brent GA. Nonthyroidal illness syndrome: Evaluation of thyroid function in sick patients. *Endocrinol Metab Clin North Am*. 2002;31(1):159–172.

64. Arem R, Cusi K. Thyroid function testing in psychiatric illness: Usefulness and limitations. *Trends Endocrinol Metab.* 1997;8(7):282–287.

65. De Groot LJ. Dangerous dogmas in medicine: The nonthyroidal illness syndrome. *J Clin Endocrinol Metab.* 1999;84(1):151–164.

66. Bocchetta A, Mossa P, Velluzzi F, et al. Ten-year follow-up of thyroid function in lithium patients. *J Clin Psychopharmacol.* 2001;21(6):594–598.

67. Benedetti MS, Whomsley R, Baltes E, et al. Alteration of thyroid hormone homeostasis by antiepileptic drugs in humans: Involvement of glucuronosyltransferase induction. *Eur J Clin Pharmacol.* 2005;61(12):863–872.

68. Surks MI, DeFesi CR. Normal serum free thyroid hormone concentrations in patients treated with phenytoin or carbamazepine: A paradox resolved. *JAMA.* 1996;275(19):1495–1498.

69. Little KY, Garbutt JC, Mayo JP, et al. Lack of acute d-amphetamine effects on thyrotropin release. *Neuroendocrinology.* 1988;48(3):304–307.

70. Vescovi PP, Pezzarossa A. Thyrotropin-releasing hormone-induced GH release after cocaine withdrawal in cocaine addicts. *Neuropeptides.* 1999;33(6):522–525.

71. Cooper DS. Subclinical hypothyroidism. *N Engl J Med.* 2001;345(4):260–265.

72. Jorde R, Waterloo K, Storhaug H, et al. Neuropsychological function and symptoms in subjects with subclinical hypothyroidism and the effect of thyroxine treatment. *J Clin Endocrinol Metab.* 2006;91(1):145–153.

73. Chueire VB, Romaldini JH, Ward LS. Subclinical hypothyroidism increases the risk for depression in the elderly. *Arch Gerontol Geriatr.* 2007;44(1):21–28.

74. Cole DP, Thase ME, Mallinger AG, et al. Slower treatment response in bipolar depression predicted by lower pretreatment thyroid function. *Am J Psychiatry.* 2002;159(1):116–121.

75. Abulseoud O, Sane N, Cozzolino A, et al. Free T4 index and clinical outcome in patients with depression. *J Affect Disord.* 2007;100(1-3):271–277.

76. Ladenson PW, Singer PA, Ain KB, et al. American Thyroid Association guidelines for detection of thyroid dysfunction. *Arch Intern Med.* 2000;160(11):1573–1575.

77. Beckett GJ, Toft AD. First-line thyroid function tests—TSH alone is not enough. *Clin Endocrinol (Oxf).* 2003;58(1):20–21.

78. Wardle CA, Fraser WD, Squire CR. Pitfalls in the use of thyrotropin concentration as a first-line thyroid-function test. *Lancet.* 2001;357(9261):1013–1014.

79. Chong JY, Rowland LP, Utiger RD. Hashimoto encephalopathy: Syndrome or myth? *Arch Neurol.* 2003;60(2):164–171.

80. Anglin RE, Rosebush PI, Mazurek MF. The neuropsychiatric profile of Addison's disease: Revisiting a forgotten phenomenon. *J Neuropsychiatry Clin Neurosci.* 2006;18(4):450–459.

81. Arlt W, Allolio B. Adrenal insufficiency. *Lancet.* 2003;361(9372):1881–1893.

82. Thomsen AF, Kvist TK, Andersen PK, et al. The risk of affective disorders in patients with adrenocortical insufficiency. *Psychoneuroendocrinology.* 2006;31(5):614–622.

83. Sonino N, Fava GA. Psychiatric disorders associated with Cushing's syndrome: Epidemiology, pathophysiology and treatment. *CNS Drugs.* 2001;15(5):361–373.

84. Papanicolaou DA, Yanovski JA, Cutler GB Jr, et al. A single midnight serum cortisol measurement distinguishes Cushing's syndrome from pseudo-Cushing states. *J Clin Endocrinol Metab.* 1998;83(4):1163–1167.

85. Reynolds E. Vitamin B12, folic acid, and the nervous system. *Lancet Neurol.* 2006;5(11):949–960.

86. Lindenbaum J, Savage DG, Stabler SP, et al. Diagnosis of cobalamin deficiency: II. Relative sensitivities of serum cobalamin, methylmalonic acid, and total homocysteine concentrations. *Am J Hematol.* 1990;34(2):99–107.

87. Stabler SP, Allen RH, Savage DG, et al. Clinical spectrum and diagnosis of cobalamin deficiency [see comments]. *Blood.* 1990;76(5):871–881.

88. Hvas AM, Nexo E. Diagnosis and treatment of vitamin B12 deficiency. An update. *Haematologica.* 2006;91(11):1506–1512.

89. Solomon LR. Disorders of cobalamin (Vitamin B12) metabolism: Emerging concepts in pathophysiology, diagnosis and treatment. *Blood Rev.* 2007;21(3):113–130.

90. Savage DG, Lindenbaum J, Stabler SP, et al. Sensitivity of serum methylmalonic acid and total homocysteine determinations for diagnosing cobalamin and folate deficiencies. *Am J Med.* 1994;96(3):239–246.

91. Carmel R. Reassessment of the relative prevalences of antibodies to gastric parietal cell and to intrinsic factor in patients with pernicious anaemia: Influence of patient age and race. *Clin Exp Immunol.* 1992;89(1):74–77.

92. Abou-Saleh MT, Coppen A. Folic acid and the treatment of depression. *J Psychosom Res.* 2006;61(3):285–287.

93. Meyer JM, Lehman D. Bone mineral density in male schizophrenia patients: A review. *Ann Clin Psychiatry.* 2006;18(1):43–48.

94. Howard L, Kirkwood G, Leese M. Risk of hip fracture in patients with a history of schizophrenia. *Br J Psychiatry.* 2007;190(2):129–134.

95. Furlan PM, Ten Have T, Cary M, et al. The role of stress-induced cortisol in the relationship between depression and decreased

bone mineral density. *Biol Psychiatry*. 2005; 57(8):911–917.

96. Meaney AM, O'Keane V. Bone mineral density changes over a year in young females with schizophrenia: Relationship to medication and endocrine variables. *Schizophr Res*. 2007; 93(1-3):136–143.

97. Heller HJ, Sakhaee K. Anticonvulsant-induced bone disease: A plea for monitoring and treatment. *Arch Neurol*. 2001;58(9):1352–1353.

98. Diem SJ, Blackwell TL, Stone KL, et al. Use of antidepressants and rates of hip bone loss in older women: The study of osteoporotic fractures. *Arch Intern Med*. 2007;167(12):1240–1245.

99. Haney EM, Chan BK, Diem SJ, et al. Association of low bone mineral density with selective serotonin reuptake inhibitor use by older men. *Arch Intern Med*. 2007;167(12):1246–1251.

100. Ovsiew F, Jobe T. Neuropsychiatry in the history of mental health services. In: Ovsiew F, ed. *Neuropsychiatry and mental health services*. Washington, DC: American Psychiatric Press; 1999:1–21.

101. St. Louis ME, Wasserheit JN. Elimination of syphilis in the United States. *Science*. 1998;281(5375):353–354.

102. Young H. Syphilis. Serology. *Dermatol Clin*. 1998;16(4):691–698.

103. El-Ad B, Lavie P. Effect of sleep apnea on cognition and mood. *Int Rev Psychiatry*. 2005;17(4):277–282.

104. Ovsiew F. Seeking reversibility and treatability in dementia. *Semin Clin Neuropsychiatry*. 2003;8(1):3–11.

105. Peppard PE, Szklo-Coxe M, Hla KM, et al. Longitudinal association of sleep-related breathing disorder and depression. *Arch Intern Med*. 2006;166(16):1709–1715.

106. Meltzer HY, Cola PA, Parsa M. Marked elevations of serum creatine kinase activity associated with antipsychotic drug treatment. *Neuropsychopharmacology*. 1996;15(4):395–405.

107. O'Dwyer AM, Sheppard NP. The role of creatine kinase in the diagnosis of neuroleptic malignant syndrome. *Psychol Med*. 1993;23(2):323–326.

108. Cournos F, McKinnon K, Sullivan G. Schizophrenia and comorbid human immunodeficiency virus or hepatitis C virus. *J Clin Psychiatry*. 2005;66(Suppl 6):27–33.

109. Landon BE, Wilson IBMcInnes K, et al. Physician specialization and the quality of care for human immunodeficiency virus infection. *Arch Intern Med*. 2005;165(10):1133–1139.

110. Matthews AM, Huckans MS, Blackwell AD, et al. Hepatitis C testing and infection rates in bipolar patients with and without comorbid substance use disorders. *Bipolar Disord*. 2008;10(2):266–270.

111. National Institutes of Health Consensus Development. National Institutes of Health Consensus Development Conference Statement: Management of hepatitis C: 2002–June 10-12, 2002. *Hepatology*. 2002;36(5B):s3–s20.

112. Geerts WH, Pineo GF, Heit JA, et al. Prevention of venous thromboembolism: The Seventh ACCP Conference on Antithrombotic and Thrombolytic Therapy. *Chest*. 2004;126(Suppl 3):338 S–400 S.

113. McCall WV, Mann SC, Shelp FE, et al. Fatal pulmonary embolism in the catatonic syndrome: Two case reports and a literature review. *J Clin Psychiatry*. 1995;56(1):21–25.

114. Pendleton R, Wheeler M, Rodgers G. Venous thromboembolism prevention in the acutely ill medical patient: A review of the literature and focus on special patient populations. *Am J Hematol*. 2005;79(3):229–237.

115. Lacut K, Le Gal G, Couturaud F, et al. Association between antipsychotic drugs, antidepressant drugs and venous thromboembolism: Results from the EDITH case-control study. *Fundam Clin Pharmacol*. 2007;21(6):643–650.

116. Liperoti R, Pedone C, Lapane KL, et al. Venous thromboembolism among elderly patients treated with atypical and conventional antipsychotic agents. *Arch Intern Med*. 2005;165(22):2677–2682.

117. Bergstrom N, Braden B, Kemp M, et al. Multisite study of incidence of pressure ulcers and the relationship between risk level, demographic characteristics, diagnoses, and prescription of preventive interventions. *J Am Geriatr Soc*. 1996;44(1):22–30.

118. Braden B, Bergstrom N. A conceptual schema for the study of the etiology of pressure sores. *Rehabil Nurs*. 1987;12(1):8–12.

119. Hitcho EB, Krauss MJ, Birge S, et al Characteristics and circumstances of falls in a hospital setting: A prospective analysis. *J Gen Intern Med*. 2004;19(7):732–739.

120. Schwendimann R, Buhler H, De Geest S, et al. Falls and consequent injuries in hospitalized patients: Effects of an interdisciplinary falls prevention program. *BMC Health Serv Res*. 2006;6:69.

121. von Renteln-Kruse W, Krause T. Incidence of in-hospital falls in geriatric patients before and after the introduction of an interdisciplinary team-based fall-prevention intervention. *J Am Geriatr Soc*. 2007;55(12):2068–2074.

122. Ganz DA, Bao Y, Shekelle PG, et al. Will my patient fall? *JAMA*. 2007;297(1):77–86.

123. Allison DB, Fontaine KR, Manson JE, et al. Annual deaths attributable to obesity in the United States. *JAMA*. 1999;282(16):1530–1538.

124. Flegal KM, Graubard BI, Williamson DF, et al. Excess deaths associated with underweight, overweight, and obesity. *JAMA*. 2005; 293(15):1861–1867.

125. American Diabetes Association, American Psychiatric Association, American Association of

Clinical Endocrinologists, North American Association for the Study of Obesity. Consensus development conference on antipsychotic drugs and obesity and diabetes. *Diabetes Care.* 2004;27(2):596–601.

126. Marder SR, Essock SM, Miller AL, et al. Physical health monitoring of patients with schizophrenia. *Am J Psychiatry.* 2004;161(8):1334–1349.

127. Beebe LH. Obesity in schizophrenia: Screening, monitoring, and health promotion. *Perspect Psychiatr Care.* 2008;44(1):25–31.

128. Egger C, Muehlbacher M, Schatz M, et al. Influence of topiramate on olanzapine-related weight gain in women: An 18-month follow-up observation. *J Clin Psychopharmacol.* 2007;27(5):475–478.

129. Schaefer M, Leopold K, Hinzpeter A, et al. Memantine-associated reversal of clozapine-induced weight gain. *Pharmacopsychiatry.* 2007;40(4):149–151.

130. U.S. Preventive Services Task Force. *Screening for type 2 diabetes mellitus in adults,* 2003, Available from: http://www.ahrq.gov/clinic/uspstf/uspsdiab.htm, cited February 14, 2008.

131. American Diabetes Association. Standards of medical care in diabetes—2007. *Diabetes Care.* 2007;30(Suppl 1):S4–S41.

132. American Diabetes Association. Diagnosis and classification of diabetes mellitus. *Diabetes Care.* 2007;30(Suppl 1):S42–S47.

133. National Cholesterol Education Program. Third report of the National Cholesterol Education Program (NCEP) expert panel on detection, evaluation, and treatment of high blood cholesterol in adults (Adult Treatment Panel III) final report. *Circulation.* 2002;106(25):3143–3421.

134. Chobanian AV, Bakris GL, Black HR, et al. Seventh report of the Joint National Committee on prevention, detection, evaluation, and treatment of high blood pressure. *Hypertension.* 2003;42(6):1206–1252.

135. Furberg CD, Psaty BM, Meyer JV. Nifedipine. Dose-related increase in mortality in patients with coronary heart disease. *Circulation.* 1995;92(5):1326–1331.

136. Whitney CG, Farley MM, Hadler J, et al. Decline in invasive pneumococcal disease after the introduction of protein-polysaccharide conjugate vaccine. *N Engl J Med.* 2003;348(18):1737–1746.

137. Jackson LA, Neuzil KM, Yu O, et al. Effectiveness of pneumococcal polysaccharide vaccine in older adults. *N Engl J Med.* 2003; 348(18):1747–1755.

138. Pittet D, Mourouga P, Perneger TV. Compliance with handwashing in a teaching hospital. Infection Control Program. *Ann Intern Med.* 1999;130(2):126–130.

139. Pronovost P, Needham D, Berenholtz S, et al. *An intervention to decrease catheter-related bloodstream infections in the ICU.* 2006:2725–2732.

140. Won SP, Chou HC, Hsieh WS, et al. Hand-washing program for the prevention of nosocomial infections in a neonatal intensive care unit. *Infect Control Hosp Epidemiol.* 2004; 25(9):742–746.

Neuropsychiatric Approach to the Psychiatric Inpatient

FRED OVSIEW, EVAN D. MURRAY, AND BRUCE H. PRICE

T his chapter focuses on the neuropsychiatric approach to patients admitted to inpatient psychiatric units. Its goal is to help clinicians construct rational evaluations to identify organic factors in their patients' illnesses. "Neuropsychiatry" designates the psychiatric subspecialty area devoted to the psychological and behavioral consequences of organic brain disease. The term *organic* was dropped from the official nomenclature with the advent of Diagnostic and Statistical Manual of Mental Disorders Fourth Edition (DSM-IV), and wisely so insofar as the decision recognizes that the consequences of brain disease are manifold and cannot be lumped together as an "organic brain syndrome." The primary goal of the framers of recent versions of the DSM, however, was to "retire"[1] the term *organic* so as to eliminate "any implication that the nonorganic disorders are without a biological basis"[2] [p. 127].

The word has not stayed "retired," to judge by questions from colleagues. They know that some, but not all, individual patients with mental disorders can be shown to have brain disease by current diagnostic instruments: the history, the physical examination, the cognitive examination, neuropsychological examination, brain imaging, electroencephalography (EEG), examination of the cerebrospinal fluid (CSF), and so on. The continued vernacular usage acknowledges that the knowledge base and clinical skills required to diagnose and manage psychiatric patients with disorders such as epilepsy, traumatic brain injury, and autoimmune brain disease are different from those needed for the care of patients with idiopathic mental disorders. The distinctiveness of this specialty area and the overlap of neuropsychiatry with behavioral and cognitive neurology have recently been validated by the development of a credential in Behavioral Neurology and Neuropsychiatry (see http://www.ucns.org/go/subspecialty/behavioral/certification).

In asserting the distinctiveness of the neuropsychiatric approach, by no means do we deny a basis in biology to schizophrenia or depression or mania or any other idiopathic psychiatric syndrome. Neuropsychiatric understanding of organic mental disorders may well be able to cast light on the biology of the idiopathic disorders, although reasoning by similarity of phenomenology has important limits.[3] Nor do the present authors assert that once an organic factor is discovered the remainder of the case is moot. Although a neuropsychiatric evaluation may lead to a diagnosis implying a specific treatment that promptly abolishes the condition and eliminates any need for further psychiatric care, such cases are not characteristic of the present authors' practices. More commonly, the organic factors in the case feature among others that also need to be taken into account. The neuropsychiatric approach elaborated in this chapter is not meant to "scoop" other approaches and does not replace them.

Management of patients with known brain disease admitted to the psychiatric unit is discussed in Chapter 17, and the management of delirious patients is discussed in Chapter 18. General medical conditions in organ systems other than the brain commonly occur in patients with psychiatric illness and frequently contribute to psychiatric morbidity. These conditions and the appropriate general medical evaluation of the psychiatric inpatient are discussed in Chapter 4. In this chapter, the neuropsychiatric bedside evaluation (history, physical examination, and cognitive examination) and the use and interpretation of ancillary investigations (neuroimaging, EEG, CSF examination, genetic testing, metabolic testing, and neuropsychological assessment) are discussed. Guidance for neuropsychiatric evaluation in several common clinical contexts on the general psychiatric inpatient unit is then provided.

Taking the Neuropsychiatric History

Obtaining an adequate neuropsychiatric history requires an understanding of common organic factors in psychopathology and their clinical manifestations. Provided here is a sketch of these elements of the history. Fuller discussion of the comprehensive neuropsychiatric history is available elsewhere.[3-5]

Atypical features of the psychiatric history should raise the question of organic origin, although it is also true that organic mental disorders can closely mimic their idiopathic counterparts. An unusual age of onset, an unusually acute onset or rapid pace of progression, the absence of a family history in a disorder (such as bipolar mood disorder) that is highly familial, or an atypical response or lack of response to treatment should lead the examiner to pursue focused inquiry about neuropsychiatric issues. Similarly, the presence of somatic symptoms such as headache, somnolence, incontinence, or altered coordination or gait should be red flags for the diagnostician. A review of neurologic symptoms along with attention to the past medical history should form part of routine psychiatric history taking (see Table 5.1). In general, correlation of the psychiatric history with organic disease benefits from specificity in regard to the brain disease: not just "stroke," but embolic stroke involving right parietal lobe, and so on. The development of psychiatric symptoms in the context of major medical illness, such as cancer, systemic autoimmune disease, or an immunocompromised state, should not be attributed to the obvious psychosocial stress of illness without full consideration of possible organic pathogenesis.

Neuropsychiatric history taking regarding development begins with the patient's gestation. Inquiry should cover abnormalities in the mother's pregnancy, labor, and delivery and go on to include perinatal illness (such as any illness that kept the patient in the hospital immediately after birth) and early developmental milestones (such as the age of walking and talking). Childhood illnesses, especially those affecting the brain, should be reviewed. These developmental factors are of demonstrated importance in the major psychiatric disorders.[6-8] In patients with epilepsy, the diagnostician should inquire about the occurrence of febrile convulsions in childhood. The patient's school performance provides important information about intellectual capacity; not only the overall level (such as whether special education was required) but also anomalies or unevenness in performance should be ascertained. Early athletic skills provide information about developmental achievement. The patient's handedness should be established by inquiry about hand use for actions including writing, using a scissors, brushing the teeth, and so on.

Among acquired illnesses, either in childhood or adulthood, traumatic brain injury and epilepsy require special mention, because of both their prevalence and their well-established relation to psychiatric symptoms. A screening question about traumatic brain injury is appropriate for virtually every psychiatric patient. Significance of head injury is generally marked by loss of consciousness and the severity of brain trauma indicated by duration of unconsciousness and the length of time between injury and recovery of ongoing memory function (posttraumatic amnesia). Traumatic brain injury is of probable significance in the histories of patients with a number of psychiatric disorders, including (to name two that may be of surprise to psychiatrists) borderline personality disorder and perpetration of domestic violence.[9-11] More information about the psychopathology of traumatic brain injury is offered in Chapter 17. Attention to the details of the injury is important in part because attribution of psychopathology to head injury by patients and families may rest less on a demonstrable connection than on their understandable wish to find some explanation for mysterious and disabling symptoms. The clinician will have to make a judgment about the connection, a judgment that should be based on clinical data, starting with the history.

In regard to epilepsy, too, the clinician should gain specific information about the nature of the epileptic syndrome, the frequency of seizures (under best and worst control), the phenomena of the seizure itself (including auras, if present), and the treatment. Much of the psychiatric literature about epilepsy has concerned itself with temporal lobe epilepsy, but the connection of epilepsy to psychopathology is not limited to this syndrome. For example, the syndrome of juvenile myoclonic epilepsy (JME) appears to have characteristic cognitive and personality correlates.[12,13] History taking in patients with limbic epilepsy should not be confined to the symptoms typical of the major psychiatric

TABLE 5.1 SOME FEATURES IN THE HISTORY AND REVIEW OF SYSTEMS WITH LEADING IMPLICATIONS FOR NEUROLOGIC DISEASE RELEVANT TO BEHAVIOR

System	Symptom	Possible Implications (not a Comprehensive List)
General	Weight loss	Neoplasm, endocrinopathy
	Decreased energy	Systemic disease
	Fever, chills	Systemic or CNS infection
	Arthritis	Connective tissue disease, infection
Head	New or altered headache	Space-occupying lesions, many others
	History of trauma	Subdural hematoma, postconcussion syndrome
Eyes	Chronic visual impairment	Ocular or posterior hemispheric disease (visual hallucinations possible with either location)
	Episodic visual loss	Vascular disease
	Diplopia	Brainstem disease
Ears	Hearing loss	—
Nose	Loss of olfactory sensitivity	Local nasal disease, head injury, subfrontal meningioma
Mouth	Oral lesions	Nutritional deficiency, autoimmune disease, self-injury from seizure
Skin	Rash	Autoimmune disease, Lyme disease, infection
	Birthmarks	Phakomatoses
Cardiovascular	Heart disease	Risk of cerebrovascular disease
	Hypertension	Risk of cerebrovascular disease
	Arrhythmia	Risk of embolic disease
Sleep	Sleepwalking/talking	Dementia with Lewy bodies
	Daytime sleepiness	Sleep apnea, narcolepsy
Motor	Focal weakness	Stroke, neoplasia
	Gait disorder	Hydrocephalus, white-matter disease, movement disorder

CNS, central nervous system.

disorders, because more specific symptoms—such as hypergraphia, hyposexuality, and preoccupation with mystical or cosmic matters—are thought by some to be characteristic correlates of this form of epilepsy.[14,15] In general, the clinical phenomena of neuropsychiatric illness may not be fully captured in the syndromes of DSM-IV, and the examiner should be on the lookout for data beyond the usual history checklists. Fitting the organic mental disorder into a DSM category by brute force is inadvisable.

Case Vignette

A young woman was seen for neuropsychiatric consultation after an admission for video-EEG monitoring required by her poorly controlled JME. During the admission, she required detoxification from large doses of alprazolam, which she was allegedly taking for myoclonus.

(continued)

Features of "borderline personality disorder" were thought to be recognized; other diagnoses previously attributed to her were schizophrenia and bipolar mood disorder. During the neuropsychiatric inquiry, her father reported that she had always been emotionally labile and easily frustrated (quite unlike her healthy sister), and he volunteered that she had never been able to get jokes because she did not understand (he searched for the right word) "irony." She performed adequately or poorly in regular school classes and had menial jobs after high-school graduation. For several years before consultation, she had a clear depressive syndrome. No manic or psychotic phenomena could be identified. The neurologic examination was unremarkable. The cognitive examination disclosed particular difficulty with spontaneous word-list generation to a semantic stimulus and with a working memory task. These personality and cognitive features were considered typical of JME.

Especially in late-life psychiatric illness, history taking should seek evidence of cognitive impairment, which is sometimes subtle or overshadowed by florid mood or psychotic symptoms. Questions about forgetfulness, getting lost, and impairment of skills of everyday independent functioning are relevant. Of equal importance is the recognition of abnormal social behavior or personality change typical of organic brain disease. Such features are often described only by a family member and remain unrecognized by the patient. Patients may show alteration of social comportment, such as eating with the fingers at the dinner table; loss of the sense of humor; lack or coarsening of emotional responses to ordinarily affecting situations, such as the death of a relative; disinhibited sexual or other appetitive behavior; or apathy with loss of initiative without the self-denigrating ideation or pervasive low mood of the depressive state. The apathy syndrome deserves particular attention because of its similarity to depression yet phenomenological, pathophysiologic, and pharmacologic differences from that syndrome.[16]

Taking the family history can be done either disease-by-disease ("does anyone in the family have a psychiatric disorder?") or family member-by-family member (ideally constructing a family tree in the process).[5,17] The latter method is more sensitive, but the two methods can be combined in the clinical interview. Some neuropsychiatric illnesses are commonly familial (such as frontotemporal dementia), and the presence or absence of a family history is then an important clue to diagnosis.

The Cognitive Examination

On the basis of the unsystematic observations, the present authors believe that most psychiatric inpatients undergo a cognitive assessment limited to tests of orientation and perhaps memory, or at most the performance of a brief standardized screening test such as the Mini-Mental State Examination (MMSE). Not infrequently, the record of this testing is limited to a checkmark in a box labeled "memory" or "language," without further reference to how the function was assessed. In this section, the domains of cognitive function and their bedside assessment are reviewed and screening instruments and their utility and drawbacks are surveyed. The authors argue for the centrality of assessment of executive function in the hospitalized psychiatric patient and provide guidelines for its performance.

COGNITIVE MODULES AND THEIR ASSESSMENT AT THE BEDSIDE

To listen properly to the heart and interpret the heart sounds and murmurs, the examiner must understand the anatomy of the cardiac chambers and the physiology of the circulation of the blood. Similarly, the assessment of cognition depends on an understanding of brain anatomy and mental function. Rote application of routine tests—"Name the last 4 presidents"—will not allow the examiner to use information from the cognitive examination to construct a brain-based formulation of cognitive deficits. A comprehensive discussion of the anatomy of cognition and behavior is beyond the scope of this chapter but has been addressed elsewhere.[18,19]

The essential concept of cognitive modularity entails that certain domains of function are relatively independent of others, with dedicated input and output streams and the possibility of derangement separate from other deficits.[3] The concept does not necessarily imply distinct anatomic sites as the substrates of processing modules, and in fact contemporary theorists consider that individual cognitive functions depend on a distributed network of brain sites, any of which may also be involved in other processing functions ("selectively distributed processing"). Further, any probe of cognitive function results in the deployment of multiple modules; for example, a putative test of memory also requires language and focused attention. For these reasons, inference from clinical examination to brain lesion can be made only on the basis of a comprehensive assessment of multiple domains of cognition, by a process of "triangulation."

Although every cognitive examination should address multiple modules as well as nonmodular cognitive functions, a comprehensive examination cannot be recommended for every psychiatric inpatient. Not only would the time requirements be excessive and the yield unreasonably low but also the psychiatric state of the patient on admission would often preclude valid testing. The goal of initial assessment at the bedside is to identify patients with deficits relevant to their functional capacity and patients who require further evaluation. At times the assessment will have to be repeated as the patient's psychiatric state changes.

The cognitive modules assessable by bedside examination include language, memory, and visuospatial function. In addition, attention, which is subserved by a highly distributed system, should be assessed. Assessment of the cognitive state is extensively described in other texts and is merely sketched here.[4,20] Executive cognitive function has a special place in the assessment of psychiatric patients and is discussed at greater length in the next section.

Attention

Attentional function can be divided into the maintenance of sustained attention, or arousal; the capacity for focused attention, or concentration; and higher forms of attentional behavior such as the capacity for divided attention or the ability to inhibit automatic attention that verge on or form part of the concept of executive cognitive function, which is discussed in detail in the subsequent text. Arousal can be gauged by the patient's responsiveness to graded interventions: the examiner's entering the room, voice, loud voice, touch, and so on. The clinician's note should specify the intervention and the response rather than relying on terms such as *lethargic* or *stuporous*.

Although observations during the interview may yield an estimate of the intactness of the patient's attentional function, every patient should have some formal probe of attention; all other cognitive functions depend on attention to some degree. Simple tasks serve well, such as forward digit span, counting backward from 20, or giving in reverse order the days of the week or the months of the year. On the MMSE, serial subtraction of 7s or spelling "WORLD" in reverse assesses this domain. Giving the letters of "WORLD" in alphabetic order is a similar probe.[21] The patient's capacity for sustained attention to external stimuli can be assessed by asking the patient to signal each time the examiner says the letter "A" during a list of randomly produced letters: "B, A, R, L, A, A, etc." The more difficult tasks (such as giving the months in reverse) require the patient to inhibit the more usual response (in that instance, giving the months in forward order) and to that extent represent tasks of executive function.

Language

Bedside examination of language should start with attention to the patient's spontaneous speech considered as a linguistic performance. That is to say, the examiner must deliberately focus on the syntactic, semantic, and prosodic aspects of speech, as against the meaning, affect, or narrative structure of the patient's output. Spontaneous speech can be fluent, with normal length of phrases and normal prosodic contour, or dysfluent, with effortful, slowed, and agrammatic output. Word-finding difficulties, circumlocution, and paraphasic errors also should be listened for.

In addition to deliberate attention to spontaneous speech, the examiner can test naming, comprehension, repetition, reading, and writing. This discussion is confined to a brief description of such testing; full discussions can be found elsewhere.[20,22] Naming can usually be tested by confrontation, using items at hand: "what is this (sleeve, thumb, pen, etc.) called?" Comprehension should be tested by commands that require little verbal or motor output, such as yes/no questions ("am I wearing a hat?" or "is ice cream hotter than coffee?") or requests to "point to the chair" or "point to the ceiling, then to the floor." The degree of impairment of repetition of spoken language may be discrepant from that of spontaneous speech. Sparing of repetition suggests a lesion outside the perisylvian language areas; disproportionate impairment suggests a lesion in or deep to left parietal cortex. Repetition can be tested by asking the patient to repeat a series of phrases of increasing complexity, starting with single words and advancing to lengthy sentences. Testing of reading entails assessment of reading comprehension (not ability to read aloud); asking the patient to point to items after reading their printed names is a simple method. Writing can be assessed by asking the patient to construct a sentence. Before testing both reading and writing, the examiner is well advised to be sure of the patient's premorbid literacy.

A thorough language examination can help to categorize an acquired disorder of language, or aphasia, although many patients have disorders that do not fit well into any established category. Fuller discussions of the classification of the aphasias can be found elsewhere.[22,23] Language errors do not always indicate language system dysfunction, and knowledge of certain confounding phenomena should help the examiner of psychiatric inpatients. "Wild paraphasias" occur in delirium, sometimes with an apparent witty quality, such as the patient mentioned by Geschwind who called an IV pole a *Christmas tree*.[24] Disturbed writing may be an especially sensitive indicator of an encephalopathic state.[24] Cutting noted that an intermittent irrelevant remark in the midst of competent replies was characteristic of delirium.[25] Although delirious patients may produce abnormal language, they also show confusion in performance (ideational apraxia) on nonlanguage tasks, such as everyday instrumental behaviors. Patients with psychotic thought disorder, even when incoherent, may show adequate performance on structured language tasks if their cooperation can be gained.

Case Vignette

A woman in her 30s had a history of alcohol abuse and several admissions for detoxification. Approximately 8 months before consultation she presented in delirium to an emergency room (ER), where a tentative diagnosis of Wernicke encephalopathy was made. After admission, however, she developed a fever, and CSF showed a lymphocytic pleocytosis with protein elevated to 100 and normal glucose. The findings for CSF herpes simplex virus (HSV) and head computed tomography (CT) were negative. Upon discharge, she was incoherent and was sent to a nursing home, where a psychiatrist prescribed a combination of two antipsychotics on a diagnosis of "schizoaffective disorder." At neuropsychiatric consultation, examination disclosed a cooperative and socially appropriate woman who had no elementary neurologic signs. Speech output was fluent but so full of paraphasic errors, such as "spoketal" for key and "farris" for glove, as to be incomprehensible. Comprehension was severely impaired. Clinically, she had Wernicke aphasia, not the Wernicke encephalopathy that her family had been told about. Subsequently, repeat CT (magnetic resonance imaging [MRI] could not be accomplished) showed extensive damage to the left temporal lobe (see Fig. 5.1). Antipsychotics were successfully discontinued.

Memory

Every cognitive examination should include some probe of memory, both because of its sensitivity to brain disease and because of the functional importance of memory.[26] Tasks such as recalling a name

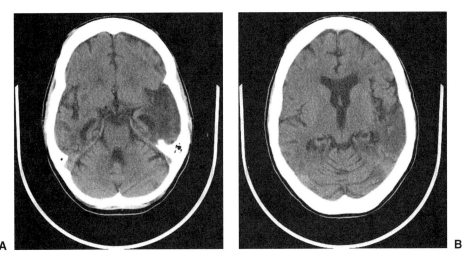

■ **Figure 5.1** Left temporal lobe encephalomalacia seen on computed tomography (CT) images at two levels.

and address after several minutes or recalling a list of several words tap into verbal memory function. However, the examiner should not ignore possible relative impairment or sparing of nonverbal memory, which can be ascertained by recall of figures or of objects hidden by the examiner in the examination room. A substantial discrepancy between verbal and nonverbal memory can be seen in patients with temporal lobe epilepsy and is of lateralizing significance.

Two forms of organic memory impairment should be emphasized. One, dependent on hippocampal mechanisms, involves rapid forgetting of material; the other, dependent on frontosubcortical mechanisms, involves impairment of retrieval. To some extent, although not so well as neuropsychological assessment, bedside evaluation can identify the form of memory impairment by using cuing strategies. While everyone is better at cued than at free recall—a multiple-choice test rather than an essay test—the discrepancy is particularly large in patients with impaired retrieval. Therefore, marked improvement in memory performance with cueing by multiple choice or by a semantic cue ("it was the name of a musical instrument") suggests dysfunction in frontal or subcortical structures.

Although relative impairment of "long-term" or "remote" memory can be identified in the neuropsychological laboratory, bedside examiners have difficulty making this distinction. Results of tests such as asking the patient to name recent American presidents have no compelling neuropsychological interpretation. Prominent forgetting of personal information, such as one's own name, with intact capacity to learn new information (as assessed by the tasks such as those described earlier) is virtually pathognomonic of psychogenic amnesia.

Visuospatial Function

Tasks of visuospatial function tap into the capacities of the "nondominant" hemisphere, typically the right hemisphere of dextrals. Failing to ascertain whether nonverbal cognitive impairment is present is particularly problematic in psychiatric settings because of the "dominant" role of the right hemisphere in affect regulation. Copying figures or the examiner's presentation of hand positions is a simple set of tasks that probe this domain.[4] Asking the patient to bisect a line drawn by the examiner or to cross out short lines arrayed within a page may reveal the hemineglect of the patient with right-hemisphere injury; this deficit also may be apparent on the clock-drawing test (see subsequent text). However, such a gross deficit as neglecting the left half of space, while not unusual in acute right-hemisphere stroke, may not be present in patients with milder or less acute damage, so these are not the most sensitive probes of visuospatial function. Patients with deficits in this domain may also show impairment in face recognition, impairment in recognizing affect in pictured scenes or vocal intonations, impairment in encoding affect into vocal output, and route-finding impairment.

Other Aspects of Modular Processing

Although what is described in the preceding text samples the classical elements of cognitive modules of long-standing interest in behavioral neurology, other aspects of cognitive processing may be disturbed with relative specificity and may be of clinical significance. Although screening for all possible deficits is impractical, awareness of other forms of impairment may lead to appropriate investigation in situations where a history of brain injury, unusual features of the psychiatric history or examination, or physical findings raise the question of additional deficits.

For example, the discussion of language disorders above addresses only disturbances of propositional discourse, not the pragmatic or affective elements of language performance. But patients with brain injury may show deficits in appreciation of emotion as coded into speech;[27] deficits in recognition of emotion in facial expression or visual scenes may occur as well. Such patients may present disturbances of affect suggestive of depression but pathophysiologically quite different from depressive states. Nothing substitutes for a broad awareness of the complex, multifarious, and at times counter-intuitive behavioral phenomena of brain disease.

SCREENING TESTS OF COGNITIVE FUNCTION

Many brief instruments have been devised to facilitate screening for cognitive deficits.[28] These instruments have the advantages of being quantitative, systematic, and repeatable across occasions and venues. They vary in their intended use, and potential users must keep in mind that the requirements for effectiveness of a brief instrument on the inpatient psychiatric unit are likely quite different from those, say, in community surveys assessing the prevalence of Alzheimer disease.

No doubt the best known instrument is the MMSE.[29] It has the advantage of being widely used and therefore easily compared across institutions. However, it has numerous limitations.[30] Of these, perhaps the most serious for the inpatient psychiatrist is its lack of any measure of executive dysfunction. The MMSE total score is also insensitive to focal brain disorders (as against delirium and dementia, its original focus) and to mild cognitive impairment. If used on the inpatient psychiatric unit, it should be supplemented by some screen for executive dysfunction. Further, any errors—even if the total score is above the standard cutoff—should be considered an indication for further evaluation, at least by additional bedside cognitive testing.

The Modified Mini-Mental State Examination (3MSE) is an expanded instrument that includes, among other additions to the MMSE, tests of executive function.[30] It contains the MMSE so that performances on the 3MSE can be compared with past or future results on the MMSE. Some instruments even simpler than the MMSE have been proposed as capable of identifying mild dementia. For example, the TE4D is an eight-item scale covering the domains of immediate recall, semantic memory, orientation, category fluency, clock drawing, and following commands.[31] The Mini-Cog assesses memory and clock drawing only.[32]

A scale developed to identify cognitive impairment related to human immunodeficiency virus (HIV) encephalopathy, the HIV Dementia Scale (HDS), focuses on the subcortical features of mental slowing, executive dysfunction, and attentional impairment characteristic of that disorder, in contrast to the MMSE and its successors, which focus more on the cortical features characteristic of Alzheimer disease.[33,34] These subcortical impairments may be especially important not to miss in patients with psychiatric disorders, because depressive states produce a picture not unlike subcortical dementia and because subcortical vascular disease may be an important cause of *de novo* psychiatric illness in late life. The HDS contains four elements: a memory task, a test of response inhibition using antisaccades, a test of psychomotor speed, and a visuoconstructional task. The antisaccade task starts with the patient looking straight ahead at the examiner's face, while the examiner places one hand in each of the patient's visual fields. The patient is asked to look at the examiner's right hand when the examiner's left hand moves, and at the examiner's left hand when the right hand moves. Looking at the moving hand represents a failure of inhibition.

Several research groups have developed broader cognitive screening instruments. For example, the Montreal Cognitive Assessment (MoCA, see http://www.mocatest.org/) probes the domains of attention, verbal fluency, language, memory, and constructional ability. The Addenbrooke's Cognitive Examination-Revised similarly explores attention, orientation, memory, language, and visuospatial function.[35]

Review of these instruments reveals that several make use of clock drawing. Drawing a clock has been touted as "the ideal cognitive screening test" because it is quick, provides a visual record of the patient's performance, is relatively insensitive to cultural variables, and is sensitive to multiple domains of cognitive impairment, including executive dysfunction.[36–38] To utilize clock drawing as an executive screen requires considering not only the visual-spatial elements of the performance (such as neglect of the left side of the clock face) but also the planning of the placement of the numbers and the setting of the hands. Scoring systems to capture these elements have been proposed. As a simple clinical procedure, the patient can be provided with a circle and asked to put in the numbers of the clock face while leaving out the hands. Then the examiner requests the patient to set the hands to "5 after 10," or some other time in which the number spoken by the examiner is not the number to which the patient must point the hand. The goal of the instruction is to see whether the patient can abstract from the concrete stimulus (the number 5) and construe it in terms of a clock face (in this instance, with the little hand of the clock pointing to the 1).

EXECUTIVE COGNITIVE FUNCTION AND ITS ASSESSMENT

Executive cognitive function refers to those aspects of mental function that deploy, monitor, and inhibit elementary cognitive functions.[39] These aspects include planning, reasoning, and judgment; deficits show themselves as perseveration, disinhibition, and poor adaptation of internal states and resources to the demands of the environment. Executive function can be measured neuropsychologically using tasks such as the Stroop test and the Wisconsin Card Sorting Test and identified at the bedside by probes such as motor sequencing tasks, tests of working memory, tests of response inhibition (such as go/no-go tapping tests or the antisaccade test mentioned earlier), and tests of verbal or design fluency. Asking a patient to name all the animals he or she can think of in 1 minute is a typical semantic verbal fluency task; an instruction to name all the words starting with a given letter creates a phonemic fluency task. Having the patient tap once when the examiner taps once and not tap at all when the examiner taps twice is a simple go/no-go test of response inhibition. Perseveration and impaired motor sequencing can be elicited by asking the patient to alternate between making a fist and forming a ring with the thumb and index finger, the Luria ring/fist test.

The Mental Alternation Test, or alphanumeric sequencing, is an oral version of the Trails B test. A patient who is able to count and able to recite the alphabet is asked to alternate numbers and letters: "1-A-2-B-3-C" is given as an example, and then the patient is asked to start at 1. Correct alternations are scored, with errors not counted; considering a score of 15 or above to be normal has been recommended.[40,41] This is a working memory test that presumptively relies on prefrontal-subcortical function. It is very simple to administer, and the expanding data about its utility are encouraging.[40–44]

Several bedside batteries of tests of executive function have been constructed. The Frontal/Subcortical Assessment Battery includes a verbal fluency task, a go/no-go task, and a motor sequencing task.[45] The Frontal Assessment Battery includes probes of abstraction, motor sequencing, verbal fluency, perseveration, response inhibition, and the grasp reflex.[46] The Behavioral Dyscontrol Scale, based on the work of the Russian neuropsychologist A. R. Luria, includes go/no-go and motor sequencing tasks, probes of perseveration and echopraxia, and the alphanumeric sequencing test described earlier.[47] The Executive Interview (EXIT-25), a copyrighted neuropsychological instrument, is somewhat more extensive, and more time-consuming, than the briefer batteries just mentioned.[48]

In addition to systematic probes, observation of the patient's behavior during the clinical evaluation can yield data regarding executive function. For example, during the interview or physical examination the patient may demonstrate echopraxia, duplicating the examiner's spontaneous gestures or mirroring the examiner's movements, or may demonstrate impersistence by failing to maintain postures or eyelid closure ("peeking"). Executive function is multidimensional, that is, no single test fully interrogates executive function, so that one, several, or even all commonly used tests can be normal in the presence of executive dysfunction.

The reason that executive cognitive function is of special importance in the cognitive examination is its correlation with autonomous functioning outside the clinical setting. Executive dysfunction is associated with functional decline and behavioral disturbance in dementia,[49] with the capacity to live independently in elders,[50] and with insight and adaptive functioning in schizophrenia.[51,52] Patients with late-onset depression and executive dysfunction (often the result of subcortical white-matter disease) show poorer outcomes than patients with similar depressive states but lacking executive dysfunction.[53] No cognitive examination on the inpatient psychiatric unit is complete without attention to executive cognitive function.

The clinician should be aware, however, that real-world functioning may differ from performance on formal testing. This may be because the testing situation—quiet, structured, based on veridical perception rather than value or emotion—does not duplicate the world in which the patient lives and in fact may make up for executive deficits. This problem, so-called ecologic validity, is the stimulus for devising new methods of examination within neuropsychology.[54]

The Neuropsychiatric Physical Examination

Neurologic examination is famously complex and abstruse. Yet to rely solely on mental state findings to disclose contributions to psychopathology from organic brain disease is to practice psychiatry with one hand tied behind one's back. Interpretation of imaging and other findings from the laboratory should always be in the context of the history and examination. Proficiency at an examination focused on cerebral systems relevant to behavioral derangements should be gained by the inpatient psychiatrist through a combination of study, instruction by experts, repeated practice, and comparison of one's own findings with those of other examiners of one's patients and with data from imaging and other investigations. Achievement of expertise in this narrow domain is a reasonable goal for the practitioner.[55] In this chapter, certain tools relevant to inpatient psychiatric evaluation are highlighted. Doing so is not meant to discourage examiners from comprehensive evaluations, but a full discussion of the many aspects of the neurologic examination—even a full discussion of those relevant to behavioral disorders—is beyond the scope of this chapter. Some elements of the general physical examination are discussed in Chapter 4, with citations of texts of physical examination and of published efforts toward focused physical examination of psychiatric patients. A more comprehensive discussion of the neurologic examination has been published elsewhere.[56]

The physical examination of the psychiatric inpatient should include attention to dysmorphic features, including so-called minor physical anomalies. This term refers to subtle developmental disturbances centering on the head, face, hands, and feet. Abnormal head circumference, facial asymmetry, low set or asymmetric ears, a high-arched or broad and flat palate, and unusual patterns of palmar creases are some of the commonly assessed features.[4] Strabismus and a sharp angulation of the external ear ("cuspidal ear") have recently been stressed.[57] Such anomalies have been most extensively studied in schizophrenia but are associated with psychosis more generally.[58,59] Recognition of developmental anomalies is crucial to the differential diagnosis of developmental disability syndromes.

In the everyday neurologic examination, testing of olfaction is often omitted. However, few other probes interrogate the orbitofrontal regions, and the olfactory nerve runs along this surface. In traumatic brain injury or subfrontal meningioma, for example, anosmia may point to damage in this region. Testing should be accomplished with odorants such as floral scents that do not stimulate the trigeminal nerve. One of the present authors uses scented lip balms, which are readily available and easy to carry, as test odors. Although olfactory sensitivity (threshold for detection) and olfactory identification (naming of the scent) can be distinguished and have different anatomic correlates, testing of this complexity requires specialized equipment and a more extended evaluation. For ordinary bedside purposes, noting whether the patient can recognize the presence of the odorant, with or without naming it, suffices.

In the neuro-ophthalmologic examination, assessment of eye movements is particularly relevant in psychiatric inpatients. For example, every alcohol-abusing patient should be examined for nystagmus on admission as an element of assessing for Wernicke encephalopathy, a commonly missed diagnosis.[60] Saccadic and smooth-pursuit movements need to be examined separately. Abnormalities of these eye movement systems as well as of lid movements have an important place in diagnosing neurodegenerative diseases.[4] The spontaneous blink rate is decreased in parkinsonian states and often increased in acute psychosis.

Facial weakness of central supranuclear origin characteristically spares the forehead; both upper and lower face are weak in lower motor neuron facial weakness. In assessing movement of the face, the examiner must keep in mind the presence of two systems, pyramidal and nonpyramidal, in the control of facial expression. Paresis of voluntary facial movement (i.e., to command) with relative preservation of spontaneous facial movement is not infrequent in patients with lesions in pyramidal regions. The opposite disturbance—intact movement of the muscles of facial expression on voluntary effort with paresis seen in spontaneous emotional expression—is seen with lesions involving nonpyramidal areas, such as the temporal lobe. Therefore in temporal lobe epilepsy, a dissociated facial paresis for spontaneous movement provides lateralizing information about the epilepsy.[61] Asymmetry of facial expression may be present at rest in these patients as well.[62]

Speech disorders, although hard to describe perspicuously in text, can often be identified easily by the experienced examiner. The scanning speech of cerebellar disease, the strangled quality of speech pyramidal disease, the slurring and nasal air escape of bulbar weakness, and the hypophonic speech of extrapyramidal disease have diagnostic value.

Detailed testing of individual muscle strength with the intent of identifying focal peripheral lesions is generally not within the province of the inpatient psychiatrist; examination of the motor system should focus on central motor systems. As discussed in subsequent text, examination of gait is essential in identifying motor impairment. Screening for pyramidal weakness can be performed using the pronator sign (the patient holds the arms outstretched, palms up, fingers together, with eyes closed; the weak extremity drifts down and pronates and the fingers spread) and the Barré sign (the patient holds the arms outstretched with wrists flexed, palms forward, fingers abducted, "like stopping traffic"; the weak extremity shows loss of wrist and finger extension and of finger abduction).[63,64] "Stickiness" and reduced amplitude in repeatedly tapping the thumb to the index finger and slowness of repeated foot tapping are other manifestations of a pyramidal deficit.[64,65]

Muscle tone is the resistance felt by the examiner when the examiner moves the patient's limb. In pyramidal disorders, tone is increased in the flexors of the upper extremity and the extensors of the lower extremity; hence the typical hemiparetic posture and gait of flexed arm and circumducted leg. The examiner feels this increase of tone in the affected muscles, but the antagonists of these muscles do not show increased tone. The increase in tone is more evident with rapid than with slow movements. This pattern is known as *spasticity*. It is to be differentiated from *rigidity*, the pattern typical of extrapyramidal disease, for example, disease of the basal ganglia. Patients with rigidity show increased muscle tone in both agonists and antagonists, throughout the range of motion and independent of velocity. Both of these patterns of increased tone are different from *paratonia* (paratonic rigidity or Gegenhälten). This form of hypertonus is associated with diffuse or frontal brain disease; patients show erratic, "pseudoactive" increased tone, seemingly unable to relax. Paratonia usually refers to the intermittent opposition to passive movement. However, facilitory paratonia can be demonstrated by repeatedly flexing and extending the patient's arm at the elbow and releasing the arm at the point of maximum extension; in the abnormal state, the patient's arm continues to flex, against gravity, actively continuing the previously passive movement.[66]

Cerebellar disease is characteristically manifested by impairment in the rate, force, or timing of movement execution. The resulting ataxia can be shown by asking the patient to touch the examiner's finger with his or her index finger, then his or her own nose, then back to the finger, and so on; to run the heel down the shin of the opposite leg repeatedly; and to pronate and supinate the upper extremity repeatedly ("like you are screwing in a light bulb").

All of these deficits—pyramidal, extrapyramidal, and cerebellar—are sensitively demonstrated in gait testing. In fact, patients may lack appendicular ataxia but demonstrate gait ataxia alone when the lesion involves the cerebellar vermis (which, because of its limbic connections, is also a structure with significant behavioral correlates).[67] If at all feasible, every patient should be asked to walk as part of the examination. After observing ordinary walking, the examiner should stress gait by asking the patient to walk on the toes, then on the heels, then tandem ("like you are on a tightrope"), and then perhaps on the outside edge of the feet ("like a bow-legged cowboy"). These maneuvers may reveal subtle weakness (heel and toe walking), ataxia of gait (tandem walking), or posturing of the upper extremities (any of the stressed gaits) associated with pyramidal or extrapyramidal lesions. Parkinsonian gait (flexed station, reduced arm swing, short steps on a narrow base) can be distinguished from the similar gait disturbance seen in cerebrovascular disease ("arteriosclerotic parkinsonism" or "lower-half parkinsonism"), in which legs are extended and stiff, the base may be widened, and the upper extremities are relatively spared.[68,69] Because the latter pattern of gait is associated with subcortical white-matter disease, it is a common, although sometimes subtle, feature of presentations of late-life depressive or psychotic disorders associated with small vessel disease due to hypertension.

Sensory testing, although of course a standard element of the neurologic examination, is not infrequently difficult or unreliable in acutely ill psychiatric patients. When possible, testing of sensitivity to pin, light touch, vibration, and temperature in the extremities can be carried out. In patients suspected to have a cortical lesion, testing of cortical sensation (two-point discrimination, graphesthesia, stereognosis) should be carried out. Recognition of distal sensory loss representing a peripheral neuropathy can be crucial in directing attention to, for example, cobalamin (B_{12}) deficiency, alcohol abuse, or (a few times in one's career) metachromatic leukodystrophy or acute intermittent porphyria. A reasonable screen for proprioceptive sensory loss in the patient unable to cooperate for more detailed testing is the Romberg test. The Romberg sign refers to a substantial decrement in postural stability upon closing the eyes while standing erect with feet together.[70] The patient who is unstable even with eyes open does not show the Romberg sign and may have a cerebellar or other nonsensory disorder.

Abnormal movements are of considerable neuropsychiatric importance for several reasons. First, pathways involved in movement organization overlap substantially with those that organize emotion. Second, and of course related to the underlying neurobiology, movement disorders often have psychiatric correlates (and vice versa): obsessive compulsive disorder with tic disorders, depression in Parkinson disease, and so on. Third, psychiatrists cause movement disorders frequently: acute dystonia or parkinsonism with antipsychotic drugs, myoclonus with serotonergic drugs, tardive dyskinesia, and others. Therefore, the psychiatrist should have considerable expertise in recognizing and differentiating the common disorders of movement and should be familiar with their psychiatric correlates.[4,71]

Tremor is a rhythmic oscillation of a body part; except in the case of tongue tremor this is oscillation around a joint. Rest tremor occurs with body part fully relaxed; characteristically it is slow (3 to 5 Hz). Postural tremor occurs with the maintenance of posture, such as with the arm outstretched. The term *parkinsonism* refers to the tetrad of akinesia (reduction, slowness, or aspontaneity of movement), rigidity, rest tremor, and postural instability. This may occur in idiopathic Parkinson disease, may be induced by dopamine-blocking drugs, or may be part of a "parkinson-plus" syndrome in certain other basal ganglion diseases. Dystonia refers to relatively fixed abnormal postures. The dystonic movement may be elicited by movement (action dystonia), sometimes quite specific movements (such as writer's cramp elicited by writing or dystonic leg movements elicited by walking but not running), and may be relieved by specific sensory tricks (*le geste antagoniste*). Myoclonus is a jerky, arrhythmic movement, which can arise with varying pathophysiologies from various levels of the neuraxis. Asterixis is a momentary loss of postural tone, electrophysiologically the inverse of myoclonus. Both multifocal myoclonus and asterixis are features of an encephalopathic state; bilateral asterixis is nearly pathognomonic of encephalopathy and therefore differentiates delirium from acute functional psychosis with near-certainty. Tics are abrupt movements experienced subjectively as suppressible, albeit at the cost of mounting inner tension. Simple tics may appear similar to myoclonus whereas the most complex tics are hard to distinguish, clinically or conceptually, from compulsions. Tics differ electrophysiologically from behaviorally identical movements produced voluntarily; this finding corresponds to the subjective sense that they are actions chosen in response to an impulse, can be suppressed, yet are not fully voluntary—in these respects like scratching an itch, as patients often report. Akathisia refers to subjective restlessness coupled with excessive movement of the lower extremities, characteristically most sensitively seen as shifting from foot to foot ("marching in place") in the standing position or foot tapping in the seated position. The excessive movement of akathisia differs from that of anxiety by being limited to the lower extremities; the finger tapping, hand wringing, and so on of anxiety are not present in akathisia.

No neurologic examination, even a screening examination, is complete without attention to reflexes: muscle stretch reflexes, or tendon jerks, and pathologic reflexes. Absence of a tendon jerk suggests peripheral nerve or radicular disease. Exaggeration of tendon jerks suggests contralateral corticospinal tract disease when the lesion is at or above the decussation of the pyramids in the medulla. The plantar reflex is elicited by stroking the lateral aspect of the foot from back to front while the patient's leg is extended at the knee. The extensor response—the Babinski sign—consists of extension of the hallux often (but not always) with fanning of the other toes. It must be distinguished from a triple-flexion synergy including hip, knee, and ankle flexion and from the "striatal toe," which involves hallux extension without fanning of the other toes (seen in basal ganglion disease). When present, the Babinski sign is a specific indicator of corticospinal tract disease. It represents disinhibition of a primitive reflex pattern that ordinarily comes under pyramidal control early in development.

Other disinhibited primitive reflexes are commonly sought but, in many cases, are less specific for disease (i.e., are often present in normal adults, especially elders). Of these the most useful is the grasp reflex, which is elicited by stroking the patient's palm from proximal to distal while the patient is distracted or instructed not to grip the examiner. The abnormal response, namely flexion of the fingers and adduction of the thumb, points to contralateral medial frontal disease.[72,73] A more extreme version of this pattern is groping, which involves active movements of the hand in pursuing a stimulus. Similar behavior can be seen in the oral region related to an abnormal suck reflex and in the visual sphere, with disinhibited pursuit of a visual stimulus, particularly the human face.

A considerable neuropsychiatric literature addresses so-called neurologic soft signs, and several batteries are available to quantitate patients' performances.[74] The term comprises a variable set of findings thought to index brain dysfunction, albeit in a way that is not localizable or pathognomonic despite being reliable. Poor performance on batteries of soft signs is characteristic in schizophrenia, in which this deficit is associated with symptom severity, course, treatment response, neuropsychological function, and volume reduction in certain brain structures.[4] However, soft signs are also present in many other psychiatric disorders.[75] The signs considered include gait disturbance, disordered complex motor performances (such as on the Luria ring/fist test or finger tapping), other motor impairments (such as mirror movements), sensory integration deficits (such as abnormal stereognosis or graphesthesia), and primitive reflexes. From a neuropsychiatric point of view it appears extremely likely that this disparate group of probes interrogates different brain structures and functions, and a more specific clinical approach is preferable.

Neuroimaging

The advent of contemporary structural neuroimaging—CT of the brain in the 1970s and MRI in the 1980s—revolutionized the process of neurologic diagnosis. Functional imaging has not had the same impact on care of patients with brain disease as CT and MRI. The exciting prospects for understanding idiopathic psychiatric disorders through research methods relying on structural and functional imaging have been widely reviewed.[76,77] However, such studies characteristically report findings and their interpretation in groups of patients, and almost never does the clinician find guidance for the use of the imaging modalities in the individual patient. Because patients with known organic brain disease (e.g., traumatic brain injury by history) are customarily excluded from the study population, little advance in the understanding of organic psychiatric disorders can be expected from the large majority of psychiatric neuroimaging research projects.

STRUCTURAL BRAIN IMAGING

CT of the brain makes use of computerized reconstruction of data obtained from multiple perspectives around the head and at multiple levels ("slices") through the brain. Images provide excellent visualization, in the axial plane, of the hemispheres and ventricular system and often less-adequate visualization of the posterior fossa; bony injury and collections of blood are generally well visualized. The use of contrast material allows identification of areas of breakdown of the blood–brain barrier as well as often of abnormal vasculature (aneurysm and arteriovenous malformation). For many purposes on a psychiatric unit, the use of contrast material (enhancement) is not necessary, and the iodinated contrast material used risks allergic reaction or renal injury, especially in the dehydrated patient. In those situations in which enhancement of CT would be advantageous (such as looking for a tumor), MRI is generally the preferred modality. A major advantage of CT is that it is quick, so that even a relatively agitated patient can be scanned. It is adequate to rule out hemorrhage, such as subdural hematoma after trauma, and is generally the preferred modality when acute trauma is the prevailing issue.

MRI relies on the differential responses of different tissues to radiofrequency pulses, and it provides images in three planes (axial, coronal, and sagittal) with far better visualization of white-matter pathology and of the posterior fossa than CT. For most nonemergent indications on the psychiatric unit, MRI is preferable. However, the noise, enclosed space, and length of time required for MRI may make it infeasible for an acutely ill psychiatric patient. The presence of a potentially mobile ferromagnetic object in the patient's body—including permanent eyeliner as well as certain surgical clips or prosthetic valves—constitutes a contraindication to the use of MRI. The contrast agent used in MRI is not iodinated and is safer than CT contrast material (although certain risks remain); enhanced studies again reveal areas of blood–brain barrier breakdown and therefore are particularly important when inflammatory conditions are under consideration (multiple sclerosis, sarcoidosis, vasculitis, etc.). A gradient-echo (T2*) image sequence is particularly sensitive to old hemorrhage and therefore should be employed in the evaluation of past traumatic brain injury (to show otherwise undetectable areas of contusion) and considered in that of dementia (to show microbleeds, consequences of hypertension like white-matter damage but independently associated with cognitive impairment).[78]

The choice of modality and the need for contrast enhancement should be judged by a clinician familiar with the strengths and weaknesses of the available options and familiar as well with the clinical issues at hand. Just as important, the clinician must judge the urgency with which an imaging study is needed and whether, for example, an acutely psychotic patient could have imaging done some weeks later when more stable behaviorally. In an acute psychiatric setting, the major risks of imaging studies may well be behavioral: the patient must go off the locked and secure unit and face an uncomfortable and potentially disturbing test. The use and interpretation of imaging studies depend on the clinical context, and the authors recommend against substitution of near-routine imaging for taking a history and performing an examination.

Several newer techniques reveal additional information about brain injury. Diffusion-weighted imaging (DWI) demonstrates regions of abnormal diffusion of water. Of great utility in acute cerebrovascular disease, it is of limited importance in the evaluation of psychiatric illness, with the exception of its role in the diagnosis of Creutzfeldt-Jakob disease.[79] Diffusion tensor imaging (DTI) allows identification of damage to white-matter pathways because axonal damage alters the directionality of diffusion of water.[80,81] In traumatic brain injury, for example, DTI may reveal damage not visualized by other MRI sequences.[82,83] Magnetization transfer imaging (MTI) similarly may detect abnormal white-matter signal in regions not identified as abnormal by routine MRI sequences, for example, in multiple sclerosis or traumatic brain injury.[80,84] DTI and MTI are not universally available to psychiatric inpatients and do not at present have a defined role in their evaluation.

FUNCTIONAL NEUROIMAGING

Three modalities of functional neuroimaging are available to the clinician.[81] Single photon emission computed tomography (SPECT, also called *single-photon emission tomography*, or *SPET*, in the United Kingdom) relies on the distribution of a radionuclide tracer to identify areas of overperfusion or underperfusion and by inference hypo- or hypermetabolism. This inference rests on the assumption of tight coupling between metabolism and perfusion, a reasonable assumption in the normal brain though less solid in the damaged brain. The scan is usually performed a few hours after the injection, so this technology has the advantage that patients who are incapable of being scanned at a point of interest—such as because of movement during a seizure—can be injected at that point but scanned later when technically feasible. The resolution of SPECT is poor compared with the other functional modalities. The technique is not quantitative, that is, the abnormality of a given region must be inferred from comparison with other regions rather than from quantitative measures.

Positron emission tomography (PET) produces images of much better resolution in both time and space at the cost of considerably greater technical difficulty. An on-site cyclotron to generate isotopes is required. However, with the increased use of PET in oncology, the availability of the technology for neurodiagnostic purposes may increase. As with SPECT, PET uses the emission of radiation from injected sources to track blood flow, with metabolism inferred from perfusion by ^{15}O or directly measured with ^{18}F fluorodeoxyglucose. In addition, PET tracers are available that bind to receptors related to neurotransmitters, such as the dopamine transporter. The demonstration of an increased or decreased number of these sites is potentially useful in the differential diagnosis of degenerative basal ganglion disease, such as the parkinsonian syndromes.

The utility of SPECT and PET in psychiatric diagnosis is controversial. The evidence suggests that perfusion SPECT studies are helpful in identifying the temporoparietal hypometabolism of early Alzheimer disease, the frontotemporal hypometabolism of frontotemporal dementia, or the occipital hypometabolism of dementia with Lewy bodies (DLB), but evidence is scant for an incremental contribution by SPECT to diagnostic accuracy after utilization of other modes of evaluation. This situation may change with the advent of voxel-by-voxel analysis (rather than brute inspection) and the development and use of receptor ligands. SPECT imaging using a dopaminergic ligand to identify a subclinical lesion of the nigrostriatal system adds substantially to diagnostic accuracy in DLB and in the differential diagnosis of parkinsonian syndromes.[85,86]

The sensitivity of SPECT is not so much in question as its specificity, that is to say the correlation of SPECT abnormalities with clinical phenomena. For example, in patients with systemic lupus, SPECT findings may be abnormal in patients who have no clinical evidence of neuropsychiatric involvement.[87] Because SPECT abnormalities can be found in patients with idiopathic psychiatric disorders, such findings cannot be used to demonstrate an organic basis for patients' deficits. In general, the present authors' impression is that perfusion SPECT is of limited applicability in the neuropsychiatric evaluation of patients presenting with noncognitive psychological symptoms.

PET is generally considered to be useful in demonstrating lobar hypometabolism in frontotemporal dementia and is Medicare-approved for this indication, although again clear evidence of its value-added in dementia diagnosis is not available except perhaps in the situation of prediction of conversion to Alzheimer disease from mild cognitive impairment.[81] Although PET certainly has applications in epilepsy, and while its potential contribution to the understanding of the pathophysiology of idiopathic psychiatric syndromes is considerable, its utility in neuropsychiatric evaluation on the inpatient unit is limited.

Functional magnetic resonance imaging (fMRI) offers excellent spatial and temporal resolution along with the advantage of requiring no injection of radiotracer. As a research tool in the neurosciences, its future is bright. At present, no role of fMRI for psychiatric diagnosis is established.

Electrophysiologic Evaluation

EEG entails recording, through electrodes on the scalp, the spontaneous electrical rhythms of the brain and their alteration by simple probes, such as sleep, hyperventilation, and photic driving. The derived data can be processed to produce maps of brain activity. In addition, brain responses to stimuli, "event-related" or "evoked" potentials (EPs), can be recorded electrophysiologically.

EEG has utility in several situations on the inpatient unit. However, the EEG is not a suitable tool to screen for organic disease; it should be ordered only to answer a specific question raised by the clinical findings. Although some data suggest that nonspecific, nonepileptic EEG abnormalities carry prognostic significance in patients with idiopathic psychotic disorders,[88] in most settings the utility of such EEG data is limited.

One situation in which EEG data can be crucial is identifying an encephalopathic state as against an acute idiopathic psychosis, especially when the clinical features of delirium are equivocal. Under these circumstances, a slowed EEG has moderate sensitivity and very high specificity for organic disease.[89]

EEG is also a crucial diagnostic test in the patient suspected of having or known to have seizures. However, the diagnosis of epilepsy remains a clinical diagnosis, in that the sensitivity of the EEG for epilepsy is relatively low.[90] Very roughly, a single EEG recorded without sleep or sleep deprivation in a patient with epilepsy shows an epileptic abnormality only a third to a half of the time, and even after multiple EEG studies the sensitivity is <90%. The sensitivity is lowest in patients who have had only a single seizure or who have well-controlled or infrequent seizures. In as many as half the epileptic patients with a negative first EEG, epileptic abnormalities are detected when sleep is recorded or when the EEG is recorded after sleep deprivation. After the second or third EEG the additional yield of further EEGs is low. Therefore, a reasonable approach in inpatients whose history and examination raise the question of epilepsy is to obtain a routine EEG and, if this is unrevealing, to obtain an EEG after sleep deprivation and with a period of recording during sleep.

True epileptiform abnormalities in the EEG are rare in healthy subjects, so that an EEG accurately read as showing spikes is highly specific for epilepsy. However, over-reading (i.e., misreading) of the EEG is not rare, including the overinterpretation of patterns once thought to be associated with psychopathology but now construed by most experts as normal variants (such as 14 and 6 per second positive spikes).[91] The inpatient psychiatrist must cast a critical diagnostic eye on EEG reports said to implicate epilepsy as the cause of behavioral abnormalities, especially if the clinical picture is equivocal or not suggestive.

Quantitative electroencephalography (QEEG) is a tool beset with methodological problems. Despite an extensive research database, some of which demonstrates statistically significant power of QEEG to discriminate between diagnostic categories, unequivocal evidence that QEEG adds to discriminations that can be made by other means is lacking.[92] In the authors' view, QEEG remains largely a research tool at present, albeit in some respects a promising one.[93,94]

Magnetoencephalography, the recording of magnetic fields rather than electrical fields, has great promise but, in the authors' view, little if any current utility in inpatient psychiatry, except insofar as it plays a role in the evaluation of epilepsy.[95,96] Recording directly from the cortex or deep structures is beyond the scope of this chapter.

Evaluation of the peripheral nervous system by electromyography and nerve conduction studies plays an occasional role in neuropsychiatric diagnosis. For example, peripheral neuropathy is a feature of some disorders that also involve the central nervous system, such as metachromatic leukodystrophy, acute intermittent porphyria, and cobalamin deficiency.

Polysomnography (PSG) interrogates brain activity and the function of multiple other body systems in the course of overnight sleep. It is crucial in the diagnosis of many sleep disorders, including sleep apnea, which is highly prevalent and psychiatrically significant (along with having substantial cardiovascular consequences), as is discussed in Chapter 4. Sleep-disordered breathing is common in patients with depression and appears to contribute to depressive symptom severity. It also is a potentially remediable cause of worsened cognitive function in patients with dementing disorders. Sleep apnea often is suspected because of a bed partner's report of altered breathing patterns or snoring, but in the inpatient environment such observations can and should be made by night nurses. Nocturnal disturbed behavior may represent rapid eye movement sleep behavior disorder (RBD), which can be caused by antidepressants but which when idiopathic commonly is associated with a progressive synucleinopathy, for example, DLB.[97] Because DLB can present with psychotic or mood symptoms in advance of parkinsonism, the additional presence of RBD can be an important clinical clue for the psychiatrist. PSG (and the properly trained polysomnographer to interpret the study) would ideally be available to inpatient units to pursue such clinical suspicions during the admission.

Examination of the Cerebrospinal Fluid

Examination of the CSF should be undertaken only in selected circumstances on the psychiatric unit, but in those circumstances it provides crucial information.

One such situation is the acutely psychotic or delirious patient, especially if febrile, in whom infectious disease is suggested by the history and examination. If, for example, herpes simplex virus encephalitis (HSVE) cannot be excluded by the history and examination, the patient should have lumbar puncture and examination of the CSF for the HSV genome by polymerase chain reaction (and should be treated for presumptive HSVE while the result is pending). Similar considerations apply in the immunocompromised patient, where the index of suspicion for infection must be high, even in the absence of typical signs such as fever and leukocytosis.

Another circumstance in which CSF examination is relevant is the patient with a positive syphilis serology (discussed in Chapter 4). If active neurosyphilis is under diagnostic consideration, the CSF yields crucial information that determines whether treatment should be for latent or active syphilis, which require different antibiotic regimens.

Case Vignette

A middle-aged construction worker was laid off because of aberrant behavior. Cognitive impairment was evident when he tried to resume work. A neurologist performed blood tests and diagnosed syphilis; the patient was treated with three injections of benzathine penicillin. His cognitive impairment progressed, and he became agitated and psychotic. He was admitted psychiatrically and treated with several psychotropic drugs. His psychiatric symptoms eased, but he remained severely cognitively impaired. He was eventually referred to an infectious disease specialist, who performed a lumbar puncture and prescribed a course of intravenous penicillin some 8 months after the original treatment for syphilis. His cognitive decline stabilized but was not ameliorated.

In the patient with systemic autoimmune disease, CSF examination is a crucial part of the workup for brain involvement.[98] Of particular importance in this situation is measurement of CSF immunoglobulins (Igs) with calculation of the IgG index; an elevated IgG index and the presence of oligoclonal bands indicate intrathecal synthesis of Igs. CSF examination is not routinely required in the differential diagnosis of dementia, but in the young or atypical case or if consideration of neoplastic or infectious origin is suggested by the history, the threshold should be low for lumbar puncture.

Measurement of putative biomarkers for Alzheimer disease in CSF is currently controversial but promising in the differential diagnosis of degenerative dementia and the prediction of decline in patients with mild cognitive impairment or the healthy elderly.[99,100]

Metabolic Testing

Late adolescence and early adulthood—the characteristic age of onset of the idiopathic psychotic disorders—also is a period during which certain uncommon diseases, many generally thought of as pediatric diseases with a late onset, can appear.[101–103] Some of these are metabolic disorders in which the pathophysiology is well established, the gene known, the diagnostic test specific, and—in some crucial cases—specific treatment effective. For example, Wilson disease must not be missed, because treatment is highly effective and the untreated outcome disastrous. Although these disorders feature cognitive and sensorimotor dysfunction, at times the psychiatric symptoms can be the leading edge of the clinical picture. The clinician must be alert for the (at times) less prominent motor and cognitive symptoms and use them as a clue to disease diagnosis and a guide to the diagnostic strategy. A few of the relevant disorders are tabulated in Table 5.2.

Genetic Testing

Genetic testing on the inpatient psychiatric unit is useful only in a few situations. As discussed in Chapter 3, commercially available pharmacogenetic tests may be helpful in guiding therapy under certain circumstances. Despite the advances in psychiatric genetics, genetic testing is not helpful diagnostically in the major idiopathic psychiatric illnesses. The genetic approach to the developmentally disabled patient is discussed in a later section of this chapter.

Genetic testing is occasionally definitive in the evaluation of a dementing patient. Identifying the triplet-repeat expansion of Huntington disease is the best-known example. Other dementing disorders diagnosable by available genetic tests include familial forms of prion disease and cerebral autosomal dominant arteriopathy with subcortical infarctions and leukoencephalopathy (CADASIL). Mitochondrial disorders can also be diagnosed genetically, and these can rarely present psychiatrically.[104] Deafness, short stature, diabetes, and myopathy are other features that may be present in patients with mitochondrial disorders and provoke consideration of genetic testing. Although genetic abnormalities

TABLE 5.2 SELECTED METABOLIC DISORDERS THAT CAN PRESENT PSYCHIATRICALLY

Disease	Psychiatric Manifestations (Cognitive Impairment and Personality Change Possible in all)	Nonpsychiatric Manifestations	Key Diagnostic Test (Genetic Tests Available for Some)
Adrenoleukodystrophy	Psychosis, mood disorder	Pyramidal signs, peripheral neuropathy, visual loss, endocrinopathy	Very long-chain fatty acids
Cerebrotendinous xanthomatosis	Psychosis	Cerebellar and pyramidal signs, peripheral neuropathy, cataracts, diarrhea	Cholestanol
Homocystinuria	Psychosis, depression	Stroke, mild developmental disability, marfanoid habitus, ectopia lentis	Plasma amino acids
GM2 gangliosidosis (adult Tay-Sachs disease)	Mood disorder, psychosis	Pyramidal and cerebellar signs, lower motor neuron signs	Hexosaminidase A
Metachromatic leukodystrophy	Schizophrenia	Peripheral neuropathy, cerebellar, and pyramidal signs	Arylsulfatase A
Neimann-Pick type C	Psychosis, mood disorder	Ataxia, movement disorder, vertical supranuclear ophthalmoplegia	Cholesterol studies in cultured fibroblasts, sea-blue histiocytes in bone marrow
Neuronal ceroid lipofuscinosis (Kufs disease when adolescent onset)	Depression	Extrapyramidal and cerebellar signs	Electromicroscopy of skin, rectal, or brain tissue for lipofuscin deposits
Porphyria (acute intermittent and variegate)	Delirium	Peripheral neuropathy, abdominal pain	Urine porphobilinogen during attack
Wilson disease	Psychosis (rare)	Movement disorder, Kayser-Fleischer rings, liver disease	Urinary copper excretion, serum ceruloplasmin

have been recognized in the frontotemporal dementias, these tests are not yet widely available. Assessing the apolipoprotein E status of a dementing patient suspected of Alzheimer disease is not currently recommended,[105] although developments in analysis of CSF amyloid and tau protein may lead to additive diagnostic value for apolipoprotein E testing, as mentioned earlier. The Fragile X premutation can present with mood and anxiety symptoms and with executive dysfunction in midlife.[106]

Neuropsychological Assessment

Neuropsychological assessment has the capacity to make precise quantitative determinations of cognitive function across the entire array of domains. In the hands of an expert neuropsychologist, this information can be used to assist with diagnosis, identify areas of impairment of independent functioning, and facilitate communication with patients and their families about matters that are often hard to discuss. The assistance the neuropsychologist can lend to conveying the patient's diagnosis and deficits to the family (often in conjunction with an occupational therapist who has evaluated the patient's skills in activities of daily living) can be of special importance with a family that is struggling to understand a newly impaired family member and to figure out what the family must do to help after discharge. Sometimes families have previously been told a diagnosis of idiopathic psychosis or mood disorder and have to reorganize their thinking when a brain disease diagnosis is made; some of these families do not easily accept the clinician's presentation of a new diagnosis. In such situations, the neuropsychological data can be very helpful.

The neuropsychologist should be regarded by the inpatient psychiatrist as a valuable potential consultant, and the neuropsychological report should be considered the response to a consultation. One implication of this view is that—as neuropsychologists always tell their consultees—the more precise the consultation question posed to the neuropsychologist, the more useful the consultation.[107]

However, for a number of reasons neuropsychological evaluations cannot replace bedside evaluations and can be used only in selected circumstances in the inpatient setting. First, neuropsychological assessment is time consuming and expensive. It cannot be used routinely. Second, the extensive data obtained by neuropsychological testing are most valuable when the patient is behaviorally stable. Data representing one point on a rapidly varying course may be impossible to interpret or misleading. The test data often are most useful if obtained when the patient is at his or her best. For example, in a patient whose cognitive state may arise partly from depression and partly from subcortical vascular disease—a common clinical situation—the neuropsychologist may be as unable as anyone else to predict how much is which; only treating the depression and testing the patient later will answer the question. Although at times the data may strongly suggest a particular organic diagnosis (such as Alzheimer disease in a depressed patient), at least as often the presence of psychiatric symptoms will confound the consultant just as it confounds the consultee. The neuropsychological data, like all medical test data, must be seen in the context of a clinical situation that the directly responsible clinician should know best. Despite the great value of neuropsychological data, the neuropsychological consultant cannot be expected, alone, to answer the question of whether organic disease is present.

Clinical Contexts

FIRST-EPISODE PSYCHOSIS

A rational strategy on evidence-based principles for ruling out organic disease in first-episode psychosis has yet to be constructed. One reason is that—surprisingly, considering how common and important the issue is—few data are available to allow an estimate of the incidence of organic disease in this population. One frequently quoted study found 15 cases (5.6%) due to organic disease among 268 patients with a first episode of psychosis.[108] However, the population studied was composed of patients referred by other psychiatrists, who may well have avoided referring patients whom they suspected or knew to have organic disease, and the study protocol did not include a systematic screen for organic disease. Indeed, to the authors' knowledge there is no study of consecutive cases with first-episode psychosis with all cases subjected to a standard battery of investigations including contemporary neuroimaging.

This dearth of evidence has allowed some authors to recommend an extensive battery of tests for all patients with a first episode of psychosis.[109] However, assessing very long chain fatty acids in all first-episode patients, for example—as Coleman and Gillberg recommended among many other tests on the grounds that some of the rare cases of late-onset encephalopathic adrenoleukodystrophy have been reported to show schizophrenia-like manifestations—seems not only a prescription for wild goose chases but also unnecessary if the patient has normal white matter on MRI, which would seem on the face of it a much more reasonable screening test. Even a highly specific test will produce a high rate of false positives if the disease being tested for is sufficiently uncommon in the population. For this reason alone, a more rational screening strategy is appropriate. In addition, cost and the risk of deflection of attention from the patient's psychosocial predicament argue for a more sparing strategy.

As discussed in the previous chapter, a simple battery of laboratory tests is reasonable for all admissions, and the first-episode patient is not an exception. Therefore, such patients should have a complete blood count, a chemistry panel (including fasting glucose, electrolytes, renal function tests, creatine kinase, liver enzymes, and albumin), a lipid panel, thyrotropin and free thyroxine, cobalamin, a serum pregnancy test in women of reproductive potential, and urine toxicology. The diagnostician should have a low threshold for testing for syphilis, HIV, hepatitis C, and tuberculosis. All these tests, however, are more likely to reveal concurrent than causal conditions. Other testing should be chosen on the basis of an attentive history, physical examination, and cognitive examination. By "attentive" the present authors mean that the diagnostician must be familiar with the diseases that can present as psychosis.[110]

Some metabolic disorders that can present psychiatrically and that are susceptible to diagnosis by specific testing were discussed earlier. Disorders known to present with psychosis include homocystinuria, metachromatic leukodystrophy, adrenoleukodystrophy, cerebrotendinous xanthomatosis, GM2 gangliosidosis, and (rarely) Wilson disease.

The use of EEG for screening purposes is inappropriate; EEG should be obtained only if epilepsy or delirium is under consideration. In the authors' view, patients with a new psychotic illness should have neuroimaging, by preference MRI, early in their course, although the present authors recognize that data to support the recommendation are not compelling. From an expert review, the National Institute for Clinical Excellence in the United Kingdom came to the opposite conclusion, namely that imaging should be obtained only when specifically indicated by the history and examination, while the reviewers acknowledged that the studies generally did not precisely address the question at hand (see http://www.guideline.gov/summary/summary.aspx?doc_id=12284 .uk/GuidelinesFinder/ViewResource.aspx?resID=280852). However, these reviewers estimated that MRI would influence management in 5% of cases. Given the difference in availability of MRI between the United Kingdom and the United States and the gravity of the situation, this appears in the American environment sufficient reason to obtain MRI routinely. However, in the absence of indications to the contrary from the history and examination, imaging is not urgently necessary, and often deferring the test until the patient is behaviorally more stable than during the initial admission is the wisest course.

CATATONIA

Catatonia is a behavioral syndrome with mutism and markedly reduced motor activity as its key features, although definitions vary and by some definitions neither is essential for its diagnosis.[4] Other motor and behavioral features include stereotypies, grimacing, echophenomena, catalepsy (waxy flexibility or posturing), and negativism. If reduced motor activity is absent—the excited form of catatonia—then these features become necessary for the diagnosis. Whether the additional presence of such distinctive elements of the catatonic syndrome has differential diagnostic implications—for example, makes an organic etiology more or less likely—is not established. The syndrome is best understood as a final common pathway of dysfunction that can occur with various etiological factors, much as delirium is understood; by no means should catatonia be equated to a form of schizophrenia (indeed mood disorder is the more common correlate) or associated solely with idiopathic psychiatric disorders. Catatonic symptoms arise commonly in Tourette syndrome and autism spectrum disorders.[111,112] A broad range of organic etiologies should be considered in the catatonic patient, including metabolic abnormalities, infection, inflammatory disease (such as cerebral lupus), drug toxicity (including neuroleptics and the neuroleptic malignant syndrome as well as serotonergic drugs and the serotonin syndrome), drug withdrawal (especially from benzodiazepines or dopaminergic agents), and hydrocephalus.

Case Vignette

A middle-aged woman was transferred to an academic medical center psychiatric unit from a community hospital psychiatric unit so that she could be treated with electroconvulsive therapy (ECT) for catatonia. The history included past diagnoses of depression with suicide attempts and of polysubstance abuse. She had recently been out of town and was reported by her family, with details unknown to them, to have been using heroin. She had presented to a community hospital ER confused and been admitted to a medical service, where a limited workup including CT but not MRI had been unrevealing. She was then transferred to a psychiatric unit, where the psychiatrist understood that she had been "medically cleared."

(continued)

By that time she had lapsed into a minimally mobile and minimally communicative state; she was described as moving her lips as if talking to herself and giggling occasionally. She failed to respond to benzodiazepines over the course of a week.

Initial examination at the university hospital revealed tachycardia, tachypnea, and fever. She was mute but appeared awake; she appeared to look at the examiner but did not respond to commands. The neurologic examination showed spasticity but no other abnormalities. Further neuropsychiatric evaluation was delayed when immediate workup of her abnormal vital signs led to laparotomy for an acute abdomen, due to a perforated sigmoid thought to have occurred during the colonoscopy she underwent at the referring hospital. However, when MRI was feasible, it disclosed extensive white-matter hypersignal (see Fig. 5.2). EEG showed generalized slowing. The final diagnosis was heroin-induced leukoencephalopathy.[113] She gradually improved over the course of weeks.

Catatonic features are common in psychiatric inpatients: Taylor and Fink estimated that 10% of patients meet criteria for catatonia during a psychiatric admission,[114] a perhaps surprisingly high estimate but one broadly confirmed by subsequent data.[115] The relative frequency of idiopathic and secondary catatonia is not well established. In an important study from an English district general hospital—the authors claimed that their population represented an epidemiologically valid sample—25 catatonic patients were consecutively identified, of whom 5 (20%) had an organic cause.[116] The presence of previous remitting episodes of catatonia is obviously reassuring as regards an organic diagnosis, but of course relapsing and remitting metabolic disorders also exist. All patients should be examined for the presence of signs (systemic and cerebral) not attributable to the catatonic state. In a patient with a first episode of catatonia, laboratory screening for potential metabolic or infectious causes should be undertaken. Ammonia, plasma amino acids, and urinary organic acids are straightforward tests if a urea cycle or other metabolic disorder is suspected.[103,117] Using the EEG to screen for encephalopathy in this setting is reasonable, as is obtaining MRI in patients with a first episode of catatonia. Any suggestion of an infectious cause should lead to examination of the CSF.

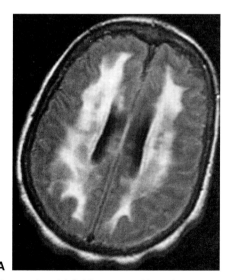 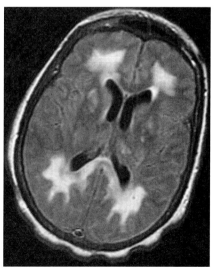

A   B

■ **Figure 5.2** Axial fluid attenuated inversion recovery-magnetic resonance imaging (FLAIR-MRI) at two levels disclosing extensive leukoencephalopathy.

Management of catatonia requires close attention to supportive care. Patients are at risk of dehydration, deep venous thrombosis with pulmonary embolus, aspiration, and other potentially life-threatening complications of immobility and impaired oral intake. These issues are discussed further in Chapter 4. Because both dehydration and catatonia itself are risk factors for neuroleptic malignant syndrome (which some see as a lethal variant of catatonia),[114] antipsychotic drugs should be used in catatonic patients only with great caution. Pharmacologic treatment of catatonia starts with parenteral benzodiazepines, for example lorazepam 1 to 2 mg IM q8 h. This approach is often strikingly successful after the first dose. If it is unsuccessful, ECT remains likely to be effective, although obtaining consent or court permission to act without consent may be a substantial obstacle to the use of this treatment in this setting (see Chapters 7 and 10). Other proposed pharmacologic approaches include amantadine, memantine, divalproex, topiramate, and second-generation antipsychotics.[118,119]

LATE-ONSET DEPRESSION OR PSYCHOSIS

The occurrence of late-onset forms of idiopathic mental disorders is well established. For example, schizophrenia with a genetic basis and clinical manifestations similar to those in late-adolescent onset cases can develop in midlife and afterward.[120] The present authors are not aware of a study in which an epidemiologically valid sample of patients presenting with depression or psychosis with onset in midlife or late life was subjected to a standard and comprehensive evaluation to allow an estimate of the prevalence of causative organic disease in an unselected population. Nonetheless, it is a reasonable clinical operating principle to have a higher suspicion of organic causation in patients with late-onset psychiatric disorders, even if the other clinical features of the disorder are not obviously organic.

On this principle, the evaluation should be more comprehensive in the patient with a late-onset syndrome. Beyond the history and examination, patients presenting with late-onset depression as well as psychosis should routinely undergo neuroimaging, by preference with unenhanced MRI (unless findings in the history and examination suggest otherwise). In addition, laboratory studies for metabolic disorders such as hypothyroidism and cobalamin deficiency should be carefully scrutinized.

The most common finding in the MRI of patients with late-onset depression is undoubtedly white-matter disease, so-called leukoaraiosis, often referred to by radiologists presumptively as *small-vessel disease*. Interpretation of the relationship of this finding to depression has been controversial. Despite negative studies, a review of the evidence suggests that white-matter disease is causatively associated with late-onset depression (although causation in the opposite direction may well also exist).[121] This "vascular depression" may have clinical differences from its idiopathic counterpart, of which the most important neuropsychiatrically is the presence of executive dysfunction. In addition, gait disorder (the lower-half parkinsonism described earlier) and incontinence are features of this condition.[122] The prognosis for these patients is poorer than for those without abnormal imaging results; the depression is more treatment resistant and liable to relapse. Late-life depression is discussed further in Chapter 16.

DEVELOPMENTAL DISABILITIES

The psychiatric evaluation of adult patients with developmental disabilities is described in Chapter 17. Whether, and how, to evaluate such adult patients for an etiology of the disability is not well established. It seems highly likely that the yield in adulthood of investigation for etiology would be lower than in childhood, many of the diagnosable cases having been diagnosed over time. On the other hand, many patients presenting to a psychiatric service in adulthood have never had a thorough evaluation for the cause of developmental disability. The evaluation in childhood depends in large part on the recognition of syndromal features of known disorders, such as the fetal alcohol syndrome, fragile X syndrome, Down syndrome, and so on.[123] It is widely accepted that children should additionally undergo MRI and chromosomal studies, including molecular-genetic studies and probes for subtelomeric deletions as indicated clinically.[123,124] A history of obstetric complications, while relevant to the assessment, should not preclude genetic studies, because those complications may themselves be a consequence of preexisting genetic abnormalities.

Bodensteiner and Schaffer argued that similar principles apply to adults: adults as well should have a neuroimaging study, by preference MRI, and chromosomal analysis, along with specific molecular genetic tests as suggested by the clinical findings.[125] Others might argue that arriving at an etiologic diagnosis in such patients is irrelevant to psychiatric management. Probably evaluation should be individualized and the decision shared with responsible family members. At times, however, the genetic workup may yield information that is of substantial significance to the understanding of the case.

Case Vignette

A woman aged 21 was referred for evaluation of psychosis. Her mother reported that she had been developmentally normal until an ear infection at age 7, at which time she had undergone brain surgery. Subsequently she required special education. In high school she developed auditory hallucinations, delusions, social withdrawal, and odd behavior; she was treated with antipsychotic drugs with limited benefit. The mother reported that she had been declining in function for several weeks. In the outpatient consultation, she held her head in her hands and was nearly mute. Her mother explained that she acted this way when she had severe headaches, which had begun 5 months earlier. The neurologic examination was limited because of incomplete cooperation. The fundi could not be visualized. She showed stereotypies of her upper extremities but no pyramidal, extrapyramidal, or cerebellar deficits. Urgent CT did not disclose a space-occupying lesion or evidence of increased intracranial pressure—or evidence of past craniotomy. Subsequent MRI disclosed dysgenesis of the left temporal lobe and a large cavum of the septum pellucidum (see Fig. 5.3). Chromosomal analysis showed a 22q11.12 deletion, well known to be associated with psychosis.[126] The developmental history as provided was concluded to be spurious. On follow-up she displayed a severe, treatment-resistant schizophrenic illness and at no time complained of headache.

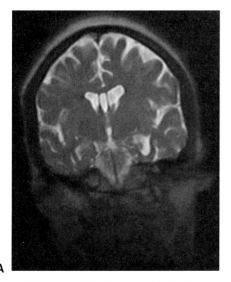 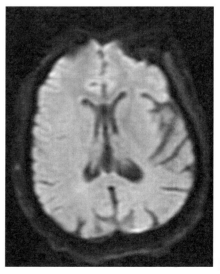

A   B

■ **Figure 5.3** Coronal T2 **(A)** and axial fluid attenuated inversion recovery (FLAIR) **(B)** magnetic resonance (MR) images. Note the enlarged left temporal horn in **(A)** and the abnormal left temporal sulcal pattern in **(B)**. Both images show the cavum of the septum pellucidum.

Autism is associated with a wide variety of disorders notably including tuberous sclerosis and fragile X syndrome. Epilepsy occurs in one third or more of persons with autism and should be considered as a cause of mental or behavioral disturbances in this population.[127] Asperger syndrome or high-functioning autism should be considered in patients with apparent personality abnormalities (notably in the schizoid realm) especially in conjunction with Tourette syndrome, obsessive compulsive disorder, and bipolar disorder.

Conclusions

The experienced and knowledgeable psychiatrist can recognize atypical aspects of the patient's history or mental state, such as an unusual age of onset or the lack of a family history of mental disorder when such would be expected; these should suggest a more thorough evaluation for organic disease. However, the psychiatrist must realize that organic mental disorders can closely resemble their idiopathic counterparts, with no striking or distinctive phenomenologic clues to their organic origin. Further, a normal elemental neurologic examination does not exclude disease in limbic, paralimbic, or prefrontal regions; the clinical picture with disease in these regions may be limited to cognitive and behavioral alterations. Similarly, negative studies on brain imaging, EEG, and routine laboratory tests do not always exclude organic causes of psychiatric symptoms. Finally, treatment response is similar for idiopathic and organic symptoms, so organic disease is not excluded by an expectable response to pharmacotherapy.

In summary, only thoughtful consideration and integration of all the data can allow the clinician to make a confident diagnosis as regards organic causation of psychopathology. It has been emphasized in this chapter that the diagnostic process rests crucially on a history, cognitive examination, and physical examination performed by a clinician familiar with the mental and behavioral manifestations of brain disease. On this solid foundation, the growing neuroscientific laboratory armamentarium can be brought to bear for the benefit of the psychiatrically ill.

REFERENCES

1. Spitzer RL, First MB, Williams JB, et al. Now is the time to retire the term "organic mental disorders". *Am J Psychiatry*. 1992;149(2):240–244.
2. Spitzer RL, Williams JB, First M, et al. A proposal for DSM-IV: Solving the "organic/nonorganic" problem. *J Neuropsychiatry Clin Neurosci*. 1989;1(2):126–127.
3. Ovsiew F. Neuropsychiatric approach to the patient. In: Sadock BJ, Sadock VA, eds. *Comprehensive textbook of psychiatry*, 9th ed. Philadelphia: Lippincott Williams & Wilkins; in press.
4. Ovsiew F. Bedside neuropsychiatry: eliciting the clinical phenomena of neuropsychiatric illness. In: Yudofsky SC, Hales RE, eds. *American psychiatric publishing textbook of neuropsychiatry and behavioral neurosciences*. Washington, DC: American Psychiatric Publishing; 2007:137–187.
5. Ovsiew F. Taking the history in behavioral neurology and neuropsychiatry. In: Arciniegas D, Anderson CA, Filley C, eds. *Behavioral neurology and neuropsychiatry*. Cambridge, UK: Cambridge University Press; in press.
6. Verdoux H, Sutter AL. Perinatal risk factors for schizophrenia: Diagnostic specificity and relationships with maternal psychopathology. *Am J Med Genet*. 2002;114(8):898–905.
7. Rantakallio P, Jones P, Moring J, et al. Association between central nervous system infections during childhood and adult onset schizophrenia and other psychoses: A 28-year follow-up. *Int J Epidemiol*. 1997;26(4):837–843.
8. Franzek EJ, Sprangers N, Janssens ACJW, et al. Prenatal exposure to the 1944–45 Dutch 'hunger winter' and addiction later in life. *Addiction*. 2008;103(3):433–438.
9. Kim E, Lauterbach EC, Reeve A, et al. Neuropsychiatric complications of traumatic brain injury: A critical review of the literature (a report by the ANPA Committee on Research). *J Neuropsychiatry Clin Neurosci*. 2007;19(2):106–127.
10. Rosenbaum A, Hoge SK, Adelman SA, et al. Head injury in partner-abusive men. *J Consult Clin Psychol*. 1994;62(6):1187–1193.
11. Streeter CC, Van Reekum R, Shorr RI, et al. Prior head injury in male veterans with borderline personality disorder. *J Nerv Ment Dis*. 1995;183(9):577–581.
12. Pascalicchio TF, de Araujo Filho GM, da Silva Noffs MH, et al. Neuropsychological profile of patients with juvenile myoclonic epilepsy: A controlled study of 50 patients. *Epilepsy Behav*. 2007;10(2):263–267.
13. Trinka E, Kienpointner G, Unterberger I, et al. Psychiatric comorbidity in juvenile

myoclonic epilepsy. *Epilepsia.* 2006;47(12): 2086–2091.

14. Blumer D. Evidence supporting the temporal lobe epilepsy personality syndrome. *Neurology.* 1999;53(5 Suppl 2):S9–12.

15. Devinsky O, Najjar S. Evidence against the existence of a temporal lobe epilepsy personality syndrome. *Neurology.* 1999;53(5 Suppl 2): S13–S25.

16. Habib M. Athymhormia and disorders of motivation in basal ganglia disease. *J Neuropsychiatry Clin Neurosci.* 2004;16(4):509–524.

17. Razvi SSM, Bone I. Draw a pedigree during the neurological consultation. *Pract Neurol.* 2005; 5(1):38–45.

18. Heimer L. *Anatomy of neuropsychiatry: the new anatomy of the basal forebrain and its implications for neuropsychiatric illness.* Amsterdam: Boston Academic Press/Elsevier Science; 2008.

19. Mesulam MM. From sensation to cognition. *Brain.* 1998;121(Pt 6):1013–1052.

20. Hodges JR. *Cognitive assessment for clinicians,* 2nd ed. Oxford, New York: Oxford University Press; 2007.

21. Leopold NA, Borson AJ. An alphabetical 'WORLD'. A new version of an old test. *Neurology.* 1997;49(6):1521–1524.

22. Rohrer JD, Knight WD, Warren JE, et al. Word-finding difficulty: A clinical analysis of the progressive aphasias. *Brain.* 2008; 131(1):8–38.

23. Alexander MP. Aphasia I: Clinical and anatomic issues. In: Farah MJ, Feinberg TE, eds. *Patient-based approaches to cognitive neuroscience.* Cambridge: MIT Press; 2006:181–198.

24. Geschwind N. Disorders of attention: A frontier in neuropsychology. *Philos Trans R Soc Lond B Biol Sci.* 1982;298(1089):173–185.

25. Cutting J. The phenomenology of acute organic psychosis. Comparison with acute schizophrenia. *Br J Psychiatry.* 1987;151(3):324–332.

26. Budson AE, Price BH. Memory dysfunction. *N Engl J Med.* 2005;352(7):692–699.

27. Ross ED. The aprosodias. In: Farah MJ, Feinberg TE, eds. *Case-based approaches to cognitive neuroscience.* Cambridge: MIT Press; 2006:259–269.

28. Cullen B, O'Neill B, Evans JJ, et al. A review of screening tests for cognitive impairment. *J Neurol Neurosurg Psychiatry.* 2007;78(8): 790–799.

29. Ridha B, Rossor M. The mini mental state examination. *Pract Neurol.* 2005;5(5):298–303.

30. Malloy PF, Cummings JL, Coffey CE, et al. Cognitive screening instruments in neuropsychiatry: A report of the Committee on Research of the American Neuropsychiatric Association. *J Neuropsychiatry Clin Neurosci.* 1997;9(2):189–197.

31. Mahoney R, Johnston K, Katona C, et al. The TE4D-Cog: A new test for detecting early

dementia in English-speaking populations. *Int J Geriatr Psychiatry.* 2005;20(12):1172–1179.

32. Borson S, Scanlan J, Brush M, et al. The mini-cog: A cognitive 'vital signs' measure for dementia screening in multilingual elderly. *Int J Geriatr Psychiatry.* 2000;15(11):1021–1027.

33. Power C, Selnes OA, Grim JA, et al. HIV dementia scale: A rapid screening test. *J Acquir Immune Defic Syndr Hum Retrovirol.* 1995;8(3):273–278.

34. van Harten B, Courant MN, Scheltens P, et al. Validation of the HIV dementia scale in an elderly cohort of patients with subcortical cognitive impairment caused by subcortical ischaemic vascular disease or a normal pressure hydrocephalus. *Dement Geriatr Cogn Disord.* 2004;18(1):109–114.

35. Mioshi E, Dawson K, Mitchell J, et al. The Addenbrooke's Cognitive Examination Revised (ACE-R): A brief cognitive test battery for dementia screening. *Int J Geriatr Psychiatry.* 2006;21(11):1078–1085.

36. Fuzikawa C, Lima-Costa MF, Uchoa E, et al. A population based study on the intra and inter-rater reliability of the clock drawing test in Brazil: The Bambui Health and Ageing Study. *Int J Geriatr Psychiatry.* 2003;18(5):450–456.

37. Juby A, Tench S, Baker V. The value of clock drawing in identifying executive cognitive dysfunction in people with a normal mini-mental state examination score. *CMAJ.* 2002;167(8):859–864.

38. Shulman KI. Clock-drawing: Is it the ideal cognitive screening test? *Int J Geriatr Psychiatry.* 2000;15(6):548–561.

39. Stuss DT, Alexander MP. Is there a dysexecutive syndrome? *Philos Trans R Soc Lond B Biol Sci.* 2007;362(1481):901–915.

40. Billick SB, Siedenburg E, Burgert W, et al. Validation of the mental alternation test with the mini-mental state examination in geriatric psychiatric inpatients and normal controls. *Compr Psychiatry.* 2001;42(3):202–205.

41. Salib E, McCarthy J. Mental Alternation Test (MAT): A rapid and valid screening tool for dementia in primary care. *Int J Geriatr Psychiatry.* 2002;17(12):1157–1161.

42. Grigsby J, Kaye K. Alphanumeric sequencing and cognitive impairment among elderly persons. *Percept Mot Skills.* 1995;80:732–734.

43. Grigsby J, Kaye K, Busenbark D. Alphanumeric sequencing: A report on a brief measure of information processing used among persons with multiple sclerosis. *Percept Mot Skills.* 1994;78:883–887.

44. Jones BN, Teng EL, Folstein MF, et al. A new bedside test of cognition for patients with HIV infection. *Ann Intern Med.* 1993; 119:1001–1004.

45. Rothlind JC, Brandt J. A brief assessment of frontal and subcortical functions in dementia. *J Neuropsychiatry Clin Neurosci.* 1993;5(1): 73–77.

46. Dubois B, Slachevsky A, Litvan I, et al. The FAB: A frontal assessment battery at bedside. *Neurology.* 2000;55:1621–1626.

47. Grigsby J, Kaye K, Robbins LJ. Reliabilities, norms and factor structure of the Behavioral Dyscontrol Scale. *Percept Mot Skills.* 1992; 74(3 Pt 1):883–892.

48. Royall DR, Mahurin RK, Gray KF. Bedside assessment of executive cognitive impairment: The executive interview. *J Am Geriatr Soc.* 1992;40:1221–1226.

49. Tsoi T, Baillon S, Lindesay J. Early frontal executive impairment as a predictor of subsequent behavior disturbance in dementia. *Am J Geriatr Psychiatry.* 2008;16(2):102–108.

50. Royall DR, Chiodo LK, Polk MJ. An empiric approach to level of care determinations: The importance of executive measures. *J Gerontol A Biol Sci Med Sci.* 2005;60(8):1059–1064.

51. Katz N, Tadmor I, Felzen B, et al. The Behavioural Assessment of the Dysexecutive Syndrome (BADS) in schizophrenia and its relation to functional outcomes. *Neuropsychol Rehabil.* 2007;17(2):192–205.

52. Aleman A, Agrawal N, Morgan KD, et al. Insight in psychosis and neuropsychological function: Meta-analysis. *Br J Psychiatry.* 2006; 189(3):204–212.

53. Alexopoulos GS, Kiosses DN, Heo M, et al. Executive dysfunction and the course of geriatric depression. *Biol Psychiatry.* 2005; 58(3):204–210.

54. Goldberg E, Bougakov D. Neuropsychologic assessment of frontal lobe dysfunction. *Psychiatr Clin North Am.* 2005;28(3):567–580.

55. Glick TH. Toward a more efficient and effective neurologic examination for the 21st century. *Eur J Neurol.* 2005;12(12):994–997.

56. Murray E, Price BH. The neurological examination. In: Stern TA, Rosenbaum JF, Fava M, et al. eds. *Massachusetts general hospital comprehensive clinical psychiatry*, 1st ed. Philadelphia: Mosby, Elsevier Science; 2008.

57. Yoshitsugu K, Yamada K, Toyota T, et al. A novel scale including strabismus and 'cuspidal ear' for distinguishing schizophrenia patients from controls using minor physical anomalies. *Psychiatry Res.* 2006;145(2–3):249–258.

58. Waddington JL, Brown AS, Lane A, et al. Congenital anomalies and early functional impairments in a prospective birth cohort: Risk of schizophrenia-spectrum disorder in adulthood. *Br J Psychiatry.* 2008;192(4):264–267.

59. Lloyd T, Dazzan P, Dean K, et al. Minor physical anomalies in patients with first-episode psychosis: Their frequency and diagnostic specificity. *Psychol Med.* 2008;38(1):71–77.

60. Sechi G, Serra A. Wernicke's encephalopathy: New clinical settings and recent advances in diagnosis and management. *Lancet Neurol.* 2007;6(5):442–455.

61. Jacob A, Cherian PJ, Radhakrishnan K, et al. Emotional facial paresis in temporal lobe epilepsy: Its prevalence and lateralizing value. *Seizure.* 2003;12(1):60–64.

62. Lin K, Carrete H, Lin J, et al. Facial paresis in patients with mesial temporal sclerosis: Clinical and quantitative MRI-based evidence of widespread disease. *Epilepsia.* 2007; 48(8):1491–1499.

63. Weaver DF. A clinical examination technique for mild upper motor neuron paresis of the arm. *Neurology.* 2000;54(2):531–532.

64. Teitelbaum JS, Eliasziw M, Garner M. Tests of motor function in patients suspected of having mild unilateral cerebral lesions. *Can J Neurol Sci.* 2002;29(4):337–344.

65. Miller TM, Johnston SC. Should the Babinski sign be part of the routine neurologic examination? *Neurology.* 2005;65(8):1165–1168.

66. Beversdorf DQ, Heilman KM. Facility paratonia and frontal lobe functioning. *Neurology.* 1998;51(4):968–971.

67. Schmahmann JD, Sherman JC. The cerebellar cognitive affective syndrome. *Brain.* 1998; 121(Pt 4):561–579.

68. FitzGerald PM, Jankovic J. Lower body parkinsonism: Evidence for vascular etiology. *Mov Disord.* 1989;4:249–260.

69. Thompson PD, Marsden CD. Gait disorder of subcortical arteriosclerotic encephalopathy: Binswanger's disease. *Mov Disord.* 1987;2:1–8.

70. Pearce JMS. Romberg and his sign. *Eur Neurol.* 2005;53(4):210–213.

71. Lang AE, Jankovic J. Movement disorders: diagnosis and assessment. In: Bradley WG, Daroff RB, Fenichel G, et al. eds. *Neurology in clinical practice.* Philadelphia: Butterworth-Heineman, Elsevier Science; 2008.

72. Hashimoto R, Tanaka Y. Contribution of the supplementary motor area and anterior cingulate gyrus to pathological grasping phenomena. *Eur Neurol.* 1998;40:151–158.

73. Schott JM, Rossor MN. The grasp and other primitive reflexes. *J Neurol Neurosurg Psychiatry.* 2003;74(5):558–560.

74. Sanders RD, Keshavan MS. The neurologic examination in adult psychiatry: From soft signs to hard science. *J Neuropsychiatry Clin Neurosci.* 1998;10(4):395–404.

75. Assadi SM, Noroozian M, Shariat SV. et al. Neurological soft signs in mentally disordered offenders. *J Neuropsychiatry Clin Neurosci.* 2007;19(4):420–427.

76. Malhi GS, Lagopoulos J. Making sense of neuroimaging in psychiatry. *Acta Psychiatr Scand.* 2008;117(2):100–117.

77. Zipursky RB. Imaging mental disorders in the 21st century. *Can J Psychiatry.* 2007; 52(3):133–134.

78. Werring DJ, Frazer DW, Coward LJ, et al. Cognitive dysfunction in patients with cerebral microbleeds on T2*-weighted gradient-echo MRI. *Brain.* 2004;127(Pt 10):2265–2275.

79. Kallenberg K, Schulz-Schaeffer WJ, Jastrow U, et al. Creutzfeldt-Jakob Disease: Comparative Analysis of MR Imaging Sequences. *AJNR Am J Neuroradiol.* 2006;27(7):1459–1462.

80. Belanger HG, Vanderploeg RD, Curtiss G, et al. Recent neuroimaging techniques in mild traumatic brain injury. *J Neuropsychiatry Clin Neurosci.* 2007;19(1):5–20.

81. Small GW, Bookheimer SY, Thompson PM, et al. Current and future uses of neuroimaging for cognitively impaired patients. *Lancet Neurol.* 2008;7(2):161–172.

82. Kraus MF, Susmaras T, Caughlin BP, et al. White matter integrity and cognition in chronic traumatic brain injury: A diffusion tensor imaging study. *Brain.* 2007;130(10):2508–2519.

83. Rutgers DR, Toulgoat F, Cazejust J, et al. White matter abnormalities in mild traumatic brain injury: A diffusion tensor imaging study. *AJNR Am J Neuroradiol.* 2008;29(3):514–519.

84. Lin X, Tench CR, Morgan PS, et al. Use of combined conventional and quantitative MRI to quantify pathology related to cognitive impairment in multiple sclerosis. *J Neurol Neurosurg Psychiatry.* 2008;79(4):437–441.

85. Walker Z, Jaros E, Walker RWH, et al. Dementia with Lewy bodies: A comparison of clinical diagnosis, FP-CIT single photon emission computed tomography imaging and autopsy. *J Neurol Neurosurg Psychiatry.* 2007;78(11):1176–1181.

86. Scherfler C, Schwarz J, Antonini A, et al. Role of DAT-SPECT in the diagnostic work up of Parkinsonism. *Mov Disord.* 2007; 22(9):1229–1238.

87. Castellino G, Padovan M, Bortoluzzi A, et al. Single photon emission computed tomography and magnetic resonance imaging evaluation in SLE patients with and without neuropsychiatric involvement. *Rheumatology (Oxford).* 2008;47(3):319–323.

88. Manchanda R, Norman R, Malla A, et al. EEG abnormalities and 3-year outcome in first episode psychosis. *Acta Psychiatr Scand.* 2008;117(4):277–282.

89. Boutros NN, Struve FA. Electrophysiological testing. In: Yudofsky SC, Kim HF, eds. *Neuropsychiatric assessment.* Arlington: American Psychiatric Publishing; 2004:69–103.

90. Pillai J, Sperling MR. Interictal EEG and the diagnosis of epilepsy. *Epilepsia.* 2006;47:14–22.

91. Benbadis SR. Errors in EEGs and the misdiagnosis of epilepsy: Importance, causes, consequences, and proposed remedies. *Epilepsy Behav.* 2007;11(3):257–262.

92. Coburn KL, Lauterbach EC, Boutros NN, et al. The value of quantitative electroencephalography in clinical psychiatry: A report by the Committee on Research of the American Neuropsychiatric Association. *J Neuropsychiatry Clin Neurosci.* 2006;18(4):460–500.

93. Hunter AM, Cook IA, Leuchter AF. The promise of the quantitative electroencephalogram as a predictor of antidepressant treatment outcomes in Major Depressive Disorder. *Psychiatr Clin North Am.* 2007;30(1):105–124.

94. Bolwig TG. EEG and psychiatry: Time for a resurrection. *Acta Psychiatr Scand.* 2008; 117(4):241–243.

95. Reite M, Teale P, Rojas DC. Magnetoencephalography: Applications in psychiatry. *Biol Psychiatry.* 1999;45(12):1553–1563.

96. Georgopoulos AP, Karageorgiou E, Leuthold AC, et al. Synchronous neural interactions assessed by magnetoencephalography: A functional biomarker for brain disorders. *J Neural Eng.* 2007;4(4):349–355.

97. Boeve BF, Silber MH, Saper CB, et al. Pathophysiology of REM sleep behaviour disorder and relevance to neurodegenerative disease. *Brain.* 2007;130(11):2770–2788.

98. Ovsiew F, Utset T. Neuropsychiatry of the rheumatic diseases. In: Yudofsky SC, Hales RE, eds. *American psychiatric publishing textbook of neuropsychiatry and clinical neurosciences,* 4th ed. Washington, DC: American Psychiatric Publishing; 2002:813–850.

99. Stomrud E, Hansson O, Blennow K, et al. Cerebrospinal fluid biomarkers predict decline in subjective cognitive function over 3 years in healthy elderly. *Dement Geriatr Cogn Disord.* 2007;24(2):118–124.

100. Schoonenboom NSM, van der Flier WM, Blankenstein MA, et al. CSF and MRI markers independently contribute to the diagnosis of Alzheimer's disease. *Neurobiol Aging.* 2008;29(5):669–675.

101. Forsyth RJ. Neurological and cognitive decline in adolescence. *J Neurol Neurosurg Psychiatry.* 2003;74(Suppl 1):i9–i16.

102. Sedel F, Baumann N, Turpin JC, et al. Psychiatric manifestations revealing inborn errors of metabolism in adolescents and adults. *J Inherit Metab Dis.* 2007;30(5):631–641.

103. Golomb M. Psychiatric symptoms in metabolic and other genetic disorders: is our "organic" workup complete?. *Harv Rev Psychiatry.* 2002; 10(4):242–248.

104. Mancuso M, Ricci G, Choub A, et al. Autosomal dominant psychiatric disorders and mitochondrial DNA multiple deletions: Report of a family. *J Affect Disord.* 2008;106(1–2):173–177.

105. Statement on use of apolipoprotein E testing for Alzheimer disease. American College of Medical Genetics/American Society of Human Genetics

Working Group on ApoE and Alzheimer disease. *JAMA*. 1995;274(20):1627–1629.

106. Bourgeois JA, Cogswell JB, Hessl D, et al. Cognitive, anxiety and mood disorders in the fragile X-associated tremor/ataxia syndrome. Gen Hosp Psychiatry. 2007 Jul–Aug;29(4):349–356.

107. Ovsiew F, Bylsma FW. The three cognitive examinations. *Semin Clin Neuropsychiatry*. 2002;7(1):54–64.

108. Johnstone EC, Macmillan JF, Crow TJ. The occurrence of organic disease of possible or probable aetiological significance in a population of 268 cases of first episode schizophrenia. *Psychol Med*. 1987;17(2):371–379.

109. Coleman M, Gillberg C. A biological approach to the schizophrenia spectrum disorders. *J Neuropsychiatry Clin Neurosci*. 1997;9(4): 601–605.

110. Murray ED, Price BH. Depression and psychosis in neurological practice. In: Bradley WG, Daroff RB, Fenichel G, et al. eds. *Neurology in clinical practice*. Philadelphia: Butterworth-Heinemann, Elsevier Science; 2008.

111. Kakooza-Mwesige A, Wachtel LE, Dhossche DM. Catatonia in autism: Implications across the life span. *Eur Child Adolesc Psychiatry*. 2008. (DOI 10.1007/s00787-008-0676-x)

112. Cavanna AE, Robertson MM, Critchley HD. Catatonic signs in Gilles de la Tourette syndrome. *Cogn Behav Neurol*. 2008;21(1): 34–37.

113. Offiah C, Hall E. Heroin-induced leukoencephalopathy: Characterization using MRI, diffusion-weighted imaging, and MR spectroscopy. *Clin Radiol*. 2008;63(2):146–152.

114. Taylor MA, Fink M. Catatonia in psychiatric classification: A home of its own. *Am J Psychiatry*. 2003;160(7):1233–1241.

115. Chalasani P, Healy D, Morriss R. Presentation and frequency of catatonia in new admissions to two acute psychiatric admission units in India and Wales. *Psychol Med*. 2005;35(11):1667–1675.

116. Barnes MP, Saunders M, Walls TJ, et al. The syndrome of Karl Ludwig Kahlbaum. *J Neurol Neurosurg Psychiatry*. 1986;49:991–996.

117. Lahutte B, Cornic F, Bonnot O, et al. Multidisciplinary approach of organic catatonia in children and adolescents may improve treatment decision making. *Prog Neuropsychopharmacol Biol Psychiatry*. 2008;32(6):1393–1398.

118. Carroll BT, Goforth HW, Thomas C, et al. Review of adjunctive glutamate antagonist therapy in the treatment of catatonic syndromes. *J Neuropsychiatry Clin Neurosci*. 2007;19(4):406–412.

119. McDaniel WW, Spiegel DR, Sahota AK. Topiramate effect in catatonia: A case series. *J Neuropsychiatry Clin Neurosci*. 2006;18(2):234–238.

120. Howard R, Rabins PV, Seeman MV, et al. Late-Onset tI. Late-onset schizophrenia and very-late-onset schizophrenia-like psychosis: An international consensus. *Am J Psychiatry*. 2000;157(2):172–178.

121. Herrmann LL, Le Masurier M, Ebmeier KP. White matter hyperintensities in late life depression: A systematic review. *J Neurol Neurosurg Psychiatry*. 2008;79(6):619–624.

122. Kuo H-K, Lipsitz LA. Cerebral white matter changes and geriatric syndromes: Is there a link? *J Gerontol A Biol Sci Med Sci*. 2004;59(8):M818–M826.

123. Moeschler JB. Genetic evaluation of intellectual disabilities. *Semin Pediatr Neurol*. 2008;15(1):2–9.

124. Shaffer LG. American College of Medical Genetics guideline on the cytogenetic evaluation of the individual with developmental delay or mental retardation. *Genet Med*. 2005;7(9):650–654.

125. Bodensteiner JB, Schaefer GB. Evaluation of the patient with idiopathic mental retardation. *J Neuropsychiatry Clin Neurosci*. 1995;7(3):361–370.

126. Murphy KC, Jones LA, Owen MJ. High rates of schizophrenia in adults with velo-cardio-facial syndrome. *Arch Gen Psychiatry*. 1999;56(10):940–945.

127. Danielsson S, Gillberg IC, Billstedt E, et al. Epilepsy in young adults with autism: A prospective population-based follow-up study of 120 individuals diagnosed in childhood. *Epilepsia*. 2005;46(6):918–923.

Psychiatric Administration

L. MARK RUSSAKOFF

R egardless of where one intends to practice, it is useful for psychiatrists to have an understanding of administration beyond the experiential. If one intends to work within any organization, then it behooves the psychiatrist to have not only an understanding of administration but also certain competencies that go beyond what is taught in many residencies or found in most medical textbooks. For psychiatrists who work in inpatient settings, the need for knowledge and competencies related to administration are clearest.

The knowledge related to functioning on an inpatient unit include administrative theory, human resources, the regulatory environment, fiscal considerations, legal and ethical principles and practices, understanding small-group and large-group dynamics, and the structuring of inpatient care. The competencies involved include ability to function within disparate areas (e.g., clinical and fiscal), comfort with power and authority, teamwork, and working amongst groups. Team skills include clear communication, trusting others, being open to feedback, ability to compromise, and the ability to commit to an overarching goal (as opposed to a personal goal). There are several texts which summarize the various administrative areas pertinent to psychiatry.[1–4]

Administrative Theory

Administrative theory attempts to address the domains of administration and management: planning, organizing, staffing, directing, coordinating, reporting, and budgeting.[5] Some of these areas deal with individual dynamics, group dynamics, and the impact of social settings. The psychiatrist may have an advantage over other administrators in already having been schooled in some of these areas. On the other hand, a psychiatrist who does not appreciate that individual psychologies do not fully explain the functioning of individuals in groups and organizations will be handicapped by that lack of understanding.

There is a stunningly large array of books and treatises on administration and management. This should not be taken as a reason to exempt oneself from learning about the area but rather as evidence of its complexity. Although mental health professionals are educated in the areas of individual and group dynamics, the education rarely extends into large group, intergroup, and organizational dynamics.[6] Knowledge in all five areas may be necessary in order to fully understand a situation.

Many books on management purport to be the final answer even as they fail to address all the tasks that need to be included. It seems that the approaches that claimed to be "scientific" were proposed during periods of relative stability.[7,8] As all organizations—not-for-profit, for-profit, manufacturing, service, financial, local, national, international, and global—have found themselves in turbulent times, each theory has failed to anticipate all the trends and resultant challenges and to provide enlightenment on those challenges. Although there had been a search for a science of management and administration, there has been an evolving acceptance that there will be no grand unifying theory. "Contingency theory" suggests that one simply pick the theory that seems to fit the situation best. However, no guidance is provided as to how to select which theory fits best. Theories that stress only one or two perspectives are unlikely to endure in their ability to capture the elements important in a rapidly changing world.

There are attempts to bring together multiple perspectives into a coherent whole. One of the most popular, probably because it integrates multiple perspectives with modern information systems technology, is the balanced score card.[9] This model has evolved as the business environment has changed.[10,11] Paralleling the familiar multidisciplinary treatment plan, it suggests that minimally an organization identify goals and objectives in four domains: fiscal, internal business processes (quality and efficiency), customer satisfaction, and learning and growth (staff development). This model contrasts with many other ones in that it raises at least these four domains to priority status. However, the knowledge regarding management and administration is fragmentary and its value linked to the specific organizational circumstances to which it is to be applied. Whereas some of the proposed principles appear to be universal, others are constrained by context.

Some of the principles that were articulated in mid-20th century are now accepted as truisms. For example, as a general approach to management of people, the traditional "command and control" approach is rarely endorsed, except in an emergency situation.[12,13] The command and control model assumes that individuals need clear direction and oversight, that without such oversight they are likely to slack, and that most people view work as a burden. Current models encourage a positive view of supervisees and their attitudes toward their work, resulting in a collaborative relationship between supervisor and supervisee.[13] Furthermore, the importance of focusing on the institution's goals and objectives, and orienting one's efforts toward those goals, is generally accepted practice.[12] This approach is the familiar "management by objectives" (which also finds expression in the structure of multidisciplinary treatment plans).

Familiarity with basic concepts relevant to administration helps clarify one's thinking regarding administrative puzzles. An understanding of leadership—its basis, the types, and situational aspects—helps one understand dynamics more effectively. As with administrative theory, literature on leadership abounds.[14,15] Different styles of leadership are suitable for different situations, and understanding the theories can help decide when to utilize each.[8,16] Having a cognitive understanding of the different types of leadership helps one develop the skills utilized by each of them. Motivation of individuals—its basis, categories, and relationship to organizational structure—is central to effective administration.[17–19] No single theory fully explains what motivates individuals in organizations. Again, some familiarity with the various approaches can help supervisors and supervisees understand their responses to work situations. It may also permit the design of more effective systems. Alternatively, it may help identify the proper source of low morale. In general, most administrators utilize a style of leadership that attempts to engage and enlist others, as opposed to casting forth edicts. Sometimes one needs to go through a progression, moving from the inspirational, to the transactional, and then the punitive mode.

Choice of Administrative Theory Model to Match a Situation

Case Vignette

The hospital had a chronic problem with discharge summaries not being dictated and signed on time. The standard was that the signed discharge summary must be in the chart within 30 days of discharge. Regulations of the state and The Joint Commission (TJC, previously known as the *Joint Commission of Accreditation of Healthcare Organizations* [JCAHO]) were clear as to how many undictated charts were acceptable; the hospital's delinquency rate easily ran ten times over the maximally acceptable number. The policy of the hospital was that if a medical staff member was delinquent in dictating and signing discharge summaries, then doctor's privileges would be suspended. However, the actual process was that when a patient from a suspended doctor sought admission, a surgery, or other care by that

(continued)

physician at the hospital, the medical director would be called at all hours of the day and night and be pressured to unsuspend that doctor's privileges. The sanction had no teeth.

The medical director, expecting that the hospital would be cited for the delinquency rate during its next TJC survey, went to departmental meetings, quarterly meetings of the medical staff, and grand rounds. Initially, the presentation was simply a verbal urging to finish the work, noting "it's the right thing to do." Secondarily, the director began to present data at such meetings, showing how much the threshold was exceeded. In response, medical staff members complained of the difficulty in dictating charts: charts being whisked off the unit too soon, poor access to charts after the patient was discharged, and obstacles to doing the dictations. In response to this feedback, changes were made in the time in which charts were removed from units, medical records were scanned and available within 48 hours of discharge, and the dictation system was modernized and made more user friendly.

The number of undictated charts remained constant and far over the acceptable threshold. Further rounds of talks were made by the medical director. It was suggested that the problem must be "a few bad apples." Upon review of the charts, it appeared that delinquency in doing dictations of discharge summaries was widespread, including senior and respected members of the medical staff. Department directors were informed who in their departments was delinquent, and the directors asked to speak to those members. The rate of delinquency remained the same.

The medical director took the issue to the Medical Board. Members of the Board wrung their hands but felt that they could not take any stronger stand on the issue, feeling that censuring a peer for merely not dictating or signing a chart on time was excessive and misguided. Members clearly harbored negative feelings about paperwork in general, especially as more and more was being required by various regulatory agencies. The problem remained; the medical director anguished over the failure of the Board to act, especially knowing that it guaranteed a citation at the next TJC survey, something that would reflect badly on the medical director as well as on the hospital.

A serious incident occurred at the hospital, unrelated to delinquency of charts. The State Department of Health came to the hospital to investigate. In the process of the investigation, they noted the excessive rate of delinquent charts and stated unequivocally that the problem must be rectified promptly.

Armed with the directive from the state, and with a deadline to respond to the state, the medical director stepped away from the approach of attempting to align medical staff members with the goal and into a command and control style. Citing the authority of the state, while noting the large number of medical staff members with delinquent charts, the medical director stated that the worst ten offenders would be targeted beginning in the following month and that their privileges would be actually suspended! The suspension would be for real and not ended until all of their dictations were complete. Those physicians would need to find other physicians to cover their patients and other responsibilities at the hospital. The names of the suspended physicians would be prominently posted in the corridor. Delinquency notices would be reviewed and updated weekly. The Medical Board reluctantly approved the program.

The delinquency rate plummeted to well below the threshold! The medical director was not vilified by the medical staff. The state was impressed with the results. When TJC came to survey a couple of years later, the delinquency rate was minimal. The change was permanent, although there are always a few physicians whose names are posted.

Hospitals are constituted of complex, overlapping—and oftentimes conflicting—hierarchical bureaucracies that operate in a highly regulated and competitive environment. "Hierarchical" implies that power is not evenly distributed, that some individuals and departments have more power than others. "Bureaucracy" implies structure as well as rules for interacting among components of the structure.[20] These rules coordinate the performance of certain activities and are the policies and procedures of the organization. One of the complicating factors in professional organizations is that other rules may also apply, such as professional ethics, which may appear to conflict, or may in fact conflict, with organizational rules. The regulations that affect hospitals come from a broad array of sources, many of which are indifferent to potential conflicts. The competitive and regulatory environment has resulted in many hospitals teetering at the edge of fiscal solvency. Hospitals are frequently one of the largest local employers and have large budgets, but the net excess margin or profit is typically very small, if any. Competition amongst providers has led to various alliances and contracts meant to insulate the institution from the payers—commercial insurers and managed care. It is not uncommon now for negotiations between provider groups (hospitals or doctors) and insurers to reach impasses, and letters are sent to patients that the providers will not accept their insurance as of a certain date. Each side accuses the other of greed and the negotiations often do not reach a settlement until the last moment. These events do little to curry favor with the patients who have a foot on each side of the battle—their providers and their costs to bear.

No law dictates that rules and hierarchies within an organization make sense or are functional. In fact, the overlapping of the structures may create inherent tensions. Hospitals are constituted of separate departments with different tasks and needs: fiscal, human resources, supportive services, and clinical staff. The clinical staff is usually divided by profession and discipline. The interplay within and among the departments directly affects the clinician and patients. Lack of knowledge regarding administrative theory and thus how the dynamic processes play out often leads to erroneous conclusions about events and then to personal distress. Better awareness of the structure, function, and dynamics of organizations can render one's experience comprehensible and facilitate more effective choices and decisions. As a result, it is also likely to improve patient care.

Failure to understand administration may lead to incorrect conclusions regarding patients, staff, and components of the organization. The interplay between patient behavior, staff behavior, and administration is well documented in such classics as *The Mental Hospital, The Psychiatric Hospital as a Small Society*, and *The Sharing of Power in a Psychiatric Hospital*.[21-23] Although these works are dated, there is no reason to believe that problems and processes similar to what they describe are not operative currently. In fact, there has probably been a loss of knowledge of milieu and hospital dynamics as clinicians are currently pressed with taking care of sicker patients and processing them more quickly. Much more attention is paid in residency training to neuropharmacology and genetics than to organizational dynamics as they affect patients and staff.

Another area in which an appreciation of administration is important is in personnel management. If one does not appreciate the need for the human resources department to have policies and procedures for corrective actions to be taken with staff, then the administrative personnel are easily vilified for not responding quickly enough to dysfunctional staff behaviors. If one does not understand the nature of the budgeting process, then it is easy to declare inappropriately that the administration is unsupportive and cheap, but one will also be ineffective in obtaining resources one needs. These situations are common and often contribute to avoidable disgruntlement amongst staff.

Progressive discipline is the process in which attempts are made to rectify problems while protecting the rights of both employer and employee. It entails counseling as well as increasing sanctions of greater severity in order to achieve a desired goal. Counseling by the supervisor to help the employee achieve the goals is a critical component. The focus should be on salvaging an employee in trouble, not punishment. However, if the employee does not improve sufficiently to meet the agreed-upon standard, then termination of employment is the ultimate step. Institutions should have explicit steps to guide supervisors along the process.

PROGRESSIVE DISCIPLINE: TIME AND ATTENDANCE

Case Vignette

The psychiatrist's position was as director of an inpatient unit. Rounds were held each morning at 9 AM, where all patients' care was reviewed. Clinical challenges were discussed and treatment planning sessions scheduled. The job description was explicit about the need to be at rounds each morning.

The psychiatrist began to call in, unable to be at rounds. Rounds would be delayed until the psychiatrist could be present. On several days, the psychiatrist did not come in until the early afternoon, without informing the staff of the further delay. Unit function was disrupted. When the psychiatrist was present, there were no problems with the psychiatrist's work. The issue was called to the attention of the director of the department. The director of the department began to sit in at rounds. This led to improved attendance, and the director stopped attending after 2 weeks.

However, shortly thereafter the problem resurfaced. The director met with the psychiatrist, who described childcare needs that "occasionally" caused the lateness. The unit was not an acute care unit, and it was noted that an occasional lateness would not materially affect the work of the unit. The department director agreed that one lateness a week would be within acceptable range. It was agreed that the psychiatrist would have a better time and attendance record.

The excess lateness persisted. The director was again informed and spoke to the psychiatrist. The psychiatrist minimized the frequency of absences. The director asked that the psychiatrist sign in on the unit; the psychiatrist agreed.

Over the course of 4 weeks, the psychiatrist was on time only four times, and many of the lateness were a matter of hours! The psychiatrist acknowledged the problem and promised to be prompt. They discussed the problems that contributed to the lateness and how they might otherwise be handled. The sheets of sign-in times and a note describing the counseling were placed in the psychiatrist's personnel file.

The psychiatrist continued to be late. The director met again with the psychiatrist and counseled the psychiatrist as to the fit between the job requirements and the psychiatrist. The psychiatrist agreed to submit a resignation and did so.

Shortly after the psychiatrist resigned, the psychiatrist filed a complaint of discrimination. The complaint was found to be without merit.

Many agencies have authority that affects inpatient services. Such agencies include accrediting ones (TJC, Centers for Medicare and Medicaid Services [CMS], State Office of Mental Health, State Department of Health) as well as safety agencies (Occupational Safety and Health Administration [OSHA], Fire Department). Inpatient services have interactions with insurance companies, social service agencies, the courts, schools, residential programs, outpatient clinics, partial hospital programs, and day treatment programs. They are likely to deal with programs for substance abusers and the developmentally disabled. The rules that apply to each system differ, and at times the interests of the agency may be at odds with or seem incomprehensible to the inpatient unit. An appreciation of the administrative differences and needs can lessen tensions and facilitate communication. On the other hand, at times there is a firewall that others may want inpatient providers to bridge, but such bridging may not be appropriate. Whereas an appreciation of the competing interests may be helpful, it may not resolve the issues and ill will and complaints may arise despite the best of efforts.

Inpatient Unit Structure

Commonly an inpatient psychiatric unit is run by a psychiatrist in concert with a nurse-manager. The psychiatrist director may be full time, geographic full time, or part time. Whereas in the past it was not uncommon for a unit chief to be salaried and not carry patients, this model has been replaced largely by the model in which billable hours generate the unit chief's salary. If other psychiatrists care for patients on the unit, the unit chief is expected to monitor the performance of the other psychiatrists through direct observation as well as various quality assurance activities. This model is cost effective, but does create certain potential complications. It is quite difficult to stand back from one's work and observe objectively the ramifications of one's actions and inactions. The same processes that befall the supervisees may affect the supervisor. The challenge is to create a system that is sufficiently open to permit reflection on what is occurring on a unit and to have a nondefensive discussion of the processes. Unit chiefs need to be able to tolerate disagreements and criticisms without resorting to counterattacks. Issues and challenges need to be seen dispassionately and discussed. Such an objective discussion is most likely to occur if there are team meetings in which controversies and problems can be aired.

There is a natural tension between the medical and nursing staff: nurses are present 24 hours a day and doctors are present for a few hours only; doctors write orders and determine who is admitted or discharged. Very often, strong opinions are deeply held, not necessarily with factual information to support them. The unit chief may relate to the nursing staff in different ways—from the extreme of abdication of oversight (leaving all nursing decisions to the discretion of the nurses) to attempts at tyrannical control (micromanaging of all of the nurses' activities). It is a challenge to exercise oversight of the nursing activities, acknowledging their unique skills and competencies, while providing insight, guidance, and consultation at the same time. Adoption of either of the polarized solutions (abdication or tyrannical control) may work temporarily but is likely to implode.

The staff is from various disciplines—social work, nursing, activities therapy, psychiatry—and reports to discipline leaders, yet at the same time the unit itself is likely to be run as a interdisciplinary team, in theory if not in fact. This type of dual reporting structure is referred to as *matrix management*.[24] Dueling discipline chiefs can vicariously create or contribute to unit tensions.

Having obtained a professional degree is not a credential for working on a interdisciplinary team. On the contrary, some have asserted that the traditional training of physicians is to be a team of one. People differ in their ability and comfort working collaboratively with others. Working collaboratively in a team is a skill that must be developed if one is to be successful working in any organization, and especially on an inpatient psychiatric unit where one is surrounded by intense emotions. The skills needed to work in a team can be developed as one works on a unit. However, these skills will not be developed if one is unaware that one lacks the skills one needs, and often such skills are not developed without an active effort.

Power and authority are not equally shared within hospitals. Physicians are given major responsibilities from which they cannot exempt themselves. Examples of this authority are the privilege to admit and discharge, the privilege to write treatment orders, the responsibility to assess for dangerousness, and to hospitalize involuntarily if necessary. This power inequality often contributes to tensions amongst the staff. Staff with the least power and authority, typically mental health workers, are often recruited from the less privileged in society, contributing to tensions that may play out on the unit. If power is tightly held and not shared amongst staff, then the resulting resentments and tensions are likely to fuel major problems. If power is shared inappropriately, then this may harm patients, the institution, or the staff.

It is the task of the leaders of the unit to empower all employees such that the differential power that results from licensure and discipline is not the primary concern of the workers. Empowerment involves acknowledging the contribution that all team members make to the functioning of the hospital, namely providing high-quality care to patients. Whereas professionals may have other sources of pride in their work, the paraprofessional staff will depend largely on the professionals as the source of acknowledgement. Team meetings can be a convenient site in which that acknowledgement is made. Appropriate acknowledgement of the work of the staff in the regular course of business will help offset those rare occasions in which one has to exercise authority in an unpopular manner, for instance not discharging a manic patient whom the staff perceive as simply manipulative and disruptive.

Patients with borderline personality disorder challenge staff on a regular basis. They regularly seek out schisms within the staff, drive wedges into those schisms, and create new ones. All staff need to be familiar with the process of splitting because the process will involve all clinical staff at one time or another. In the administration of a unit, the unit chief needs to be sensitive to such actions and be prepared to diagnose the process so as to be able to intervene. The unit chief may be drawn in to some of the conflicts, and a well-functioning team can act as a way to observe the process and intervene. In order for this to occur, the team must be functioning before the crisis occurs; an *ad hoc* team will be a team in name only.

Teamwork is as much art as science.[25-27] One cannot prescribe the attitudes necessary to work on a team, but they can be described. These attitudes and skills can be demonstrated in team meetings, and learning by modeling is common. Demonstrating trust in the judgment of others, being open to feedback, keeping the focus on the overarching goal of the team—all will contribute to better team membership and functioning. Persons who are excessively suspicious and mistrustful and those with very rigid beliefs about social roles may not be able to function as effective team members. Individuals who grew up in cultures in which authority is never questioned, where such questioning is seen as disrespectful, can often be educated about a participative culture in which questioning is common. On the other hand, team members need to acknowledge legitimate authority and appreciate that their having an alternative opinion does not necessarily mean that a decision will be made as they wish. In some situations, the team as a whole may make the decision, but not all decisions can be decided by the team as a whole. Some decisions are the province of a particular discipline. Many critical decisions in inpatient psychiatry are made with limited time to work them through and with only partial information. The decision to discharge a patient who has been disruptive is never an easy one and typically a lightening rod for staff disagreements and resentments. Similarly, the decision to retain a patient involuntarily can reveal staff conflicts. It is obviously best if there are clear lines of communication and regarding authority amongst the staff before such conflicts erupt.

Alignment and Assignment: Removal of an Obstacle for Admissions

Case Vignette

The not-for-profit hospital was located in an area where psychiatric beds were relatively numerous. Nevertheless, the census of the unit was lower than that of other local hospitals. The director was told to solve the problem. During regular business hours, the emergency room (ER) and admissions were covered by salaried psychiatrists. Off-hours, salaried psychiatrists, and private practitioners shared call. Call was taken from home, assuming that the doctor could get to the ER within half an hour. A call room was available but rarely used.

A review of the low census indicated that the process of referral for admission was encumbered, especially off-hours. Most of the admissions occurred during regular business hours, yet most referrals were made off-hours. The daytime referral process appeared to work better than the off-hours process. During business hours the departmental office would be called and the day duty doctor, who was on site, would be called by the secretary. Off-hours, the duty doctors were almost never on site. The referral calls were received by a number of people: the ER staff, the hospital operators, and the inpatient unit staff. Depending on

(continued)

who was called, the request was triaged differently. Only the duty doctor was authorized to acknowledge the availability of beds or accept a patient. Because the duty doctor was not on site, the delays were often extensive.

The process was changed. A central referral number was installed, answered by secretarial staff during business hours and the inpatient unit staff off-hours. If there were empty beds, the off-hours staff would inform the caller. If it were a patient calling and inquiring about admission, the inpatient staff would tell the patient to proceed to the ER. If the patient showed up in the ER, the patient would be evaluated by the staff, and if appropriate the psychiatrist called to come in and evaluate the patient. Transfers from other facilities still required authorization by the duty doctor, as required by state law.

The census increased significantly. The encumbered process of making an inquiry off-hours was rectified. The disinclination of the duty doctors to see patients had created a roadblock for admissions. Patients had been discouraged to come to the ER. By facilitating referrals and the arrival of patients to the ER, appropriate patients were admitted, and the hospital developed a reputation of being "user friendly;" the income of the hospital increased.

Quality Improvement Activities

Health care providers are under great pressure to improve quality of care. There is a general impression that the current system is inefficient and ineffective. Cross-national comparisons are interpreted to support these assertions. The Institute of Medicine produced a report in 1999 *To Err is Human*, which called attention to "unnecessary deaths." This report sharpened to focus on patient safety. Business, as exemplified by the Leapfrog Group, and independent professional groups, as exemplified by the Institute for Healthcare Improvement (IHI), have combined with regulators (TJC) and payers (Medicare) to change the way medicine is practiced and make it more cost effective and safer. The Leapfrog group promoted the use of hospitalists and intensivists. The IHI completed its 100,000 Lives campaign (December 2004 to June 2006), enlisting 2,000 hospitals in its efforts. This resulted in the wide adoption of rapid response teams to handle problematic situations before there were crisis situations. The IHI has now launched its 5 Million Lives campaign (December 2006 to December 2008), focusing on preventing deaths and morbidities through targeting nosocomial infections, high-alert medications, surgical complications, pressure ulcers, congestive heart failure, and governance structure. Hospitals are under pressure to sign on to various national goals that purport to promote better health care. Hospitals that either do not sign on or perform badly on the performance measures may fair poorly in the market, especially as more information is released to the public on performance measures. TJC findings, which were previously confidential, are now being published.

All inpatient services are required by TJC and other regulators to measure the quality of care provided and to have a performance improvement (PI) program. The regulations that surround these activities are in constant flux. Historically these activities have not been warmly embraced by most psychiatrists. Psychiatrists have often articulated the idea that what they do cannot be captured by the trivial and mundane measures proposed to assess quality. However, over the last 30 years the culture of medicine has changed, and the need to find measures of quality of care is a given.

The earliest quality assurance activities were centered upon quality-control activities, now seen as utilization management: medical necessity of admission, continued length of stay, high-volume activities, problem-prone activities, and high-risk activities. Clearly some of these elements were proxies to limit the cost of care—unnecessary admissions and prolonged hospital stays. Programs would regularly assess the adequacy of admitting histories and physicals, documentation of the need for the admission and continued stay, documentation of seclusion and restraint, and parameters of the use of electroconvulsive therapy (ECT). The focus was on the processes of care: adequacy of the psychiatric evaluation, documentation of the treatments, and documentation of disposition planning. Many felt that one could focus only on processes and not on outcomes because outcomes were either too far removed from the interventions or too hard to characterize in advance. The lack of use of reliable, quantitative scales in the general practice of psychiatry contributed to the sense that measurement was a fiction, performed solely for the purpose of satisfying the regulators. Because the bulk of inpatients suffer from chronic and recurrent disorders, problems in outcome were seen as inherent in the illnesses and unrelated to the quality of the interventions.

In the 1980s, health care, driven by the JCAHO, borrowed various quality improvement activities from Japanese industry.[28] The premise was that quality can be measured and then improved. The hope was to move away from quality-control approaches—find "the bad apple"—and move to a concerted effort to improve the quality of care. The focus would be on the processes of care so as to design processes that would ensure high-quality outcomes. The approach was to look for deviations from expected outcomes. There was a strong push to use statistics as a tool for quality improvement. Because of this pressure to produce graphs and statistics, the focus of most of these activities in hospitals was on activities that could be quantified. The expectation was that these quality assessment tools would be easily transferable to medical care evaluation and that the quality of care would be measured and then improved. Before that time, most quality assurance activities were qualitative.

The first of these statistics-based, JCAHO-mandated activities was termed *continuous quality improvement* (*CQI*), but that label was replaced by "PI," as CQI was a phrase from one of the quality gurus (Deming) and the choice of that phrase seemed to endorse his approach to the exclusion of others; PI was seen as neutral. A veritable industry developed around PI activities.

Teams were created to examine clinical areas of interest and to analyze where problems in care emerged. The teams collect the data supporting or contradicting their analysis. Changes would be made in accordance with the data and the process iterated. The model "Plan-Do-Check-Act" was the byword of CQI. The model has been expanded, and now most facilities have PI programs that use multiple teams to examine care processes and look for means to improve them.

In 1997 TJC introduced the requirement to report on various outcome and performance measurements, titled the Oryx program. These requirements have now been incorporated into their standards. Since 2004, the accreditation survey process has been unannounced, so that instead of a flurry of activity occurring just before the survey is due, the organization has to be in continuous readiness. Additionally, interim self-assessments are required to be submitted to TJC.

Areas invariably included in current quality improvement activities include the use of seclusion and restraints, conduct of ECT, and medication management. Seclusion and restraint have joined with suicide as events that represent treatment failures and which require close examination to see if there were ways in which the situation or patient could have been managed differently and to prevent the failure. Previously clinicians may have viewed seclusion or restraint as a relatively uncommon but inevitable and necessary intervention; the perspective now is that seclusion and restraint represent institutional and treatment failures. The only acceptable rate of these interventions is zero. Surveyors from the TJC and state licensing agencies regularly review documentation of incidences of seclusion and restraint, with special emphasis on the required documentation, which is quite explicit. It is critical for staff to appreciate that the rigid time frames defined in regulations are not to be taken lightly; accreditation of the facility may be jeopardized by a cavalier attitude. If this appreciation is gained primarily by blaming the accrediting agencies, then the motivation to perform the required tasks tends to be poor and conformance a problem. The regulations do force administrators to embrace the cultural shift that seclusion and restraint are not just another treatment intervention but do represent a problem in the treatment of the individual. The cultural shift to the position that seclusion and restraint can be avoided by other clinical interventions is possible and has occurred at many facilities, including large state facilities that do not have an abundance of clinical staff.

There has been a shift away from process measures to outcome measures.[29] Process improvement is only as good as the outcomes that are produced. Many have been dissatisfied with the results of PI programs on the actual health of the treated population. This shift is clearest in other areas of medicine, such as the treatment of acute myocardial infarction (MI). CMS has instituted a series of quality measures for hospitals, such as administration of aspirin and β-blockers to patients with acute MI upon arrival to the hospital. The results of these measures are now published and available on the Internet. Newspapers sometimes pick up these stories about how local hospitals have fared in these current competitive endeavors. Sensitive to the ramification of poor publicity from faring poorly on such measures, hospitals now must focus their resources and attention on the items to be measured, so that they will compare favorably. It remains to be seen whether such attention simply shifts resources from one area to another or whether the pressure to perform well on the quality measures pushes up the level of care overall.

There is pressure to report on measures that are used across agencies so that there can be comparisons amongst agencies. The American Psychiatric Association (APA) formed a task force to suggest various quality indicators across the spectrum of care.[30]

At the time of the writing of this chapter, CMS is promoting "Pay for Performance" programs (P4P), but at this date they do not affect inpatient psychiatric care. Professional groups, including the APA, have been consulted to develop objective measures of quality of care for which Medicare would provide a premium, currently 1.5%. The current outpatient psychiatric measure is that a person treated for major depression is prescribed an antidepressant. Although this is clearly a crude measure, it does signal a commitment to seek out ways to align quality measurement and fiscal performance. One of the tasks of the psychiatric administrator is to keep abreast of these developments and to help the staff accommodate to the changes without fueling their anger.

Although many clinicians see the PI activities as either irrelevant or superficial, for the institution they are crucial for survival. All staff need to cooperate with the endeavors, despite the fact that these mandates never come with more money. The clinicians will need to shoulder more responsibilities in the quality area over time. However, many spend more time criticizing the quality programs than attempting to find more relevant measures that could be examined. The successful psychiatric administrator will appreciate the trends, understand the requirements, and articulate a vision of quality improvement that enlist the cooperation of the psychiatric staff in performing the required tasks. Administrators who talk only about the budget and not about the quality of care rendered will ultimately alienate the staff and contribute to poor morale.

Many of the currently used quality indicators focus on the use and effects of psychotropic medication. With the lawsuits against the pharmaceutical manufacturers regarding metabolic effects of atypical antipsychotics, the drug companies have sponsored large number of educational activities directed at providers to educate them and thereby off-load risk. Because atypical antipsychotics are very frequently prescribed for inpatients, a monitor of the patient's metabolic status at admission and the metabolic effects of the drugs is sensible and not difficult to do in general hospitals. This would parallel the routine use of abnormal involuntary movement scale (AIMS) assessments in the days of typical antipsychotics.

Legal and Forensic Issues

Psychiatric admissions are governed by the specific laws of each state. There are typically regulations about who may sign themselves, or someone else, into a psychiatric unit. Because these laws differ from state to state, it behooves the inpatient psychiatrist to be familiar with the laws of his or her state.

For instance, in New York State, a patient who meets medical necessity criteria for admission may come to the unit as an informal, voluntary, or involuntary patient. There are several types of involuntary patients. An *informal* patient is admitted in a manner similar to a general medical patient and broadly assumes the same right as a general medical patient to leave the hospital at his or her own discretion, even against medical advice. An informal patient does not sign a specific request to be admitted to the psychiatric unit. If an informal patient wishes to leave the hospital at any time, that wish is expected to be effected. There is a provision for the conversion of such a patient to involuntary status, if clinically indicated.

A *voluntary* patient makes a written request for admission. Just as in informal patient, such a patient may be discharged at his or her request. However, a voluntary patient may be retained for up to 72 hours for observation if the patient is deemed to be possibly imminently dangerous to himself or herself or to others. Within 72 hours, the hospital must either release the individual or petition the court for involuntary retention. This provision of the 72-hour holding and observation period distinguishes the legal status of the informal from the voluntary patient.

There are several means of a patient becoming an *involuntary* patient, depending on who petitions for the admission. In New York State, involuntary patients, as well as voluntary patients who are being held against their wishes, have the right to a court hearing to decide on the appropriateness of their admission and continued stay.

Because it is a serious breech of one's constitutional rights to be involuntarily admitted, the court system takes the entire process quite seriously. Clinicians need to appreciate that this "mere paperwork" is the guardian of the patients' constitutional rights and not to be taken lightly. Judges have been known to release patients because the paperwork was not dated and timed properly. Clinicians need to be sensitive to this issue because they cannot depend on a judge's taking a more clinical point of view. This means that the unit chief needs to review the paperwork on admissions. If ER physicians or house doctors are involved in completing the paperwork for involuntary admissions, they may not fill in all the areas—time of completion, for instance—and thereby invalidate their work. It is ultimately the unit chief's obligation to educate the other doctors or otherwise to ensure that the paperwork is done correctly.

Confidentiality of medical records is a priority at all sites of health care. Inpatient facilities will have policies and procedures to safeguard the confidentiality of patients' records. The passage of the Health Insurance Portability and Accountability Act (HIPAA) of 1996 introduced federal requirements that must be addressed. Because some of the rules regarding release of information are arcane, inpatient staff must be familiar with their hospitals' policies and procedures, which would be tailored to all the relevant laws. One of the requirements of HIPAA is the "minimum necessary" rule, that is, only that amount of information should be released to meet the specific need. This rule often means that a new document tailored to the request must be prepared. It does not mean that misleading information should be released, such as altering diagnoses or omitting diagnoses that are relevant.

HIPAA regulations do permit the release of information without written authorization in order to treat the patient or for the payment of health care bills. Not infrequently, health care providers are too cautious about the release of information, such as when a patient is referred from one agency to another and a call is placed to inquire as to the most recent medications or other immediate concerns. The proper care of the patient needs to be the central concern and guiding principle. Rules of confidentiality are there to protect patients, not interfere with their obtaining care. HIPAA permits the release of health care information without written authorization for the purpose of treatment. Failure to provide information to the ER in which the patient has been taken because one does not have a written authorization is a misinterpretation of the law. Which lawsuit do you want to defend—the one in which the patient was improperly treated because information was withheld from another provider or the allegation of violation of confidentiality by having provided appropriate and pertinent information to that provider?

Treatment over objection is another area in which the psychiatrist and other clinical staff need to be familiar with the local law. In New York State, a distinction is made in law between the need to be in the hospital and the need to be medicated against one's will. That is, a patient who meets the criteria for involuntary admission does not automatically meet the criteria for involuntary administration of medication. The law does permit the administration of medication over objections in an emergency, but the concept is articulated that emergencies are brief; continued involuntary administration of medication treatment beyond the period of the emergency is not permitted without a court order. To continue to medicate a patient against his or her will, the hospital must seek court authorization. The patient has a right to a court hearing to decide this issue. Psychiatrists who go to court should familiarize themselves with the process and the legal requirements in order to properly assist their patients. It is not rare for the judges assigned to these hearings to be inexperienced in issues of mental health law; such judicial assignments do not appear to be coveted ones. As a result, sometimes the judges act as if it were a criminal trial and apply criminal, not civil, standards of evidence. The better prepared the expert psychiatric witness is, the more predictable the outcome. Courtrooms are not venues for academic dissertations or vague impressions but thrive best on specific observations combined with terse clinical logic, clear conclusions, and clear recommendations.

Psychiatric Care Management

The overall management of patients on the unit is the responsibility of the staff psychiatrists. By federal and many state regulations, each patient has a multidisciplinary evaluation, which culminates in a multidisciplinary treatment plan, which the psychiatrist is required to sign. These requirements are predicated upon the belief that the treatment of a psychiatric patient requires input from several disciplines, which must coordinate their efforts in order to treat the patient effectively.

Because multidisciplinary treatment plans are mandated, and because little training has occurred in psychiatric residencies regarding their clinical use, they are often the stepchild of treatment. They are signed in a pro forma manner, treated as a bureaucratic annoyance. However, the treatment plan can be a real tool in treating the individual patient as well as managing the staff. Most individuals admitted to the inpatient service have complicated conditions through either comorbidity or their psychosocial situations. The treatment plan can be an effective tool for focusing the efforts of the team on the activities most relevant to the care of the patient. This opportunity is lost if the members of the team rush through the process to treat the chart. The treatment planning process, done as a team, can be the site of work to minimize the effects of splitting, educate the staff regarding the relevant disorders, build team morale, and professionalize staff. This process is not one way: the staff educates the psychiatrist as to the nuances of the patient's condition, how the patient appears the other 23 hours, and how to best manage this individual.

Inpatient work is teamwork. All members need to possess or develop team skills as described in the preceding text. Staff members want to feel that they are partners in providing care, not customers or servants of the psychiatrist. Psychiatrists who are focused on being at the top of the hierarchy and who cannot see themselves as partners with the staff will suffer from attacks from below. These attacks are likely to occur regardless, but will be omnipresent if one is perceived as arrogant and controlling. The participative style of leadership is more helpful than the authoritarian style in developing an atmosphere that is conducive to the free exchange of ideas in the team and the evolution of sustenance of mutual respect.[8]

The comments in the preceding text do not mean that the psychiatrist is simply the traffic cop of communications. Psychiatrists do need to lead and direct the program. The issue is one of balance: too forceful a style will ride roughshod over the staff. It may work initially but will inevitably lead to resistance and challenge. Additionally, too forceful a stance will undermine the development of the staff: just put the question to the doctor, we do not have to think!

Whereas much of the work of the staff development can be done in team meetings, while doing the treatment planning, it is necessary to have staff meetings too. These staff meetings need to be directed to some of the bureaucratic issues of a hospital, but some time should be reserved for staff development. With a new staff psychiatrist, on a unit with only one psychiatrist, this kind of work probably needs to be done weekly. On a unit with more than one psychiatrist, the usual frequency of meetings should suffice. As the staff members get to know each other and how they operate, the frequency of the meetings can be decreased. At a minimum, such meetings should occur every 2 months, with the option to schedule more urgent meetings. The advantage of meeting every 2 months is that it allows issues to be discussed that will otherwise smolder and poison the unit atmosphere.

Controversial issues on inpatient units often have to do with adequacy of medication of patients, responses to disruptive behaviors of patients, and dealing with family members or significant others. It is important for staff to understand the pharmacologic management of patients. Although nursing staff are on the front lines with the patients often for 8- to 12-hour shifts, the psychiatrist may see the patient only briefly. Although the psychiatrist may feel that he or she has a handle on how difficult the patient is to manage, there is often the sense from the staff that "if the doctor only knew how bad it was the doctor would give him Haldol." The only antidote to such a reaction is to communicate and overcommunicate with the nursing staff about the medication plan and why more or different medicines are not indicated. Likewise, manic patients are often perceived by inexperienced staff as simply troublesome, not ill.[31] Their intrusive, manipulative behaviors are often perceived as warranting punitive responses, including administrative discharge. It is within the purview of the psychiatrist to educate staff about the "manic game," which then increases the staff's professionalism and sense of competence. Because staff turnover is likely to be high at the mental health worker level, this education occurs not just once but repeatedly.

Recruitment Issues

There is a dearth of mental health professionals, especially psychiatrists and psychiatric nurses. There is a persistent flow of projections that indicate that there are not enough psychiatrists to treat all those in the country with psychiatric illnesses. Although nurse practitioner programs in psychiatry have developed, there are functions that they cannot perform as well as few graduating. It is an administrative responsibility to assist in the recruitment of staff to one's unit and their retention. Rural areas are particularly hard pressed to recruit psychiatrists.

Psychiatric administrators need to have an awareness of the local recruitment issues. From this appreciation, and in coordination with the human resources department, one should have plans regarding future staffing and recruitment. There are no easy solutions to the staffing problem. Sometimes the federal government can assist with loan-forgiveness programs for physicians if the area is designated a health professional shortage area.

Because of the difficulty recruiting psychiatrists, use of physician extenders, such as nurse practitioners in psychiatry and physician assistants, is growing. Their scopes of practice differ from state to state. For instance, in New York State a nurse practitioner in psychiatry may be privileged to admit and discharge patients, prescribe psychotropic medications, and perform therapy as long as there is a collaborative agreement with a psychiatrist. There are limitations in law as to how many nurse practitioners a physician may have collaborative agreement with. A well-trained nurse practitioner could work on an inpatient psychiatric unit performing almost all the functions of a psychiatrist.

It is now common outside of major metropolitan areas for emergency psychiatric services to be provided by nonpsychiatrists, that is psychiatric social workers, psychiatric nurses, and psychologists. A psychiatrist may be on call for backup purposes. The inadequate supply of trained professionals to deal with the mental health needs of society is likely to persist. A psychiatric administrator must be mindful of these staff shortages and be forward thinking as to how to meet the clinical need with the staff available.

Managed Care

Most psychiatric patients with employer-sponsored insurance have a managed mental health benefit. There is growing pressure in some states to bring Medicaid into managed care, including the mental health benefit for the seriously and persistently mentally ill. For institutions that care for commercially insured individuals, managed-care negotiations are a primary concern.

Many managed-care companies require precertification of the admission. Several of the large carve-out companies have contracts with a limited number of institutions, and it behooves the admitting personnel to ascertain whether the patient may be hospitalized at their facility. It has not been declared to be an Emergency Medical Treatment and Active Labor Act (EMTALA) violation to require transfer of a patient from a facility that has psychiatric services and a bed but not a contract with the insurer to another facility that has a contract. Failure to precertify risks nonpayment for the hospitalization or the patient being served with a large bill. Likewise, if one wants to transfer a patient, one often needs to do the precertification. Typically the reviewers appear to be working off a checklist, the details of which can be ascertained by their questions. If the admission or continued stay is denied, and the clinician feels that the admission or continued stay is necessary, then the clinician is obliged to appeal the decision. Discharge of a patient against the firm judgment of the clinician because of fiscal considerations has been grounds for malpractice suits against clinicians. It is cheaper to take the potential loss of income from the denial than to defend or pay for a malpractice suit. The care of the patient needs to be primary.

Managed-care reviewers typically require a finding of imminent dangerousness for justification of admission. It is the presence of this dangerousness in the context of a person with a mental disorder that constitutes "medical necessity." Where the issue is absolutely clear, such a decision is medically essential. In the absence of an incontrovertible act—such as a suicide attempt that necessitates an intensive care unit (ICU) admission after which the patient expressed regret at being alive—there is a need to convey to the reviewer the legitimacy of the inpatient admission. Clinicians should be trained as to how to do such assessments and to convey the findings in a manner that is intelligible and acceptable to reviewers. The decision is dichotomous: admit or not admit. The information has to be presented in a manner that clearly comes down on the side of the decision one is requesting. However, as soon as the imminence is dissipated, the expectation is that the patient will be discharged to a lower level of care. Clinicians need to be sensitive to this approach and therefore document the necessity for continued stay clearly. From the clinical and fiscal points of view, it is more important to document the clinical necessity for continued stay than the nuances of improvement. Notes written to celebrate small improvements but that ignore the reasons that justify continued stay will be interpreted as indicating that the patient is ready for discharge. Those improvements can be emphasized with the patient and the family, who will appreciate them.

REFERENCES

1. Talbott JA, Hales RE, eds. *Textbook of administrative psychiatry: new concepts for a changing behavioral health system*, 2nd ed. Washington, DC: American Psychiatric Press; 2001.
2. Rodenhauser P, ed. *Mental health administration: a guide for practitioners*. University of Michigan Press; 2000.
3. Reid WH, Silver SB, eds. *Handbook of mental health administration and management*. New York: Brunner-Routledge; 2003.
4. Greenblatt M. *Anatomy of psychiatric administration:the organization in health and disease*. New York: Plenum Press; 1992.
5. Russakoff LM. Administrative theory. In: Reid WH, Silver SB, eds. *Opere citato*. Brunner-Routledge; 57–73.
6. Kreeger L, ed. *The large group: dynamics and therapy*. Itasca: Peacock Publishers, Inc.; 1975.
7. Taylor FW. *The principles of scientific management*. Mineola: Dover Publications; 1998.
8. Likert R. *The human organization: its management and value*. New York: McGraw-Hill; 1967.
9. Kaplan RS, Norton DP. *The balanced scorecard: translating strategy into action*. Boston: Harvard Business School Press; 1996.
10. Kaplan RS, Norton DP. *The strategy-focused organization*. Boston: Harvard Business School Press; 2001.
11. Kaplan RS, Norton DP. *Alignment*. Boston: Harvard Business School Press; 2006.
12. Drucker PF. *Management: tasks, responsibilities, practices*. New York: Harper & Row; 1974.
13. McGregor D. *The human side of enterprise*. New York: McGraw-Hill; 1960.
14. Bass BM. *Bass and Stogdill's handbook of leadership: theory, research and managerial applications*. New York: Free Press; 1990.
15. Yukl G. *Leadership in organizations*, 5th ed. Upper Saddle River: Prentice Hall; 2002.
16. Vroom VH, Jago AG. *The new leadership: managing participation in organizations*. Englewood Cliffs: Prentice-Hall; 1988.
17. Mayo E. *The human problems of an industrial civilization*. Boston: Macmillan; 1933.
18. Herzberg F. *Work and the nature of man*. Cleveland: World Publishing; 1966.
19. Maslow AH. *Maslow on management*. New York: John Wiley & Sons; 1998.
20. Mintzberg H. *Structuring in fives*. Englewood Cliffs: Prentice-Hall; 1983, 1993.
21. Stanton AH, Schwartz MS. *The mental hospital: a study of institutional participation in psychiatric illness and treatment*. New York: Basic Books; 1954.
22. Caudill W. *The psychiatric hospital as a small society*. Cambridge: Harvard University Press; 1958.
23. Rubenstein R, Lasswell HD. *The sharing of power in a psychiatric hospital*. New Haven: Yale University Press; 1966.
24. Davis SM, Lawrence PR. *Matrix*. Reading: Addison-Wesley; 1977.
25. Katzenbach JR, Smith DK. *The wisdom of teams*. New York: HarperCollins; 1993.
26. Katzenbach JR, Smith DK. *The discipline of teams*. New York: John Wiley & Sons; 2001.
27. Lencioni P. *The five dysfunctions of teams*. San Francisco: Jossey-Bass; 2002.
28. Deming WE. *Out of the crisis*. Cambridge: MIT Center for Advanced Engineering Study; 1982.
29. IsHak WW, Burt T, Sederer LI, eds. *Outcome measurement in psychiatry: a critical review*. Washington, DC: American Psychiatric Press; 2002.
30. APA Task Force in Quality Indicators. *Quality indicators: defining and measuring quality in psychiatric care for adults and children*. Washington, DC: American Psychiatric Press; 2002.
31. Janowsky DS, Leff M, Epstein RS. Playing the manic game. *Arch Gen Psychiatry*. 1970;22:252–261.

CHAPTER 7

Legal Issues in Inpatient Psychiatry

GABOR VARI, MACE BECKSON, AND ROBERT WEINSTOCK

T he legal aspects of inpatient care often are not fully understood by or seem daunting to psychiatrists. The goal of this chapter is to provide an overview of legal issues involved in inpatient psychiatric care. Topics include hospital admission, informed consent, confidentiality, subpoenas, special considerations with suicidal and homicidal patients, legal issues involving involuntary administration of medication, and seclusion and restraint. Some of the details in this chapter are specific to the law in the state of California. The principles discussed, however, apply across states; most states have laws that address these issues. Practitioners should be aware of local laws because many of the legal principles discussed in this chapter vary state by state.

Admission

In the past, mentally ill patients had few rights. Patients were committed to mental hospitals by psychiatrists on the advice of families. Even when legal rights were recognized in theory, the problems patients had in legal representation in the absence of public defenders to handle such cases often made the theories hollow. Psychiatrists generally are most concerned with patient welfare or doing what is in the best interests of the patient. However, in recent decades the law has been less concerned with patient welfare and more concerned with balancing the patient's autonomy (civil liberties) with public safety. To the dismay of psychiatrists and families, patient welfare receded into the background in terms of justifying involuntary hospitalization.[1]

Two current theoretic concepts provide the state with justification for involuntary admission: police power and *parens patriae*. The principle of police power dictates that an individual's freedom may be restricted when he is deemed to be an acute danger to himself or others. *Parens patriae* (doing what is best for a patient much like a parent might do) is in conflict with the patient's right to autonomy. *Parens patriae* comes into play though only when the patient lacks competence to make his or her own decisions. In the past when psychiatrists had more authority to do whatever they thought best, they often ignored patients' autonomy and ordinary right to make their own decisions even if not the best ones. Concern for public safety and reluctance to take risks led psychiatrists to hospitalize patients for lengthy periods. Because of this, courts and legislation have had to balance these conflicting considerations. Many psychiatrists believe that the pendulum has swung too far in the direction of patients' rights as opposed to patient welfare. In many circumstances, a cumbersome legal bureaucracy more often interferes with treatment than provides meaningful patient protection. It can be unnecessarily wasteful of psychiatric and judicial time.[1] Often there are lengthy legal proceedings over a few extra days' hospitalization.

Case Vignette

Mr. A was a 45-year-old homeless man with a history of schizophrenia. He was brought to the emergency room by local police after they responded to a disturbance call. When the police encountered Mr. A, he was found walking in a residential area, breaking car windshields with a baseball bat and yelling "Jesus is Lord, savor his sword." A citizen attempted to intervene, and Mr. A postured aggressively threatening to kill him if he did not back away. When police arrived Mr. A did not respond to verbal redirection and swung his bat at officers. In the emergency room, psychiatric evaluation revealed a markedly tangential thought process and psychomotor agitation. The patient was clearly responding to internal stimuli. He had a record of multiple previous similar presentations to mental health facilities. He refused voluntary admission, and was, therefore, admitted to the inpatient unit as a danger to others.

In this case, Mr. A's involuntary admission was based on the psychiatrist's diagnosis of an active mental illness (in this case, a psychotic disorder) as well as danger to others. The patient's threatening behavior in the field was used as evidence. By using "danger to others" to justify Mr. A's admission and subsequent hold and evaluation period, the psychiatrist invoked the principle of police power. In this case police were actually involved, but the principle of police power may be invoked in the absence of involvement of law enforcement. Mental health professionals who are certified by the state to hospitalize patients involuntarily have the explicit legal power to deem a patient a danger to self or others and therefore place the patient on an involuntary hold using the concept of police power in some jurisdictions. In others after a short period of detainment the psychiatrist must apply to the court for civil commitment.

Case Vignette

Mr. B was a 47-year-old man with a history of bipolar disorder brought into the emergency room by his brother for recent worsening of manic symptoms. His brother stated that he found the patient wandering on the streets after days of looking for him; he had been missing for more than a week. The patient had stopped taking his lithium 2 weeks earlier. The patient appeared disheveled and was malodorous. On examination, Mr. B demonstrated pressured speech, grandiosity, and flight of ideas. He was able to attend, was alert and oriented four times, and clearly denied suicidal and homicidal ideation. When asked about plans to provide for his own food, clothing, and shelter, the patient replied, "A man, a plan, a canal, panama, palindromes, palindromes, motherfucker, what!" After repeated questioning the patient was still unable to provide a logical plan should he leave the emergency room. His brother said that he was unable to care for the patient in his current condition. The patient refused to consent to admission and was therefore admitted to the inpatient unit on the grounds of inability to care for himself. In states such as California such inability to provide for basic needs is called *grave disability*.

In this case, Mr. B was clearly not deemed to be a threat to himself or others and therefore police power could not be used to justify involuntary admission. The legal principle behind this admission is *parens patriae*. The principle of *parens patriae* (literally "father of the country"), like that of police power can outweigh a patient's right to freedom. In contrast to police power, this principle emphasizes the paternalistic duty of the state; that is, the state at times can deem that a patient is not able to provide for his or her own basic needs due to a mental illness and, by means of detention, can provide for the individual. In this situation, the patient is deemed to be negligent toward himself or herself rather than an active threat.

When a patient is deemed to be a danger to himself or herself, a danger to others, or unable to provide for himself or herself because of a mental illness, then the patient meets criteria for involuntary admission to a psychiatric unit. Because the US Supreme Court determined that "clear and convincing" is the minimum standard for civil commitment the burden of proof in some jurisdictions can be as high as "beyond a reasonable doubt,"[2] but it must now be at least "clear and convincing."[3,4] The patient ordinarily should first be offered a voluntary hospitalization. In some states such as California there is a system other than civil commitment in which the patient is not held as a result of a judicial order. Instead the patient is hospitalized by means of a hold instituted by a mental health professional, and the patient files a writ of *habeas corpus* to the court to be released. It is unclear what standard of proof applies under this framework, but it often is treated as if the standard is one of a preponderance of the evidence. It therefore is very important to know the specific jurisdiction and its laws.

In some states such as California, courts do not care whether a patient has the capacity to consent to even psychotropic medication so long as the patient consents. Expediency trumps common sense here because incompetent consents in reality are meaningless. However, there is legal precedent for finding against the hospital. In Florida, a patient was voluntarily admitted after consenting to hospitalization while actively psychotic, thinking he was signing into heaven, and lacking the decision-making capacity to agree to this hospitalization.[5] This Florida case decided by the US Supreme Court was based on a Florida statute requiring that a patient being voluntarily admitted be competent to consent to hospitalization and treatment. The Court found that the hospital had deprived the patient of the due process that an involuntary hospitalization legal proceeding would provide. In most states a judge would be petitioned early in the process to continue to hold, evaluate, and treat the patient. If the judge gives such an order for continuing assessment and treatment, then the process is known as *civil commitment*. In other states like California, physicians place the patient on a continuing hold after the initial assessment and treatment, and the patient has a right to go to court for a writ of *habeas corpus* to be released. In some states a guardian *ad litem* is appointed to make decisions on the patient's behalf.

On inpatient medical and surgical wards, a patient may be deemed to lack decision-making capacity with regard to consenting to medical treatment. Procedures are more informal in some states, such as California, with courts encouraging doctors and family to work out what is best. Courts may need to be involved only in cases of conflict. A surrogate decision maker should be identified. Ordinarily, this is the closest relative or the person who is designated previously by the patient in an advance directive. Ideally, the surrogate decision maker should be familiar with the patient's general wishes and be able to exercise substituted judgment on the patient's behalf (what the patient would have decided if competent). If that is not known, then doing what is thought to be in the patient's best interest is the next best standard. If no such surrogate can be found then physicians may petition the court to act as the patient's temporary surrogate or, in circumstances when this is not immediately practical, may form a consensus amongst a team of physicians to act temporarily on behalf of the patient until a surrogate decision maker can be assigned. In an emergency, it generally is advisable if at all possible to have two physicians agree with the planned emergency medical treatment.

If a patient is admitted voluntarily to a psychiatric ward for treatment, this technically means that the patient may leave the psychiatric ward at any time unless the patient meets the criteria for involuntary hospitalization and can be detained. Should the patient request immediate discharge while admitted on a voluntary basis, a psychiatrist should evaluate the patient within a reasonable amount of time. That time is defined in some jurisdictions by statute. If the evaluation reveals that the patient meets criteria for involuntary hospitalization, then the patient may be placed on a hold at this time or a petition filed for civil commitment. However, if the patient no longer meets criteria for hospitalization, then the patient cannot be kept against his or her will on the psychiatric unit. Some jurisdictions think such "involuntary" voluntary hospitalizations deprive patients of their rights to a judicial review and prefer patients who would not be allowed to leave be hospitalized involuntarily even if they are willing to be hospitalized. Because jurisdictions differ in the details about these procedures, the clinician must be familiar with the details of the local laws. Some policies may even differ between counties in the same state about procedures not specifically addressed in state law.

Treatment against the Patient's Will

In some states, including California, Massachusetts, Illinois, and New York, detaining a patient involuntarily for assessment and treatment does not automatically authorize involuntary treatment with psychotropic medication. This can often cause a dilemma for psychiatrists, nurses, and the ward milieu because many patients are hospitalized precisely because their behavior is felt to be grossly dangerous or out of control. Therefore, in these jurisdictions, a patient hospitalized because the need for treatment of mental illness was felt to trump the right to freedom under current civil law nonetheless cannot receive involuntary psychotropic medication absent an emergency.[6] In such states, in cases of medication refusal, a separate legal proceeding determines whether the patient lacks the capacity to refuse psychotropic medication.

In states with this requirement, involuntary treatment is allowed temporarily when there is clear evidence that a patient poses imminent danger to himself or herself or to others and there is an acute emergency. Frequent examples include agitated psychotic or manic patients and self-harm behaviors or suicide attempts in patients hospitalized for depression, mania, psychosis, or personality disorders. Involuntary psychotropic medication can be administered in the absence of an acute danger after the required legal proceeding. In many other states involuntary hospitalization automatically authorizes all psychiatric treatment against the patient's wishes, even psychotropic medication. Some states, though, have separate procedures for electroconvulsive therapy (ECT).

Often, problems with patient refusal of medication can be avoided by strictly following the principle of informed consent. This topic will be discussed in more detail later; briefly, informed consent for medication refers to full disclosure of a medication's risks, benefits, side effects, and alternatives. The informed consent process is a dialogue in which the psychiatrist discusses medication choice with the patient. Especially when patients are held in the hospital against their will, it is important to convey an air of cooperation. If the psychiatrist focuses on strengthening the therapeutic alliance and engages the patient fully in the informed consent process, the likelihood of medication adherence is higher. If the patient experiences side effects or otherwise does not tolerate or wish to continue with the medication, the patient is more likely to try other medications or engage in dialogue if there is a strong therapeutic alliance. Voluntary acceptance of medication usually is best regardless of the legal ability to administer it involuntarily. It also obviates the need for additional legal proceedings, which may be necessary when patients refuse. It also is more likely to result in patient compliance after discharge.

When a patient refuses treatment it is important to understand why the patient is refusing. Often, a severely ill patient refuses medication for a legitimate reason, such as a bothersome side effect. Assuming that patients are refusing medication because of psychosis or lack of insight is a common error in inpatient practice. It is important to attempt a dialogue with the patient so as to understand the reasons for refusal. The patient may have legitimate concerns about side effects of a specific medicine, such as weight gain. Often the concern can be accommodated by using a medicine low in the specific side effect that bothers the patient.

If the patient is unable or unwilling to participate in the initial informed consent process or later in the treatment course decides to stop complying, the psychiatrist must carefully evaluate the clinical picture in order to decide how to proceed. In such circumstances, informed consent must be obtained at a later time if the patient regains the capacity to give informed consent. Psychiatrists may forget to do this.

Case Vignette

Ms. C was a 42-year-old woman with borderline personality disorder and multiple somato-form disorders who had been admitted 3 days earlier on a hold for danger to self after she had attempted suicide by cutting superficially on her wrists and taking 10 pills of sertraline 100 mg. She was monitored briefly in the emergency room and had no significant medical sequelae of her overdose. Her wrists were treated with Neosporin and gauze bandages. Ms. C was well known to the hospital and the treating psychiatrist; this was her fourth hospi-talization in the last 6 weeks. She had many episodes of low-risk self-injurious behavior. She reported having tried to hurt herself because her therapist recently left on vacation. She had failed multiple selective serotonin reuptake inhibitor (SSRI) trials and after detailed discussion about possible medication trials she was agreeable to starting a low-dose antipsychotic. After 2 days on this medicine, the patient refused to continue taking it. She complained of headache, stomach upset, and worsening of irritable bowel syndrome symptoms. Recom-mendations to wait through the side effects or try a new medicine were refused. She was able to explain the risks of refusing psychotropic treatment including decompensation and death. She denied current suicidal ideation, had been calm and cooperative on the ward, and demanded discharge. Her hold for involuntary hospitalization was to expire later in the day. She no longer met the legal criteria for involuntary hospitalization and appeared to have the capacity to consent to or refuse psychotropic medication.

Case Vignette

Mr. B, the manic patient described earlier, had been admitted to the ward on a hold for grave disability. His lithium was restarted in combination with an atypical antipsychotic. After 3 days he was sleeping more and was less hyperactive, but he remained manic and psychotic. He had also been placed on an additional 14-day hold as he remained gravely disabled and was unwilling to stay in the hospital. On hospital day 4 he refused lithium and the antipsychotic. Asked why he was refusing the medication, the patient began hopping on one foot and recited, "Able was I, ere I saw Elba" in falsetto. He was considered at high risk for elopement.

The above-discussed vignettes present some common therapeutic dilemmas faced by inpatient psychiatrists. In both vignettes, the patients are refusing medication and wish to leave the hospital. For Ms. C, discharge and more comprehensive outpatient treatment planning may best suit the patient's interests. It is unlikely that a petition to the court for involuntary medication will be successful as the patient demonstrated decision-making capacity. Additionally, even if the court did grant the petition, the patient would be unlikely to remain compliant once an outpatient. Moreover, the patient appears no longer to meet the criteria for involuntary hospitalization.

With Mr. B, the psychiatrists are confronted with a patient who is manic and psychotic and is now refusing medication. He does not demonstrate decision-making capacity and continues to remain gravely disabled. The patient should continue to be offered routine medication. If he continues to refuse treatment, this should be documented along with his concomitant mental status. In this scenario, the treating psychiatrist in states that require this would likely petition the court in order to treat the patient with psychotropic medication against his will. If the court grants the petition then the patient may receive intramuscular injections against his will if he first refuses the offering of oral medication. Frequently, patients will take oral medicines they have previously refused once the court has found that they may be given injections against their will.

Guardianship or Conservatorship

A common clinical experience in inpatient psychiatry is the phenomenon of repeated admissions for a chronically seriously mentally ill patient, a phenomenon discussed in detail in Chapter 13. These admissions are frequently in the setting of severely limited psychosocial supports (e.g., homelessness and few friends or family) and poor medication compliance. This experience is frequently a frustrating one for health care providers. It is also typically financially burdensome for hospitals and, if many of these types of patients live in a given catchment area, can significantly tax mental health resources which are already stretched very thin in some areas.

Case Vignette

Mr. D, a 38-year-old homeless man with schizophrenia, was hospitalized on a hold for grave disability after he was brought by police who had found him wandering through a busy intersection. He was grossly disheveled, emaciated, malodorous, and sunburned. On contact with police, he spoke illogically about Neptune, Poseidon, and the Toronto Maple Leafs. He was well known to the hospital and staff and had been hospitalized eight times over the last 12 months in this hospital alone, and a review of mental health records demonstrated multiple stays at other hospitals. During his recent hospitalizations his psychotic symptoms resolved with routine antipsychotic administration. Each time he was discharged with apparently intact reality-testing yet inevitably failed to follow up with outpatient psychiatric follow-up, stopped taking his medicines, became psychotic, and was brought in by police shortly thereafter.

In order to deal with chronically relapsing seriously mentally ill patients, states either have long-term civil commitments or have implemented systems such as a limited guardianship, guardian *ad litem*, a committee, or a mental health conservatorship. A guardian or conservator has fiduciary responsibility for the patient to make decisions regarding the patient's placement, finances, and, if approved by the court, medical decisions and psychiatric treatment decisions including psychiatric hospitalization. The patient need not consent to treatment; frequently conservatorship terms require that the conservator consent to the specific treatment on behalf of the patient. The spirit of conservatorship is to place the patient in "the least restrictive environment." Typically, however, individuals who have such a clearly demonstrable level of persistent grave disability require fairly restrictive living and treatment accommodations. Although in the past, mentally ill patients were considered incompetent for all purposes the presumption generally now is that they are competent for most civil purposes unless specifically adjudicated to be incompetent for a specific purpose.

Court hearings can be part of the process for conservatorships, writs of *habeas corpus*, guardianships, and conservatorships. Hearings in the psychiatric ward as well as hearings in a courthouse proper can seriously disturb the doctor–patient relationship. Inpatient psychiatrists and inpatient staff should be familiar with not only the logistics of conservatorship procedures but also the collateral psychological toll it can take on patients and, secondarily, the ward milieu.

Dementing illnesses in the elderly are not considered serious mental illnesses in some jurisdictions in the same vein as schizophrenia and bipolar disorder. For individuals who are gravely disabled or unable to care for themselves by virtue of a dementia, inpatient psychiatrists in some states must pursue probate conservatorship of the person and/or estate. In some states, including California, this form of conservatorship helps with discharge planning as severely demented patients can be placed in more appropriate locked units and can also provide the patient's family (if applicable) with the ability to manage the patient's estate. This is especially relevant if psychiatric treatment is not in question because in California probate conservators cannot place the patient in a mental hospital, but they can place patients in other facilities including locked ones. Some states use terms such as *limited guardianships* or *committees*.

Suicide Risk Management

Suicide is the number one cause of malpractice lawsuits against psychiatrists. Of the approximately 30,000 suicides annually in the United States, some 5% to 6% occur in the hospital.[7] There are examples of hospitals being found liable when patients complete suicide on psychiatric wards,[8] patients suffer harm after eloping from the ward,[9] and patients commit suicide after alleged negligent release.[10] Inpatient suicides usually occur within the first week of admission.[11] In addition, suicide is more common during shift changes and in the days and weeks following discharge.[12] Liability is based on the suicide being foreseeable. When a suicidal patient has been hospitalized, whether on a voluntary or involuntary basis, the hospital and staff have been put on notice and have a duty, greater than with outpatients, to take reasonable steps to protect such an inpatient from self-harm. The performance of the attending clinician, inpatient staff, and hospital may be at issue; most common are the failure to assess risk properly or, having assessed the risk, failure to take proper protective action, such as failure to implement the appropriate level of supervision and monitoring based on the risk assessment.[13] In addition, liability may be incurred through failure to plan and implement appropriate treatment interventions, premature discharge, and failure to arrange for appropriate outpatient treatment, including level of care (e.g., partial hospitalization, intensive outpatient treatment, or traditional outpatient treatment).

Increased risk for inpatient suicide has been associated with a history of suicide attempt[14] as well as mood disorders, family history of psychiatric illness, and documentation of suicide risk in the medical record.[15] Simon and Gutheil,[16] in a review of 100 cases of suicide in litigation, identified a recurrent pattern of characteristics of suicide victims: hard-working, middle-management, family men between the ages of 30 and 50; in their first psychiatric hospitalization; suffering from a major depressive episode, single, severe, with melancholic features and psychotic features; with prominent anxiety or agitation; hopeless; withdrawn and detached from relationships; with no therapeutic alliance; denying psychiatric illness; denying current suicidal ideation, intent, plan, or attempt; poor adherence to treatment; avoidance of activities; pressing for discharge; unable to work or perceived threat to job; ready access to guns; and with financial constraints to treatment. (See also, chapter 2.)

Each state has laws regarding the involuntary hospitalization and treatment of suicidal patients. When a suicidal patient is unwilling to remain in the hospital on a voluntary basis, the available legal interventions should be utilized as appropriate. In situations of uncertainty, erring on the side of safety as part of a good-faith effort to protect the patient is advisable. The trier of fact, such as a judge, will make the ultimate determination of whether there are adequate grounds to maintain involuntary hospitalization. Furthermore, the trier of fact has immunity from lawsuits, while the clinician may not. In many states there can be immunity for the discharge itself and for the acts of the patient after discharge if the patient is released by a psychiatrist from involuntary hospitalization. These laws were adopted to encourage release from involuntary hospitalization, but there may be exceptions to this immunity or other theories of liability. Also, such immunity does not extend to acts such as suicide committed while in the hospital, to voluntary patients, or in many states to patients released by clinicians other than a psychiatrist.

Since 1995, the Joint Commission on Accreditation of Healthcare Organizations (JCAHO) has compiled statistics on "sentinel" (i.e., serious adverse) events, including inpatient suicides.[17] As of September 30, 2007, JCAHO had reviewed 4,693 sentinel events reported by its accredited organizations; inpatient suicide was the second most common type of sentinel event, comprising 12.2% of the total. Root cause analysis of the inpatient suicides most commonly identified problems with "assessment," followed by "environmental safety/security." Environmental safety and security are almost automatically implicated in the event of a successful suicide: for example, if a patient has committed suicide by hanging, the most common means of inpatient suicide, then the utilized feature of the environment (e.g., bathroom grab bar, door knob, etc.) becomes a root cause. In recent years, there has been an increasing focus on implementing safety features in inpatient units, such as utilizing breakaway shower rods, recessed shower heads, concealed pipes, small mesh-covered ventilation, piano-type door hinges, unbreakable mirrors and glass, and windows that cannot be opened. However, no hospital can be made suicide-proof and relying entirely on the environment to prevent suicide is folly.[12] Although a hospital is expected to make the environment reasonably safe, determined patients can be inventive and a completed suicide often reveals a new environmental hazard, resulting in additional modification of the environment. Nevertheless, such modifications do make the means of suicide less readily available. Similarly, it is generally prudent to remove belts, bras, shoelaces, and sharps and to maintain a strict contraband policy; control and count utensils and razors; detect "cheeking" and hoarding of pills; and keep cleaning solutions locked away from suicidal patients. A guiding principle should be the balancing of suicide risk and related precautions with patient dignity and autonomy.[18]

Of greater importance in the prevention of suicide are the appropriate assessment of suicide risk and the determination and implementation of an appropriate treatment plan, all of which must be documented in the medical record. The clinical risk assessment is based on the history; a timely and complete psychiatric examination; observations; and collateral information obtained from family and friends; as well as available previous records, such as faxed discharge summaries. Treatment team meetings on a regular and as-needed basis provide an opportunity to bring together data from multiple vantage points, thereby assisting in the accurate assessment of risk. As noted by Simon,[12] suicide risk assessment is an ongoing process, not an event, and should be done on admission, at discharge, and at significant clinical junctures, such as changes in levels of suicide precautions. As patients generally improve gradually, sudden improvement may be feigned in order to obtain discharge or may reflect a decision to commit suicide.[12] Risk factors for suicide, as well as protective factors against suicide, are identified and an assessment of risk is made.[19] On the basis of this assessment, a treatment plan is devised with the goal of reducing dynamic risk factors and mobilizing protective factors, thereby reducing the overall immediate risk of suicide. A suicide prevention contract should not be relied upon as a means to reduce risk. Treatment interventions, along with appropriate level of supervision, are the mainstay of reducing suicide risk.[12] The inpatient hospital provides an intensive evaluation and therapeutic milieu with around-the-clock management that can quickly implement treatment.[20] An important function of the inpatient hospitalization of the suicidal patient is stabilization and return to the independent functioning required for outpatient treatment. Important goals are improved autonomy, efficacy, and self-control.[20]

Appropriate supervision and monitoring is based on the suicide risk assessment and may include, in increasing intensity, nursing checks every 15 minutes, continuous line-of-sight observation, 1:1 observation at arm's length, and four-point hard leather restraints. As with environmental safety, monitoring alone cannot be relied upon to prevent inpatient suicide, and determined patients have successfully committed suicide on 1:1 observation. In a study of 76 inpatient suicides, 9% were on 1:1 observation or with a staff member at the time. In addition, 1:1 observation causes loss of privacy, and may result in embarrassment, humiliation, increased hopelessness, and elevated suicide risk.[12] Furthermore, maintaining patient control by overutilizing suicide precautions, such as placing a patient on long-term 1:1 observation or keeping a patient in continuous physical restraints, would be countertherapeutic, promoting regression, dependence, and lack of self-control. Therefore, treatment of short-term risk factors and the underlying psychiatric disorder are crucial in reducing suicide risk and preventing suicide. In addition to treating the underlying mood or psychotic disorder, aggressive targeted treatment of anxiety, panic, agitation, and insomnia is very important. Detoxification from alcohol and drugs of dependence is similarly very important. A period of observation off individual safety precautions before discharge is prudent. When a voluntary patient requests a discharge against medical advice (AMA), a risk assessment should be performed, with involuntary hospitalization considered as appropriate. AMA discharges should be accompanied by documentation of discussion with the patient of the risks of discharge and the benefits of hospitalization and an assessment of the patient's capacity and understanding.[21] Before the discharge of a suicidal patient, verified removal of firearms by family members is important.[18]

In the present managed care environment, it is common for inpatient psychiatrists to feel pressured to discharge suicidal patients at the behest of insurance companies. Insurers will often initiate physician to physician review of the medical necessithy of the current hospitalization. At times they will deny payment of further hospitalization because MDs employed by insurance companies will declare that patients no longer meet criteria for inpatient hospitalization. This trend has resulted in much shorter inpatient stays than it was 20 or even 10 years ago. It is important for clinicians to trust their own judgment and to make appropriate treatment decisions even when these decisions run contrary to the insurance companies' requests or threats of nonpayment. In the management of the suicidal patient, if the inpatient physician believes that a patient remains suicidal and a significant threat to himself or herself, then the physician should allow his or her own medical and ethical judgment to trump the financially motivated judgment of the insurer. This may result in the provision of services that the insurer does not cover. However, it would be the best patient-care choice, and a money-saver in the event of a suicide and subsequent law suit.

Violence Risk Management

Violence or the potential for violence due to a mental disorder may be the basis for an inpatient hospitalization. As with suicidal patients, a clinical risk assessment for violence must be made based on all sources of information that are reasonably obtainable. Treatment interventions geared toward reducing risk of violence should be implemented including an appropriate level of supervision and monitoring. While maintaining immediate safety, an appropriate diagnostic assessment must be made such that treatment of the underlying disorder may be accomplished, thereby reducing violence risk. Several instruments have been developed that may aid in inpatient violence risk assessment.[22,23] Many risk factors for inpatient violence have been postulated including anger regulation problems, interpersonal style, disturbed mental state,[24] and earlier onset of illness.[25] Additionally, long-term hospitalizations, diagnoses of borderline personality disorder or antisocial personality disorder, frequent medication changes, use of multiple sedating medications, and a past history of violence all seem to correlate positively with risk of violence on the inpatient unit.[26]

The initial interview is an important time to gather information about risk factors for violence. In addition to standard static and dynamic risk factors, interviewers should pay attention to the quality of the therapeutic alliance in the interview. A poor therapeutic alliance during the initial interview is a predictor of violence during that stay.[27] Another group found that hostility during the initial assessment is a predictor of verbal aggression but not necessarily physical violence.[28]

While waiting for treatment to reduce the severity of the psychiatric disorder, use of sedative medication, seclusion, or restraint may be effective interventions to reduce the potential for violence and injury to the patient and staff. The environment must be reasonably safe and free of obvious potential weapons; contraband must be identified and removed. (See also, chapter 12.)

Hospitalization of the potentially violent patient serves to protect intended victims, although notification of intended victims may be advisable legally or clinically, or in rare instances required by the jurisdiction. Involuntary hospitalization may be required; the laws vary by jurisdiction and should be known to the inpatient psychiatrist. Probable cause is a common legal standard. In situations of uncertainty, erring on the side of safety to prevent harm is preferable, and the trier of fact will determine whether the patient may be held against his will. Failure to assess the risk of violence appropriately or failure to intervene when there is high risk may result in liability for the hospital and staff. Premature discharge or failure to make appropriate postdischarge plans may be additional sources of liability.[29,30] However, practitioners should note that a history of inpatient psychiatric hospitalization does not raise an individual's risk for violent behavior above that of the general public.[31] Violent patients may have criminal records, be on parole or probation, or even have a warrant for their arrest. Patient confidentiality precludes contacting law enforcement unless the jurisdiction has a Tarasoff-type requirement that is best satisfied in a particular case by contacting law enforcement.[32–34] This requirement is in reference to the landmark *Tarasoff* case, which ultimately established a duty for psychotherapists to take reasonable steps to protect third parties in cases in which the therapist deems the patient an immediate and realistic threat to that person.

"Duty to protect" has been interpreted differently in different jurisdictions, although practitioners frequently erroneously refer to the *Tarasoff* decisions as creating a "duty to warn." Most states including

California allow for alternative protective options to a "Tarasoff warning." Not all jurisdictions have Tarasoff-type obligations. The inpatient psychiatrist has no duty to report violent crimes previously committed by a patient; indeed, to do so would be a violation of confidentiality. Reporting a past crime is not a legal requirement. There is no ethical or legal rationale to report such a patient solely for punishment and not to prevent future violence. Although controversial and generally involving situations of double agentry in which the patient's and the hospital's interests conflict, many practitioners believe law enforcement may be contacted to report an act of intentional violence on the inpatient unit. These usually involve situations that result in patient or staff injury and which is not the result of paranoia or delusion caused by a mental disorder; typically, such acts are done by patients with antisocial traits.

Case Vignette

Mr. E was a 24-year-old man with a history of opiate dependence who was admitted to the inpatient psychiatric ward voluntarily for opiate detoxification. Given his history of multiple failed detoxifications, drug use in prison, and having a friend bring him contraband heroin while detoxing in the past, he was thoroughly searched. A male staff member examined the patient while he was disrobed and went through his belongings to ensure that there was no contraband. He had intermittent symptoms of withdrawal in the first few days of admission and at times appeared lethargic with pinpoint pupils and absent withdrawal symptoms. On hospital day 7, he was found in the bathroom shooting up heroin. On detailed questioning, the patient revealed that he had smuggled a minute amount of heroin in with him by taping a small plastic bag to his scrotum which went undetected during the search.

In addition to preventing violence and suicide, inpatient wards are also charged with protecting patients from their own and other patients' impulsive behavior. For instance, manic patients are frequently sexually preoccupied and may seek sexual activity with patient peers, staff, or physicians. Ward staff and clinicians should monitor this type of behavior and make reasonable attempts to preclude this activity. Frequent verbal redirection may be necessary at times. Ideally, coed wards are structured such that men and women are housed in mutually inaccessible hallways, meeting only in common areas, but psychiatric units are often not so designed. Ward staff should be generally vigilant and should specifically closely monitor any patient who may pose a risk of sexual assault or other sexual misbehavior. Ward staff should also not overlook the possibility of impulsive same-sex sexual activity. Hospitals may be liable if they are found negligent in cases of transmission of sexually transmitted diseases or unintended pregnancy that result from such behavior.

Clinicians who are ultimately found liable are liable not for making the "wrong" decision but rather for failing to demonstrate and document a careful consideration and evaluation of clinical data justifying their decision within the standard of care, that is, negligence. Documentation of an adequate risk assessment is generally sufficient to demonstrate that this evaluation has taken place. In especially high-risk cases, clinicians are encouraged to obtain consultation from a colleague, preferably one with significant experience and expertise with the disorders at hand. Thorough documentation and consultation are the most important steps that clinicians can take in limiting their own liability in high-risk inpatient psychiatric cases.

Informed Consent

In the past, the patient–doctor relationship was seen primarily as paternalistic, with physicians prescribing or performing procedures as they saw fit for the patient. It actually was not until the end of the 19th century that consent was required. After the severe abuses of medicine by the Nazis and the Nuremberg trials, the doctrine of informed consent developed. At first, the standard was the malpractice standard: what other physicians were doing. In the 1970s this changed to a "reasonable man" standard. In *Cobbs v. Grant*[35] and *Canterbury v. Spence*,[36] courts decided physicians needed to provide the information that a reasonable patient would want to know to make an informed decision. The current standard is referred to as a *reasonable patient* standard. Ideally the information a specific patient would want to know should be provided, but because of the difficulty in determining this, the minimum standard is to provide the information a reasonable patient would consider material.

The conceptualization of the patient–doctor relationship has evolved into a more collaborative one, with patients having more input into their treatment based on personal preferences. Emphasis on informed consent has been key to the evolution of the patient–doctor relationship.

The burden is on the physician to ensure that informed consent is obtained before initiating a treatment course for a medical disorder. This should be documented in the chart. Many inpatient facilities have a patient sign a sheet that details the risks, benefits, and potential side effects of and alternatives to individual treatment modalities. However, because most patients do not read a consent form carefully or retain much of what is in it, a meaningful discussion of the risks and benefits is the crucial element in informed consent. Written informed consent forms are helpful but do not themselves demonstrate true informed consent.

Informed consent is made up of three elements: information, voluntariness, and competency. First, the patient must be clearly informed of risks, benefits, and potential side effects of and alternatives to a particular treatment recommended by the physician. Patients need not be informed of every possible adverse outcome or every possible treatment alternative, but they should be made privy to potential side effects and alternatives that a "reasonable patient" would want to know. Frequency of occurrence and seriousness are important considerations in determining what should be discussed.

Some physicians are concerned that detailed discussion of potential adverse outcomes of a recommended treatment may discourage patients from accepting it. However, patients who feel that they are fully informed develop more trust in their physicians and are more willing to accept treatment recommendations even with full explication of potential side effects or complications. Many malpractice cases rest on the plaintiffs' arguing that they suffered a significant injury that they did not foresee because the physician did not explain the potential for this adverse outcome. This is to say that a procedure or medication was administered without fully informed consent.

A second component of informed consent is voluntariness. In order for a patient to provide informed consent, he or she must be willing to undergo the recommended treatment course free of coercion. Voluntary psychiatric patients should give informed consent to treatment including medication. However, in some states, including California, there generally is no concern that consent to psychiatric treatment be competent. The only concern is that the relevant information be provided and that the patient consent whether or not it is a competent consent. Some counties in California do prefer that the consent to hospitalization be competent and the patient otherwise be held involuntarily such that their legal rights are protected. Other California counties want patients who are incompetent to consent to treatment to be nonetheless allowed to sign in voluntarily just so long as they consent. Some states, including Florida, require that the consent to both hospitalization and treatment be competent. It is essential to know the law and interpretation of the law not only in your state but sometimes in your specific county.

The third component of informed consent is competency. Competency is a legal term, so commonly in psychiatric practice the concept of decision-making capacity is used instead. However, so long as it is clarified that a psychiatrist's opinion about a patient's competence or lack of it does not make the patient legally competent or incompetent, it is possible to refer to the psychiatrist's opinion about a patient's competence to make treatment decisions. Psychiatrists should evaluate individual patients for decision-making capacity by assessing the patient's capacity to weigh the risks and benefits of a specific procedure. This means that the psychiatrist decides whether the patient has an ability to understand his or her diagnosis, why the treatment is being recommended, and the potential risks, benefits, and side effects of and alternatives to the treatment. The patient should also have an appropriate understanding of the potential consequences of declining the treatment.

In addition to understanding, the term *appreciate* is generally used in assessing decision-making capacity. Appreciate includes a broader affective understanding than pure cognitive understanding. Although the term *appreciate* may ultimately need to be assessed in cognitive terms, it still is a useful term to clarify that more than a simplistic cognitive understanding may be necessary for decision-making capacity in some contexts. The ability to reason is also necessary in reaching a competent decision in some contexts. Decision-making capacity is evaluated during a specific time for a specific treatment. For example, if a patient is deemed not to possess the capacity to make a decision about complex surgery, this does not mean that he or she lacks decision-making capacity to accept or decline a less complex medical treatment or psychotropic medication. In other words, the determination of decision-making capacity must be performed individually for different components of the patient's treatment. In some jurisdictions such as California, Massachusetts, and New York, in order to treat patients with psychotropic medicines against their will, as discussed earlier, the patient must be found to lack competence to give informed consent in some type of legal procedure.

Exceptions to informed consent also exist. There are times in treatment when the need for immediate treatment trumps the individual's right to autonomy and the patient need not be fully informed. In the concept of therapeutic privilege, the potential side effects of a medicine may not be volunteered to a patient who is too agitated and psychotic to understand and weigh the risks and benefits of a medicine or procedure. This privilege for the physician must be used cautiously. Patients even if mentally ill are presumed to have a right to give or withhold informed consent to treatment. Material information for a decision cannot be withheld just because a patient might refuse. Additionally, there is an obligation to discuss this with a patient as soon as the patient regains capacity to weigh the risks and benefits. Often physicians fail to do this, or doctors may change. Psychiatrists risk liability in such circumstances for failure to obtain informed consent when the patient becomes competent to give informed consent.

On the inpatient ward, agitated patients who are at immediate risk for harm to themselves or others should be treated in an emergency with psychotropic medication for their agitation regardless of consent. Sometimes, though, involuntary treatment can be avoided by redirection to a quiet area for decreased stimulation. Sometimes in emergencies, there can be a takedown with seclusion and restraints often thought by the law to be less intrusive than psychotropic medication because it is not mind altering, although most clinicians see things differently. In these emergency situations, consent need not be obtained, although there are frequently guidelines and regulations pertaining to more restrictive measures such as seclusion and restraint.

Seclusion and Restraints

When a patient is agitated and not redirectable and there is imminent risk of harm to the patient, other patients, or staff, seclusion and restraint are sometimes employed. Consistent with contemporary focus on patient's rights, patients should be treated and their agitation best addressed with the least restrictive alternative. Seclusion and restraint should typically be used only in emergency circumstances and only when less restrictive alternatives, such as verbal redirection or sending patients to their rooms, have already been exhausted. Restraint and seclusion should never be used for punitive purposes. In prisons there often are pressures for a psychiatrist to condone seclusion, restraint, and psychotropic medication used as a punishment. Psychiatrists must resist such pressures in prisons and certainly in hospitals. These interventions play an important role in the management of the agitated patient as well as in decreasing stimulation in the ward milieu.

State and local statutes vary in regard to definitions of seclusion and restraints, documentation and monitoring requirements, and indications and contraindications. Practitioners are advised to be familiar with the requirements of their local jurisdiction regarding administration of seclusion and restraints.

The Joint Commission mandates that institutions have their own policies in place governing patient assessment and monitoring, type of restraints used, length and frequency of restraint or seclusion use, and physician orders and nursing documentation. Staff and physicians should copiously document the clinical justification for using seclusion or restraints, including the failure of less restrictive alternatives. Patients should regularly be monitored by physicians and nursing staff to ensure that they remain medically stable; morbidities associated with restraints include circulatory obstruction if restraints are administered too tightly, aspiration if the patient is kept horizontal, and respiratory suppression depending on which medicines were administered. Frequent monitoring assists in providing good patient care and also limits institutional liability exposure in this area.

Physicians are required to write an order for restraint or seclusion before the patient being secluded or restrained or immediately thereafter in emergencies. Additionally, the physician must evaluate the patient within a reasonable amount of time of entering seclusion or restraint to ensure patient safety. States may specify these time limitations. If patients are going to be placed in restraint, they should typically be medicated first. The medicine should be administered by mouth if the patient is willing or intramuscularly while the patient is restrained if the patient is uncooperative. Medicines are administered primarily to decrease agitation. Additionally, sedating medicines may be helpful in preventing the patient from fighting against restraints and thereby reduce risk of harm to self or others.

Keep in mind that there are exceptions to this general rule. For example, if neuroleptic malignant syndrome (NMS) is suspected to play a role in the agitation of a delirious patient then neuroleptics should not be administered in the course of placing the patient in seclusion or restraints. If the patient has an elevated creatine kinase (CK) in the setting of possible NMS, restraint may be relatively contraindicated as it could result in further CK elevations if the patient struggles. Additionally if delirium of unclear etiology is suspected to play a role in the agitation then benzodiazepines should be withheld as they have a propensity to exacerbate delirium.

Case Vignette

Mr. B remained manic and psychotic. He entered the dayroom and screamed, "Madam I'm Adam! Madam I'm Adam!" repeatedly and began jumping on furniture and stepping on and slightly injuring other patients. He did not respond to verbal redirection and remained agitated and noninteractive with staff. The resident physician was paged and agreed with nursing staff that the patient required an emergent intervention. The patient's current behavior, imminent danger to self and others, and lack of responsiveness to alternative treatment modalities were thoroughly documented. An order was written for seclusion and restraint. He was taken down, placed into restraints, and administered a combination of haloperidol, lorazepam, and diphenhydramine. He was placed in the seclusion room for de-escalation as well. The resident physician performed a physical examination and documented it. Nursing staff frequently monitored the patient to ensure his safety. After a few hours, he was allowed out of restraint and seclusion and interacted appropriately with staff and other patients.

Confidentiality

Patients admitted to a psychiatric ward have a right to confidentiality. On admission, patients should sign a release of health information form listing all parties to whom they permit the release of information regarding their health and admission. Absent such a release, under typical circumstances, staff and physicians should refrain from divulging any health information to any inquiring third party without the patient's permission. Indeed, employees should be trained to neither confirm nor deny even the presence of specific patients on the ward at any given time. In some jurisdictions, patient permission is needed even to contact family members and friends to get information necessary for the assessment. In most jurisdictions, involuntary hospitalization for assessment and treatment alone authorizes contacting third parties to collect necessary information.

Steps should also be taken to ensure patients' anonymity from one another. In some jurisdictions, charts may not have patients' full names visible from the outside. Identifiers such as social security numbers or medical record numbers should also not be plainly visible to patients or visitors. Many psychiatric wards have bulletin boards listing patients' names with their corresponding physician, therapist, social worker, and other support staff. Names on this list should be first name only and when patients of the same name are on the ward then the minimal additional distinguishing information should be provided.

There are exceptions to this rule of confidentiality. Some states permit breaking confidentiality to notify family of the inpatient hospitalization of their relative or to obtain information about an involuntarily hospitalized patient. Other jurisdictions, including California, require patient permission before doing this. When there is sufficient evidence that an inpatient is planning to harm another specific person, then clinicians in many jurisdictions may elect to execute their *Tarasoff* duty by informing the police or the intended victim, or both, of the specific threat including the patient's identity. In some jurisdictions, such confidentiality violations are not permitted. Confidentiality requirements also do not pertain to civil commitment proceedings, writs of *habeas corpus* from a mental hospital, or civil commitment procedures. In other words the patient need not consent to allow the physician to divulge specific clinical information at a civil commitment hearing or a hearing for a writ of *habeas corpus* for release from the hospital.

It is important to understand the difference between confidentiality and privilege. Confidentiality is an ethical requirement of the physician often reinforced by statute. Privilege is the patient's right to keep information out of a court or legal proceeding. Only a patient intentionally or by his actions can give up this privilege. The doctor cannot violate this privilege without patient permission or unless specifically ordered by a judge to do so.

It is important not to hand over records automatically in response to a subpoena. If the records are privileged, as treatment records are, the person requesting them may have no right to them without the patient's permission. It is important to check with an attorney or malpractice carrier. A subpoena means only that the person requesting the information has told a judge the information was relevant. It does not mean that the judge has considered competing privilege considerations or that the requesting person has a legal right to the information or records. Also, even in the absence of privilege, lack of relevance is a reason to keep sensitive or embarrassing information out of the courtroom. Often a treating psychiatrist may wish to enlist the help of the patient's attorney or the psychiatrist's or hospital's attorney to keep privileged or irrelevant information out of court.

A subpoena must be responded to but not necessarily by doing what is asked. There could even be liability for handing over information in response to a subpoena in violation of the patient's privilege. Psychiatrists sometimes fail to consider that the privilege is the patient's and not the doctor's. Unless specifically ordered to hand over the records by a judge after considering privilege issues, there can be liability for violating the patient's privilege. There are even greater protections for drug treatment records or reproductive counseling or reproductive health care. Care must always be taken before handing over any records without the patient's permission.

Conclusion

This chapter has aimed to cover basic legal issues that face the inpatient psychiatric clinician. Topics covered have included legalities of hospital admission, informed consent, confidentiality, subpoenas, special considerations with suicidal and homicidal patients, involuntary administration of medication, and seclusion and restraints. This chapter is not intended to be a comprehensive and exhaustive reference on each of these issues but rather a primer with basic principles of these topics. Clinicians are strongly encouraged to be cognizant of these various legal concepts as they pertain to inpatient psychiatric practice; a fundamental understanding of these concepts should aid in reduction of liability as well as more thorough and comprehensive delivery of patient care. Clinicians are also encouraged to familiarize themselves with their local and state statutes pertaining to individual aspects of inpatient psychiatry as these may significantly vary from one jurisdiction to another. Consultation with experienced practitioners, forensic psychiatrists, attorneys, and risk-management experts is often important.

REFERENCES

1. Stone AA. *Mental health and the law: a system in transition.* New York: Jason Aronson Inc; 1976.
2. *Lessard v. Schmidt.* 349 F. Supp 1078,1972:851–852.
3. *Fasulo v. Arafeh.* 378, A.2d., 1977:553.
4. *Addington v. Texas.* 441, U.S. 418, 1979:852–853.
5. *Zinermon v. Burch.* 494, U.S. 113, 1990:854–855.
6. *California Welfare and Institutions Code Section 5332(b).*

7. Busch KA, Clark DC, Fawcett J, et al. Clinical features of inpatient suicide. *Psychiatr Ann.* 1993;23:256–262.

8. *Winger v. Franciscan Medical Center*, 701 N.E.2d 813 (Ill. App. 1998).

9. *Rohde v. Lawrence General Hospital*, 614 N.E.2d 686 (Mass. App. 1993).

10. *Bell v. New York City Health and Hospitals Corporation*, 456 N.Y.S. 2d 787 (N.Y. 1982).

11. Qin P, Nordentoft M. Suicide risk in relation to psychiatric hospitalization. *Arch Gen Psychiatry.* 2005;62:427–432.

12. Simon RI. *Assessing and managing suicide risk: guidelines for clinically-based risk management.* Washington, D.C.: American Psychiatric Publishing; 2004.

13. Bongar B. *The suicidal patient: clinical and legal standards of care.* Washington, D.C.: American Psychological Association; 2002.

14. Bostwick JM, Pankratz VS. Affective disorders and suicide risk: a re-examination. *Am J Psychiatry.* 2000;157:1925–1932.

15. Sharma V, Persad E, Kueneman K. A closer look at inpatient suicide. *J Affect Disord.* 1998; 47:123–129.

16. Simon RI, Gutheil TG. A recurrent pattern of suicide risk factors observed in litigation cases: Lessons in risk management. *Psychiatr Ann.* 2002;32:384–387.

17. Joint Commission on Accreditation of Healthcare Organizations. http://www.jointcommission. org/NR/rdonlyres/D7836542-A372-4F93-8BD7-DDD11D43E484/0/SE_Stats_9_2007.pdf. [Cited: December 28, 2007]. [Online]

18. Sokolov G, Hilty DM, Leamon M, Hales RE. Inpatient Treatment and Partial Hospitalization. In: Simon RI, ed. *The American psychiatric publishing textbook of suicide assessment and management.* Washington, DC: American Psychiatric Publishing; 2006.

19. American Psychological Association. *APA practice guidelines for the treatment of suicidal behavior.* 2003.

20. Chiles JA, Strosahl KD. *Clinical manual for assessment and treatment of suicidal patients.* Washington, DC: American Psychiatric Publishing; 2005.

21. Gerbasi JB, Simon RI. When patients leave the hospital against medical advice: Patients' rights and psychiatrists' responsibilities. *Harv Rev Psychiatry.* 2003;11:333–334.

22. Ogloff RP, Michael D. The dynamic appraisal of situational aggression: An instrument to assess risk for imminent aggression in psychiatric inpatients. *Behav Sci Law.* 2006;24(6):799–813.

23. Abderhalden C, Needham I, Dassen T, et al. Predicting inpatient violence using an extended version of the Brøset-Violence-Checklist: Instrument development and clinical application. *BMC Psychiatry* 2006 Apr 25;6:17.

24. Doyle M, Dolan M. Evaluating the validity of anger regulation problems, interpersonal style, and disturbed mental state for predicting inpatient violence. *Behav Sci Law.* 2006;24(6):783–798.

25. Chang JC, Lee CS. Risk factors for aggressive behavior among psychiatric inpatients. *Psychiatr Serv.* 2004;55(11):1305–1307.

26. Soliman AE, Reza H. Risk factors and correlates of violence among acutely ill adult psychiatric inpatients. *Psychiatr Serv.* 2001;52(1):75–80.

27. Beauford JE, McNiel DE, Binder RL. Utility of the initial therapeutic alliance in evaluating psychiatric patients' risk of violence. *Am J Psychiatry.* 1997;154(9):1272–1276.

28. Troisi A, Kustermann S, Di Genio M, et al. Hostility during admission interview as a short-term predictor of aggression in acute psychiatric male inpatients. *J Clin Psychiatry.* 2003;64(12):1460–1464.

29. *Ewing v. Goldstein*, 15 Cal Rptr. 3d 864 (Cal. Ct. App. 2004).

30. *Ewing v. Northridge Hospital Medical Center*, 16 Cal Rptr. 3d 591 (Cal. Ct. App. 2004).

31. Steadman HJ, Mulvey EP, Monahan J, et al. Violence by people discharged from acute psychiatric inpatient facilities and by others in the same neighborhoods. *Arch Gen Psychiatry.* 1998;55:393–401.

32. *Tarasoff v. Regents of University of California*, 551 P.2d 334 (Cal. 1976).

33. *Tarasoff v. Regents of University of California*, 529 P.2d 553 (Cal. 1974).

34. Weinstock R, Vari G, Leong GB, et al. Back to the past in California: A temporary retreat to a Tarasoff duty to warn. *J Am Acad Psychiatry Law.* 2006;34(4):523–528.

35. *Cobbs v. Grant* 150 US App DC 263; 464 F2d 772, 780, aff'd. 409 US 1064.

36. *Canterbury v. Spence*, 464 F.2d 772, 1972:863.

CHAPTER 8

Psychiatric Education on the Inpatient Unit

CYNTHIA A. PRISTACH AND SUBHDEEP VIRK

T he hospital has traditionally been the main training site for medical students, residents, nurses and other health care professionals. As the practice of medicine has evolved, other venues for training have emerged, and more psychiatric care is being provided in ambulatory settings.[1] Nevertheless, the inpatient hospital setting remains an important training site with many opportunities for teaching and learning.

Strengths of Training in an Inpatient Setting

The inpatient setting offers a rich environment for studying psychopathology, learning pharmacotherapy, and beginning skills in psychotherapy. Hospitalized patients are generally the most severely ill, suffering from psychosis, mania, and suicidal behaviors. Students and residents are able to participate in their treatment in a safe, controlled environment with direct, regular on-site supervision by an attending psychiatrist. They have an opportunity to interact with patients and the supervising attending free of the time constraints typical of other treatment settings, such as outpatient clinics or the emergency department. Given that inpatient-based clerkships have predominated in medical education since the late 19th century,[1] there is a hospital culture, including nursing and administrative staff, that encourages education in this setting. Attending psychiatrists serve as role models, especially because they are more involved in direct patient care than in the past, in part due to state and federal regulations.[2] Unlike many other educational settings, students and residents participate directly in the process of evaluation, diagnosis, and treatment of the patient under supervision. Because hospital stays are shorter, there is an emphasis on rapid, accurate diagnosis and treatment planning, as well as the need to establish relationships with severely ill patients.[3] Students and residents participate as members of an interdisciplinary treatment team of health care professionals, including nurses, psychologists, social workers, occupational therapists and recreational therapists, an experience that may not be replicated elsewhere. In acute inpatient settings, families are typically involved, and their inclusion in treatment planning gives residents and medical students a chance to learn basic family assessment and intervention methods. In the inpatient setting, residents and medical students encounter problems that are unique to the discipline of psychiatry, such as the legal and ethical issues of involuntary commitment and treatment.

Perhaps the greatest strength of having residents train in the inpatient setting is that it encourages integration of their identities as physicians, even as they begin to assume their new roles as psychiatrists. As part of the Accreditation Council on Graduate Medical Education (ACGME)[4] "Patient Care" competency, psychiatry residents are expected to perform physical and neurologic evaluations on their patients, and be able to integrate their findings to establish a clinical diagnosis. Depending on the training site, residents might be expected to assume complete management of their patient's acute and chronic medical and neurologic problems, or work in conjunction with a medical consultant. At the very least, residents must be proficient in the diagnosis and treatment of organic mental disorders such as delirium and dementia, as well as pharmacologic and medical complications associated with other psychiatric illnesses. This early opportunity to integrate the roles of physician and psychiatrist is best done in the inpatient setting, and can be further enhanced in later rotations, such as consultation/liaison or emergency psychiatry.

Weaknesses of Training in an Inpatient Setting

Many factors have influenced the education of health care professionals, including psychiatrists. For example, the advent of managed care has had a tremendous impact on how and where clinical care is delivered, length of stay, treatment planning, and supervision of trainees. Inpatient admission is no longer an option for many patients, depending on their diagnosis and degree of lethality. Some insurance companies allow only patients with overt suicidal ideation or attempts to be admitted and many allow only brief stays. As a result, students and residents see the most severely ill patients with whom contact is usually brief due to shortened length of stays.[5] Criteria for admission are now more stringent, and patient problems are generally narrower in scope and not likely to mirror the kinds of issues residents will face in actual practice settings.[6] Patients must demonstrate severe pathology or symptoms, such as active suicidal ideation or acute psychosis, in order to be deemed appropriate for admission. In reality, most residents will practice in outpatient settings where patients are more likely to present with anxiety, mood, adjustment, or personality disorders. Most medical students will pursue training in specialties other than psychiatry, where patients present with more subtle psychiatric symptomatology which they may have difficulty recognizing if their training in psychiatry is limited to treating patients with psychopathology typical of those seen in inpatient settings. Because of shorter lengths of stay, medical students and residents may not have the opportunity to see their patients progress to the point of full recovery from their illnesses, or to develop relationships which enable them to focus on psychological factors influencing the patient's illness.[2]

Because of the acute nature of the patients' illnesses, treatment modalities in the inpatient setting are often limited. Medication, rather than psychotherapy, is the norm, and students get a distorted view of available psychiatric interventions. They may lose sight of the importance of the therapeutic alliance in treatment, and the value of psychotherapy, even for chronically ill patients. For medical students in particular, their impression of mental illness may be skewed such that they might perceive it in a negative light. Students have less of an opportunity to observe that even patients with severe illnesses can have productive and satisfying lives, a fact that is often lost because of short length of stays.

Case Vignette

A patient with paranoid schizophrenia is assigned to a third year medical student. The patient is convinced that Osama bin Laden was in her house, and she needed to contact the White House and FBI. During a discussion with the student, she becomes so upset that she needs to be restrained and medicated. The student is shocked by the intensity of the patient's psychosis, and confides to a friend that he does not think psychiatry is the specialty for him.

Faster turnover of patients and increased clinical caseloads for psychiatric attending physicians result in less time to educate students and residents.[7] Requirements for documentation by attending physicians, as well as concerns about liability issues are additional factors which limit time spent with residents and students.[8]

Emotional Aspects of Working in an Inpatient Setting

Care of patients in the inpatient setting can be particularly stressful for students and residents, especially residents who are at the beginning of their training. Beginning residents from all specialties experience stressors unique to starting residency training. These include defining one's role as a physician, managing significant clinical demands with limited clinical experience, balancing training and personal needs, and forging a satisfactory relationship with supervisors and peers. For psychiatry residents in particular, there are unique obstacles to training, which are not experienced by residents from other specialties. The "beginning psychiatry training syndrome," a typically transient and potentially valuable adaptive response, has been described and characterized as having temporary neurotic symptoms, psychosomatic disturbances, and symptomatic behavior.[9] While the "syndrome" was first recognized at a time when psychotherapy was a mainstay in the treatment of psychiatric inpatients, the basic tenets are applicable even now regarding the emotional turmoil faced by beginning residents, and even medical students. Residents rotating on inpatient units usually have limited experience, yet are confronted by patients with the most severe illnesses. Residents must learn to recognize psychopathology, and assume significant responsibility for treatment of their patients, including psychological treatment. It is in the inpatient setting that residents first learn to process their own emotional response to patients and begin to define their role as a psychiatrist[9] while maintaining their medical identity.

Case Vignette

A first-year resident is assigned to treat a 78-year-old woman admitted with symptoms of mania. She also has congestive heart failure and diabetes, which is poorly controlled. Despite repeated discussions with his supervisor, the resident fails to obtain a medicine consultation with the result that he devotes most of his time to the medical, rather than the psychiatric care, of the patient. When confronted with the issue during supervision, he admits that he feels more comfortable treating the patient's medical problems, and is not really sure how to deal with her mania. He is able to see that he is torn between his identity as a physician, and his new role as a psychiatric resident.

Emotional distress experienced by beginning psychiatry residents is part of normal professional development. Programs should monitor residents for stress, and can aid personal growth by incorporating professional development seminars, or experiential or T-groups into the curriculum. These may be especially useful to encourage beginning residents to forge relationships with their peer group and provide a forum to discuss the stresses associated with training in the inpatient setting.[10]

Educational Methods in the Inpatient Setting

Fortunately, the inpatient psychiatric unit remains a vibrant entity for education of health care professionals. With some creativity and flexibility, many of the traditional methods of teaching in the inpatient setting remain valuable for training.

INTERDISCIPLINARY TREATMENT TEAM

Participation on an interdisciplinary treatment team is an excellent experience for students and residents. The interdisciplinary health care model typically involves members from two or more disciplines working together in a collaborative relationship to provide health care to a patient. Information is assimilated and shared, members recognize and appreciate the skills and contributions of other disciplines, and share the risk of decision making for the patient.[11] Residents must learn to be participants, as well as leaders, and to negotiate role ambiguity with other specialists, such as nurses, psychologists, occupational therapists, and social workers.[3] By gradually having the resident and student take a more active role on the team, the attending psychiatrist can model and teach professionalism, consensus building, and communication skills. As members of all disciplines share their observations of and experiences with patients, students and residents learn to incorporate these findings into their view of the patient and to modify the treatment plan. Teaching can be done by all members, each of whom has their own theoretic and practical viewpoint regarding psychiatric assessment and care.

Case Vignette

A resident starts an inpatient rotation on an eating disorders unit. He meets a newly assigned patient in the dining room during breakfast. The patient insists they leave the dining room before she has eaten in order to have more privacy, so the resident brings the tray to the patient's room. The staff becomes infuriated with the resident, and accuses him of siding with the patient and encouraging splitting. The issue is discussed in team meeting where all staff express their concerns. The resident is included in the revision of the treatment plan.

TREATMENT TEAM MEETINGS

The treatment team meeting generally serves to make clinical care and treatment decisions, to review patient progress, and to teach relevant clinical issues. Such meetings ensure that all members of the treatment team are aware of the main concerns and treatment issues for each patient.[12] A variation of the treatment team meeting is chart rounds. Chart rounds typically include the interdisciplinary treatment team where the patient's history is briefly reviewed, pertinent medical and psychiatric issues and treatment are discussed, along with discharge planning. The opinion of all members of the treatment team is respected, including input from medical students and residents. Medical students, in particular, are often impressed with the large role they play in their patient's care. Chart rounds is also an excellent time for the attending psychiatrist to review progress notes and orders written by students and residents and to teach good written communication skills. Proper documentation should emphasize content (including adequate but concise description of psychopathology and discussion with patient), medicolegal issues (especially in cases of lethality), and legibility. Progress notes should also respond to advice from consultants[13] and address pertinent medical problems or laboratory abnormalities.

WALK-ROUNDS

Borrowing from other specialties where inpatients are treated, walk-rounds are a valuable teaching tool. Actual teaching at the bedside has declined in all specialties in the past number of years, for a variety of reasons. Time constraints, increased reliance on technology, and concerns about patient privacy are just some of the reasons why this teaching tool is so little used. Bedside teaching may in fact be more difficult and challenging to the attending psychiatrist, requiring adequate knowledge, good observation skills, and sensitivity to the needs of the patient and learners.[14] However, walk-rounds give medical students and residents a chance to directly observe the attending psychiatrist interact with and evaluate the patient. Professionalism, communication skills, and treatment of the patient that is kind and compassionate are just a few of the areas that can be taught at the bedside. Evaluations of patients are usually brief, but can be used to elicit psychopathology and assess symptom severity, demonstrate therapeutic interventions, or determine medication response or side effects. It is important to avoid marginalizing the patient during the encounter and to include him or her in the discussion of symptoms or illness. For the supervising psychiatrist, this is an excellent opportunity to model good interpersonal and communication skills, as well as patient education. Walk-rounds can also be used for the attending to observe the student's or resident's interaction with the patient and provide direct, immediate feedback regarding their psychotherapeutic interaction.[15] Conducting walk-rounds with the entire interdisciplinary team is more complicated, but allows inclusion of the patient in the treatment planning process, especially when social issues are part of the discussion.

FORMAL CASE PRESENTATIONS

Another educational strategy in the inpatient setting is the use of formal case presentations by residents or medical students. A patient with an unusual symptom complex, medical complication, or difficult treatment issue can be selected and presented by a student or resident. All or part of the treatment team can participate, providing a chance for discussion and education for members of all disciplines. The formal case presentation can be used to demonstrate and integrate the biopsychosocial and psychodynamic aspects of a patient's problems and to incorporate these into the treatment plan.[2] While the discussant might be the attending psychiatrist, the experience can be greatly enriched by including a guest faculty who is a general psychiatrist, subspecialist (e.g., addiction, geriatric psychiatrist) or from a completely different discipline (e.g., internal medicine, neurology). In addition to the benefit of the consultation, such interdisciplinary conferences enable the attending to instruct the student or resident in the art of written and oral presentation skills.

EVIDENCE-BASED MEDICINE

Evidence-based medicine focuses on data derived from clinical research to make treatment decisions, rather than reliance on clinical experience or intuition.[16] By using evidence-based approaches to patient care, residents learn to analyze data and integrate findings into clinical practice. In the inpatient setting it is not difficult to generate questions that are relevant and directly applicable to the clinical situations that confront the student. Faculty play a key role in teaching evidence-based medicine, especially when they act as enthusiastic role models, have the necessary knowledge and skills to engage in it, and value its utility.[17] Evidence-based medicine taught in the classroom setting has been shown to improve knowledge of trainees. However, instructional methods that incorporate the approach into routine clinical practice have been found to improve knowledge as well as skills, attitudes, and behaviors of trainees.[18] Admittedly, teaching evidence-based approaches in the clinical setting rather than the classroom requires more effort and time, but the rewards of behavioral change are substantial, with the potential to improve patient care.

Evidence-based approaches can be applied during direct patient contacts, in treatment team meetings, formal case presentations, and psychiatric interviewing. Direct encounters with patients, such as on walk-rounds, can serve as the stimulus to introduce evidence-based material. For example, when evaluating a patient with treatment-resistant depression, the attending psychiatrist can request that the resident or student appraise the literature on the topic, and later use the information to discuss treatment options with the patient. By doing so, the attending demonstrates how to incorporate evidence into the clinical decision-making process to improve patient care.

The treatment team meeting is another venue where evidence-based approaches can be modeled and taught. When questions about a particular treatment approach or issue arise, residents or students can be asked to appraise the literature on the topic and report back to the group for discussion and clinical integration.[19]

Case Vignette

A young woman is admitted to the inpatient unit with frank psychosis and mood lability. She had been on clozapine in the past with excellent results, but clozapine was discontinued 1 month earlier when she experienced arterial thrombosis. The attending and resident are both uncertain whether or not clozapine can be restarted; the resident undertakes a literature search to determine the risks of clozapine use in the patient, as well as treatment recommendations. The resident finds several articles on the topic, and presents them to the treatment team, as well as to his fellow residents at a morbidity and mortality conference.

Using evidence-based medicine to teach interviewing skills is more complex, but models have been developed that teach patient-centered interviewing. Interview topics such as patient education, breaking bad news, and management of somatization disorders can successfully incorporate evidence-based material while using a patient-centered technique.[20]

THE PSYCHIATRIC INTERVIEW

While the inpatient service is a busy place with rapid patient turnover, it remains an ideal setting to teach the psychiatric interview. The ability to conduct a thorough interview is an essential element of psychiatric residency training, and is included in the core competency "Interpersonal and Communications Skills" as outlined by the ACGME.[4] For medical students, psychiatric interviewing is considered a core skill of the clerkship, and students are expected to be competent at conducting a psychiatric diagnostic interview.[21] As such, attending staff needs to recognize its importance and devote adequate time and attention to this area.

Distinction has been made between doctor-centered interviewing, which focuses on symptom and data collection, and patient-centered interviewing which focuses on the needs, emotions, concerns, and requests of the patient. These data are integrated into a comprehensive understanding of the patient's illness.[22] Realistically, hospitalization of a patient necessitates the establishment of a diagnosis and treatment plan. However, obtaining an accurate diagnosis need not preclude conducting an interview in a therapeutic and empathic manner while establishing a therapeutic alliance. Ideally, residents and medical students should be taught to (a) build a therapeutic alliance, (b) obtain a psychiatric database, (c) interview for diagnosis, and (d) negotiate a treatment plan with the patient.[23] Evidence-based guidelines for teaching patient-centered interviewing have been developed[20] and successfully used to apply the biopsychosocial model to patient assessment and treatment. The guidelines have applicability in the assessment of psychiatric inpatients, as well as patients in primary care settings.

Techniques to teach interview skills are varied and will depend on the time available. Residents and students should first observe the supervisor interview a patient. This allows the expert interviewer to demonstrate styles of communication, such as open-ended and closed-ended questions, techniques for interviewing difficult patients (e.g., the manic or uncooperative patient), time management, and rapport-building techniques (e.g., empathic validation). It is essential to also focus on the process of the interview, and not just the psychopathology of the patient.[24] Of importance when teaching interviewing is the giving of feedback. Only through practice and constructive feedback is interviewing truly learned, and unless students and residents interview patients while directly observed by the supervisor, it is unlikely that they will become skilled interviewers. Feedback should be immediate and precise, so the learner is able to incorporate criticism directly into practice[21,25] and should focus on communication and diagnostic and management skills.[15] Giving constructive feedback to medical students in particular regarding their interviewing ability requires skill and delicacy, because criticism may be felt more personally by them than when they are practicing more concrete tasks.[26] Involving the entire group of trainees in the interview process is generally helpful, especially in providing feedback and support. Peer involvement has been found to increase motivation to learn and perform better, and is seen by students as supportive and constructive.[24]

Case Vignette

A third-year female medical student is interviewing a newly admitted man with paranoid schizophrenia in front of the group. When the student asks the patient about his sexual preference, the patient becomes slightly agitated and begins to say very sexual things to the student.

(continued)

The student tries to change the subject, avoids eye contact with the patient, and eventually ends the interview abruptly. The supervising attending takes over, focusing on the patient's social history and mental status examination. The patient becomes calmer and more organized. The attending later discusses psychological issues and interview techniques pertinent to patients with psychosis. The student's own feelings about the interaction are also addressed.

In conjunction with interviewing, residents and students must be taught how to properly conduct a mental status examination. This examination involves the systematic evaluation and organization of information about the patient's current psychological functioning.[27] The mental status examination is the psychiatrist's tool to elicit psychopathology in a systematic and comprehensive manner. As with interviewing, practice and constructive feedback are the keys to conducting a thorough examination, and students should first watch an experienced clinician examine a patient, and then be observed by the supervisor. Part of the teaching process should involve guiding the student to integrate findings from the mental status examination with information elicited during the interview. Case formulation, differential diagnosis, and treatment planning can be incorporated into the teaching session.

Feedback regarding the interview process, including mental status examination, can be given using checklists completed by the patient[28] or by the supervisor or peers. Patient checklists tend to focus on rapport-building techniques and professionalism, while supervisor or peer checklists focus on interview techniques as well as rapport. Checklists have the advantage of being more objective and give the interviewer specific written feedback about performance. Nevertheless, observation of the trainee's interview has the added benefit of improving patient care. Traditional supervisory methods, in which trainees give a verbal report or case presentation regarding patients they have seen, have been criticized for reliance on observations and reports given by relatively unskilled students or residents. Studies comparing differences in data collected, psychiatric diagnoses, and treatment outcomes reveal significant differences between trainees and clinical supervisors.[29–31] Careful observation of the trainee's interview is important to help the trainee to formulate an accurate diagnosis and treatment plan for the patient.

Though perhaps more complicated, an effective way to teach interviewing is through the use of videotaped interviews. Taped interviews that are purchased or made in-house can be used to discuss interview techniques and serve as a stimulus for discussion about other topics such as diagnosis, psychodynamic issues, transference/countertransference, and treatment. There are many advantages to using videotaped interviews. These include the ability to choose the topic to be discussed, including level of difficulty, to match technique to a particular clinical scenario or diagnostic category, and to stop at any point in time to discuss what is happening in the interview and entertain other options or interventions. Although anxiety-provoking for the student, the chance to be videotaped while interviewing a patient is an excellent learning experience. Although observation of the flow and content of the interview is important, the interviewer's reaction to the patient, mannerisms, facial expression, and body language are important aspects to be covered as well, and can serve as a springboard for discussion about psychodynamic issues. The interview can be critiqued individually by the supervisor, or with a group of students. While supervision of videotaped interview sessions has the advantage of convenience of viewing time for supervisor and trainee, the disadvantage is that there is no way to offer immediate treatment interventions to the patient. In addition, the process may be seen as intrusive by the patient or the student.[32] When developing videotapes on-site, precautions must be taken to ensure that patient consent is obtained, confidentiality is maintained, and the tapes are stored in a secure location where access is limited.

PSYCHOTHERAPY

For the most part, psychotherapy is conducted primarily in outpatient settings. Despite shorter lengths of stay and more severe diagnoses of patients, there are many advantages to teaching psychotherapy in the inpatient setting. Compared to outpatients, inpatients are on-site, so the supervisor can interact with and evaluate them on a daily basis. Hospitalized patients are usually more regressed and demonstrate striking psychopathology, including transference phenomena. Because of the intensity of the interaction with their patients, residents are able to self-reflect regarding their own feelings and behaviors toward their patients. Being on-site, the supervising attending can regularly assess the impact of the resident's work on the patient and the milieu, and residents and students can observe therapeutic interactions between other treatment team members and their patients.[33]

Case Vignette

A resident is assigned to treat an elderly man who was a college physics professor at a major University. The patient did important research, but is now delusional with dangerous behavior. The patient displays some memory problems and has delusions that "gases are pumped in by enemies." The resident is kind and empathic, but fails to conduct thorough testing of the patient's memory, or question the patient about his behavior before admission. When the case is discussed with the inpatient psychotherapy supervisor, the resident is initially defensive, but later admits that the patient reminds her of her own physics professor, and that she feels guilty to be part of the process that will institutionalize the patient. A discussion about transference/countertransference ensues.

Given that inpatients have unique issues including the reason for their hospitalization, diagnosis, and legal status, the process of psychotherapy must be modified to meet their needs. Supportive psychotherapy is particularly well suited for the treatment of inpatients. Ideally, residents should receive didactic instruction regarding the principles and techniques of supportive psychotherapy as part of their curriculum. Having a solid knowledge base enables them to practice supportive psychotherapy during individual sessions with selected patients. Residents and students must learn to establish a therapeutic alliance while promoting themselves as "real objects" who enhance reality while working toward specific, definable goals. Supervision is essential, either by the ward attending or an outside supervisor, and the supervisor should see the patient briefly as well. Supervision should guide the learner with session and treatment planning, and monitor transference and countertransference reactions. Unlike the outpatient clinic, therapy within the hospital setting is a much more public event which often occurs in the open milieu and is reported to the treatment team.[34] Because of this, residents and students have the advantage of receiving input from various members of the treatment team with different theoretic orientations. In settings where faculty and staff have the expertise, cognitive behavioral and psychodynamic psychotherapy can be employed, and residents can gain experience with these techniques. For short-term psychodynamic psychotherapy, emphasis must be on establishing a therapeutic alliance, modifying the treatment to account for impaired ego functioning and the unique qualities of treatment setting, as well as issues related to separation and discharge.[35] As with supportive psychotherapy, the resident or student must have solid grounding in the theoretic framework for the psychotherapies before they can successfully practice them in conjunction with regular, frequent supervision.

For medical students in the inpatient setting, it is important to distinguish between talking with the patient in a reality-based manner and psychotherapy. Students sometimes confuse their daily interactions and interventions with the patient as being a form of psychotherapy, which minimizes the complexity and skill involved in its execution. Because of this misinterpretation, they tend to rightly devalue psychotherapy, as well as the profession. It is important for the supervising psychiatrist to clarify this point, and ideally, allow the student to observe a psychotherapy session with a patient.

GROUP THERAPY

Trainees have numerous opportunities to learn and participate in group activities on inpatient units. Depending on the individual institution, inpatient group therapy offered to patients includes cognitive behavioral therapy, dialectical behavioral therapy, occupational and recreational therapy, milieu psychotherapy, psychoeducation group, family therapy, multisystemic therapy, general psychotherapy, and psychoanalytic/psychodynamic psychotherapy. Other group meetings include community meetings, family meetings, peer advocate meetings, and parent training. Groups are typically conducted by members of the interdisciplinary treatment team.

Working in the hospital permits observation and evaluation of family interaction patterns. Treatment team members are able to develop an alliance with families and to educate them about the mental illness, treatments, and resources in the community. Trainees should be taught to modify their interview techniques to match family styles, and understand differences between inpatient and outpatient interventions. Inpatient family intervention generally involves the patient and their family together in one or more family sessions. The goal of family interventions is to favorably affect patient course of illness and treatment by increasing the family's and patient's understanding of the illness and decreasing the stress on the patient. Students should be introduced to the process, goals, and techniques of inpatient family interventions including individual family therapy, multiple family-group therapy, conjoint couples group, and family psychoeducational workshops (family survival skills workshop or family support group).[36] Given the flexibility and diversity of different types of staff/family interactions that is possible on the inpatient unit, trainees can have experiences ranging from alliance building to formal family therapy sessions geared for change.

Trainees also get acquainted with the purpose and importance of occupational and recreational therapy, which provides therapeutic activity groups including health promotion, education and discussion groups, music appreciation, relaxation, creative art and writing, cooking, healthy living, and physical activities. Having residents and students participate directly in group activities allows them to assess patients' social skills and to develop these through therapeutic interactions in groups. Occupational therapy also involves the evaluation of the patient's ability to solve problems of daily living associated with disability, including limitations in occupational performance, and at a minimum, students should gain an appreciation for this type of therapy.

General therapy groups run by nursing staff and other members of the mental health team explore relationships of the patients with their peers and hospital staff, and conflicts and anxieties that arise in their interpersonal relationships. The group therapist provides a structure by directing the flow of content and affect. This may include introduction of material, asking catalytic questions, and focusing the content.[37]

After gaining some experience observing group therapy, residents should be encouraged to serve as coleader or lead specific groups, such as community meetings. These are usually held once or twice weekly for 30 to 45 minutes on the unit, and are attended by all patients, nursing staff, and members of the treatment team. These meetings can provide a setting in which the patients and staff members come to terms with community problems. Free communication and information exchange are emphasized. Community meetings can also be used to address administrative issues or activity planning, and to inculcate values, norms, and attitudes deemed therapeutic. Therefore, these can be viewed as one of the devices for implementing and maintaining a therapeutic culture.[38]

Training Residents from Other Specialties on Inpatient Units

The need to train residents from other medical specialties in mental health has been widely recognized and recommended. The ACGME requires behavioral science/mental health training for residents from a number of specialties including Emergency Medicine, Internal Medicine, Family Medicine, Obstetrics and Gynecology, and Pediatrics. The ACGME also requires that resident trainees from all specialties be able to demonstrate competency in effective listening skills, communication and counseling, and education of parents and families.[4] Historically, most programs utilized ambulatory care settings to train nonpsychiatric residents. However, with current advances in the field of psychiatry and the implementation of evidence-based treatments, such as short-term psychotherapy, pharmacotherapy, and electroconvulsive therapy, the inpatient setting offers advantages in providing a diverse educational experience for trainees. Although differing opinions exist as to what should be emphasized in psychiatric education, it is essential that, at a minimum, psychiatric educators prepare primary care physicians for the inevitable scientific advances in the field and to train them in basic psychiatric care with an emphasis on diagnostic and therapeutic skills.

The current resident curriculum in primary care specialties includes a minimum of 1 month on a psychiatric service during training. Participation in a psychiatric inpatient service allows primary care residents to gain experience in the timely diagnosis and treatment of psychiatric patients and to perform an effective mental status examination.[39] Residents should become familiar with common types of psychiatric disorders, including mood, psychotic, and personality disorders. Training is designed so that primary care residents gain the necessary confidence to assess, treat, and provide care to a severely mentally ill patient population. Residents from other specialties get experience in conducting supportive counseling and the ability to discuss emotionally difficult issues with their patients. Consultations on the inpatient unit provide exposure to the interface between medicine and psychiatry. Seminars that review the implications of comorbid psychiatric illness in combination with various medical disorders are beneficial and help trainees to recognize when to request a psychiatric consult or referral.

A study by Leigh et al. examined mental health and psychiatry training in primary care residency programs. The study found that while specialty-specific differences in satisfaction exist, not all primary care residents have the same needs, and it may be necessary to develop specialty-specific primary care psychiatry training programs. For example, it might be more important for internal medicine residents to receive training in recognition and treatment of delirium and dementia, for obstetrics and gynecology residents to receive training in disorders of pregnancy and the postpartum period, and for pediatric residents to be trained in the diagnosis and treatment of eating disorders. This can be accomplished by utilizing specialty adult and child/adolescent inpatient units.[40,41]

Training Students from Other Specialties on Inpatient Units

The inpatient setting is an excellent venue to train students from other professions including psychology (both Ph.D and Psy.D students), social work, and nursing.

The Committee on Accreditation (CoA) of the American Psychological Association sets guidelines for the doctoral graduate training program, which, through didactic and experiential training in the science and practice of psychology, affords the student the opportunity to learn the basic competencies necessary to provide psychological services to patients. The psychology internship is a year-long experience which builds on the professional skills and competencies acquired during doctoral training, and gives the psychology student the opportunity to take responsibility for carrying out major professional functions, tasks, duties, and roles under appropriate supervision. Postdoctoral residencies in professional psychology provide education and training in preparation for the practice of professional psychology at an advanced level of competency in a substantive practice area.[42] Inpatient programs provide the means whereby students can acquire and demonstrate substantial understanding of and competence in the breadth of psychology.

Social work education, from baccalaureate to doctoral levels, employs educational, practice, scholarly, interprofessional, and service delivery models to orient and shape the future of the profession in the context of expanding knowledge, changing technologies, and complex human and social concerns. The Council on Social Work Education (CSWE) Educational Policy and Accreditation Standards (EPAS) sets forth basic requirements of the curricular content and educational context to prepare students for professional social work practice.[43] Beyond the basic requirements of EPAS, individual programs should focus on areas relevant to their institutional and program mission, goals, and objectives. Although these do not specify mandated training on the inpatient units, it can be an advantageous placement for trainees.

Similarly, nursing students have certain educational goals and objectives that must be achieved on inpatient units. These include admission assessment (such as collecting data related to the patient's danger to self or others, chief complaint and symptoms, mental status, and any other pertinent information), and being able to formulate a diagnosis based on data obtained. Nursing students must also become familiar with accepted classification systems, such as those developed by the North American Nursing Diagnosis Association,[44] the Nursing Diagnosis Classification, the International Classification of Diseases, or the Diagnostic and Statistical Manual of Mental Disorders Fourth Edition-text revision (DSM-IV-TR). Nursing students should participate in interdisciplinary team meetings and participate in all unit or facility activities, maintaining a therapeutic milieu within the context of activities. Nursing students play a large role in assisting patients with activities of daily living, including meals, hygiene, exercise, community groups, outings, and adjunct therapies. In addition, nursing students, under the supervision of the nurse or the instructor, can administer prescribed medications to patients. They can also participate in other groups such as wellness group, anger management, stress reduction, or life management.[45]

Research on Inpatient Units

The ACGME recommends that residency programs provide the opportunity for residents to participate in scholarly activities, including research. The general psychiatry training criteria state "Graduate medical education must take place in an environment of inquiry and scholarship in which residents participate in the development of new knowledge, learn to evaluate research findings, and develop habits of inquiry as a continuing professional responsibility."[4] Research is considered a significant component for the growth and development of the practicing physician and can assist with the understanding of scientific methodology and enhance critical thinking skills. Therefore, participation in research is strongly encouraged. The National Institute of Mental Health has recognized the dire shortage of psychiatric clinician investigators. In order to address the problem, it commissioned the Institute of Medicine in 2003 to conduct a study entitled "Research Training in Psychiatry Residency: Strategies for Reform." The committee concluded that barriers to research training span three categories: regulatory, institutional, and personal factors. Recommendations include calling for research literacy requirements and research training curricula tailored to psychiatric residency programs of various sizes. The role of senior investigators and departmental leadership is emphasized in the report as is the importance of longitudinal training (e.g., from medical school through residency and fellowship).[46]

In the last decade, research in the area of psychiatry, behavioral sciences and neuroscience has advanced and developed exponentially. Application of evidence-based medicine in the decision-making process for diagnosis and treatment has become increasingly important. One of the key areas for conducting research has been the inpatient unit. Some institutions have designed specialized research or clinical trials units, which are an ideal environment for research training for students from all specialties. Other hospitals conduct research on general adult and child units, which provides opportunities for trainees to be actively involved with the research and interdisciplinary treatment teams. The structure of the research team allows for solid research to be done and also exposes learners to research-oriented role models and mentors. Participation on a research team gives residents and students multiple opportunities to present their work and be involved with a variety of projects throughout their training. For research conducted on general psychiatry units, involvement of the interdisciplinary inpatient team has the added advantage in that it can evaluate all aspects of the research and treatment, including biological, psychological, and social factors influencing the patient's care. Ideally, residents who participate in research projects during their training will have better critical appraisal skills, clinical reasoning, and life-long learning skills, which will translate into improved clinical care. Research training is also an asset for students applying to residency training programs and for residents applying for fellowships or academic careers.

An essential component of research education in an inpatient setting must include the resident becoming familiar with the principles, ethics, design, and methods of research. Trainees can be involved in all facets of the research from its initiation. They can participate in subject recruitment, including inclusion and exclusion criteria, the process of informed consent, and the collection, analysis and interpretation of data. With additional training, students gain expertise in the use of rating scales and clinical assessment instruments (such as the Clinical Global Improvement [CGI] scale, the Hamilton Depression [HAM-D] Scale, the Positive and Negative Symptoms Scale [PANSS] and the Abnormal Involuntary Movement Scale [AIMS]) and structured psychiatric interviews (such as the Schedule for Affective Disorders and Schizophrenia [SADS] and the Structured Clinical Interview for DSM-IV Disorders [SCID-R]). There is an opportunity to evaluate patients with a standard set of instruments and physical procedures on admission, and follow up their progress using research protocols. Also in this setting, residents get clinical experience and confidence using investigational psychopharmacologic agents. Trainees should also be encouraged to review the medical literature, develop their own projects, present their data, and prepare a manuscript, case report, or case series.

Conclusions

Although inpatient psychiatric units have undergone many changes in the recent past, they remain an excellent resource for teaching psychiatry to medical students, residents and students from other specialties. Participation on an interdisciplinary treatment team, involvement in individual and group psychotherapy, and learning interview techniques and formal case presentation skills are just of a few of the experiences available to students and residents in the inpatient setting. With creativity and resourcefulness, educators can optimize the educational environment to establish a challenging learning environment, which can generate enthusiasm for the field.

REFERENCES

1. Pessar LF. Ambulatory care teaching in the psychiatry clerkship. *Acad Psychiatry*. 2000;24: 61–67.
2. Hogan EA, Sharp J, Miller M. Inpatient residency training in a time of change. *Harv Rev Psychiatry*. 1998;6:49–52.
3. Houghtalen R, Guttmacher L. Facilitating effective residency education on short-term inpatient units. *Psychiatr Q*. 1996;67:111–125.
4. Accreditation Council for Graduate Medical Education. *Essentials of accredited residencies in graduate medical education*. www.acgme.org, 1999.
5. Druss B, Bruce ML, Jacobs S, et al. Trends over a decade for a general hospital psychiatry unit. *Adm Policy Ment Health*. 1998;25:427–435.
6. Crowder M, Jack RA. Educational opportunities and inpatient psychiatry. *Psychiatr Med*. 1987;4: 417–429.
7. Brodkey A, Sierles F, Woodard J. Use of clerkship learning objectives by members of the Association of Directors of Medical Student Education in Psychiatry. *Acad Psychiatry*. 2006;30:150–157.
8. Summergrad P. General hospital inpatient psychiatry in the 1990s: Problems and possibilities. *Gen Hosp Psychiatry*. 1991;13:79–82.
9. Merklin L, Little RB. Beginning psychiatry training syndrome. *Am J Psychiatry*. 1967;124:193–197.
10. Hales RE, Borus JF. A reexamination of the psychiatric resident's experience in the general hospital. *Gen Hosp Psychiatry*. 1986;8:432–436.
11. Zeiss R. Interdisciplinary treatment and training issues in the acute inpatient unit. *J Interprof Care*. 1997;11:279–286.
12. Skottowe I. Teaching psychiatry in mental hospitals. *Br Med J*. 1966;2:941–943.
13. Roth LS. Writing progress notes: 10 dos and don'ts. *Curr Psychiatry*. 2005;4:63–66.
14. LaCombe MA. On bedside teaching. *Ann Intern Med*. 1997;126:217–220.
15. de Groot J, Tiberius R, Sinai J, et al. Psychiatric residency: An analysis of training activities with recommendations. *Acad Psychiatry*. 2000; 24:139–146.
16. Hoge MA, Tondora J, Stuart GW. Training in evidence-based practice. *Psychiatr Clin North Am*. 2003;26:851–865.
17. Evidence-based Medicine Group. Evidence-based medicine: A new approach to teaching the practice of medicine. *JAMA*. 1992;268:2420–2426.
18. Coomarasamy A, Khan K. What is the evidence that postgraduate teaching in evidence-based medicine changes anything? A systematic review. *Br Med J*. 2004;329:1017–1027.
19. Richardson W, Dowding D. Teaching evidence-based practice on foot. *Evid Based Nurs*. 2005; 8:100.
20. Smith RC, Marshall-Dorsey AA, Osborn GG, et al. Evidence-based guidelines for teaching patient-centered interviewing. *Patient Educ Couns*. 2000;39:27–36.
21. Sierles F, Pessar L, Brodkey A. Psychiatric clerkships. In: Kay J, ed. *Handbook of psychiatric education*. Washington, DC: American Psychiatric Publishing; 2005.
22. Smith RC. *The patient's story: integrated patient-doctor interviewing*. Lippincott Williams & Wilkins; 1996.
23. Carlat D. *The psychiatric interview*. Philadelphia: Lippincott Williams & Wilkins; 2005.
24. Lovett L, Cox A, Abou-Saleh M. Teaching psychiatric interview skills to medical students. *Med Educ*. 1990;24:243–250.
25. Nuzzarello A, Birndorf C. An interviewing course for a psychiatry clerkship. *Acad Psychiatry*. 2004;28:66–70.
26. McIlwrick J, Nair B, Montgomery G. "How am I doing?" Many problems but few solutions related to feedback delivery in undergraduate education. *Acad Psychiatry*. 2006;30:130–135.
27. MacKinnon RA, Michels M, Buckley PJ. *The psychiatric interview in clinical practice*. Washington, DC: American Psychiatric Publishing; 2006.
28. Black A, Church M. Assessing medical student effectiveness from the psychiatric patient's perspective: The medical student interviewing performance questionnaire. *Med Educ*. 1998;32:472–478.
29. Jaynes S, Charles E, Kass F, et al. Clinical supervision of the initial interview: Effects on patient care. *Am J Psychiatry*. 1979;136: 1454–1457.

30. Muslin HL, Thurnblad RMG. The fate of the clinical interview: An observational study. *Am J Psychiatry*. 1981;138:822–825.

31. Spitzer R, Skodol AE, William JBW, et al. Supervising intake diagnosis. A psychiatric "Rashomon." *Arch Gen Psychiatry*. 1982;39:1299–1305.

32. Salvendy J. Supervision of the initial interview: A choice of methods. *J Psychiatr Educ*. 1987;11:121–126.

33. Silver D, Book H, Hamilton J, et al. Psychotherapy and the inpatient unit: A unique learning experience. *Am J Psychother*. 1983;37:121–129.

34. Prosen M, Ross D. Inpatient Psychotherapy. In: Lion JA, Adler WN, Webb WL, eds. *Modern hospital psychiatry*. New York: W.W. Norton & Company; 1988.

35. Liebenluft E, Goldberg R. Guidelines for short-term inpatient psychotherapy. *Hosp Community Psychiatry*. 1987;38:38–43.

36. Sederer L. *Inpatient psychiatry: diagnosis and treatment*. Baltimore: Williams and Wilkins; 1991.

37. Kibel H. A conceptual model for short-term inpatient group. *Am J Psychiatry*. 1981;138:74–80.

38. Klein R. The Patient-staff community meeting: A tea party with the mad hatter. *Int J Group Psychother*. 1981;31:205–211.

39. Hodges B, Inch C, Silver I. Improving the psychiatric knowledge, skills and attitudes of primary care physicians, 1950–2000: A review. *Am J Psychiatry*. 2001;158:1579–1586.

40. Leigh H, Stewart D, Mallios R. Mental health and psychiatry training in primary care residency programs. Part I. Who teaches, where, when and how satisfied? *Gen Hosp Psychiatry*. 2006;28:189–194.

41. Leigh H, Stewart D, Mallios R. Mental health and psychiatry training in primary care residency programs. Part II. What skills and diagnoses are taught, how adequate, and what affects training directors' satisfaction? *Gen Hosp Psychiatry*. 2006;28:195–204.

42. American Psychological Association. *Guidelines and principles for accreditation of programs in professional psychology*. American Psychological Association Committee on Accreditation; www.apa.org/ed/accreditation, 2000.

43. *Educational policy and accreditation standards. Council on Social Work Education*. www.aswe.org/CSWE, 2004.

44. North American Nursing Diagnosis Association (NANDA). www.nanda.org, 2006.

45. Ford M, Karshmer J, Hales A. Using standards of practice and key clinical points for teaching psychiatric-mental health nursing. *Nurs Educ*. 2000;25:149–152.

46. Yager J, Greden J, Abrams M, et al. The Institute of Medicine's report on research training in psychiatry residency: Strategies for reform-background, results, and follow up. *Acad Psychiatry*. 2004;28(4):267–274.

Clinical Contexts

CHAPTER 9

Hospital Treatment of Depression and Mania

STAN D. ARKOW, SUSAN TURNER, AND DAVID A. KAHN

T he hospital treatment of depression and mania has undergone major changes in recent decades as the use of medication and psychotherapy has become more specific and sophisticated, and as reimbursement has been reduced. The senior authors of this chapter have collaborated for more than 25 years in running a 24-bed inpatient teaching unit at an academic medical center and have witnessed the evolution of care from the open-ended stay to the era of managed care. When the authors of this chapter began working together, lengths of stay were 4 to 6 weeks, with gradual discharge through passes and test visits home. The authors now discharge the average patient in 11 days, and their emphases are controlling immediate threats to safety, clarifying diagnosis, and initiating treatment to the point where the patient and family are ready to engage in outpatient care.

An organized and streamlined approach that anticipates as many of the complications as possible is required in order to treat mood disorders effectively on an inpatient unit. Diagnosis, institution of treatment, monitoring symptom resolution and impediments to this improvement, as well as appropriate disposition planning remain the major tasks of the inpatient team.

General Considerations

STAGING THE PHASE OF TREATMENT AT ADMISSION

Major depression and bipolar disorder tend to have recurrent courses that begin in the early adult decades of life, with future episodes only partially prevented by ongoing treatment. At the time of admission, it is helpful to conceptualize three stages based on the patient's placement in this life course because each sets up a specific goal for the hospital stay in addition to the generic goal of safe, appropriate treatment.

- First episode with no prior diagnosis or treatment: *Make the correct diagnosis and educate the patient and family*
- Recurrent episode with a known diagnosis, but currently receiving no care: *Identify barriers to ongoing care*
- Recurrent episode or relapse despite continuous treatment (including the first episode of mania in a patient previously treated only for depression): *Systematically evaluate prior diagnoses and treatments*

In all these stages, hospitalization provides safety and a care-intense structure to relieve extreme suffering. Hospitalization can also motivate the treatment team, patient, and family to identify vital information that will aid in diagnosis and treatment. Although each stage presents unique needs, the process of engaging patients and their families as partners in care remains, perhaps, the most important overarching goal in assuring that the inpatient stay has a lasting impact on the future course of illness.

The First-Episode Patient

Diagnosis and education are the key tasks in the hospital care of the first-episode patient. An initial hospitalization for suspected depression or mania may come about through referral from primary care physicians, psychiatrists who have conducted an initial evaluation in the outpatient setting, or the emergency room. From the clinician's perspective, the probable or definite diagnosis of a mood disorder may be clear, or at least may lead the possibilities in differential diagnosis. The patient on the other hand, especially in mania and sometimes in depression, may not understand what is happening. The buildup of symptoms may go on for several months before a patient comes to clinical attention; especially in mania weeks or months of negotiation by the worried family or outpatient clinician may precede actually getting the patient into the hospital.

Apart from obvious presentations where depression is the chief complaint and patients readily give the diagnostic history, the illness may present in ways that only later, on evaluation, give rise to the diagnosis of depression. Some examples include expressions of suicidality, or a suicide attempt; unexplained medical signs and symptoms, including pain, weight loss, or somatic preoccupations; or a state of feeling emotionally overwhelmed, sometimes presented as a "normal" reaction to adverse life events, but accompanied by marked difficulty functioning in everyday life.

Unlike depression, "mania" is almost never the patient's chief complaint, although insomnia or agitation may be. More often, a manic episode, even one leading to hospitalization, does not even present with subjective distress on the part of the patient apart from anger at feeling coerced into treatment. As in depression, the initial diagnosis is sometimes clear to the clinician, but examples of less obvious presentations in which diagnosis emerges over time include first episodes of paranoid psychosis, violent or aggressive behavior, rapidly escalating patterns of substance abuse, or physical complaints of insomnia and exhaustion. In addition, complaints of depression and suicidality with extreme agitation or anxiety may herald an unrecognized mixed state.

In taking the history, participation of family members or others who know the patient well is essential, balancing appropriate confidentiality against the imperative to build alliances with others who will be essential in providing key information and supporting aftercare. In the case of newly admitted depressed patients, history is typically influenced by their current mood state which may negatively color perceptions, as well as recall difficulties due to poor concentration. The patient may view his or her emotions as entirely appropriate to dismal experience, real or distorted. By the same token, getting a history from an acutely manic patient on first admission can be challenging to even a skilled psychiatrist because of unwillingness to cooperate, as well as distractibility, sheer energy, and behavioral dyscontrol.

Of specific interest in the history for newly diagnosed or suspected mood disorders is the past history of subsyndromal mood episodes or enduring personality styles that were below diagnostic thresholds, unrecognized episodes of dysthymia or hypomania, or even frank undiagnosed major depression or mania. Nonbipolar depression is a diagnosis of exclusion, that the currently depressed patient has never been manic or hypomanic. Up to 20% of depressed patients become manic when treated with unopposed antidepressants, and delays of up to 10 years before accurate diagnosis of bipolar disorder are not uncommon. A brief structured interview, even using a formal tool such as the Mood Disorder Questionnaire, can be helpful to be sure this base is covered in the assessment.[1] Family history of bipolarity may also place a depressed person at risk for conversion to mania and is therefore vital to obtain.

As in all psychiatric patients, a history and workup is undertaken for differential diagnosis from states due to general medical conditions, medicines, or substances of abuse. Comorbid psychiatric conditions that affect treatment are common, especially substance abuse, anxiety, and personality disorders.

Once the psychiatrist is convinced that a mood disorder is in fact the correct primary diagnosis the process of education, explaining what is happening, the rationale for medication, goals of psychotherapy in the hospital, and what time course to expect for improvement and recovery can begin. During the hospital stay, patients and families can be mobilized to gather extensive information regarding areas such as family history and prior undiagnosed mood episodes. The first mood episode is a crucial time to provide the realistic hope that recovery is expected, tempered by the reality that there may be a process of trial and error before an ideal regimen is found. Patients must be educated about how long to continue treatment to prevent relapse of the current episode or recurrence of future episodes.

The first hospitalization is the time to look at other aspects of the patient's situation that will help the psychiatrist understand the context of the illness, tailor aftercare and near-term life decisions, and motivate the patient to follow through with what may become many years, if not a lifetime, of preventive treatment. Such factors include, of course, the common comorbidities such as substance use disorders, anxiety, and personality disorders, as well as interpersonal stresses broadly. Patients are encouraged to think psychologically about themselves in ways that are not necessarily geared toward pathology but also take into account strengths, personality styles, and life goals as these interact with their mood disorders.

The Patient in a Recurrent Episode of a Known Diagnosis, Not Currently Receiving Care

Understanding barriers to care is the key goal in the hospitalization of the patient with a severe, recurrent episode of a known diagnosis of bipolar disorder or depression but who is not under care at the time of admission. Why has this happened now and what can be done to prevent it from happening again? What is discovered will set the tone for the major psychological work of the hospital stay, above and beyond the issues in treating the episode itself. These barriers can be explored in a manner as systematic as the history taken in the first episode to establish the diagnosis of mania or depression.

First, several psychiatric issues must be considered. Inadequate prior treatment may have left residual symptoms that reduced motivation for ongoing care. There may be comorbid conditions interfering with treatment, such as a personality disorder or substance abuse. Side effects of medicines may have led to nonadherence.

Second, attitudes toward illness may have impeded care. Denial and lack of insight may be part of the disease process itself as well as parts of a psychological defensive structure. Classic components include enjoying positive aspects of mania or being hopelessly pessimistic in depression. Secondary gain of illness represents another unconscious dimension of care rejection. Fear of stigma in the social world of the patient or a negative and critical family attitude toward mental illness and the need for treatment may also discourage care.

Third, there may have been inadequate past psychoeducation, with a lack of knowledge about signs and symptoms of a new episode of mania or depression, and lack of information about the importance of continuation treatment in reducing future episodes. Lastly, there may be problems in the care delivery system available to the patient, either because of lack of financial resources or lack of access to knowledgeable providers with the proper expertise.

The treatment team evaluates the contribution of these factors to "dropping out" from care. The easiest part of care is recognizing the mood disorder, obtaining prior treatment history, and reinstituting appropriate medication. If medication side effects or an incomplete prior response are the culprits, alternative regimens should be used; if previous medicines worked but other factors led to nonadherence, the inpatient team will need to expend great effort addressing the root cause of the disconnect. Psychosocial work and psychoeducation will be paramount in reducing barriers to long-term well-being.

The Patient with a Recurrent Mood Episode Despite Continuous Treatment

To this category belong patients who may be admitted either emergently or electively for mania, depression, or patterns of continuous cycling that have become resistant or refractory to treatment. True episodes of prolonged mania are rare but enormously consuming of hospital resources such as one-to-one security, use of seclusion and restraint, and effects on other patients on the inpatient unit. Most patients with treatment-refractory mood disorder suffer from chronic depression, both in bipolar illness and recurrent major depressive disorder. Patients may experience considerable demoralization and disability, increasing the risk of family stress, divorce, unemployment, and a further slide toward suicidality. Apart from the usual indications for inpatient care (safety, inability to function, intensity of suffering), the hospital care of these patients uses the full involvement of the round-the-clock staff to achieve interlocking goals revolving around four issues for systematic reevaluation: diagnosis, adequacy of previous medication, adverse effects of medication, and psychosocial management. In effect, the inpatient stay is in part an extended consultation.

First, diagnostic reevaluation can proceed at several levels. There may be episode features such as psychotic symptoms that have been overlooked requiring the use of antipsychotics or electroconvulsive therapy (ECT). Underlying diagnosis may be changed, such as reclassification from nonbipolar to bipolar disorder, agitated depression to mixed episode, or mood disorder to schizoaffective illness or schizophrenia. One may be able to identify a complicating comorbid psychiatric disorder diagnosis whose symptoms overlap with the mood disorder, but which needs focused treatment in order for mood disorder treatment to succeed, for example, substance abuse, anxiety disorders, attention deficit hyperactivity disorder, or personality disorders. Finally, inpatient workup and treatment may be needed for a complex medical condition that overlaps with a mood disorder or complicates its treatment, such as many central nervous system disorders, autoimmune diseases, heart disease, or pregnancy.

Second, the psychiatrist should reevaluate the adequacy and effects of prior medication treatment by a detailed, chronologic review: Were doses and durations of treatment appropriate? Were all suitable medicines actually tried? Was abandonment of a medicine because of a side effect truly warranted—were doses lowered, or antidotes tried? Physicians can make an enormous effort in the hospital to unearth this information by systematically obtaining prior treatment and pharmacy records, especially before an elective admission, and then treat through the gaps. They can also retry promising, but poorly tolerated, medicines at lower doses, or promising, but inadequately dosed, medicines at higher levels, both with close side effect and safety monitoring. In conducting this review, a structured psychopharmacology treatment interview[2,3] and the visual technique of "life charting" are often helpful aids.[4]

Third, the present authors use the hospital to eliminate some or all medicines in the polypharmacy regimens that may accumulate in treatment-resistant patients, a step that can provoke great anxiety in patients and psychiatrists alike, for fear of worsening the situation. One reason to "clear the decks" is to rule out side effects that resemble psychiatric symptoms, such as extrapyramidal or cognitive side effects mimicking depression. Another common objective is eliminating antidepressants from the regimen of a patient with bipolar disorder who may be experiencing paradoxical worsening of depression or mood cycling.

Fourth, it is important to reevaluate the outpatient psychosocial management. Are there major life stressors that have gone unaddressed? Major losses (e.g., a spouse, a child or parent, a therapist, a home, a job) are associated with relapses into both mania and depression. As an example, in the 6 months after the death of a prominent psychiatrist in the authors' area, several of his former patients were admitted to the authors' unit. Almost none of them, on admission, identified his death as a stressor, yet all of them recognized its importance as the treatment proceeded. On occasion, the patient may be receiving the wrong type of psychotherapy, however well intentioned. Psychotherapy can intensify mood symptoms, such as marital or family therapy that inadvertently creates greater conflict. Tactfully exploring a meaningful but misguided therapeutic relationship may be a factor in understanding apparent treatment-resistant mood states. Instituting more constructive approaches and dealing with potentially explosive family conflicts may be needed while the patient is in the safe environment of the hospital. It is also common for patients to have not received specific, evidence-based approaches such as cognitive behavior therapy that are not widely available in community-based outpatient centers.

Finally, treatment-resistant cases may be seen where appropriate new treatment has been started recently before the patient enters the hospital but has not had sufficient time to bear fruit. All that may be needed is confirmation of the approach without undertaking an overhaul.

Treatment of Specific Mood States

MANIA

General Management

Acutely manic patients are, perhaps, the most difficult of all psychiatric patients to treat due to the complexity of both psychological and pharmacologic management. Full cooperation with treatment is rare. Mania is accompanied by impairments in judgment, insight, observing ego, impulse control, anxiety and frustration tolerance, and often in reality testing itself. Therefore, the clinicians may find themselves treating a patient who not only does not want their help, but also can be nasty, belligerent, irritating, and even litigious. Often admitted involuntarily, they may insist on a court review of their admission. Not uncommonly, medicines are refused and may not be given over objection if the patient is not imminently out of control of impulses. With treatment at a standstill, a court order may be needed.

Case Vignette

Mr. W is a 28-year-old, single, unemployed male attorney with no children whose family lives in the Midwest. Each of his previous two psychiatric hospitalizations for bipolar disorder type I was followed by nonadherence with the treatment plan resulting in aggressive, violent behavior. Recently, he punched one person on the street, attempted to hit several others, and threatened to rape his psychiatrist. He was admitted to the inpatient unit floridly manic and psychotic.

Medication was begun using valproic acid, clonazepam, and quetiapine, with rapid de-escalation of his manic symptoms. On day 6 of his admission, still experiencing a thought disorder and psychomotor agitation but able to contain his behaviors appropriately, Mr. W began to refuse medicines about half the time. Without any working alliance, court-ordered treatment over objection was contemplated. He threatened a lawsuit. In consultation with the unit chief, the authors reviewed the current residual symptoms, which included impaired judgment and poor impulse control. With the history of treatment nonadherence and violence, they decided that a partial hospitalization program was an insufficient plan. Court-mandated treatment was then obtained. On return from court, Mr. W refused valproic acid initially. Once the court order was read and the patient told he would be medicated intramuscularly, if needed, he agreed to take the medicines.

The team social worker contacted the family and arranged their help in Mr. W's treatment. They visited the patient, having never seen him in an acute manic episode before and although shocked, began the process of educating themselves about the illness. Final discharge plans included the patient's attendance to a partial program near his family in the Midwest. Upon discharge, the patient was most appreciative for the team's efforts in helping him grapple with his illness.

When a manic patient arrives on the floor, these psychological and pharmacologic difficulties must be expected. In addition to a detailed history of his or her symptoms and a diagnostic formulation, the mental status examination must carefully focus on mood symptoms such as irritability, cognitive distortions (loose associations or flight of ideas or delusions), perceptual abnormalities (hallucinations), suicidal or homicidal thoughts, plans and actual current or past attempts, loss of impulse control, or deficits in insight or judgment. On admission, the alliance with such patients does not exist and will develop over time only as the psychopathology resolves. Unskilled clinicians and trainees often mistake compliance shortly after admission for a developing alliance. The experienced clinician recognizes that manipulation, as well as deception, are part of the manic patient's presentation. When treatment has been given over objection, patients' reactions are complex. When they recover, many agree that coercion was justified[5] even if they remain ungrateful.[6]

Nursing assessment in conjunction with the physician's evaluation is crucial at this juncture to facilitate patients' integration into the milieu. Issues such as room assignment for ease in monitoring and a level of observation (e.g., frequent checks or close observation by an individual staff member) must be decided. Medication and dosing frequency as well as other aspects of the treatment plan should be clear to all staff members. This point cannot be stressed enough. Manic patients, often threatening and frightening to staff, may bully other patients on the unit, for example, determining which television shows will be watched or taking whatever food they may see and want. Early communication between team members is crucial to treating the current psychopathology without any individual believing that the patient would be better left alone (often a countertransference pitfall that hardly serves the patient).

Although inpatient psychiatrists may be busy off the unit for hours at a time with other duties, the nursing staff, floor attendants, and activities therapists are on the front lines, interacting with the patients more closely and continuously assessing their overall condition. A manic patient who is about to lose control will more likely be identified by these staff members, who must be prepared at all times to defuse the situation. De-escalating interventions can include verbal reassurances, "time-outs" in the patient's own or quiet room, and offers of p.r.n. medication. At times a "show of force" with the possibility of restraint or seclusion may be necessary. Formal programs exist to train nursing and security staff in managing the aggressive patient;[7] the nature of the threat and the number of staff members available and formally trained in "take-down" techniques are factors in whether to call for security backup. These issues are discussed further in Chapter 12.

Social work involvement is essential from the moment the patient arrives on the unit. Relatives and/or significant others need to be contacted to clarify history and the emergence of symptoms, as well as to clarify comorbid conditions and family psychiatric history. Family members should be seen as close to admission as possible, allowing an alliance to develop. Healthier family members may help implement treatment later in the hospital course if the patient is nonadherent with those recommendations. In addition, enabling behaviors by relatives and friends which impede treatment can also be identified early. The limited available research on inpatient family therapy suggests that the focus should be psychoeducation and that benefits are more pronounced in female patients.[8]

For the newly presenting case as well as in the questionable diagnostic cases, it is sometimes difficult to distinguish hypomanic or mixed mood states (and on occasion even manic states) from severe character pathology with borderline features. Overlapping behaviors include irritability, controlled but aggressive behavior, flirtatiousness, seductiveness, sexually inappropriate behavior, manipulativeness, sarcastic devaluation of others, and oppositional behavior. Many of these interpersonal maneuvers have been described by others[9] and make for challenges in treatment second to none.

Case Vignette

Ms. N is a 26-year-old college graduate with depression, irritability, and behavioral deterioration, admitted for medication washout and ECT. She began having symptoms of anxiety in her mid-teens and entered psychotherapy. By college, she had periods of depression, and exhibited difficulties with unstable relationships, occasional substance abuse, and irresponsible spending, with subjective improvement on escitalopram. Two years later, sequential trials of other antidepressants were attempted because of relapse while still taking medicines. These were ineffective, apart from a brief period of euphoric hypomania that ended with a recurrence of depression. Her treatment was not changed because there was no consensus as to her diagnosis, and antidepressant trials with some variations continued for another year.

Psychopharmacologic consultation led to a diagnosis of bipolar II disorder. Lithium was begun, with intermittent trials of lamotrigine, carbamazepine, and atypical antipsychotics. Antidepressants were restarted several times. Ms. N developed a pattern of transient improvement with worsening relapses, accompanied by anxiety and difficulty concentrating. She showed patterns of overly intense attachments and subsequent angry endings in both romantic and platonic relationships. Questions were raised about the diagnosis of bipolar II versus borderline personality disorder. Olanzapine plus lithium were the only medicines that reliably provided partial relief. Weight gain created further anger, then hopelessness. She quit her job because of depressive symptoms and alternately pleaded for advice from friends and expressed anger with their responses.

Ms. N was hospitalized, taken off all medicines, and after anxiety and tearfulness increased, ECT was begun. Her behavior rapidly grew worse with mood lability, demanding behavior, and episodes of physically aggressive behavior when she did not get her way. She agreed to only one ECT treatment at a time, always threatening to sign out of the hospital, which never occurred. She refused all communication with her parents and "fired"

(continued)

her psychiatrists. She required several injections of chlorpromazine to contain aggressive behavior. Consensus of staff members was a diagnosis of a mixed episode of bipolar disorder, accelerated by years of antidepressant exposure, rapid cessation of lithium, and absence of any effective mood-stabilizing medication while awaiting the effects of ECT to take hold. Dramatic improvement in her mood, behavior, and insight was observed after six ECT treatments. She was anxiety-free and expressed an appreciation of the efforts of her parents and doctors. She agreed to continue the acute ECT course as an outpatient and to begin dialectic behavior therapy to address her problems of instability in relationships and work, though after leaving the hospital some limit-testing behavior with her parents and needy dependence on her friends persisted.

The hospital played an indispensable role in her recovery. It allowed the team to stop her medication, a step that everyone had been afraid to take without a complete safety net; containment of behavior that was increasingly damaging to key relationships; confirmation of a serious underlying diagnosis of bipolar disorder; and initiation and continuation of a treatment that she otherwise would not have cooperated with, but for which she was subsequently grateful.

With this vignette in mind, one can see how challenging it is for staff to treat these patients when, at times, they are being verbally or physically abused by the patient. Educating new staff members about bipolar patients, reviewing the countertransferences generated toward bipolar patients, and discussing psychopathology with staff is very helpful in easing the strong feelings such patients engender in staff members. After the patient has improved and is ready for discharge, reviewing the resolution of symptoms and focusing on the most annoying and disruptive behaviors as well as on the feelings each staff member may have experienced as they cared for this patient has great educational and clinical value.

Pharmacotherapy

The pharmacotherapeutic approach to mania is to try and "get it right" the first time by combining medicines in aggressive doses in order to maximize the odds of rapidly stabilizing mood, thinking, and behavior. The American Psychiatric Association (APA) practice guideline for bipolar disorder[10] recommends the combination of lithium or divalproex, or potentially carbamazepine, with an antipsychotic, preferably an atypical. Any antidepressants the patient had been taking should be stopped, on the assumption that they may be causing the episode.

Monotherapy Versus Rational Polypharmacy

As to how antimanic drugs should be used, some practice guidelines[11,12] recommend monotherapy with lithium or divalproex, especially in nonpsychotic mania, supplementing with a benzodiazepine for sleep. However, only approximately 50% of patients respond to standard short-term (e.g., 3-week) monotherapy trials of mood stabilizers in clinical trials, and the outcome measures are not necessarily geared toward reaching discharge criteria from the hospital. Similar statements apply to second-generation antipsychotics, all of which are U.S. Food and Drug Administration (FDA)-approved for acute mania, and similar overall to lithium and divalproex in controlled clinical trials. There are many situations where monotherapy with any of the approved agents is the most appropriate course of action, including patients with past histories of rapid response to monotherapy; significant medication side effects; past histories of uncertain medication response to multiple agents where clarity is now needed; complex medical illness; or relatively mild-to-moderate severity.

An alternative approach is to begin cases with combination treatment of either lithium or divalproex, plus an antipsychotic, enhancing the likelihood of a rapid result. A recent meta-analysis found that while both types of agents were superior to placebo, the antipsychotics as a group were slightly more effective acutely than lithium or divalproex, and that the combination strategies were superior to monotherapy with lithium or divalproex.[13] Combination treatment had more side effects, but the overall benefits were highly significant. The study authors concluded that second-generation antipsychotics had fewer depressive and extrapyramidal side effects compared to haloperidol, but they were equivalent in efficacy.

The authors, as well as others, prefer second-generation over first-generation antipsychotics for initial treatment in mania, whether in monotherapy or combination, although they note that comparisons between classes on long-term effectiveness and costs have not been conducted in bipolar disorder. The authors turn to first-generation antipsychotics when second-generation antipsychotics fail, or when emergency sedation is needed with intramuscular injection of haloperidol or chlorpromazine (see Rapid Dosing in the subsequent section).

Rapid Dosing

An important aspect of inpatient treatment is the availability of close monitoring to facilitate rapid dosing of antimanic medication. Divalproex is given in a loading up to 30 mg per kg per day in divided doses, achieving therapeutic blood levels within days and shortening clinical response time over standard gradual titrations. Lithium does not lend itself to such a strategy, but the authors find that it is safe and tolerable to begin young, healthy patients on an average dose of 900 mg per day with frequent monitoring and adjustments to achieve therapeutic levels. Carbamazepine and oxcarbazepine are more difficult to give in rapid doses due to central nervous system side effects. Among antipsychotics, the authors do not hesitate to give within the first 24 hours 10 to 20 mg of olanzapine, 300 to 400 mg of quetiapine, or 2 to 4 mg of risperidone. However, they have found that such rapid dosing of ziprasidone or aripiprazole can result in higher rates of acute extrapyramidal side effects. Because further sedation may be needed to induce sleep or control aggression and agitation, a benzodiazepine is often supplemented further, such as clonazepam or lorazepam starting at 2 to 4 mg over 24 hours and sometimes going much higher.

For emergency treatment with intramuscular treatment, chlorpromazine or haloperidol continues to be used unless contraindicated by history of severe extrapyramidal reactions, in which case olanzapine is the choice. The second-generation antipsychotics olanzapine, ziprasidone, and aripiprazole are all available for intramuscular use, but are more costly, and in the case of the latter two less sedating than desirable, in the authors' view, for emergencies. Frequent extrapyramidal reactions have also been seen with intramuscular ziprasidone or aripiprazole, requiring antiparkinsonian treatment.

Choice of Medication

The next consideration is whether subtypes of manic symptoms respond preferentially to one or another medicine. Consensus-based guidelines[11] have suggested that divalproex may be preferred over lithium in patients with dysphoric or mixed mania, and when there is a history of rapid cycling. This theory has not been carefully tested for acute mania, and appears not to stand up in long-term treatment of rapid cycling.[14] Surprisingly, psychosis itself may not even be a consistent predictor of preferential response to antipsychotics compared to other antimanic medication.[15]

It is enormously helpful to attend to previous histories of antimanic treatment, both for efficacy and side effects. Of increasing concern are experiences of excessive weight gain with olanzapine, counterbalancing the evidence that olanzapine is among the most efficacious antipsychotics for acute treatment.[11] To a lesser extent, risperidone and quetiapine share this problem. Because of many options with less likelihood of this side effect, including even first-generation antipsychotics, the authors try to follow the wishes of patients with previous weight gain to try alternatives.

Treatment-Resistant Mania

There are no ideal formulas for patients with mania who do not improve with aggressive doses of the combinations the authors have been discussing, or who enter the hospital having broken through carefully administered outpatient treatment (apart from being sure that any antidepressants are stopped). Anecdotal evidence and consensus guidelines[11,12] suggest various triple combinations (e.g., lithium and divalproex plus an antipsychotic). Carbamazepine has numerous drug interactions, resulting in preference by many clinicians for the related compound, oxcarbazepine. The authors note that there is far less experience and evidence regarding its efficacy.[16] Although more difficult to administer and requiring consent and cooperation, clozapine[17] and ECT[18] are well established in treatment-resistant mania.

Safety Issues

Aggressive dosing of multiple medicines—lithium, divalproex, antipsychotics given orally by injection, and benzodiazepines—often increases staff members' anxiety about safety, leading to hesitation in giving not only the prescribed dosage but also "as needed" or p.r.n. medication to control belligerent and dangerous behavior. During well-staffed weekday shifts, standing doses may be easily adjusted by adding p.r.n. doses, and more effort can be made to apply psychosocial techniques to moderate agitation. During more thinly-staffed evening and night shifts, and on weekends, with less overall unit structure, elective doses may decrease and symptoms escalate. A night doctor on call who may not know the patient well may be called. Moreover, if extra medicine has to be given intramuscularly, it may require a second antipsychotic, perhaps from the first-generation, on top of one the patient is already taking by mouth.

Therefore, the stage is set for potential medical complications especially during off-hours, when increasing doses of medicine may be given for the aggressive, potentially violent, manic patient. Blood pressure can fall. High dosages of intramuscular antipsychotics may create a need for benztropine for extrapyramidal side effects. Anticholinergic delirium can ensue, with confusion and disorientation that may be hard to distinguish from mania itself. Seclusion and/or restraint to manage erratic, overly intrusive behavior may be accompanied by dehydration. The risk of neuroleptic malignant syndrome increases in agitated, secluded, dehydrated patients, especially those on multiple antipsychotics. This pharmacologic balancing act is one of many trying aspects in the acute treatment of mania.

Case Vignette

Ms. S is a 57-year-old single, childless, unemployed woman with a 30-year history of bipolar disorder, type I, with >20 psychiatric admissions for acute mania, always in the context of medication nonadherence. She was admitted emergently for out of control behavior, which included screaming behavior, irritability, throwing objects in her home, and paranoid thoughts about family and friends.

Treatment began in the emergency room with olanzapine 20 mg, lorazepam 4 mg, and divalproex sodium 500 mg. On arrival to the inpatient floor, Ms. S began screaming at both staff and other patients. She continued to escalate, and in the course of the evening received two injections of haloperidol 5 mg, lorazepam 2 mg, and benztropine 1 mg. Later in the night, frightened that she had been kidnapped, she began screaming and lunged at the nurse's aide with her. The doctor on call prescribed chlorpromazine 25 mg, of which she received four injections over 8 hours until she slept.

The next morning she was lethargic but combative, as well as confused and disoriented. On medical evaluation, she was febrile, tachycardic, and hypotensive and found to have a urinary tract infection. Serum creatine phosphokinase was elevated but this was determined to be due to the intramuscular injections and not to neuroleptic malignant syndrome. She was diagnosed with delirium due to infection and anticholinergic toxicity. She cleared cognitively and became more cooperative over the next 48 hours after treatment with antibiotics and a standing regimen of chlorpromazine 500 mg per day by mouth in divided doses. She was eventually discharged to a day hospital on olanzapine 20 mg per day and lorazepam 3 mg per day.

Education about Medication

Inpatient pharmacotherapy further can make use of distinct features of the milieu to improve both response and, it is hoped, adherence to eventual outpatient treatment. These features include intensive opportunities to educate, detect and manage side effects, and work through reluctance to take medicine. The hospital setting provides unique opportunities in all three areas to maximize medication effectiveness. A related topic is terminology. "Mood stabilizer" has become ambiguous because of the multiple classes of medication approved by the FDA for short-term or long-term management of mania and bipolar disorder. To facilitate clear psychoeducation, the authors would advise that the unit staff adopt a consistent approach to using or not using the term with patients and families, and decide how to talk about the array of classes and individual medicines. One approach is to use "mood stabilizer" as a function, not for a specific medicine or class, and talk about this property as it relates to different phases of illness—stabilization from "above" for mania, from "below" for depression, and long-term stabilization. The goal is to educate with a clear vocabulary about why medicines are combined and how they may be added or subtracted over time as phases of bipolar illness wax and wane.

DEPRESSION

General Management

Depressed patients present in a variety of ways. They may be withdrawn, sullen, and psychomotorically retarded with little in the way of verbal output. Often indifferent to their surroundings, they may be only passive participants in their overall care. Others may demonstrate great irritability and anxiety, verbalizing worry and fear about the future and hopelessness. Still others, with a depressive episode as well as character pathology, may enter the hospital in a crisis involving work or relationship instability. Any of these may present with suicidal thoughts, plans, or an actual attempt. The purpose of the inpatient setting is to provide a safe environment to permit workup and treatment and support a return of basic functioning. Unlike mania, where the authors often aim for substantial episode resolution before discharge, many depressed patients are discharged before treatment has taken full effect given the long delay in antidepressant response. Instead, the goals are to ameliorate acute problems of safety and motivation, and safely initiate appropriate care. The authors note that the calculus is somewhat different after a suicide attempt in the context of major depression, where substantial episode resolution should be achieved before discharge.

Assessment

Although most depressed patients are treated as outpatients, the presence of complicating factors is often what tips the balance toward the need for hospital admission. As examples, these include stressful interpersonal losses or disruptive events that provoke and intensify underlying mood disorders (and may have partly resulted from the mood disorder in the first place); medical problems that contribute to depression directly or make the use of medication more difficult; new or recurrent substance abuse; and significant unstable character pathology that interferes with functioning or with outpatient treatment relationships. Family stress from independent causes, or from the experience of living with the depressed member, may also create a downward spiral. Although suicidal thoughts and attempts are an obvious final common pathway to the hospital, these other factors may contribute to demoralization and exhaustion in the patient, family, or provider and lead to the hospital for reevaluation and intensification of treatment.

Suicidality

Suicidal risk must be carefully evaluated in depressed patients upon arrival to the unit. The mental status examination and history from all sources should include assessment of current and past thoughts, plans, attempts, and lethality. Complications that predict suicide potential should be sought, including psychosis, substances of abuse, character pathology, and medical illness.[19] Demographically, being single and male are amongst the highest predictors of intent in hospitalized patients.[20] Family history of mood disorder, substance abuse, suicide attempts, and completions must be elicited as these also may be relevant to the patient's risk. Notes indicating "patient contracts for safety" are often seen from outpatient providers or from emergency department (ED) physicians, but must never deter the staff's own evaluation and judgment. The overall risk assessment will influence the level of observation needed, such as a one-to-one observation (specifying if this means within arms length or only visual range), frequent checks, and a room assigned closer to the nursing station.

Completed suicides are a rare but highly significant and disturbing event on an inpatient unit. Delusions in depression appear to be an especially strong risk factor.[21] Suicidal gestures and attempts, while still uncommon, are a constant concern, despite all attempts to "sanitize" the environment with restrictions on clothing and possessions and expensively customized room fixtures and architecture. Patients have cut their wrists with plastic utensils, paperclips, broken pieces of plastic, even with the serrated edges of the towel dispenser. Head banging, attempted drowning in the sink, and hiding of pills and other objects in bathroom and bedroom nooks and crannies have all been tried. Strangulation by hanging with bedsheets or clothing such as a bra made for especially severe, almost successful attempts. The risk can decrease as treatment begins, family members become involved in the treatment, patients become educated about their illnesses, and a somewhat tenuous, but initial alliance develops.

Case Vignette

Mr. B was a 35-year-old, married, high-functioning partner in a law firm, with two young children. He had no history of any mood disorder or other medical conditions, although his father had suffered from a number of depressive episodes. Over the last 6 months he had increasing neurovegetative symptoms in the context of increasing demands at the office. His wife began drinking more than usual, creating difficulties at home. Three months before, he was called by the Federal Bureau of Investigation FBI to testify about transactions at his firm concerning a client. He became convinced that his actions at work were being monitored, and he would be arrested and disbarred. Colleagues tried to reassure him about the reasons for the FBI investigation having nothing to do with the patient, all to no avail. After weeks of worry, he decided that death would spare his family the humiliation he was sure would transpire. After overdosing on over-the-counter pills in a hotel room, he called his wife, and was admitted to the intensive care unit ICU of a general hospital.

After medical stabilization, the patient was started on a tricyclic antidepressant TCA and an atypical antipsychotic on the general medical service. He indicated increased hopefulness and a wish to live. One-to-one observation was discontinued. Notes indicated the patient was contracting for safety. Days later, the patient tried to inject air into his intravenous in a further attempt to kill himself. He was transferred to the authors' unit for continued treatment of this psychotic depression.

Here is a case of a first-episode, psychotic depression in a patient with a family history of mood disorder, no personal history of suicide attempts, no medical comorbid conditions, and no substance abuse, who, in a paranoid delusional state, "contracted for safety." He appeared to be improving, only to again reattempt suicide on the medical unit. The removal of one-to-one observation on the inpatient unit is a difficult judgment to make, requiring a balance between patient safety with increasing independence and financial constraints. On the authors' unit, they often discontinue one-to-one observation in a graduated manner, starting with the day shift, then to evenings and finally nights, moving patients from individual to group observational status (i.e., must be in a common area) before permitting full independence.

Vigilance regarding suicide should continue through discharge, a time when anxiety can heighten symptoms.

Complicated Patients

Depressed individuals with persistent alcohol abuse and/or character pathology are among the most difficult patients to treat. Frequently admitted in crisis, their character issues that have interfered with continuing outpatient care surface early in the hospital, and now interfere with the institution of new pharmacologic and psychological interventions. The focus of the patient's treatment often turns to what the staff is not doing for them rather than a self-reflective process of understanding how they have come to be in crisis. Engaging such patients and helping them transition to meaningful outpatient care is the core of hospital treatment. Medication for nonspecific insomnia, anxiety, or "mini" psychosis and detoxification from substances of abuse may help the patient engage in psychotherapeutic and psychosocial interventions. However, during the days before relief begins, the patient may threaten to leave, insist on medication changes, or insist on receiving craved prescription drugs of abuse such as opiates, benzodiazepines, or stimulants. Similar to the manic patient, these depressed patients sorely try the staff. They are needy and demanding and staff may feel berated or devalued. Splitting behaviors and defense mechanisms, either fundamental to the patient's character pathology or exacerbated in the regressed state of the depressive episode, may cause disagreement in the approach to treatment by the staff. These staff conflicts may persist even after medication or ECT has been initiated for the depressive component of the picture.

Here is a vignette of a potentially tumultuous situation that was defused sufficiently to allow treatment.

Case Vignette

Ms. Q was a 48-year-old professor of literature at a prestigious university, admitted for depression, acute suicidality, and alcohol abuse. She had a 30-year history of recurrent depression and a 20-year history of alcohol abuse, with one prior admission for "depression, detox, rehab." She had been married 25 years to a man significantly less successful in her academic field. She was admitted for 3 months of worsening alcohol abuse, depression, and acute suicidal thoughts.

Six weeks before admission she discovered that her husband had been having an affair since the second year of their marriage. He told her that she was too much of a "self-absorbed fool to realize it." After 10 years of sobriety, she abruptly resumed drinking one to two bottles of wine nightly. Her mood began to "crash" and she was unable to teach her classes. After being confronted by the dean about frequent absences and erratic behavior in the classroom, she drank 1.5 bottles of wine, took a cab to a local bridge with the plan of jumping. She called her psychiatrist and admission was arranged. On the second day of her admission she complained vehemently about the food and the lack of attention from staff and requested discharge. The inpatient psychiatrist engaged her by empathizing with the series of blows the patient had endured—her marriage, her job and now, as an inpatient, her sense of autonomy and a level of control over her life. Confrontation of the inability to accept responsibility for the circumstances she found herself in helped this patient to agree to continued stay to begin a broader look at the many psychodynamic and psychosocial issues in her life. She was successfully detoxified, and ultimately did well with antidepressant medication and referral to an outpatient psychiatrist able to work with her intensively on her characterological problems.

Pharmacotherapy

Major Depressive Episodes in the Nonbipolar Patient

The authors of this chapter will first consider previously untreated patients, or patients who have had distant past episodes and have a recurrence while off medicine. For those who are not psychotic and do not appear to have bipolar I or bipolar II disorder, treatment follows standard parameters such as those outlined in the APA practice guideline for depression,[22] or the types of protocols embodied in recent research programs on the real-world effectiveness of antidepressants.[23] Barring medical contraindications, they generally begin with a selective serotonin reuptake inhibitor (SSRI) (fluoxetine, sertraline, citalopram, escitalopram, paroxetine) or a combined serotonin norepinephrine reuptake inhibitor (SNRI) (duloxetine, venlafaxine). Other antidepressants of similar efficacy, such as bupropion and mirtazapine, are completely acceptable alternatives when particular properties weight the balance, such as promoting sleep and appetite with mirtazapine, or avoiding weight gain and sexual dysfunction with bupropion.

Knowing that these will take several weeks to work, the authors try to achieve rapid symptom relief (agitation, insomnia, and anxiety), by simultaneously prescribing a benzodiazepine, typically clonazepam (longer acting) or lorazepam (shorter acting), or trazodone, or a low-dose, sedating second-generation antipsychotic such as quetiapine. Within the inpatient milieu, using these additional medicines at adequate doses to help restore basic physical functions such as relief of physical anxiety, insomnia, and loss of appetite can be extraordinarily helpful.

Less often used nowadays, but especially worth considering in the hospital, are TCAs or monoamine oxidase inhibitors (MAOIs). Most patients with onset of depression since the mid-80s have not tried them. Some tricylics have a distinct advantage of having the dose determined accurately with therapeutic blood level monitoring. The authors utilize this to achieve rapid therapeutic doses, often within a week, taking advantage of the hospital setting to monitor for side effects such as orthostatic hypotension, tachycardia, and anticholinergic side effects. Similarly, the nonselective MAOIs, phenelzine and tranylcypromine, can be started with careful patient education regarding dietary restrictions. The new transdermal formulation of selegiline, a selective MAOI-B that at lower doses requires no tyramine-free dietary restriction, is another option.

The recently reported Sequenced Treatment Alternatives to Relieve Depression (STAR*D) results suggest there is value in early pursuit of combination therapy (two antidepressants) or augmentation (an antidepressant plus a second drug without primary antidepressant effects), rather than prolonged sequential monotherapy trials.[24] Following this logic, when a patient comes to the hospital having only recently started an antidepressant that has not yet worked on an outpatient basis, the physicians often find it reasonable simultaneously to maximize the dose of the first treatment while adding a second antidepressant from a different class (e.g., adding bupropion to an SSRI or venlafaxine), increasing the odds of response while using the hospital milieu to monitor the greater potential for side effects.

For patients already receiving combination antidepressants, or with histories of such trials as outpatients, augmenting strategies such as thyroid hormone or lithium may be used. These have recently been revalidated for outpatients as being modestly helpful, with thyroid being the more tolerable of the two.[25] A less evidence-based approach, but one that is often found rapidly helpful, is augmentation of SSRIs and SNRIs with stimulants such as methylphenidate or mixed amphetamine salts. The authors find stimulants especially useful in patients who are fatigued or feel a flattened mood, often despite lengthy medication treatment before entering the hospital. Second-generation antipsychotics are another augmentation strategy that they sometimes use even in the absence of psychosis, agitation, or anxiety, although the evidence for their utility purely as augmentation is inconclusive at best.[26]

Psychotic depression poses further challenges because of the well-documented findings that antidepressants alone are insufficient treatment.[22] In this condition, the authors add a full therapeutic dose of a second-generation antipsychotic to a standard antidepressant (generally a combined SNRI or a tricylic antidepressant). They recommend ECT if psychotic depression is dire, if prior appropriate combined antidepressant and antipsychotic therapy has failed, or when suicide risk is high.

Bipolar Depression

For major depressive episodes in bipolar disorder, there is little clear evidence to guide the approach, even in relatively treatment-naïve patients. Experts agree that depressed patients with bipolar I disorder should always receive a mood stabilizer known to prevent mania, although opinion is more divided regarding this need in bipolar II disorder, especially if depression is the main problem over time.[11,27] The only approved medicines for acute treatment of major depression in bipolar disorder are the combination of fluoxetine and olanzapine (marketed as Symbyax),[28] and more recently quetiapine.[29] Each has disadvantages; there are concerns with both about weight gain and sedation, and about the possibility of cycling induction with long-term fluoxetine exposure. Because of growing awareness that traditional antidepressants pose risks of cycling even when used with mood stabilizers, lamotrigine, while indicated only for long-term prevention in bipolar disorder, has become a popular approach for acute bipolar depression. It has been shown to be somewhat effective both as monotherapy[30] and when added to an established mood stabilizer[31] in bipolar I depression. The APA and the consensus-based guidelines suggest beginning with either lithium or lamotrigine as monotherapy, or in combination when there is a strong history of bipolar I disorder as lamotrigine alone is not protective against mania. It is noted, however, that due to the required slow titration of lamotrigine, taking 6 weeks to reach a target dose of 200 mg per day, results may not be seen until well after discharge. This underscores the need to seek symptom stabilization through other means in the milieu and with other simultaneously administered medicines (e.g., to treat insomnia and anxiety).

In more severe bipolar depression, the physicians often begin a standard antidepressant along with lithium, or add an antidepressant for a patient who has broken through maintenance therapy on a mood stabilizer. Prospectively gathered data, such as that recently published by the Systematic Treatment Enhancement Program for Bipolar Disorder (STEP-BD)[32] add to the doubts on the utility of antidepressants in this situation. In a group of patients with an average of ten previous episodes, remission rates and times to remission were similar whether placebo or an antidepressant was added to a mood stabilizer, although switch rates to mania were higher with antidepressants. Among commonly used antidepressants, venlafaxine is associated with higher switch rates, and bupropion lower, with sertraline intermediate in risk.[33] There is a subset of approximately 15% of bipolar depressed patients who improve and do not switch on antidepressants (added to a mood stabilizer) in the first 2 months of treatment, who then tend to remain well by continuing antidepressants.[34] Unfortunately this group cannot be identified in advance by any clinical characteristics other than previous history. The authors have no information on whether results are improved by combining a mood-stabilizing antimanic agent with both lamotrigine and a traditional antidepressant, although that is another approach they have seen increasingly used.

Apart from antidepressants and lamotrigine, the conservative approaches include using higher doses of lithium, or adding a second mood stabilizer (e.g., augmenting lithium by adding divalproex) which may be just as effective as adding a standard antidepressant. Second-generation antipsychotics other than quetiapine have not been systematically studied as antidepressants, but offer another approach that at least will not cause cycling.

What should the inpatient clinician do, pressed for time but with no clear evidence to support a best practice? First, individualize to the patient's prior history of response or exacerbation of bipolar disorder symptoms with antidepressants. Second, use the safety of milieu to try a different approach if prior history is a series of disappointments: the clinicians can choose either to initiate treatment with an antidepressant and observe for signs of early switching to mania or stick to combinations of mood stabilizers. They can try to introduce cognitive or family-based psychotherapies if they have not been explored, or just address precipitating psychosocial stressors in a supportive manner in the hope of speeding a "spontaneous" remission without dramatically changing medication—a course that studies suggest happens more often than one can appreciate. The inpatient treatment of bipolar depression requires substantial guesswork and risk evaluation, with carefully, individualized follow-up after discharge to watch for cycling or relapse.

In the most apparently treatment-refractory patients, as has been outlined in the earlier discussion of stages of treatment, the most helpful first maneuver may be to carefully reduce and eliminate medicines. The inpatient environment sometimes has the effect of galvanizing the treatment team, including the referring psychiatrist, to perform a thorough review of years of medication therapy. This may lead to a retrial of medicines previously helpful, which may work again after a long hiatus, or to a novel combination that bears fruit.

Electroconvulsive Therapy

ECT is an important option for patients with depression, whether bipolar or not, as well as mixed states and sometimes mania. On the 24-bed unit, 10% of patients receive ECT. Situations where ECT should be considered earlier rather than later are the agitated elderly patient already on multiple medicines for general medical conditions, the treatment-refractory depressive patient who had multiple outpatient trials with deteriorating function and increasing despair, psychotic depression, the actively suicidal patient with a plan or recent attempt, and some pregnant patients. There are also infrequent though dramatic special situations in which ECT is the treatment of choice, as in the following case of catatonia.

Case Vignette

Patient A was a 33-year-old, single, white woman with a remote history of panic attacks and bulimia, who presented with a complicated neuropsychiatric history of several months' duration, including three hospitalizations on various psychiatric and neurologic inpatient services before transfer to the neurology close-monitoring unit for an atypical movement disorder together with an atypical psychosis. After initiation of various treatments including antipsychotics, the patient developed what was initially thought to be neuroleptic malignant syndrome, later revised to a diagnosis of lethal catatonia. Unilateral ECT was begun. The patient did extremely well with 22 treatments and was discharged on lithium, receiving a retrospective diagnosis of bipolar disorder, depressed episode with catatonic and psychotic features.

As a course of ECT can last a month or more, there are several important ways to reduce length of stay. First, whenever possible, the ECT pretreatment medical workup and anesthesia clearance is best done before admission to shorten length of stay and begin treatment on admission. Second, medicines that interfere with ECT can often be washed out before admission. These include anticonvulsants and MAOIs, although it is not clear the latter are as much a danger during anesthesia as once feared.[35] Finally, the authors try to transition to outpatient status when patients have adequate social support and symptomatic improvement to make this safe.

Light Therapy

Light therapy using one-half hour of 10,000 lux wide spectrum light may be helpful in nonseasonal depression, in some cases with dramatic results reported as an adjunct to antidepressants.[36] The authors have begun to employ this strategy on their unit, as well as in patients receiving ECT. Severely depressed outpatients may be challenged by the usual early morning schedule, but can be mobilized by the inpatient nursing staff. Its effectiveness requires further study.

Psychosocial Interventions in the Therapeutic Program

In addition to general management, daily physician supportive interviews, and biological interventions, the present authors provide depressed and bipolar patients with multimodal psychosocial therapies. Occupational therapy runs 16 groups weekly on the floor including grooming, crafts, life skills, current events, socialization, and daily walks. Recreation therapy similarly runs an additional 18 hours of activities, which include stress management, creative expressions, movement, supervised computer time with Internet access, goal setting, bingo, and ping-pong. Exercise therapists meet with patients individually and in groups in an on-floor exercise room (with treadmill, stair climber, universal gym equipment) 7 hours weekly. Psychologists and social workers run substance abuse and depression psychoeducation/psychotherapy groups as well as a group for family and friends of patients with an affective disorder. Additional groups currently include pet-assisted therapy and a chaplain-run spirituality group. This program is individualized by diagnosis (manic or depressed), stage in the course of illness, and level of education.

The authors hear more feedback about this aspect of the program than about any other treatment modality. A patient satisfaction survey conducted by their hospital showed that of all activities offered on their inpatient unit "social/recreational therapy" was felt to be the most helpful with 87.5% ranking it first. And it is often in the context of psychosocial therapies that a patient begins to understand the illness and its impact on his/her life. The authors believe that these therapies, geared to reducing demoralization and promoting healthier thinking and functioning, are crucial in being able to discharge depressed patients well before the time course typically required for an antidepressant to have significant effects. Both verbal and activities groups provide valuable feedback regarding symptoms and functioning. The ability to control behavior, affect, and language is often judged better when patients are observed in a variety of tasks requiring more or less structure than in brief mental status interviews.

All of the modalities create opportunities to reflect behavior back to the patient to promote change, in a manner that is more immediate than in outpatient settings. This constant reinforcement of how one is perceived by others, a reinforcement more effectively provided in a group setting rather than individual interventions, is the foundation of insight.

Case Vignette

Mr. C is a 31-year-old man, a single, recently fired investment salesman living on the opposite end of the country from his family, admitted for the fourth time with florid mania characterized by grandiosity and paranoid delusions. While acutely manic, he wielded a knife at his fiancée, threatening to kill her for an affair he believed her to be having with a movie star. He had been chronically noncompliant with medication for 7 years and has been frequently unemployed. Within 8 days he de-escalated on lithium carbonate and risperidone, but then demanded immediate discharge. He stated that the hospital team "overreacted and overmedicated" him and denied having a mental illness. The turning point came in a psychoeducation group in which he scoffed at the idea of medication for himself or others. He mocked his peers as "dupes" until they begin to relate to him who he was, what he had said and done while manic. Although this feedback from staff never had any impact, hearing it from other patients left him deeply affected and ultimately convinced. Despite having no memory of the events while he was manic, he was able to trust what they told him and to acknowledge that "something is wrong." At a meeting to which his family flew in, he agreed to partial hospitalization and to allow his fiancée to have contact with his psychiatrist because "I need another set of eyes. I can't trust my own right now."

There is significant evidence that psychosocial interventions are extremely effective in improving adherence and reducing relapse rates in outpatient populations with bipolar disorder.[37] These interventions can reduce relapse in bipolar patients by almost 40% compared to standard treatment alone.[38] Another examination of treatment nonadherence in mood disorders found that in unipolar depression, 8% to 10% of patients never fill the prescription for antidepressant medicine on discharge and, within 1 month, 68% are medication nonadherent. The use of an SSRI had no effect on these patterns of nonadherence. Similarly, among bipolar patients >50% become either nonadherent or intermittently adherent during the maintenance phase of illness.[39] The authors see the inpatient unit as the place to begin interventions to improve adherence.

Psychoeducation groups focused on diagnosis and medication can answer questions that patients are sometimes reluctant to pose to a psychiatrist. In these settings, patients can turn to peers to confirm or validate information offered by their psychiatrist. Clinicians often misunderstand the concerns that lead to nonadherence. In one study,[39] researchers polled bipolar patients and clinicians about reasons for stopping lithium. There was low level of concordance between reasons that clinicians suspected and those cited by patients. But there was a high concordance between patients, whether or not they had been adherent to treatment before admission. Individual counseling from psychiatrists is important, but contact with peers who are struggling with the same illness can have a superior impact.

Acknowledgment

The authors thank Cindy J. Aaronson, M.S.W., Ph.D., for editorial assistance.

REFERENCES

1. Hirschfeld RM, Williams JB, Spitzer RM, et al. Development and validation of a screening instrument for bipolar spectrum disorder: The Mood Disorder Questionnaire. *Am J Psychiatry.* 2000;157:1873–1875.
2. Oquendo MA, Barca-Garcia E, Kartachov A, et al. A computer alogorithm for calculating the adequacy of antidepressant treatment in unipolar and bipolar depression. *J Clin Psychiatry.* 2003; 64:825–833.
3. Sackeim HA. The definition and meaning of treatment-resistant depression. *J Clin Psychiatry.* 2001;62(Suppl 16):10–17.
4. Denicoff KD, Smith-Jackson EE, Disney ER, et al. Preliminary evidence of the reliability and validity of the prospective life-chart methodology (LCM-p). *J Psychiatr Res.* 1997;31:593–603.
5. Borgeat F, Zullino D. Attitudes concerning involuntary treatment of mania: Results of a survey within self-help organizations. *Eur Psychiatry.* 2004;19:155–158.
6. Gardner W, Lidz CW, Hoge SK, et al. Patients' revisions of their beliefs about the need for hospitalization. *Am J Psychiatry.* 1999; 156:1385–1391.
7. Morrison EF. An evaluation of four programs for the management of aggression in psychiatric settings. *Arch Psychiatr Nurs.* 2003;17:146–155.
8. Spencer JH Jr, Glick ID, Haas GL, et al. A randomized clinical trial of inpatient family intervention, III: Effects at 6-month and 18-month follow-ups. *Am J Psychiatry.* 1988;145:1115–1121.
9. Janowsky D, Leff M, Epstein R. Playing the manic game. *Arch Gen Psychiatry.* 1970; 22(3):252–261.
10. American Psychiatric Association. Practice guideline for the treatment of patients with bipolar disorder (revision). *Am J Psychiatry.* 2002;159(Suppl 4):1–50.
11. Kahn DA, Sachs GS, Printz DJ, et al. Medication treatment of bipolar disorder 2000: a summary of the expert consensus guidelines. *J Psychiatr Pract.* 2000;6(4):197–211.
12. Suppes T, Rush AJ, Dennehy EB, et al. Texas medication algorithm project, phase 3 (TMAP-3); clinical results for patients with a history of mania. *J Clin Psychiatry.* 2003;64: 370–382.
13. Scherck H, Pajonk FG, Leucht S. Second generation antipsychotic agents in the treatment of acute mania: A systematic review and meta-analysis of randomized controlled trials. *Arch Gen Psychiatry.* 2007;64:442–455.
14. Calabrese JR, Shelton MD, Rapport DJ, et al. A 20-month, double-blind, maintenance trial of lithium versus divalproex in rapid-cycling bipolar disorder. *Am J Psychiatry.* 2005;11:2152–2161.
15. Swann AC, Daniel DG, Kochan LD, et al. Psychosis in mania: Specificity of its role in severity and treatment response. *J Clin Psychiatry.* 2004;65:825–829.
16. Mazza M, Di Nicola M, Martinotti G, et al. Oxcarbazepine in bipolar disorder: A critical review of the literature. *Expert Opin Pharmacother.* 2007;8:649–656.
17. Suppes T, Webb A, Paul B, et al. Clinical outcome in a randomized 1-year trial of clozapine versus treatment as usual for patients with treatment-resistant illness and a history of mania. *Am J Psychiatry.* 1999;156:1164–1169.
18. American Psychiatric Association. *The practice of electroconvulsive therapy: recommendations for treatment, training and privileging: a task force report of the Americna Psychiatric Association,* 2nd ed. Washington, DC: American Psychiatric Press; 2001.
19. Rihmer Z. Suicide risk in mood disorders. *Curr Opin Psychiatry.* 2007;20:17–22.
20. Kumar CT, Mohan R, Ranjith G, et al. Characteristics of high intet suicide attempters admitted to a general hospital. *J Affect Disord.* 2006;91:77–81.
21. Roose SP, Glassman AH, Walsh BT, et al. Depression, delusions, and suicide. *Am J Psychiatry.* 1983;140:1159–1162.
22. American Psychiatric Association. Practice guideline for the treatment of patients with major depressive disorder (revision). *Am J Psychiatry.* 2000;157(Suppl 4):1–45.
23. Rush AJ, Trivedi MH, Wisniewski SR, et al. Acute and longer-term outcomes in depressed patients requiring one or several treatment steps: A STAR*D report. *Am J Psychiatry.* 2006;163: 1905–1917.
24. Rush AJ. STAR*D: What have we learned? *Am J Psychiatry.* 2007;164:201–202.
25. Nierenberg AA, Fava M, Trivedi MH, et al. A comparison of lithium and T(3) augmentation following two failed medication treatments for depression: A STAR*D report. *Am J Psychiatry.* 2006;164:1519–1530.
26. Valenstein M, McCarthy JF, Austin KL, et al. What happened to lithium? Antidepressant augmentation in clinical settings. *Am J Psychiatry.* 2006;163:1219–1225.
27. Crismon ML, Trivedi M, Pigott T, et al. The Texas medication algorithm project: Report of the Texas consensus conference panel on medication treatment of major depressive disorder. *J Clin Psychiatry.* 1999;60:142–156.
28. Tohen M, Vieta E, Calabrese J, et al. Efficacy of olanzapine and olanzapine-fluoxetine combination in the treatment of bipolar I depression. *Arch Gen Psychiatry.* 2003;60: 1079–1088.

29. Calabrese JR, Keck PE, McFadden W, et al. A randomized, double-blinded, placebo-controlled trial of quetipine in bipolar I or II depression. *Am J Psychiatry*. 2005;162: 1351–1360.

30. Calabrese JR, Bowden CL, Sachs GS, et al. A double blind placebo-controlled study of lamotrigine monotherapy in outpatients with bipolar I depression. *J Clin Psychiatry*. 1999;2:79–88.

31. Nierenberg AA, Ostacher MJ, Calabrese JR, et al. Treatment-resistant bipolar depresion: A STEP-BD equipoise randomized effectiveness trial of antidepressant augmentation with lamotrigine, inositol or risperidone. *Am J Psychiatry*. 2006;163:210–216.

32. Sachs GS, Nierenberg AA, Calabrese JR, et al. Effectiveness of adjunctive antidepressant treatment for bipolar depression. *N Engl J Med*. 2007;356:1711–1722.

33. Leverich GS, Altshuler LL, Frye MA, et al. Risk of switch in mood polarity to mania or hypomania in patients with bipolar depression during acute and continuation trials for venlafaxine, sertraline and bupropion as adjuncts to mood stabilizers. *Am J Psychiatry*. 2006;163:232–239.

34. Post RM, Leverich GS, Nolen WA. A re-evaluation of the role of antidepressants in the treatment of bipolar depression: Data from the Stanley Foundation Bipolar Network. *Bipolar Disord*. 2003;5:396–406.

35. Doleric TJ, Habl SS, Barnes RD, et al. Electroconvulsive therapy in patients taking monoamine oxidase inhibitors. *J ECT*. 2004; 20(4):258–261.

36. Termin M, Termin JS. Light therapy for seasonal and nonseasonal depression: Efficacy, protocol, safety, and side effects. *CNS Spectr*. 2005;10(8):1–17.

37. Scott J, Gutierrez MJ. The current status of psychological treatments in bipolar disorders: A systematic review of relapse prevention. *Bipolar Disord*. 2004;6:498–503.

38. Scott J, Colom F, Vieta E. A meta-analysis of relapse rates with adjunctive psychological therapies compared to usual psychiatric treatment for bipolar disorder. *Int J Neuropsychopharmacol*. 2006;10:123–129.

39. Lingam R, Scott J. Treatment non-adherence in mood disorders. *Acta Psychiatr Scand*. 2002;105(3):164–172.

CHAPTER 10

Electroconvulsive Therapy

WALTER KNYSZ, III AND C. EDWARD COFFEY

T he use of convulsive therapies in the treatment of major mental illness dates back to the use of camphor in the 16th century.[1] The use of electricity to induce a therapeutic seizure first occurred in 1938 and provided the benefit of being shorter acting and more reliable.[1,2] Electroconvulsive therapy (ECT) was first used in the United States in 1940, with many technical advances since that time.[1-4] ECT has a strong safety record and in some patients is better tolerated than psychotropic medication.[1-3] The efficacy of ECT for specific disorders has been well established in the medical literature, and ECT may work more rapidly than alternate forms of treatment.[1-6] When used to treat an acute episode of a mood disorder, ECT may be started on either an inpatient or outpatient basis (the grounds for this decision are discussed in subsequent text), and when used to protect against relapse/recurrence it is typically performed as an outpatient procedure.[2,4] Like many other treatments in medicine, the exact reasons for the effectiveness of ECT are uncertain.[1,4] It is known, however, that the benefits of ECT depend on producing a seizure and that technical factors related to how the seizure is produced are also important.[1-4] Research continues in attempts to understand better the biochemical processes responsible for the efficacy of ECT and to refine further the technical aspects of the procedure.

Indications

ECT is most often considered when patients do not respond to adequate medication trials, a situation commonly encountered on an inpatient psychiatric unit. Other reasons include a lack of tolerance to medication side effects, prior response to ECT, patient preference, and clinical circumstances that require rapid response for medical and/or psychiatric reasons. These situations include, but are not limited to, clinical deterioration, suicidality, and catatonia, all of which are also commonly seen on an inpatient psychiatric unit.[1-6]

A substantial body of literature documents the efficacy of ECT in the treatment of mood disorders.[1-6] This includes the treatment of unipolar depression (single and recurrent), bipolar depression, mania, and mixed states. Treating a patient with bipolar disorder depression with ECT may produce a "manic switch." In such cases, treatment would continue in a similar manner, as ECT can be effective in treating both bipolar depression and mania.

ECT can also be effective in treating psychotic disorders such as schizoaffective disorder, schizophreniform disorder, and schizophrenia.[2,7-10] Particular consideration should be given to ECT in the setting of catatonia, when a psychotic episode develops over a short period of time, and when a patient has successfully responded to ECT in the past.[1-6,11,12]

In addition to the primary psychiatric disorders listed in the preceding text, ECT may also be efficacious in the treatment of patients with serious affective and psychotic symptoms due to medical conditions, although the data to support this indication are less clear. There is also some suggestion that ECT may be effective in treating some medical conditions such as Parkinson disease, intractable seizures, and delirium.[1-6,13-20]

Of particular relevance in an inpatient setting, ECT can be effective in treating neuroleptic malignant syndrome (NMS) as well as catatonia (regardless of the etiology).[21-26] However, before treating a patient with NMS with ECT the vital signs should be stabilized. As the offending antipsychotic agent is discontinued in patients having NMS, and rechallenging them with an antipsychotic at a later point in time is not without risk, ECT has the added benefit of potentially being effective in the treatment of the underlying psychiatric disorder as well as treating the NMS.[1-6]

Pre-Electroconvulsive Therapy Evaluation

The pre-ECT evaluation consists of several components, including a neuropsychiatric and medical evaluation performed by a clinician experienced in ECT, a general medical evaluation performed by an anesthesiologist, initiation of the informed consent process, and preparation of the patient and family for the treatment. The goal of the neuropsychiatric evaluation is to determine the indication for ECT; establish a baseline for outcome measures including a baseline of cognitive functioning; and screen for, identify, and develop a plan to manage any medical conditions that would increase the risk of the procedure. These goals are accomplished by taking a thorough medical and neuropsychiatric history, including an interview and review of available records, and performing a thorough neuropsychiatric examination.[1-6]

A thorough psychiatric evaluation should identify whether an indication for ECT is present. This includes a diagnostic evaluation as well as review of previous medication trials (including dose, duration, efficacy, and side effects), response to previous courses of ECT, and identification of a need for rapid and definitive response to treatment.[1-6]

The identification of outcome measures and the collection of objective data at baseline as well as periodically during the treatment course are essential. This is true of psychiatric symptoms and functioning as well as of cognitive functioning.[1-6] The APA Task Force Report (2001) summarizes the use of a number of standardized rating scales that may be utilized in addition to the clinical interview.[2] Assessment tools used in physicians' practice include the Montgomery-Asberg Depression Rating Scale (MADRS), the Bech and Rafaelsen Mania Rating Scale, the Carroll Self-Rating Scale for Depression, the Global Assessment of Functioning (GAF) scale, the Social and Occupational Functioning Assessment (SOFA) scale, and the Karnofsky scale. The present authors also use the Mini Mental State Examination (MMSE) to track cognitive status during a treatment course. Additionally, the present authors administer the CogniStat before and at the conclusion of an index course as it may provide further detail about a patient's cognitive status and is relatively easy to administer. Further clinical perspective may be gained from interviewing family or friends over the course of treatment.[6]

Screening for medical risk factors cannot be overemphasized. Although ECT is generally a very safe procedure, the risk of morbidity and mortality increases in the context of comorbid medical risk factors. Appropriate management of these medical risk factors is essential to minimizing this risk. This is especially true in an inpatient setting as these patients are likely to have more severe medical and psychiatric problems. When screening for risk factors, the clinician should pay special attention to the neurologic and cardiopulmonary systems, as ECT produces transient but significant changes in cerebral and cardiovascular physiology. A patient with a history of significant cardiac disease, such as ischemia or heart failure, requires careful evaluation. Stabilization of these conditions is required before proceeding with treatment, and the treatment technique may need to be modified. A thorough neurologic examination should also be performed. If any abnormalities are discovered, further evaluation including neuroimaging may be required. A patient with a history of significant skeletal disease may require x-rays of the spine and a patient with significant pulmonary disease likely requires a chest x-ray. A patient's dentition should also be examined and note taken of any loose or chipped teeth and the presence of dentures.[1-7]

The patient should also be asked about a history of problems with anesthesia as well as a family history of such problems.[1-4,6,7] In addition, as the use of succinylcholine in patients with prolonged immobility increases the risk of hyperkalemia-related fatal arrhythmias, the presence of prolonged patient immobility should be determined and communicated to the anesthesiologist and an alternate muscle relaxant considered.[3,5] This is especially relevant in an inpatient setting, for example when treating patients with NMS, catatonia, or significant psychomotor retardation or akinesia.

Before beginning ECT, the patient should also be evaluated by the anesthesiologist in order to identify any factors that may increase a patient's risk when undergoing general anesthesia. This includes assessment of the cardiopulmonary systems and of dentition. The anesthesiologist should not only evaluate the patient and communicate any concerns to the other members of the ECT treatment team but also go through the informed consent process with the patient.[1–7]

In the event a patient is found to have a significant or unstable medical condition consultation with an appropriate medical specialist may be required.[1–7] A request for "clearance" is not advisable as the concept of clearance is not as helpful as that of risk assessment. Rather, the consultant should be asked to comment on the additional risks for an individual patient and asked for guidance in managing medical conditions before and during a course of ECT.[2] This includes any guidance involving medication used to mitigate or reduce risk around the time of the procedure,[1–7] for example, the use of inhalers before ECT for a patient with chronic obstructive pulmonary disease, adjustment in an antihypertensive regimen in a patient with poorly controlled hypertension, or adjustments in insulin dosing the mornings of treatment in a patient with difficult to control diabetes.

There are no routine laboratory tests required as part of the pre-ECT evaluation, although the authors recommend obtaining a baseline electrocardiogram (ECG) and serum electrolytes, especially potassium given the variety of arrhythmias that can arise in the setting of hyperkalemia and hypokalemia and the potential for succinylcholine to elevate serum potassium levels. Certainly, appropriate tests should be obtained to further define medical risk factors identified during the history and physical. Although ECT is generally considered safe during pregnancy, it is important to determine whether women of childbearing age may be pregnant because certain modification in the ECT procedure will be required.[5]

At the time of consultation, as well as during the treatment course, decisions regarding concurrent use of psychotropic medication will need to be made. Before beginning ECT, medicines such as anticonvulsants used for mood stabilization, benzodiazepines used for anxiety, and any other medicine that raises seizure threshold are generally tapered and discontinued. If benzodiazepines are deemed necessary then short-acting agents are preferred and their administration generally held for at least 24 hours before each treatment. Antipsychotic medicines may be used as they tend to lower seizure threshold. Lithium should also be tapered and discontinued before starting ECT as its use concurrently with ECT has been associated with severe adverse reactions including prolonged seizure duration and confusional states.[1–7]

Whether to discontinue antidepressant medication is less clear. The authors recommend that antidepressants also be tapered and discontinued before beginning ECT, as there is no conclusive evidence that the combination increases clinical efficacy in the treatment of depression when compared to ECT alone. In addition, concurrent use of antidepressants with ECT may increase the risk of side effects. Some studies, however, suggest that there may be added benefit to combining antidepressant medication and ECT.[27–29] Future research may clarify this issue. For the present, if a patient has a primary anxiety disorder in addition to the condition for which ECT is indicated, the use of antidepressants may be continued for their anxiolytic properties.[1–6]

In addition, a risk/benefit discussion with the patient regarding electrode placement (bitemporal, bifrontal, and right unilateral) should occur before beginning treatment. Clinicians should be able to administer competently both unilateral and bilateral treatment, as the choice of electrode placement affects the risk of cognitive side effects and possibly efficacy as well. Bitemporal placement is associated with the highest risk of cognitive side effects and right unilateral with the least risk. When efficacy data are compared for the treatment of major depressive disorder, bilateral electrode placement appears superior to right unilateral electrode placement unless the stimulus dose with right unilateral placement is significantly above seizure threshold (approximately six times threshold), in which case efficacy appears to be comparable.[1–5]

Consent

Informed consent is a process that begins at the time of initial consultation and continues throughout the treatment course. In addition to ethical and legal implications, the informed consent process can be utilized to strengthen the therapeutic alliance and ease patient anxiety. Generally, written consent is obtained before the initiation of the treatment series and periodically thereafter, as defined by the applicable laws. The authors also obtain oral consent before each treatment and document that discussion in the medical record. The patient should continue to be informed of treatment progress, and any changes in medical risks should be conveyed as the treatment proceeds. Written informed consent should again be obtained before beginning the continuation/maintenance phase and periodically thereafter.[1-6]

The informed consent process begins with the patient's being adequately informed of the indications for ECT, the risks and benefits of ECT, and the risks and benefits of alternative treatments including no treatment. If specific medical risk factors are identified during the consultation process the patient may not necessarily be able to be completely informed of their risks until after further medical workup, consultation, and medical management to reduce the medical risks. The patient and the family should be given ample opportunity to have their questions answered, and the patient should be allowed the opportunity to make an informed decision free of coercion by the treatment team or family members.[1-6]

In addition to the patient's being provided adequate information to make an informed decision, a determination needs to be made regarding the patient's capacity to understand this information and to make a reasoned decision. This assessment can be particularly challenging on inpatient psychiatric units where the severity of mental illness is greatest. A balance must at times be struck between patient autonomy and ensuring patients are not deprived of potentially effective treatment. The treating ECT psychiatrist should be well versed in state and local mental health law and the petitioning of a court pursued when appropriate.[1-6]

Treatment Procedure

Because of its safety profile, ECT can generally be administered as an outpatient procedure, assuming the patient can safely manage the pretreatment protocols (e.g., NPO after midnight, administration of standing oral medications, etc.), can travel safely to and from the procedure, and has adequate posttreatment supervision at home. ECT is typically administered on an inpatient basis when the patient requires psychiatric hospitalization because of the acuity of the mental disorder. As clinical improvement occurs over the course of treatment, the patient may be discharged from inpatient care and complete the index course of ECT as an outpatient. Inpatient ECT may also be required for those patients who require close medical management before or after the procedure, or who develop unusually severe cognitive side effects and therefore cannot be cared for safely at home.[1-4]

Generally the ECT treatment team consists of a psychiatrist, an ECT nurse, and an anesthesia provider. Each facility should determine which specific disciplines (anesthesiology, nurse anesthesia, psychiatry) are privileged to provide anesthesia care during an ECT procedure. Before each treatment the patient should be seen by the psychiatrist, ECT nurse, and anesthesia provider, at which time an interval medical history should be obtained including review of medication and any change in the patient's medical status. In addition, a review of the patient's chart and medical review of systems should be performed, and there should be confirmation that the patient has remained NPO. Vital signs should also be taken and reviewed. Evaluation of the patient's psychiatric status including evaluation of outcome measures through patient interview, inpatient chart review, discussion with unit staff, and the utilization of standardized rating scales should take place. Finally, the patient should be given an opportunity to have questions or concerns addressed.[1-4]

Once the patient has been taken to the procedure area casual conversation between staff should cease. The patient should have each step of preparation explained as it occurs to help minimize anxiety. Intravenous access should be established if it has not been done already and any pretreatment medications administered. It is not uncommon to administer anticholinergic medication such as glycopyrrolate to dry out secretions or atropine in certain circumstances in which the patient may be at risk for vagally mediated bradyarrhythmia. It is recommended that patients receive atropine before their first treatment when dosage titration is used to estimate seizure threshold, as such patients are at risk of asystole should a stimulus be given and a subsequent seizure not occur. Some patients may benefit from an antiemetic before the treatment.[1-4]

A blood pressure cuff and pulse oximeter should be applied and a set of vital signs should again be obtained in the treatment room. ECG/electroencephalogram (EEG) leads as well as the stimulus pads should be applied. A "time out" should be performed according to the standards of the Joint Commission on Accreditation of Healthcare Organizations JCAHO confirming patient identity and stimulus pad location. Treatment settings on the treatment device should also be set and confirmed. Patients should receive preoxygenation with 100% oxygen at this time.[1-4]

Once the above-mentioned steps have been completed, the patient should be asked if he or she is ready to proceed, at which time the anesthetic should be administered. The short-acting barbiturate methohexital is generally the anesthetic of choice given its rapid onset, short duration of action, and tendency for smooth induction/recovery. Other agents such as etomidate, thiopental, propofol, and ketamine are sometimes used instead. Ketamine, which lowers the seizure threshold, may be particularly beneficial when a patient's seizure threshold is particularly high. It is common practice to inflate a blood pressure cuff around the right ankle (ipsilateral to right unilateral stimulation) once the patient is anesthetized and before the administration of the muscle relaxant (usually the depolarizing agent succinylcholine). This technique is used as a means to monitor the convulsive phase of the seizure as it prevents the muscle relaxant from traveling to the foot.[1-4]

As the anesthesia and muscle relaxant begin to take effect, the anesthesiologist begins ventilating the patient using a mask and 100% oxygen with a goal of hyperventilation to ensure adequate preoxygenation. Hyperventilation has the added benefit of lowering the seizure threshold. The need for intubation is uncommon. Once complete muscle relaxation has been achieved a bite block should be placed to protect dentition. This is followed by the application of the electrical stimulus. Following the stimulus, the convulsion, the seizure morphology and duration, the ECG, and regular vital signs (e.g., after 30 seconds, 1 minute, 3 minutes, and 5 minutes) should be monitored. Restimulation should be performed if indicated. Seizures generally last 30 to 90 seconds. Although a prolonged seizure (>3 minutes) is rare, this should be promptly treated with additional intravenous barbiturate anesthetic or a benzodiazepine.[1-4]

Given the sympathetic surge and outflow of catecholamines that occur during a seizure it is expected that the patient will become transiently hypertensive and tachycardic. It is usually not necessary to treat these elevated vital signs and caution should be used when considering such action to avoid inducing hypotension. If an antihypertensive agent is to be used, a short-acting β-blocker such as esmolol is generally preferred. Careful postprocedure monitoring of vital signs is essential.[1-4]

As the patient emerges from anesthesia in the postictal state, dialogue among staff and patient stimulation should be minimized. In the rare instance of an emergent delirium a short-acting benzodiazepine such as midazolam may be used intravenously. Once the patient is awake with stable vital signs and able to maintain adequate oxygenation without ventilatory assistance, the patient may be transferred to the recovery area where regular monitoring of vital signs and mental status recovery should be performed.[1-4]

Generally, the patient is ready for discharge from the recovery area back to the inpatient unit within an hour of the treatment, at which point the patient generally is alert and fully oriented. The patient may feel tired and may want to sleep in the hours following the treatment. However, the patient should generally be allowed to participate in milieu activities as tolerated. Any complaints of headache or muscle soreness should be evaluated but generally respond well to typical doses of acetaminophen or ibuprofen. The treating ECT psychiatrist should be contacted with any questions or concerns about the treatment or subsequent patient complaints.[1-4]

Outcome Evaluation

As previously mentioned, it is important to determine appropriate outcome measures before beginning treatment. Monitoring of these outcome measures should be performed at regular intervals, such as at weekly intervals during the index phase and at every continuation/maintenance treatment. It is advisable to have the assessment take place on days in between treatments or in the morning just before treatment. It is useful to use both clinician-rated and patient-rated standardized scales in addition to subjective patient, family, and clinician impressions.[1-4,6]

It is common for an index course of ECT to last between 6 and 12 treatments with treatments typically being administered 3 days a week. Some treatment courses may be shorter and others longer depending on the clinical circumstances. The use of a predetermined fixed number of treatments is not supported in the literature and should not take the place of reasoned clinical judgment. So long as a patient is showing clinical improvement, it is reasonable to continue with treatments 3 days a week. Once clinical improvement plateaus, it is advisable to begin tapering the treatments as opposed to abruptly discontinuing treatment. The index course may be continued and the taper begun even after the patient has been discharged from the inpatient setting. This requires, however, close coordination between the inpatient, outpatient, and ECT treatment teams.[1-4]

No matter what the modality of treatment, psychotropic medication or ECT, most patients require some form of continuation (to prevent relapse) and possibly maintenance (to prevent recurrence) therapy. The decision to use ECT for continuation/maintenance therapy is best made between the patient, outpatient psychiatrist, and ECT consultant. Continuation/maintenance ECT is a clinically reasonable option and in many cases is preferable to reverting to medicines that were either not efficacious or not tolerated in the first place. Continuation/maintenance ECT is routinely performed as an outpatient procedure and once the initial taper is completed (over the course of approximately 2 months) it is commonly administered every 4 to 6 weeks.[1-4]

Adverse Effects

Certain cognitive side effects are routinely encountered, such as mild confusion and disorientation upon awakening from the procedure. This side effect is related both to the anesthesia and to the postictal state and typically resolves within an hour.[1-4]

The cognitive side effect that has received the most attention is memory loss. ECT results in two types of memory loss. The first involves rapid forgetting of new information (anterograde amnesia). For example, patients may have difficulty remembering conversations or material that they have read. Patients can be reassured that this type of memory loss is mild and short-lived and typically lasts for no more than a few weeks after completion of a course of ECT.[1-5]

The second type of memory loss is retrograde in nature and typically affects episodic (personal) memories. Some patients may experience gaps in their memory for events that occurred in the weeks or months (and less commonly years) before the treatment course. This retrograde memory loss also is typically mild and improves following the completion of a course of ECT, although some patients may experience permanent gaps in memory for events that occurred close in time to the treatment.[1-5]

Patients should be reassured that memory loss is not necessary to obtain benefit from the treatment. Furthermore, many psychiatric disorders treatable with ECT can also have cognitive impairment associated with them, such as problems with attention and concentration and the "pseudodementia" associated with depression. Consequently, it is not unusual to find a patient's cognition improved after the psychiatric disorder is successfully treated with ECT.[1-5]

As previously mentioned, the present authors administer the CogniStat before and at the conclusion of an index course. The present authors recommend administering an instrument such as the MMSE on at least a weekly basis during an index course as well as before each continuation/maintenance treatment. If possible, the cognitive assessment should be performed at least 24 hours after the most recent treatment.[2] Should cognitive concerns arise, further standardized assessment may be considered.

The risk of cognitive side effects is influenced by a number of factors, one of which is the location of the stimulus electrodes. Bitemporal stimulation is associated with the highest risk, and right unilateral is associated with the least risk. Bifrontal electrode placement may also have a more beneficial cognitive side effect profile, although fewer studies have examined this issue. Another factor is the time interval between treatments, with more treatments and a greater frequency of treatments being associated with higher risk of cognitive side effects. The risk of cognitive side effects diminishes as the treatments are spread out over time during the continuation/maintenance phase.[1-5]

Other factors that can contribute to the risk of cognitive side effects include stimulus waveform (sine wave greater than brief pulse), the size of the dose of anesthesia, and escalating stimulus dose relative to seizure threshold. In addition, the use of psychotropic medication during a course of ECT can increase the risk of cognitive side effects. Finally, patients with preexisting neurologic disorders and cognitive impairment are at increased risk of cognitive side effects.[1-5]

Patients sometimes ask if ECT causes brain damage. They should be reassured that the scientific evidence strongly speaks against this possibility. The amount of electricity that reaches the brain is too small to cause electrical injury.[1] Furthermore, although prolonged seizures lasting hours may result in neural damage, there is no evidence that a brief seizure like the one induced with ECT does.[2-4] Finally, neuroimaging research has shown no evidence of injury to the brain associated with ECT.[3,4]

As previously mentioned, other side effects of ECT can include anesthetic-related nausea (which can be treated with an intravenous antiemetic), headache, and muscle soreness (both of which can be treated with nonsteroidal anti-inflammatory medication). Of note, muscle soreness is generally most common after the first treatment and is likely related to the actions of the depolarizing muscle relaxant.[1,2]

Conclusion

In summary, ECT is a safe, rapid and effective treatment option for a number of clinical conditions. Treatment may be started in the inpatient setting and continued on an outpatient basis, or the entire treatment course may be given on an outpatient basis. Once the index course has been completed, a decision whether to continue ECT or to revert to medication for the continuation/maintenance phase must be made. The effectiveness of this treatment depends on appropriate pre-ECT evaluation, which identifies the indication for the procedure, medical risks, and outcome measures as well as treatment technique.

REFERENCES

1. Prudic J. Electroconvulsive therapy. In: Sadock BJ, Sadock VA, eds. *Kaplan and Sadock's comprehensive textbook of psychiatry*, 8th ed. Philadelphia: Lippincott Williams & Wilkins; 2005:2968–2983.

2. American Psychiatric Association. *The practice of electroconvulsive therapy: recommendations for treatment, training, and privileging – a task force report of the American Psychiatric Association*, 2nd ed. Washington, DC: American Psychiatric Association; 2001.

3. Coffey CE, Kellner CH. Electroconvulsive therapy. In: Coffey CE, Cummings JL, ed. *The american psychiatric press textbook of geriatric neuropsychiatry*, 2nd ed. Washington, DC: American Psychiatric Press; 2000:829–859.

4. Coffey CE. Electroconvulsive therapy. In: Coffey CE, Brumback RA, eds. *Pediatric neuropsychiatry*. Philadelphia: Lippincott Williams & Wilkins; 2006:655–668.

5. Weiner RD, Coffey CE, Krystal AD. Electroconvulsive therapy in the medical and neurological patient. In: Stoudemire A, Fogel BS, Greenberg DB, eds. *Psychiatric care of the medical patient*, 2nd ed. New York: Oxford University Press; 2000:419–428.

6. Coffey CE. The Pre-ECT Evaluation. *Psychiatr Ann*. 1998;28(9):506–508.

7. American Psychiatric Association. *Practice guideline for the treatment of patients with schizophrenia*, 2nd ed. American Psychiatric Association; 2004.

8. Fink M, Sackeim HA. Convulsive therapy in schizophrenia? *Schizophr Bull*. 1996;22: 27–39.

9. Thompson JW, Blaine JD. Use of ECT in the United States in 1975 and 1980. *Am J Psychiatry*. 1987;144:557–562.

10. Thompson JW, Weiner RD, Meyers CP. Use of ECT in the United States in 1975, 1980, and 1986. *Am J Psychiatry*. 1994;151: 1657–1661.

11. American Psychiatric Association. *Practice guideline for the treatment of patients with major depressive disorder*, 2nd ed. American Psychiatric Association; 2000.

12. Weiner RD, Coffey CE. Indications for use of electroconvulsive therapy. In: Frances A, Hales R, eds. *Review of psychiatry*, Vol. 7. Washington, DC: American Psychiatric Press; 1988:458–481.

13. Carrasco Gonzalez MD, Palomar M, Rovira R. Electroconvulsive therapy for status epilepticus. *Ann Intern Med*. 1997;127:247–248.

14. Dubovsky SL. Using electroconvulsive therapy for patients with neurological disease. *Hosp Community Psychiatry*. 1986;37:819–825.

15. Faber R, Trimble MR. Electroconvulsive therapy in Parkinson's disease and other movement disorders. *Mov Disord*. 1991;6:293–303.

16. Fink M, Kellner CH, Sackeim HA. Intractable seizures, status epilepticus, and ECT. *J ECT*. 1999;15:282–284.

17. Kellner CH, Beale MD, Pritchett JT, et al. Electroconvulsive therapy and Parkinson's disease: The case for further study. *Psychopharmacol Bull*. 1994;30:495–500.

18. Kramp P, Bolwig TG. Electroconvulsive therapy in acute delirious states. *Compr Psychiatry*. 1981;22:368–371.

19. Krystal AD, Coffey CE. Neuropsychiatric considerations in the use of electroconvulsive therapy. *J Neuropsychiatry Clin Neurosci*. 1997;9:283–292.

20. Rasmussen KG, Abrams R. Treatment of Parkinson's disease with electroconvulsive

therapy. *Psychiatr Clin North Am.* 1991;14: 925–933.

21. Addonizio G, Susman VL. ECT as a treatment alternative for patients with symptoms of neuroleptic malignant syndrome. *J Clin Psychiatry.* 1987;48:102–105.
22. Casey DA. Electroconvulsive therapy in the neuroleptic malignant syndrome. *Convuls Ther.* 1987;3:278–283.
23. Davis JM, Janiak PG, Sakkas P, et al. Electroconvulsive therapy in the treatment of the neuroleptic malignant syndrome. *Convuls Ther.* 1991;7:111–120.
24. Nisijima K, Ishiguro T. Electroconvulsive therapy for the treatment of neuroleptic malignant syndrome with psychotic symptoms: A report of five cases. *J ECT.* 1999;15:158–166.
25. Ozer F, Meral H, Aydin B, et al. Electroconvulsive therapy in drug-induced psychiatric states and neuroleptic malignant syndrome. *J ECT.* 2005;21(2):125–127.
26. Troller JN, Sachdev PS. Electroconvulsive treatment of neuroleptic malignant syndrome: A review and report of cases. *Aust N Z J Psychiatry.* 1999;33:650–659.
27. Sung YF. Anesthesia strategies for the high-risk medical patient receiving electroconvulsive therapy. In: Stoudemire A, Fogel BS, Greenberg DB, eds. *Psychiatric care of the medical patient,* 2nd ed. New York: Oxford University Press; 2000:429–439.
28. Lauritzen L, Odgaard K, Clemmesen L, et al. Relapse prevention by means of paroxetine in ECT-treated patients with major depression: A comparison with imipramine and placebo in medium-term continuation therapy. *Acta Psychiatr Scand.* 1996;94:241–251.
29. Nelson JP, Benjamin L. Efficacy and safety of combined ECT and tricyclic antidepressant therapy in the treatment of depressed geriatric patients. *Convuls Ther.* 1989;5:321–329.

CHAPTER 11

Inpatient Evaluation and Management of First-Episode Psychosis

RICHARD FRASER, PETER BURNETT, AND PATRICK McGORRY

Rationale for a First-Episode Psychosis Service and Inpatient Unit

Inpatient units are often the first point of entry to mental health services for new patients and their families. Patients who need inpatient care are likely to be more disturbed, have less insight, and be at greater risk of harm or neglect than those who can be treated in an ambulatory setting. Yet the experience of hospitalization itself can be traumatic,[1] and if not handled well may impair subsequent engagement and treatment alliance.

Potential benefits of early intervention and treatment in psychotic illness include reduced morbidity, speedier recovery, better prognosis, preservation of psychosocial skills, preservation of family and social supports, and decreased need for hospitalization.[2] Other aims of an early intervention service include minimizing the use of restrictive and coercive practices, initiation of low-dose atypical antipsychotic medications, and maintenance of continuity of care.[3] A long duration of untreated psychosis (DUP) may be detrimental,[4–6] and during recent years the idea that neurotoxicity occurs during onset of illness has gained credence.[7] Intervention early on in a critical period may improve outcome by minimizing damage.[8] This is the philosophy underpinning the early-intervention ethos,[9] and inpatient units have a particularly important role to play in fostering these principles.[10]

The goals of inpatient care for first-episode psychosis (FEP) have some elements in common with other psychiatric inpatient care, and this chapter will not duplicate discussions elsewhere in this book. The authors focus on a young person's FEP inpatient service, such as the one at ORYGEN in Melbourne, Australia. The Early Psychosis Prevention and Intervention Center (EPPIC) at ORYGEN is one of the first youth-specific services and has developed an expertise in the early identification and treatment of psychosis in young people. Some of the key principles are outlined in Table 11.1.

Optimal treatment for psychosis requires a staging approach to illness.[11,12] Staging allows a more sophisticated approach to management based not only on diagnosis but also on the phase of illness.[13] A young person with a first episode of psychosis will need a very different service from an older person with established schizophrenia. Adult psychiatric services are not always geared up to engaging and treating young people with emerging psychotic disorders. Often the symptoms are not severe enough or specific enough to gain entry into mainstream services. Delay in recognition, engagement, and treatment initiation may result,[14] often with a traumatic first crisis admission when either the family support structure can no longer cope or the behavioral disturbance of the young person is so severe it cannot be ignored. There may be police involvement, restraint, and traumatization of not only the patient but also the family and those involved in the admission process. Although it is desirable to offer treatment in the least restrictive setting with home-based treatment of FEP, hospitalization is often necessary for a short period of time to assess and initiate treatment for those who are too unwell or too risky to manage in the community.

TABLE 11.1 GOALS OF INPATIENT CARE

Ensure safety
Provide comprehensive assessment
Provide effective treatment with the lowest possible doses of medication to minimize the side effects
Minimize the trauma of admission to a psychiatric unit
Instill hope and an expectation of recovery
Provide counseling and support to assist the patient come to terms with the illness and hospitalization
Involve the family in assessment, treatment, and discharge planning
Provide information about psychosis and treatment for the patient and family
Involve a case manager as soon as possible, to facilitate engagement with the community team and continuity of care
Involve a primary-care physician in care as soon as possible
Provide activities and group programs which are appropriate for young people and promote supportive social interactions

Conversely, a service set up specifically to identify proactively and engage those with FEP early on in the illness aims to minimize trauma and maximize chances of engagement and retention in therapy.[15] There is an increasing number of such services worldwide as well as specific organizations (International Early Psychosis Association, IEPA) and research centers (Early Psychosis Prevention and Intervention Center, EPPIC, Melbourne, Australia).

The incidence and prevalence of mental illness vary with age, with high rates in adolescence and young adulthood. More than 75% of all serious mental health and related substance use disorders commence before age 25 and approximately 14% of 12- to 17-year-olds and 27% of 18- to 25-year-olds experience such problems in any given year. A recent study showed that 40.8% of patients had their onset of psychosis between the ages of 15 and 19 years.[16] A youth mental health model takes into account a developmental perspective and the age-specific needs of younger people. These data relate to young people with FEP; those with a later onset of psychosis will not be addressed in this chapter (see Chapter 16).

An Ideal Setting

General adult psychiatric inpatient units typically contain 24 beds or more with one communal area. Because of the need to care for a wide variety of disorders and a patient group with predominantly long-standing mental health problems, the setting is not ideal for the patient with FEP. Patients with FEP are mainly a younger group and are unlikely to have experienced mental health inpatient facilities in the past. They are usually medication-naive, more impulsive yet unknown quantities as far as risk is concerned, and more likely to have comorbid substance use disorders. They are still developing in all areas including social and cognitive domains. As a result their needs and those of their families are different from those with established mental illness.

Consequently, the authors recommend where possible a dedicated inpatient unit for patients with FEP (including those within 3 years of diagnosis) with smaller numbers of beds—a 16-bed unit divided into two or three subunits. A separate locked area can be used for more intensive care and to provide a low-stimulus environment for up to four patients. If it is not possible to provide a dedicated unit then part of an existing ward could be used for this purpose. The FEP inpatient unit needs to be able to provide a positive initial experience of the mental health service as these first few days of contact are crucial to developing a good therapeutic alliance and maximizing the chance of retention in treatment. The environment should be as low-key and homely as possible in order to minimize "culture shock" on arrival and to promote an atmosphere of safety and healing. Attention should be paid to important personal issues including flexible visiting times for families and friends, a family room for parents to stay overnight, access to telephones, and a space to prepare snacks. Leisure facilities should include a television area, music facilities, and recreational facilities where possible. An outdoor area for exercise and fresh air is desirable. Although ward policy may not allow smoking, if this is allowed there should be a designated area for this.

Locked-door policies are generally not appropriate despite many of the patients being involuntary. Generally research supports the idea of an open ward in order to promote a less restrictive atmosphere and increased patient and family satisfaction.[17] Patients who are a serious absconding risk can be managed in the low-stimulus locked area or maintained on 1:1 observation rather than locking the whole unit.

Information regarding the inpatient unit, mental health law, the management of various disorders, and substance abuse should be provided in written form in an easily accessible location. New patients need to be oriented to the unit as soon as feasible. Clinicians must bear in mind that patients with FEP and their families may have misconceptions and fears about such places largely based on myths from the media and popular culture.

Referral Process

An acute FEP inpatient unit needs to be able to accept referrals at any time. At ORYGEN, the youth assessment team triages referrals and considers alternatives before admitting. Patients with FEP may have significant histories of substance use, legal problems, and risky behaviors that need to be identified at the point of referral. Occasionally admissions are elective, for example, to initiate clozapine treatment or for an inpatient assessment of a complex presentation.

Involuntary Admission

Many people experiencing FEP have limited or no insight. Outpatient treatment of those with aggressive or suicidal behavior may be unacceptably risky, and initiation and supervision of treatment may be difficult in the community. In such cases involuntary admission may be necessary. This process can be frightening and disempowering for the patient and family. Retraumatization may occur if there have been previous incarcerations, for example, prison or forced deportation. A clear and transparent care plan should be presented to the patient and family including information about the relevant mental health law. Families and treaters are often concerned that the therapeutic alliance will be damaged by this process, as indeed it may be, although clearly in these situations the risk of not admitting will take precedence. Providing the patient and family with clear explanations will make the team less likely to be accused of trickery or foul play. The alliance can be repaired later on. Indeed, patients and families will often agree later that the detention was necessary and appropriate.[18]

Involuntary admission should be for as short a time as possible and in the least restrictive environment. The patient's wishes should be respected wherever possible. Often negotiation of personal issues such as access to a computer, seeing visitors, or having accompanied leave from the unit can assist in allowing the patient to maintain some autonomy and control in what otherwise may be experienced as a jail sentence.

The use of community treatment orders (outpatient commitment) where available can facilitate early discharge from hospital and embraces the philosophy of treating in the least restrictive environment. In the authors' experience, if engagement and psychoeducation are addressed enthusiastically during the inpatient stay, the need for involuntary community treatment is reduced.

When to Admit

The need for hospital admission arises when the risks to self or others cannot be managed safely at home, when home support is insufficient or has been overstretched, or when lack of insight impedes assessment and treatment in the community. In a recent study at EPPIC three-quarters of the patients with FEP were admitted to an inpatient unit at some stage during the first 3 months of treatment.[19] Admission should not be seen as a failure on the part of the family or the community team. A brief spell in hospital should be framed as a chance for all key players to get to know each other better and for engagement to be nurtured.

Wherever possible, admission should be arranged before a full-blown crisis has developed and police are required to assist the process. In an integrated FEP service the patient with an evolving psychosis is already in treatment with a lower chance of unexpected crises precipitating admission. Of course sometimes a "difficult" admission cannot be avoided. In these cases it is essential that the team be aware of risks and maintain the safety of patient, family, and professionals while being mindful of minimizing trauma and stigmatization during the process.

Engagement and Interview Technique

Engagement is arguably the most important factor in ensuring an optimal outcome from treatment in FEP or indeed any illness. Adherence to medication is notoriously poor in medicine and particularly in psychiatry where insight may be compromised.[20] Special skills are required to engage a young person with FEP. Common ground needs to be sought so that patient and clinician are able to agree on the first steps forward. No particular style of interviewing works better than another, although a less interrogative approach is preferred, with active listening, frequent checking that information is correct, and use of lay language where possible. Crucially with this patient group clinicians should try to "be themselves." Young people with FEP are likely to be guarded and suspicious, may be frightened, and may be intimidated by those in authority. A genuinely caring attitude and interested demeanor helps to put patients at ease.

Wherever possible, patients need to be provided with options regarding management. This flexibility will limit their sense of lost control and foster a trusting relationship. Often when insight is impaired this ability to gain the trust of the patient allows treatment to begin and coercion to be avoided. Early on in the engagement process the clinician should respect the patient's interpretation of psychotic experiences as much as possible. Confrontation at this stage is likely to be counter-therapeutic. This stance needs to be balanced by the clinician's own judgment of the situation and the provision of relevant information and advice regarding treatment (see Table 11.2).

Assessment

The assessment process can be seen as the first step in engaging the patient and family with the service. Careful integration of the assessment process should minimize the number of clinicians involved and unnecessary duplication of data-gathering.

A comprehensive assessment includes a clinical history focusing on evolution of the psychotic episode from prodrome or at-risk mental state through transition to frank psychosis. Onset of symptoms, course, duration, and ameliorating factors are all important to consider, and collateral information from different sources including family and other professionals is required to verify and complete the picture. Possible risk factors for psychosis should be sought including family history, perinatal history, developmental history, premorbid personality, and organic factors such as epilepsy or brain injury. The latter are rare

TABLE 11.2 ENGAGEMENT TECHNIQUES

Recognize that the patient may be nervous, wary, or not want to see health professionals
Be aware that psychosis might distort patients' interactions and their ability to process information
Listen carefully to patients and take their views seriously
Acknowledge and respect patients' viewpoints
Identify common ground
Find the distress
Consider appropriate body language when interviewing patients who may be paranoid, aroused, or manic (sit side-by-side, avoid too much eye contact, allow personal space)
Be helpful, active, and flexible; negotiate
Carefully explain the procedures involved in physical or other assessments
Gather information gradually, at the same time as fostering a close relationship
Introduce key players who will take part in the patient's management
Provide good continuity of care and good communication between professionals

(Adapted from Edwards J, McGorry PD, eds. Implementing early intervention in psychosis: a guide to establishing early psychosis services. London: Dunitz; 2002.)

in this age-group but should not be overlooked. The workup for such organic conditions is discussed extensively in Chapter 5.

Exploring the history of psychiatric and medical problems together with past treatment and investigations is important. Potential precipitants of the psychotic episode should be enquired after, such as substance use and psychosocial stressors. A careful evaluation of risk is essential, particularly of suicide and violence, and must be incorporated into the formulation and management plan. Overall, the clinical history should aim to inform the treating team of "why this person, with this illness, at this time?"

Some aspects of mental state examination are worth mentioning in relation to FEP. It is important to be aware of situational and diurnal variations in presentation. The patient may conceal psychotic symptoms to avoid prolonged hospitalization or perceived unnecessary treatment. Different staff may elicit different symptoms. Presentation may alter over the course of the day. Early on patients tend to be lethargic; energy level and agitation may increase in the afternoon.

As patients with FEP are new to psychosis and are still developing cognitively their symptoms may not be classic. Early in the acute phase of illness the psychosis may be more florid, with perplexity and fear prominent features. Delusions may be fleeting and poorly formed or systematized. Equally, because of the variable presentation it may be difficult to determine with confidence what is psychosis and what is within the broad range of normal for the young person's developmental stage. Some beliefs that appear unusual to the clinician are culturally sanctioned. If the DUP has been lengthy there has been more time to develop a system around the beliefs, and the patient may experience less distress. Indeed, the family or carers may have come to accept some of these beliefs as personality-based rather than part of an illness. A shorter DUP is associated with fewer bizarre delusions, but these may be discussed quite readily with the clinician.[21]

Depressive and anxiety symptoms are extremely common and should be looked for actively. These symptoms are unwelcome for the patient and therefore can serve as the common ground on which to initiate a treatment plan in those with poor insight. Insight itself is multifactorial and requires special attention. It is not a binary construct but rather a continuum implying individuals' understanding of their well-being and the need to access appropriate treatment. Cognitive function, mood, and level of arousal all affect insight.

Cognitive functioning and the negative symptom profile need assessment as these affect the prognosis for functional recovery. Those whose cognitive functioning has been significantly impaired by the FEP are less likely to make a full functional recovery. This may be related to the possibility of direct neurotoxicity as a result of longer DUP.[22] Similarly the presence of significant negative symptoms makes a full functional recovery less likely.[23]

WARD-BASED ASSESSMENT

Although it is possible to assess a patient with FEP in a community setting, the inpatient unit provides a secure environment where risk can be managed and a more intensive assessment can be carried out. In FEP this includes a behavioral assessment, mental state assessment, and risk assessment with contributions from all members of the interdisciplinary team. An initial period of 24 to 48 hours' antipsychotic-free observation provides valuable information regarding initial presentation, evolution of symptoms, and influence of setting in order to formulate better the individual patient's illness and ensure appropriate treatment. When psychotic presentations are complicated by substance use, vague symptoms, or an unsubstantiated history this period allows for careful consideration before initiating antipsychotic drug treatment. This period is not treatment-free. Benzodiazepines are recommended for symptomatic relief of anxiety and promotion of sleep. Psychological support, good nursing care, family work, and addressing of physical health needs also occur during this time. If there is very disturbed behavior or significant aggression, emergency treatment including antipsychotic medication may be needed.

NEUROPSYCHOLOGICAL ASSESSMENTS

Neurocognitive deficits in psychosis are well documented. Patients with FEP appear to have some cognitive impairment already,[24] with further impairment occurring during the early course of the illness and then plateauing.[25] Deficits include attentional, information processing, and verbal memory and learning impairments. Brain changes observed using imaging studies correlate reasonably well with these neuropsychological deficits and indicate involvement of prefrontal and temporal regions.[26]

In recent years it has become increasingly evident that cognitive dysfunction is an important determinant of outcome variables such as work and psychosocial functioning. The degree of cognitive impairment also has an impact on insight, medication adherence, and coping skills. Consideration needs to be given to postdischarge planning when impaired memory and cognition are likely to reduce ability to manage medication, appointments, and therapy or psychoeducation.

Both nonprescribed and certain prescribed (e.g., benzodiazepines, anticholinergics) medicines are likely to cause further impairment in the already cognitively challenged and may also lead to either self-medication or nonadherence. Information needs to be provided in clear format, in lay terms, in multiple media (oral, written, and visual) and on several occasions in order to maximize impact. Involvement of family and carers where appropriate also aids in getting the message across. Atypical antipsychotic medication may ameliorate neurocognitive deficits (see subsequent text).

Intelligent quotient (IQ) and personality testing is not generally valid while a patient is acutely psychotic. Involvement of a neuropsychologist at an early stage during recovery is sometimes useful when learning problems are suspected. Premorbid level of functioning can be estimated from school or college reports and prior psychometric testing. In practice not every patient with FEP can get neuropsychological testing, but such testing can provide valuable prognostic information as well as allowing for monitoring of progress.

Ultimately, those with significant neurocognitive deficits may benefit from vocational advice as a return to previous work or college placement may not be realistic and may place undue stress on the individual. This potentially paternalistic attitude must be balanced with an open-minded view and a hopeful outlook to avoid the danger that the clinician, not the illness, prevent people with psychosis from pursuing their goals.

RISK

An initial risk assessment must be carried out at the point of admission in order to ensure safety of the patient, others, and the environment. In reality this process of assessing risk began before admission. Collateral information will have been gathered where possible. A formal risk assessment tool aids in assessment, but this should be used in conjunction with clinical judgment. Effective communication of risk is crucial in safely managing any psychiatric patient. With patients having FEP there may be more unknown variables because they are new to treatment and potentially more aggressive, agitated, substance-using, and impulsive than patients who are already in treatment. They are generally medication-naive and unlikely to have had a complete physical workup.

Suicide

Suicidal ideation is common in patients with FEP. Up to 23% experience such thoughts, and 15% have a history of previous suicide attempts.[14] Ten percent to 15% of psychotic patients eventually commit suicide with the risk highest in the first few years of illness.[27] All patients should be asked about suicidal ideation, intent, and planning. Inquiry does not increase likelihood. Gentle but focused inquiry can happen toward the end of interview once some rapport has been established. Further discussion of suicide risk assessment is offered in Chapters 2 and 9.

Risk of suicide in FEP can be increased by factors including psychosocial stress, current substance use or withdrawal, and psychotic symptoms such as command auditory hallucinations and paranoid delusions. Protective factors also need to be considered and can provide the clinician with ideas for interventions aimed at decreasing risk. Suicide risk assessment must include a discussion with the patient about how to get help on the inpatient unit should suicidal feelings arise—whom to alert and what sorts of interventions might be initiated. Suicide risk in patients with FEP is changeable, especially early on in the admission. Frequent risk assessment reviews should be carried out, especially at times of change such as lowering of level of observation or at discharge. It is not unusual for patients with FEP to expect a quick fix, so a realistic time frame needs to be negotiated in order to minimize frustration and impulsivity.

In the inpatient setting, it is important to pay attention to the history and behavior of the patient, not just what he or she says about current intent. Most of the successful inpatient suicides denied intent shortly before the act. Agitation is a reliable indicator of suicidal thinking.[28] Significantly, early intervention in psychosis has been shown to reduce suicide risk.[21,29]

Violence

Assessment of violence risk shares much with suicide risk assessment. There are static factors including history of aggression and personality as well as demographic variables such as male gender and younger age. Clinical, dynamic variables appear to be more important predictors of violence for acutely psychotic patients in the inpatient setting. These dynamic risk factors include hostility, suspiciousness, agitation, and cognitive impairment. Substance use is an important risk factor and is discussed in the subsequent text. In the FEP inpatient population, those at greatest risk of violent behavior appear to be recently admitted males.[18]

The ward environment and culture deserve special mention. Design of the ward needs to allow patients a degree of space and privacy where possible but without compromising safety, access, and visibility. When acutely unwell young people are placed together in close proximity and possibly involuntarily the chances of aggressive outbursts are increased as feelings of threat, frustration, and anger are acted out. Staff require training in managing such behavior, both preventive and acute. Locked wards where nursing and medical staff are inaccessible much of the time behind doors breed an "us and them" culture. Increasing demands for cigarettes, leave, and medication lead to frustration on the part not only of patients but also of the staff, leading to the potential for further division. Staff morale, training, and ward milieu all contribute to minimizing this effect and maximizing satisfaction amongst patients, families, and professionals. Incidents of violence need to be reported and analyzed in order to learn and adapt ward policy to prevent these behaviors from becoming entrenched. Patient violence needs to be managed proactively. Unchecked, it becomes a major source of dissatisfaction and demoralization for staff, especially nurses who bear the brunt of its effects.

Risk to environment

Acutely psychotic patients, who may be paranoid, agitated, and frightened, are at risk of harming their environment. This includes damage to property because of primary aggression (antisocial or substance-related) and also because of delusional beliefs, command auditory hallucinations, or disorganization. Management might include nursing in a low-stimulus environment, one-to-one observation level, and adequate medication such as short-term use of benzodiazepines.

Absconding

The risk of absconding from the inpatient unit is increased early on in an admission, during substance withdrawal, when insight is impaired, and when therapeutic alliance is limited. Patients who abscond tend to be younger males with frequent readmissions, paranoid and manic presentations, and comorbid substance use or antisocial personality traits.[18]

Although it may be tempting to keep wards locked to prevent elopement, in the authors' view the overall outcome is to produce an unpleasant environment that increases the risks of aggression, nonadherence, and oppositionality.[17] Therefore while initially it is advisable to err on the side of caution if there are concerns about absconding, the team should be realistic about what the actual risks are should the patient abscond and concentrate on developing an alliance rather than being unnecessarily restrictive. In the authors' experience, where possible it is usually better to negotiate leave from the unit for patients allowing them some control and hence decreasing the risk of absconding. An individualized care plan should seek to address this issue and is preferable to sweeping ward policies regarding locked wards.

Vulnerability

People with psychotic disorders are vulnerable to exploitation and victimization by others. Within inpatient units with high levels of acuity there are opportunities for vulnerable patients to become victims of violence, sexual harassment or assault, and other crime such as theft of personal belongings. Particularly vulnerable patients should be identified early and measures taken to protect them such as one-to-one nursing until they are more settled.

Nonadherence to treatment

Treatment nonadherence in FEP may be more common than in other psychiatric populations. Although not a great deal of research has been carried out in this area, estimates in the region of 60% nonadherence rates in FEP populations have been quoted.[30] Clearly this confers a significant risk of early relapse in psychotic illness, leading to further behavioral disturbance and readmission.[31] Treatment nonadherence in a young group with FEP could be interpreted as a normative response and denial of illness. Younger people are cognitively less mature and may feel immortal or beyond the usual rules of society and life. Although this is an understandable response to danger or bad news, clinicians need to address this faulty schema in order to minimize chances of nonadherence, not only to medication but also to other aspects of treatment. An initial assessment of patient attitude to treatment, explanatory model of illness, and family attitudes to treatment will help inform the clinician of likely stumbling blocks when planning and initiating treatment. Using the lowest possible dose of an atypical antipsychotic in order to minimize side effects is likely to have a positive effect on adherence, as is inclusion of the patient in formulating the management plan and involvement of family and carers early on.

Treatment nonadherence also occurs on inpatient units even with supervision of medication. It should be suspected when there is unexpected deterioration in symptoms or failure to improve.

Social/Occupational Functioning

Functional recovery in FEP has to some extent been overlooked until recently. Achieving remission from positive and negative symptoms is often the goal, and the most commonly used objective outcome measurements such as the Brief Psychiatric Rating Scale (BPRS) and the Positive and Negative Symptoms Scale (PANSS) reflect this. EPPIC data show that although >90% of FEP patients make a symptomatic recovery, only 50% make a functional recovery, that is, a return to their previous role, perhaps as a student or employee.[32] Because of the usual age of onset, FEP is likely to interfere with important developmental tasks including completion of education and starting work.

Research has shown that early psychosocial interventions improve vocational outcome.[33,34] During an inpatient stay there should be some assessment of social functioning to get an idea of premorbid abilities, support networks, and goals. Occupational therapists are able to provide assessments of functioning to guide postdischarge management, especially if independent living is a possibility. Functional aspects of recovery should begin to be addressed on the inpatient unit where resources exist for a practical evaluation of daily living skills and social strengths and weaknesses. Inpatient groups are particularly useful in alleviating boredom while assessing living skills and preparing patients for more structured programs after discharge.

Outcome Measurements

Psychotic symptoms are often the focus of attention, but other outcomes are also important including nonpsychotic psychiatric symptoms, side effects of medicines, psychosocial functioning, disability, satisfaction with services, substance use, and family burden.[2] Various tools are used to measure these outcomes, such as the BPRS, Clinical Global Impression (CGI) scale, the Liverpool University Neuroleptic Side Effect Rating Scale (LUNSERS),[35] the Quality of Life Scale (QLS),[36] and the Global Assessment of Functioning (GAF) scale.

Diagnosis

Diagnosis in FEP is not particularly stable, with approximately 25% of initial diagnoses altering over the first 6 months.[37] Nonetheless, in order to formulate a management plan a working diagnosis is necessary. The authors advocate an interdisciplinary approach using an integrated biopsychosocial model to generate this diagnostic formulation. It can be difficult to make a stable or precise diagnosis of subcategories of psychosis early on in the first episode. Symptoms and signs can change and vary in intensity. Comorbid substance use, personality disorder, and normal variations in development can obscure the underlying illness. The threshold for diagnosis of psychosis can at times appear arbitrary. At EPPIC the authors have defined it as the duration and intensity of psychotic symptoms that would indicate use of antipsychotic medication. Operationally this equates to the presence of clear-cut delusions, hallucinations, or severely disorganized speech lasting at least 1 week.[18]

Thea authors recommend using a diagnosis of "first-episode psychosis" for a number of reasons. First, instability in diagnosis early on may lead to potentially inappropriate treatments and expectations. Second, misdiagnosis may decrease patient confidence in the treating team and hinder psychoeducation. Third, the combinations of symptoms can be thought of as representing dimensions of psychopathology and treatment strategies directed thereby. As time progresses the diagnosis usually becomes clearer. The use of the broad term *FEP* is certainly not a way of avoiding diagnosis. Ultimately, once the treating team knows the patient better and symptoms have stabilized into a recognizable syndrome, a more formal diagnosis is appropriate.

The question a formulation in FEP seeks to answer is the same as for other psychiatric formulations: "Why this person at this time with this disorder?" The framework encompasses predisposing, precipitating, and perpetuating factors incorporating biopsychosocial perspectives. Specifically one is looking to gain an understanding of the individual as a unique person and to hypothesize how this illness arose and the ways in which illness and person interact. In FEP this means identifying prodrome, DUP, comorbid conditions, personality, risk factors, and protective factors as well as the acute presentation.

The key message is not to avoid making a diagnosis but rather to keep the diagnosis broad acknowledging the instability early on. Therefore, FEP is the preferred initial diagnosis, a foundation upon which the building blocks of engagement, treatment, and psychoeducation can establish a firm footing.

An additional and more sophisticated model of diagnosis in FEP proposes the use of a concept well known in other areas of medicine, clinical staging (see Table 11.3).[12] Clinical features and objective measures are linked to pathophysiology so that treatment can be focused more effectively and course predicted with greater accuracy.

Investigations

Although it is relatively unusual to elucidate an organic cause for FEP in young patients—approximately 3%[38]—a full physical examination and organic screen are still recommended at the outset, not only to inform diagnosis but also to evaluate the general physical health of the patient. The details of evaluation are discussed in Chapters 4 and 5. Basic physical examination should occur early on, and a more thorough examination can take place once the patient is settled in the inpatient unit. Higher rates of soft neurologic signs and neurodevelopmental disorders have been found in those with psychosis and may predict poorer prognosis.[39]

Neuroimaging techniques have advanced the physicians' understanding of the psychotic disorders and their biological basis. Computed tomography (CT) and magnetic resonance imaging (MRI) are the two techniques most used in diagnostic investigation of FEP. In most clinical settings a CT scan should be performed in all new presentations. If there are any suspicions of abnormalities an MRI should then be arranged (see Table 11.4).

Management

Optimal treatment of FEP integrates biological, psychological, and social interventions at the earliest opportunity.[40] The focus of treatment will vary depending on the phase of illness, for example, in the early acute phase medication will play a major role, with the introduction of psychosocial interventions once the patient is more settled. Supportive psychotherapy and gentle psychoeducation should begin at the outset. It cannot be stressed enough that treatment of FEP will provide patients with a first experience of mental health services on which they will base future contacts. If this initial experience is

TABLE 11.3 CLINICAL STAGING MODEL FRAMEWORK FOR PSYCHOTIC AND SEVERE MOOD DISORDERS

Clinical Stage	Definition	Target Populations for Recruitment	Potential Interventions	Indicative Biological and Endophenotypic Markers
0	Increased risk of psychotic or severe mood disorder; no symptoms currently	First-degree teenage relatives of probands	Improved mental health literacy, family education, drug education, brief cognitive skills training	Trait marker candidates and endophenotypes, e.g., smooth pursuit eye movements, P-50, niacin sensitivity, binocular rivalry, prepulse inhibition, mismatch negativity, olfactory deficits, etc.
1a	Mild or nonspecific symptoms, including neurocognitive deficits, of psychosis or severe mood disorder; mild functional change or decline	Screening of teenage populations, referral by primary care physicians, referral by school counselors	Formal mental health literacy, family psychoeducation, formal CBT, active substance abuse reduction	Trait and state candidates where feasible according to sample size
1b	Ultra high risk: moderate but subthreshold symptoms, with moderate neurocognitive changes and functional decline to caseness (GAF <70)	Referral by educational agencies, primary care physicians, emergency departments, welfare agencies	Family psychoeducation, formal CBT, active substance abuse reduction, atypical antipsychotic agents for episode, antidepressant agents, or mood stabilizers	Niacin sensitivity, folate status, MRI and MRS changes, HPA axis dysregulation
2	First episode of psychotic or severe mood disorder, full threshold disorder with moderate-severe symptoms, neurocognitive deficits, and functional decline (GAF 30–50)	Referral by primary care physicians, emergency departments, welfare agencies, specialist care agencies, drug and alcohol services	Family psychoeducation, formal CBT, active substance abuse reduction, atypical antipsychotic agents for episode, antidepressant agents or mood stabilizers, vocational rehabilitation	Continue with markers of illness state, trait, and progression
3a	Incomplete remission from first episode of care; could be linked or fast-tracked to stage 4	Primary and specialist care services	As for "2" with additional emphasis on medical and psychosocial strategies to achieve full remission	Continue with markers of illness state, trait, and progression
3b	Recurrence or relapse of psychotic or mood disorder which stabilizes with treatment at a level of GAF, residual symptoms, or neurocognition below the best level achieved following remission from first episode	Primary and specialist care services	As for "3a" with additional emphasis on relapse prevention and "early warning signs" strategies	Continue with markers of illness state, trait, and progression

TABLE 11.3 CONTINUED

Clinical Stage	Definition	Target Populations for Recruitment	Potential Interventions	Indicative Biological and Endophenotypic Markers
3c	Multiple relapses, provided worsening in clinical extent and impact of illness is objectively present	Specialist care services	As for "3b" with emphasis on long-term stabilization	Continue with markers of illness state, trait, and progression
4	Severe, persistent, or unremitting illness as judged on symptoms, neurocognition, and disability criteria Note: could fast-track to this stage at first presentation through specific clinical and functional criteria (from stage 2) or alternatively by failure to respond to treatment (from stage 3a)	Specialized care services	As for "3c" but with emphasis on clozapine, other tertiary treatments, social participation despite ongoing disability	Continue with markers of illness state, trait, and progression

The clinical staging model provides greater utility for testing efficacy, cost-effectiveness, risk-benefit ratios, and feasibility of available interventions. Clinicopathological correlates and predictors of illness stages can also be introduced within a neurodevelopmental framework.

CBT, cognitive behavior therapy; GAF, global assessment of functioning; HPA, hypothalmic pituitary axis; MRI, magnetic resonance imaging; MRS, magnetic resonance spectroscopy.

(Adapted from McGorry PD, Hickie I, Yung A, et al. Clinical staging of psychiatric disorders: A heuristic framework for choosing earlier, safer and more effective interventions. *Aust N Z J Psychiatry*. 2006;40[8]:616–622.)

negative, whether because of inappropriate or inadequate treatment interventions or because of unacceptable inpatient facilities, then patients will be less likely to engage in the long term and less likely to seek help voluntarily.[41] A collaborative approach to treatment, involving the patients (wherever possible) and their families or carers in decision making will foster a therapeutic alliance and provide a framework for future care.

The aims of treatment of FEP are remission of positive symptoms; prevention or early recognition and treatment of comorbid symptoms including depression, negative symptoms, mania, anxiety, post-Traumatic stress disorder (PTSD), and substance use; psychosocial recovery; and the involvement of family and carers in continuing recovery. Treatment strategies include reducing delay in accessing treatment, minimizing trauma, fostering engagement and therapeutic alliance, low-dose antipsychotic medication, developing an explanatory model of illness, crisis planning, support for family and carers, promoting functional recovery, and preventing maladaptive coping such as substance use.[2] The authors discuss these strategies in the subsequent text.

MEDICATION

As mentioned earlier, the authors recommend an initial period of 24 to 48 hours of antipsychotic-free observation. During this time benzodiazepines can provide immediate relief from symptoms such as agitation, anxiety, and insomnia, for example, diazepam 5 mg three times daily (up to 40 mg total per day).

TABLE 11.4 RECOMMENDED MEDICAL INVESTIGATIONS IN FIRST-EPISODE PSYCHOSIS

Investigations	Sequence	Comments
CBC	Baseline and yearly	Signs of infections, red blood cell anomalies (macrocytosis in chronic alcoholism)
Urea and electrolytes	Baseline and yearly	Severe dehydration
Liver function	Baseline and yearly	Liver infections, intoxication, post overdose e.g., paracetamol
Thyroid function	Baseline and yearly	Thyroid dysfunction is often associated with many psychiatric symptoms
B$_{12}$ and folate	Baseline and yearly	Alcoholism, malnutrition
Random glucose	Baseline and yearly	Higher diabetes risk in psychotic illness
Lipid profile	Baseline and yearly	Lipid abnormalities are major side effect of antipsychotic medication
Urinalysis	Baseline	—
Creatinine clearance	As clinically indicated	In young patients only if they have a history of kidney problems before treatment initiation
Urine drug screen	As clinically indicated	Useful to obtain on all new admissions
ECG	Baseline and yearly	If possible prior treatment initiation, thereafter annually or as clinically indicated (in particular exclude QTc prolongation)
Brain scan	Baseline	Suspicions of organic reason for psychosis such as Huntington disorder, multiple sclerosis, or encephalopathy
Weight and waist circumference	Baseline and as clinically indicated	Monthly measures important for the initial couple of months, at least quarterly thereafter
Electroencephalogram	As clinically indicated	If atypical presentation or history of seizures or "blackouts"

CBC, complete blood count; ECG, electrocardiogram.
(Adapted from Fraser R, Berger G, McGorry P. Emerging psychosis in young people – part 2 – key issues for acute management. *Aust Fam Physician*. 2006;35:323–327.)

TABLE 11.5 DOSE RECOMMENDATIONS IN ACUTELY ILL PATIENTS WITH FIRST-EPISODE PSYCHOSIS (FEP)

Suggested Lowest Effective Dose to Treat	Neuroleptic-Naive FEP Patients (mg/d)	Previously Neuroleptic-Treated Patients (mg/d)
Risperidone	2	2–6
Olanzapine	7.5	15–30
Quetiapine	200–300[a]	300–800
Amisulpiride	200–300[ab]	>400[b]
Aripiprazole	5–10[a]	10–30

Maintenance doses may vary on an individual basis.
[a]Optimal dose has yet to be established for drug-naive first-episode psychosis.
[b]Lower doses to treat negative symptoms only (e.g., 100 mg).
(Adapted from Fraser R, Berger G, McGorry P. Emerging psychosis in young people – part 2 – key issues for acute management. *Aust Fam Physician*. 2006;35:323–327.)

Antipsychotic Medication

The mainstay of pharmacologic treatment in psychosis is the antipsychotics. Antipsychotic medicines have proven efficacy in reducing positive (e.g., hallucinations and delusions) and negative (e.g., social withdrawal) symptoms. At EPPIC the authors recommend use of the atypical or second-generation antipsychotics (risperidone, olanzapine, quetiapine, amisulpiride, aripirazole, ziprasidone, paliperidone, and clozapine). Although the typical or first-generation antipsychotics, such as haloperidol, are effective in treating positive symptoms, they are far more likely to cause acute side effects, especially in an FEP population. In the FEP population it is essential to begin at a low dose and increase gradually to avoid unwanted extrapyramidal and other side effects with consequent early discontinuation.[42] Atypical antipsychotics also have lower incidence of tardive dyskinesia compared to the older agents and have small but encouraging beneficial effects on cognitive dysfunction. Balanced against these advantages of the atypicals is their potential to cause the metabolic syndrome and subsequent cardiovascular problems, as discussed in the subsequent text and in Chapters 3 and 4.

Table 11.5 illustrates the dosages used in FEP. Lower doses of antipsychotic medicines are required in neuroleptic-naive patients compared with those who have been previously treated. In general FEP patients need approximately half the dose of antipsychotic compared with patients with chronic schizophrenia.[43]

Before beginning treatment in FEP the clinician should explore possible misconceptions about such treatment with the patient and family. People experiencing FEP are likely to be fearful and suspicious of others and of the treatment being offered. Wherever possible a collaborative approach to treatment should be employed, providing the patient and family with choice about which medicine might be most suitable. This is likely to improve engagement and adherence. Careful explanation of the need for medication, mode of action, side effects, and recommended length of treatment should be given. This oral explanation can be backed up with written information. For those patients who are too unwell or lacking insight it might be necessary to provide a temporary rationale for taking medication such as "to help with the stress" or to aid sleep. Later on in treatment when insight improves the other actions of antipsychotics can be discussed.

Excepting clozapine and possibly olanzapine, the atypical antipsychotics have similar efficacy.[44] Therefore the choice of medicine will depend on patient preference and side effect profile. The side effect profile can be used to some advantage. For example, for those patients requiring sedation olanzapine or quetiapine are good choices. For those in whom sedation is less desirable and weight already excessive then risperidone would be justified. In sexually active males avoidance of those antipsychotics more likely to elevate prolactin, such as risperidone and amisulpiride, would be prudent.

Psychotic symptoms can take 10 to 14 days to begin to respond to treatment following initiation of antipsychotic medication and 6 weeks or even more for maximal response.[39] Scant evidence supports increasing dosage of antipsychotic rapidly, so patience is advocated. Rapid titration is likely to cause side effects[45] and make the patient wary of medication and indeed psychiatric services. The aphorism "start low, go slow" remains sound and is central to the prescribing ethos at EPPIC and similar early intervention services around the world. In this early stage of treatment benzodiazepines are extremely useful.Using more than one antipsychotic at a time should be avoided. Finding the minimal effective dose of antipsychotic is not necessarily an easy task. There is often a temptation to increase antipsychotic dose in order to speed recovery and shorten duration of hospitalization. This is a false economy and merely leads to increased side effects and longer hospital stays.[46] Table 11.6 lists recommended dose increases.

Route of administration needs to be given some consideration. Ideally the oral route is preferred. Tablets are the safest and cheapest way to administer medicines. They also allow the patient some degree of control and are clearly more collaborative and less traumatic than injections. For those who are accepting oral medication but whose compliance is questionable—for example, holding medication in the mouth and later spitting—orally disintegrating tablets are available for risperidone, aripiprazole, and olanzapine. Supervision of medication is achievable as staff need only observe the patient for a minute after medicine has been taken. Short-acting intramuscular formulations of the atypicals olanzapine and ziprasidone are now available and can be useful when it is necessary to begin treatment without patient's consent or in emergency situations. Injections should be avoided wherever possible in patients with FEP as this mode of administration is likely to be experienced as traumatic. Sometimes despite

TABLE 11.6 SUGGESTED FORTNIGHTLY INCREMENTAL DOSE INCREASES OF ANTIPSYCHOTIC MEDICATION

Suggested Dose Increases at Fortnightly Intervals	Milligram
Risperidone	1
Olanzapine	5
Quetiapine	100–200
Amisulpiride	100
Aripirazole	5–10

(Adapted from Fraser R, Berger G, McGorry P. Emerging psychosis in young people – part 2 – key issues for acute management. *Aust Fam Physician.* 2006;35:323–327.)

careful and gentle negotiation the patient still refuses treatment and is at risk of further deterioration or harm. In these cases intramuscular administration is acceptable but only in the short term and if possible with the agreement of significant family members or carers. Subsequent doses should always be offered orally so that the patient may resume some control over their medication regime and feel less coerced.

The long-acting intramuscular injection of risperidone has meant that there is now an atypical alternative to first-generation depot antipsychotics. Other atypical long-acting injections are currently being developed because this form of administration has proved effective in treating those in whom noncompliance has been proved and risk of nontreatment too high. Patients with FEP should always be given the opportunity to manage their medication using oral preparations of antipsychotics. It is not acceptable to opt immediately for a long-acting injection in order to ensure compliance before a trial of oral medication has taken place. Occasionally patients will choose the long-acting injection because of the advantages of not having to remember daily dosing, being less obvious to others that they are taking medication (stigma), and a more stable plasma level of medication.

Mood Stabilizers

Mood stabilizers such as lithium are recommended in FEP not only for manic psychosis but also for schizoaffective disorder and as an adjunct to antipsychotic medication in treating psychotic patients who present with an affective component. Lithium can potentiate the effects of antipsychotics,[47] allowing lower doses to be used. Lithium can be used to treat symptomatic aggression and overactivity in FEP and may also be neuroprotective.[48] Other mood stabilizers such as sodium valproate and carbamazepine are useful for those who present with atypical mania (e.g., dysphoric or mixed) or who will not manage the regular blood tests required for lithium treatment. Valproate also allows for lower doses of antipsychotics to be used when in combination.

Antidepressants

Up to 50% of those with FEP present with depression and anxiety.[49] Increasingly we are becoming aware that depression and anxiety are important symptoms to treat in FEP, regardless of whether the primary psychosis is affective. These symptoms often resolve once the psychosis has been treated effectively, but some patients require treatment with an antidepressant. Electroconvulsive therapy (ECT) plays an important role in treatment of FEP with severe depression and significant suicidality.[50] ECT can also be useful to treat resistant psychosis and mania where there is a need to turn things around rapidly perhaps because of catatonic features, physical exhaustion, or suicidality.[51] ECT is discussed further in Chapter 10.

THE TREATMENT-REFRACTORY PATIENT

Up to 20% of first-episode schizophrenia-like cases fail to achieve remission after adequate treatment with at least two atypical antipsychotics.[52] Noncompliance and untreated comorbidity such as substance use may perpetuate illness. If treatment refractoriness is confirmed then the authors recommend early use of clozapine, as in such cases the continuation of active illness is extremely damaging. Clozapine has been shown to be more efficacious than other atypical antipsychotics.[53] The risks of weight gain, diabetes, and cardiovascular problems as well as seizures and potentially fatal agranulocytosis all mandate that a pretreatment workup and close monitoring be carried out. Preclozapine workup should include electrocardiogram (ECG), echocardiogram, blood tests including troponin (baseline for myocarditis), fasting glucose and lipids, blood group, full blood count, and renal and liver function tests. In Australia there has been increased concern compared with the United States and United Kingdom regarding fatal myocarditis associated with clozapine therapy,[54] which is reflected in the practice of arranging an echocardiogram and ECG as part of the clozapine workup. Any abnormalities should be discussed with an internist before commencing treatment with clozapine.

Cognitive behavior therapy (CBT) (see subsequent text) and ECT (see earlier) should also be considered where treatment with clozapine is not possible. Other strategies such as combining clozapine and atypical antipsychotics or high doses of other atypicals are beyond the scope of this chapter.

PSYCHOLOGICAL INTERVENTIONS

Psychological interventions in FEP form an important part of the integrated treatment plan (see Table 11.7). Initially supportive psychotherapy provides containment while patient and family attempt to make sense of what has happened and the therapeutic alliance is nurtured. During the first week of inpatient treatment psychological assessment is carried out to place the illness in the context of the individual's experience. Challenging of delusions and hallucinatory experiences is often counterproductive early on before insight has improved, although this of course varies depending on the individual. Instead, earlier on the clinician should be seeking the common ground on which both patient and team are in agreement and can therefore begin targeting collaboratively. This common ground often includes the distress from beliefs and experiences, social anxiety, low mood, agitation, and poor sleep.

CBT can be used to treat psychotic symptoms in the acute and recovery phases[55] as well as depression, anxiety, and PTSD.[56] CBT has been shown to be helpful in increasing medication adherence[57] and reducing substance use.[58]

Once insight has improved and symptoms are less distressing other psychological interventions such as problem solving, skills training, and stress management can be implemented. Little hard evidence supports the use of psychodynamic or analytic psychotherapy in the acute and recovery phases of FEP, but this is arguably for lack of research in this area. Other therapies include cognitive analytic therapy (CAT), which has been adapted for use in psychosis and is promising.[59] Cognitively oriented psychotherapy for early psychosis (COPE) has been developed to improve adaptation to illness.[60]

The authors suggest an eclectic approach to psychological interventions, with clinicians using their skills to match the therapy with the individual.[61] The psychological interventions discussed earlier

TABLE 11.7 WHY PSYCHOLOGICAL TREATMENTS ARE NECESSARY IN PSYCHOSIS

To develop a therapeutic alliance
To promote adherence to medication
To provide emotional support in the face of disturbing subjective experiences and stigma
To specifically target individual symptom complexes, comorbidities, and maladaptive schemas
To reduce treatment resistance
To enhance coping and adaptation
To improve cognitive functioning
To improve interpersonal relationships which may be independently problematic or have been disrupted by illness
To promote vocational recovery
To provide support and care to family members including siblings
To reduce risks of suicide and aggression
To prevent relapse

can be delivered by suitably trained nursing staff, clinical psychologists, psychiatrists, or allied mental health professionals. In the inpatient setting, a supervision group for staff delivering such interventions is feasible and can prove to be an enlightening experience for ward-based clinicians because they are able to consider the patients and families they work with on a different level.

There is increasing interest in the use of CBT for treatment resistance in psychosis. There is certainly strong face validity and some evidence that CBT helps in this group of patients when used in conjunction with standard treatments such as clozapine.[62] Other important foci of psychological intervention in FEP include suicide and aggression,[63] to promote vocational recovery, to improve cognitive functioning, to reduce harm from comorbid conditions such as substance use and to prevent relapse.[64]

PSYCHOEDUCATION

A message of hope and therapeutic optimism should be conveyed to those with FEP. Helping patients begin to reframe their experiences through offering alternative explanations is part of psychoeducation. This process of making the patient an expert should begin early on in treatment and forms part of the engagement process. Clinicians should be aware that several variables affect the focus of psychoeducation, including developmental level of the individual, stage of the illness, insight, willingness to engage, family and supports available, explanatory model of illness, and comorbidity. Generally mental health literacy among psychiatric patients and their families is poor.[41] Patients and their families may have misconceptions about mental illness, treatments, and inpatient facilities. These should be sensitively explored and alternative explanations, models, and experiences offered.

At EPPIC various media are employed to provide psychoeducation for the patient and family. Staff are able to begin with oral information and discussion, backed up with written materials (translated where appropriate) and audiovisual media such as videos or DVDs. CD-ROMs (available through www.orygen.org.au) have proved to be useful tools, especially as they allow an interactive approach and patients can proceed at their own pace using a medium they are likely to feel comfortable with. Group sessions on the inpatient unit focus on various aspects of psychoeducation, including substance use and problem solving. Naturally, patients will be at different stages of recovery and this should be allowed for in the groups. More often than not those who are further down the road to recovery will be able to offer some support to those more acutely unwell. Family and carers should also be involved in this process, both on the inpatient unit and in separate family support groups.

GROUP INTERVENTIONS IN ACUTE PSYCHOSIS

Once patients are more settled it is important to provide group-based activities for socialization, sharing of experience, psychoeducation, and alleviation of boredom (see Table 11.8). Groups can be facilitated by various members of the team and may focus on issues such as drugs and alcohol, healthy living, stigma, medication, and illness models. In addition some groups may use art, music, cooking, sport, relaxation, or creative writing as a theme to encourage interaction and promote recovery. Groups with a nonpsychiatric focus may be less threatening for those patients who are more unwell. The aim should

TABLE 11.8 GROUP PROGRAMS IN ACUTE PSYCHOSIS—SPECIAL CONSIDERATIONS

Recognize that participants may have features such as distressing symptoms, impaired mental state, suspiciousness, poor concentration, and impaired social interaction
Use small groups that are less intimidating and can adapt to individuals' needs
Build a positive foundation for later participation in group programs during recovery
Tolerate the disruptions of an inpatient unit, including the "competing" requirements of doctors, nurses, other staff, and families
Try to tolerate the involvement of those who have more disruptive behavior, as a structured environment may help them to settle
Allow flexible attendance, including participants' leaving a group if they need to
Model positive social behaviors including respect, listening, and gentle firmness in ensuring safety of all participants

be for inclusion of all patients wherever possible. Family support groups too can be initiated by the inpatient unit.

Family Work

When a member of the family becomes unwell there is a systemic response to the illness that varies depending on the explanatory model, previous experiences of care, resources within the family, and other concurrent issues. When a member of the family experiences a psychotic illness this is a novel situation for many families and evokes feelings of fear, confusion, loss, sadness, and sometimes guilt or anger. The family may be overwhelmed and uncertain how to proceed.[65] Equally the family may already have first-hand experience of major mental illness, and their experience of mental health services may have been positive or negative.

If the son or daughter with FEP still lives at home, which is often the case,[66] the family may have had to call in mental health services to get help without the consent of their child. This can potentially set up a dynamic of resentment and mistrust within the family, a dynamic that needs to be addressed early on if therapy is to be effective.

Some possible fears of families about treatment are as follows:

1. Clinicians will overtly or covertly blame the family for the illness.
2. Clinicians will automatically admit the person to hospital without consultation.
3. Clinicians will fail to provide adequate follow-up after the assessment process.
4. The young person will be turned into a "zombie" by medication.
5. The young person will never forgive the family for contacting the service.

Initially it is important to collect collateral history and to corroborate information regarding illness evolution and associated risks. As the team gets to know the family better the process of debriefing and providing psychoeducation begins. As with the patient with FEP it is important that this initial experience of mental health services be a positive one as the family can provide support for the patient and encourage engagement. The inpatient unit should welcome families and carers and maintain a flexible approach to visiting and meeting times.

Where appropriate the family should be involved in treatment decisions, in order to promote a sense of regaining cohesion and to encourage involvement in what may be a serious and enduring illness. Sometimes patients will not consent to family involvement, in which case the treating team must decide whether to break confidentiality based on risk and capacity to make such decisions. Usually with gentle and careful negotiation the family can be involved. Often a nominated member of the family can be contacted who can then begin to involve the others.

A stressful family environment with critical comments, hostility, and emotional overinvolvement (high expressed emotion) has been shown to increase the risk of early relapse in schizophrenia.[67] Working with families empathically and nonjudgmentally to provide insight into the nature of the relationship between stress, the environment, and staying well is a task which should begin on the inpatient unit and continue after discharge. The sessions offered at EPPIC for families provide basic information and discussion about psychosis. Although the sessions are facilitated there is an interactive style with opportunities for families to swap stories and gain mutual support.

MANAGEMENT OF AGGRESSION AND SELF-HARM

Pointers to a high risk of aggression include previous episodes of aggression, substance withdrawal, increasing agitation, akathisia, low tolerance for frustration, and unmet needs (see Tables 11.9 and 11.10). Staff should be provided with specific training in management of aggression and violence, with regular refresher courses. They should be confident in such situations and be able to use the minimal force necessary to contain and make a situation safe. Often this might mean negotiation with the patient and not need actual physical force. Leadership and coordination are crucial (see Table 11.11).

Although violence should not be tolerated on an inpatient unit it is important to nurture a culture of thoughtfulness among staff on an inpatient unit. Staff should be encouraged to avoid knee-jerk reactions such as immediate use of intramuscular medication in incidents of aggression unless other options such as time-out fail. Restraint and seclusion may be required until the patient is able to regain self-control. These issues are discussed at length in Chapter 12.

TABLE 11.9 BEHAVIORS INDICATING IMPENDING AGGRESSION

Loud, clipped, or angry speech
Pacing
Angry facial expression
Refusal to communicate
Threats or gestures
Physical or mental agitation
Restlessness
Persecutory ideation
Delusions or hallucinations with violent content
People themselves reporting violent feelings

Use of medication combinations such as benzodiazepines and sedative atypical antipsychotics can be effective. Oral medication should be offered initially if possible before opting for the intramuscular route of administration. When restrained, patients should be closely observed. The need for seclusion must be reviewed regularly by nursing and medical staff. The management of agitation and aggression is discussed further in Chapters 2 and 12.

Management of self-harm also needs careful consideration. Those who have FEP and harm themselves probably require a different approach from someone who persistently self-harms in the context of borderline personality disorder. In FEP delusional beliefs or command auditory hallucinations may drive the behavior. Comorbidity of FEP and personality disorder such as borderline is not uncommon and can be trickier to treat. Generally, the principle of ensuring patient and ward safety should prevail initially. This may be achieved by providing containment, medication, and an increased level of observation and support by nursing staff. Psychotic patients who are self-harming may need to be managed in a secure environment until symptoms and distress are under control. These patients may be unpredictable and potentially at high risk to themselves. As they represent an unknown quantity the treating team should err on the side of caution until it is clearer what the actual risks are.

PHYSICAL HEALTH

Patients with mental illness have higher rates of physical health problems compared with the general population, as discussed in detail in Chapter 4.[68] Admission to the inpatient unit should prompt a full physical health check and, once immediate issues of safety have been addressed, appropriate

TABLE 11.10 POTENTIAL PRECIPITANTS OF AGGRESSIVE EPISODES

- Fear
  - Psychosis (e.g., delusional belief of being persecuted or threatened)
  - Anxiety
  - Decreased inhibition
  - Confusion (e.g., delirium, dementia)
  - Neurologic disorders
  - Drug or alcohol intoxication or disinhibiting medication
  - Poor impulse control (e.g., in some people with developmental disability)
- Anger
  - Humiliation
  - Rejection
  - Antisocial or borderline personality traits
  - Being ignored
  - Concerns or requests dismissed
- Stress
- Grief
- Frustration/helplessness
- Pain
- Agitation (e.g., secondary to depression)

TABLE 11.11 RESPONSES TO AGGRESSION IN AN INPATIENT UNIT

Distinguish between normal adolescent behavior and symptoms of psychosis
Redirect energy through sport activities, walks with staff, or other physical activity
Exert a high degree of self-control despite anxiety in the face of aggressive behavior
Check what the patient wants: the issue might have arisen from difficulty with a simple request such as access to a phone—control only what you need to!
Avoid looking or becoming nervous: stay calm and self-confident
Recognize real threats and withdraw when appropriate: do not be a "hero," and have the confidence to exit safely
Use a calm voice at low volume to convey simple messages
Adopt a nonthreatening posture with some eye contact but avoid staring.
Do not confront the person physically or "tower over them" (e.g., if they are seated)
Allow the individual ample "personal space"
Use an empathic, nonconfronting manner, emphasizing your desire to help
Do not turn your back
Focus on the immediate situation—the "here and now"—and the immediate needs of the individual, rather than dwelling on the past
Try not to give ultimatums
Ensure that adequate backup is available in case the situation escalates; alert police or other personnel security if appropriate and, if possible, have them located unobtrusively close by
If your safety or that of others is directly threatened, then withdraw rather than persist
Maintain as much privacy as is possible while ensuring a safe environment
If in a room, ensure you can reach the door but do not block the exit from the young person (angry people may rather leave than resort to violence)
Consider removing clothing (such as ties or necklaces) which could be used to grasp you, or items such as pens or other objects which could be used as weapons

management of any physical health problems. Smoking cessation should be addressed, and indeed as increasing numbers of inpatient units adopt a no-smoking policy[69] it is essential that patients be asked about smoking and provided with information on quitting and nicotine replacement therapy.[70] This issue is discussed further in Chapter 15.

All pharmacologic treatments have side effects. Antipsychotic medicines can cause weight gain, diabetes, metabolic syndrome, and cardiovascular problems. Patients with major mental illness may have a greater risk of diabetes and dyslipidemias independent of psychotropic medication and predating treatment.[71] Mood stabilizers also cause weight gain and other side effects including tremor and worsening of skin conditions. Clinicians should be prepared to manage medication side effects, for example, by dietary advice, exercise groups, smoking cessation counseling, and referral for specialist advice.

SUBSTANCE USE

The link between substance use and psychosis is now well established.[72] Use of illicit drugs can make teasing out complex symptomatology and assessing treatment response difficult for treating clinicians. Up to 80% of young people experiment with drugs, alcohol being the most frequently used.[73] Approximately one in three adolescents use cannabis, with approximately 10% to 15% using more than twice a week.[74] An admission to the inpatient unit can precipitate a withdrawal for those who are dependent on substances. Withdrawal needs to be managed appropriately with use of medication and withdrawal scales to monitor symptoms and ensure correct dosage. Psychoactive substances may precipitate or aggravate psychotic symptoms. As substance use disorders adversely affect outcomes in the treatment of psychotic disorders they should be treated vigorously. Antipsychotic medication may need to be prescribed in higher doses for those who are regular substance users. Counseling should be provided regarding substance use, focusing on assessing readiness for change, and risks associated with such behaviors. This information needs to be given in a nonjudgmental manner and in plain language.

Some inpatient units have a dedicated substance abuse clinician working with the team. In the authors' experience having such a clinician is a real bonus and improves detection of substance abuse disorders and continuity of care after discharge. Further discussion of comorbid substance abuse is provided in Chapter 15.

CONTINUING CARE—DISCHARGE PLANNING

A well-integrated service with a home-based treatment team linked closely to the inpatient unit is able to achieve successful shorter hospital stays. The mean length of stay in the authors' unit at ORYGEN was 10.5 days in 2003–2004. Continuing care teams work in conjunction with the inpatient unit, meeting patients and families during the hospitalization, anticipating discharges in order to ensure a seamless transition into community-based care (CBC). The case management model allows for each new patient with FEP and family to be allocated a continuing care clinician and psychiatrist while an inpatient and to receive ongoing monitoring, treatment, and psychoeducation on an outpatient basis. Through this specialist interdisciplinary biopsychosocial approach to treatment of FEP the best possible outcomes can be achieved, maximizing potential for recovery and a return to premorbid functionality. In many areas this model does not exist and cannot easily be created, in which case there should at the very least be a clear demarcation of responsibility at the time of discharge in order to minimize risk during transition of care. Primary care teams may assume responsibility and can be supported by specialist psychiatric services, perhaps by consultation, teleconference, or through the Internet.

CULTURAL ISSUES

Patients and families from different backgrounds need to have their cultural needs met. This includes use of interpreters of both language and culture. Clinicians may have difficulty judging whether beliefs are culturally normal or are delusional, so in these situations it is essential to work with someone from that particular cultural background. Written information should be available in all the languages spoken in the area covered by the inpatient unit.

RESEARCH AND TEACHING

Specialist FEP inpatient units offer a unique opportunity to study a population early in the course of psychiatric disorder. Such services should be set up to capture as much data as possible and improve physicians' understanding of the etiology, treatment, and prognosis of psychosis. Developing a culture of curiosity and research improves staff satisfaction and increases the knowledge base within the team, potentially leading to more evidence-based treatments being employed and greater creativity in planning management strategies.

Summary

Although patients experiencing FEP share some characteristics and needs with people experiencing other disorders or those at a later stage of illness, they also represent a unique group of individuals with particular vulnerabilities. They are best managed in a specialist service, with specialist inpatient facilities wherever possible. In this way it is possible to maximize the chances of a positive outcome and long-term engagement, and to minimize the risk of trauma, negative experience, and poor engagement.

REFERENCES

1. McGorry P, Chanen A, McCarthy E, et al. Post-traumatic stress disorder following recent-onset psychosis as an unrecognized post-psychotic symptom. *J Nerv Ment Dis.* 1991;179: 253–258.
2. Edwards J, McGorry PD, eds. *Implementing early intervention in psychosis: a guide to establishing early psychosis services.* London: Dunitz; 2002.
3. McGorry PD, Killackey E, Elkins K, et al. Summary Australian and New Zealand clinical practice guideline for the treatment of schizophrenia. *Australas Psychiatry.* 2003;11:136–147.
4. Bleuler E. In: Zinkin J, ed. *Dementia praecox or the group of schizophrenias.* New York: International Universities Press; 1950:1911.
5. Sullivan HS. The onset of schizophrenia. *Am J Psychiatry.* 1927;151(Suppl 6):135–139.
6. Marshall M, Lewis S, Lockwood A, et al. Association between duration of untreated psychosis and outcome in cohorts of first-episode patients. *Arch Gen Psychiatry.* 2005;62:975–983.

7. Pantelis C, Velakoudis D, McGorry PD, et al. Neuroanatomical abnormalities before and after onset of psychosis: A cross-sectional and longitudinal MRI comparison. *Lancet.* 2003;361: 281–288.

8. Birchwood M, MacMillan JF. Early intervention in schizophrenia. *Aust N Z J Psychiatry.* 1993;27:374–378.

9. McGorry PD. 'A stitch in time' … The scope for preventive strategies in early psychosis. In: McGorry PD, Jackson HJ, eds. *The recognition and management of early psychosis: a preventive approach.* New York: Cambridge University Press; 1999:3–23.

10. Harrison G, Hopper K, Craig T, et al. Recovery from psychotic illness: A 15- and 25-year international follow-up study. *Br J Psychiatry.* 2001;178:506–517.

11. Fava GA, Kellner R. Staging: A neglected dimension in psychiatric classification. *Acta Psychiatr Scand.* 1993;87:225–230.

12. McGorry PD, Hickie I, Yung A, et al. Clinical staging of psychiatric disorders: A heuristic framework for choosing earlier, safer and more effective interventions. *Aust N Z J Psychiatry.* 2006;40(8): 616–622.

13. Malla A, Norman R. Early intervention in schizophrenia and related disorders: Advantages and pitfalls. *Curr Opin Psychiatry.* 2002;15: 17–23.

14. McGorry PD, Henry L, Power P. Suicide in early psychosis: Could early intervention work? In: Kosky R, Goldney R, Hassan R, eds. *Proceedings of suicide prevention. The global contact.* New York: Plenum Press; 1998.

15. Harrigan S, McGorry PD, Krstev H. Does treatment delay in first episode psychosis really matter? *Psychol Med.* 2003;33:97–110.

16. Malla A, Payne J. First-episode psychosis: Psychopathology, quality of life, and functional outcome. *Schizophr Bull.* 2005;31(3): 650–671.

17. Middelboe T, Schjodt T, Byrsting K, et al. Ward atmosphere in acute psychiatric inpatient care: Patients' perceptions, ideals and satisfaction. *Acta Psychiatr Scand.* 2001;103:212–219.

18. Power P, McGorry PD. Initial assessment of first episode psychosis. In: McGorry PD, Jackson HJ, eds. *The recognition and management of early psychosis: a preventive approach.* New York: Cambridge University Press; 1999:155–183.

19. Wade D, Edwards J, McGorry P. Treatment for the initial acute phase of first-episode psychosis in a real-world setting. *Psychiatr Bull.* 2006;30: 127–131.

20. Nosé M, Barbui C, Gray R, et al. Clinical interventions for treatment non-adherence in psychosis: A meta-analysis. *Br J Psychiatry.* 2003;183: 197–206.

21. Melle I, Larsen T. Does early detection improve outcome? *Schizophr Res.* 2006;86(Suppl):24.

22. McGlashan TH. Duration of untreated psychosis in first episode schizophrenia: Marker or determinant of course? *Biol Psychiatry.* 1999;46: 899–907.

23. Mayerhoff DI, Loebel AD, Alvir JM, et al. The deficit state in first episode schizophrenia. *Am J Psychiatry.* 1994;151:1417–1422.

24. Brewer WJ, Edwards J, Anderson V, et al. Neuropsychological, olfactory and hygeine deficits in young men with negative symptom schizophrenia. *Biol Psychiatry.* 1996;40:1021–1031.

25. Cahn W, HulshoffPol HE, Lems EB, et al. Brain volume changes in first episode schizophrenia; a 1 year follow up study. *Arch Gen Psychiatry.* 2002; 59:1002–1010.

26. Wright IC, Rabe-Hesketh S, Woodruff PWR, et al. Meta-analysis of regional brain volumes in schizophrenia. *Am J Psychiatry.* 2000;157(1): 16–25.

27. Verdoux H, Liraud F, Gonzales B, et al. Suicidality and substance misuse in first admitted subjects with psychotic disorder. *Acta Psychiatr Scand.* 1999;10:389–395.

28. Busch K, Fawcett J, Jacobs D. Clinical correlates of inpatient suicide. *J Clin Psychiatry l.* 2003;64: 14–19.

29. Harris MG, Burgess PM, Chant D, et al. Impact of specialised first-episode psychosis treatment on suicide following initial presentation to mental health services: Retrospective cohort study. *Schizophr Res.* 2006;81(Suppl 1):307.

30. Coldham E, Addington J, Addington D. Medication adherence of individuals with a first episode of psychosis. *Acta Psychiatr Scand.* 2002;106: 286–290.

31. Viguera AC, Baldessarini RJ, Hegarty JD, et al. Clinical risk following abrupt and gradual withdrawal of maintenance neuroleptic treatment. *Arch Gen Psychiatry.* 1997;54:49–55.

32. Fraser R, Berger G, McGorry P. Emerging psychosis in young people – part 3 – key issues for prolonged recovery. *Aust Fam Physician.* 2006;35: 329–332.

33. Malla A, Norman R, Joober R. First-episode psychosis, early intervention, and outcome: What have we learned? *Can J Psychiatry.* 2005;50: 881–891.

34. Killackey E. Exciting career opportunity beckons! Early intervention and vocational rehabilitation in first-episode psychosis: Employing cautious optimism. *Aust N Z J Psychiatry.* 2006;40(11-12): 951–962.

35. Day JC. A self-rating scale for measuring neuroleptic side-effects - validation in a group of schizophrenic patients. *Br J Psychiatry.* 1995;166: 650–653.

36. Heinrichs DW. The quality of life scale: An instrument for rating the schizophrenic deficit syndrome. *Schizophr Bull.* 1984;10(3):388–398.

37. Fennig S, Craig T, Tanenberg-Karant M, et al. Comparison of facility and research diagnoses in first admission psychotic patients. *Am J Psychiatry*. 1994;151:1423–1429.

38. Johnstone E, Macmillan J, Crow T, et al. A magnetic resonance study of early schizophrenia. *J Neurol Neurosurg Psychiatry*. 1986;49(2): 136–139.

39. Lieberman JA. Prediction of outcome in first episode schizophrenia. *J Clin Psychiatry*. 1993; 54(Suppl):13–17.

40. Wyatt RJ, Damiani LM, Henter ID. First episode schizophrenia. Early intervention and medication discontinuation in the context of course and treatment. *Br J Psychiatry*. 1998;172(Suppl): 77–83.

41. Day JC, Bentall RP, Roberts C, et al. Attitudes toward antipsychotic medication: The impact of clinical variables and relationships with health professionals. *Arch Gen Psychiatry*. 2005;62: 717–724.

42. Hellewell JS, Haddad PM. Differing tolerability profiles among atypical antipsychotics. *Am J Psychiatry*. 2001;158:501–502.

43. McEvoy JP, Hogarty GE, Steingard S. Optimal dose of neuroleptic in acute schizophrenia. A controlled study of the neuroleptic threshold and higher haloperidol dose. *Arch Gen Psychiatry*. 1991;48:739–745.

44. Davis JM, Chen N, Glick ID. A meta-analysis of the efficacy of second generation antipsychotics. *Arch Gen Psychiatry*. 2003;60:553–564.

45. Remington G, Kapur S, Zipursky RB. Pharmacotherapy of first episode schizophrenia. *Br J Psychiatry*. 1998;172(Suppl):66–70.

46. Kulkarni J, Power P. Initial treatment of first episode psychosis. In: McGorry PD, Jackson H, eds. *The recognition and management of early psychosis: a preventive approach*. Cambridge University Press; 1999:184–205.

47. Christison GW, Kirsch DG, Wyatt RJ. When symptoms persist: Choosing among alternative somatic treatments in schizophrenia. *Schizophr Bull*. 1991;17:217–245.

48. Manji HK, Moore GJ, Chen G. Lithium up-regulates the cytoprotective protein BCL-2 in the CNS *in vivo*: A role for neurotrophic and neuroprotective effects in manic depressive illness. *J Clin Psychiatry*. 2000;61:82–96.

49. Whitehead C, Moss S, Cardno A, et al. Antidepressants for the treatment of depression in people with schizophrenia: A systematic review. *Psychol Med*. 2003;33:589–599.

50. Linnington A, Harris B. Fifty years of electroconvulsive therapy. *Br Med J*. 1998;297: 1354–1355.

51. Kellner C. Is ECT the treatment of choice for first break psychosis? (Editorial). *Convuls Ther*. 1995; 11:155–157.

52. Sheitman BB, Lieberman JA. The natural history and pathophysiology of treatment resistant schizophrenia. *J Psychiatr Res*. 1998;32:143–150.

53. Lieberman JA, Safferman AZ, Pollack S. Clinical effects of clozapine in chronic schizophrenia: Response to treatment and predictors of outcome. *Am J Psychiatry*. 1994;151:1744–1752.

54. Kilian JG, Kerr K, Lawrence C, et al. Myocarditis and cardiomyopathy associated with clozapine. *Lancet*. 1999;354:1841–1845.

55. Tarrier N, Lewis S, Haddock G, et al. Cognitive-behavioural therapy in first-episode and early schizophrenia: 18-month follow-up of a randomised controlled trial. *Br J Psychiatry*. 2004;184:231–239.

56. Lewis S, Tarrier N, Drake R. Integrating non-drug treatments in early schizophrenia. *Br J Psychiatry*. 2005;187:S65–S71.

57. Haddock G, Lewis S. Psychological interventions in early psychosis. *Schizophr Bull*. 2005;31:697–704.

58. Edwards J, Elkins K, Hinton M, et al. Randomized controlled trial of a cannabis-focused intervention for young people with first-episode psychosis. *Acta Psychiatr Scand*. 2006;114:109–117.

59. Ryle A, Kerr IB. *Introducing cognitive analytic therapy: principles and practice*. Chichester: John Wiley & Sons; 2002.

60. Jackson H, McGorry PD, Henry L, et al. Cognitively oriented psychotherapy for early psychosis (COPE): A 1-year follow-up. *Br J Clin Psychol*. 2001;40:57–70.

61. Cullberg J, Johannessen J. In: Gleeson J, McGorry P, eds. *Psychological interventions in early psychosis: a treatment handbook*. Chichester: John Wiley & Sons; 2004:81–98.

62. Edwards J, Maude D, Hermann-Doig T, et al. A service response to prolonged recovery in early psychosis. *Psychiatr Serv*. 2002;53:1067–1069.

63. Power P, Bell R, Mills R, et al. Suicide prevention in first episode psychosis: The development of a randomised controlled trial of cognitive therapy for acutely suicidal patients with early psychosis. *Aust N Z J Psychiatry*. 2003;37:414–420.

64. McGorry PD. In: Gleeson J, McGorry P, eds. *Psychological interventions in early psychosis: a treatment handbook*. Chichester: John Wiley & Sons; 2004:1–21.

65. Addington J, Burnett P. In: Gleeson J, McGorry P, eds. *Psychological interventions in early psychosis: a treatment handbook*. Chichester: John Wiley & Sons; 2004:99–116.

66. Addington J, Jones B, Ko T, et al. Family intervention in early psychosis. *Psychiatr Rehabil Skills*. 2001;5:272–286.

67. Leff JP, Vaughn C. *Expressed emotion in families*. New York: Guilford Press; 1985.

68. Phelan M, Stradins L, Morrison S. Physical health of people with severs mental illness. *Br Med J*. 2001;322:443–444.

69. O'Gara C, McIvor R. Smoke free psychiatric services. *Psychiatr Bull.* 2006;30:241–242.
70. Olivier D, Lubman D, Fraser R. Smoking in psychiatric inpatient units. *Aust N Z J Psychiatry.* 2007;41:574–582.
71. Ryan MC, Collins P, Thakore JH. Impaired glucose tolerance in first episode drug naïve patients with schizophrenia. *Am J Psychiatry.* 2003; 160:284–289.
72. Arseneault L, Cannon M, Witton J, et al. Causal association between cannabis and psychosis:

Examination of the evidence. *Br J Psychiatry.* 2004;184:110–117.
73. Pederson W, Skrondal A. Ecstasy and new patterns of drug use: A normal population study. *Addiction.* 1999;94:1695–1706.
74. Van Os J, Bak M, Hanssen M,et al. Cannabis use and psychosis: a longitudinal population based study. *Am J Epidemiol.* 2002;156:319–327.

CHAPTER 12

Inpatient Agitation and Aggression

EILA SAILAS, ALICE KESKI-VALKAMA,
AND KRISTIAN WAHLBECK

P eople with mental disorders are somewhat more likely to manifest violent behavior in the community than those with no history of psychiatric illness. However, demographic variables, including ethnicity and gender, predict violence better than psychiatric diagnosis.[1] A Swedish study demonstrated that violent crime rate would be reduced only by 5.2% if all those with severe mental illness were institutionalized indefinitely.[2] A history of psychiatric illness, especially in combination with substance abuse, is associated also with becoming a victim of violence.[3–5]

In psychiatric hospital care, aggression and agitation are a major concern. A frequent reaction to patient aggression is the implementation of coercive measures, often perceived as being harmful and unfair by patients and also a target for public criticism. On the other hand, patient aggression inflicts harm on providers of mental health care as well. Although major physical injuries are rare,[6] nonphysical effects create much suffering. Nurses' predominant responses to patient aggression have been found to be anger, fear or anxiety, post-traumatic stress disorder symptoms, guilt, self-blame, and shame.[7] Inpatient aggression can also be directed toward other patients, who are then vulnerable to both physical and psychological trauma. Violent patient behavior also has financial implications as it requires increased staffing.[8]

It is not necessarily easy to keep in mind the low overall risk of violent behavior by psychiatric patients and to be an advocate of reason when confronted with the everyday behavioral problems of patients in mental institutions.[9] In institutional settings, it is a challenge to maintain the safety of the patients and the staff while providing a therapeutic environment.

Agitation

An expert consensus on a precise definition of agitation in psychiatric illness is currently lacking. However, there are fairly consistent definitions in the medical literature. These include "exceeding restlessness associated with mental distress" and "excessive motor activity associated with a feeling of inner tension."[10] The word "agitation" is used not only for nonaggressive behavior such as repetitive questioning and pacing, but also for physically and verbally aggressive outbursts. It is likely that in the future it will be possible to define the parameters of psychomotor agitation and related symptoms more specifically.[11] This would be useful because agitation is a common warning signal that often precedes violence.[12]

Epidemiology of Inpatient Aggression

Official incident reports from psychiatric hospitals tend to underestimate inpatient violent behavior, and even more so self-harm and property damage.[13] The inpatient aggression prevalence rates differ substantially across studies with gross international and interhospital variation.[14] It has been estimated that 3% to 25% of psychiatric inpatients exhibit violent behavior while hospitalized.[15–17] A meta-analysis of all studies using the same method of measuring aggression found the number of aggressive incidents to vary considerably between acute admission wards, ranging from 0.4 to 33.2 incidents (average 9.3) per patient year.[18] A UK study recruiting patients with first-episode psychosis found that almost 40% were aggressive at first contact with services and more than half of these were physically violent.[19] One study estimated that in a 12-month period at an acute psychiatric hospital ward a nurse would have a one in ten chance of receiving any kind of injury as a result of patient's physical aggression.[20]

There are several explanations for the reported variation in prevalence of violent acts performed by psychiatric inpatients. The most obvious explanation is the lack of common understanding and standardization not only across different studies but also among staff as to what constitutes an act of aggression or violence.[21] Agitation is even harder to define, yet combined with the threat of violence it is the most common reason for coercive measures such as seclusion or restraint, as well as for hospitalization itself.[22] Obviously, prevalence is also dependent on the tasks and functions of the ward in question. Many of the studies measuring inpatient aggression have been carried out on high-risk wards thereby yielding skewed results. There are also major differences in local and national policies and cultures that contribute to patient and staff behavior on hospital wards. Studies of disruptive patient behavior reveal that conflict behavior is not only ubiquitous but also heterogeneous. One typology created seven categories: the angry absconder, the angry refuser, the absconding misuser, the protestor, the self-harmer, the abstainer, and the medication ambivalent. Only the first two were associated with aggressive behavior.[23]

Only a few epidemiologic studies have been done to assess the prevalence of agitation.[11] Agitation is common among emergency patients with psychoses, and it has been estimated that 21% of psychiatric emergency visits may involve agitated patients with schizophrenia.[24]

Most studies of inpatient aggression have been carried out on adult wards and have not emphasized older people in particular. The overall impression is of a high incidence of usually low-impact aggression among people with dementia.[25] There are even fewer studies about violence on child and adolescent psychiatric units. In spite of the lack of epidemiologic data, the existence of the problem is proved by the published practice guidelines on management of acute aggressive behavior in young people in inpatient treatment facilities.[26]

Measuring, Monitoring, and Reporting

Observer-rated scales have been developed for the quantitative measurement of violence during inpatient treatment. The Staff Observation Aggression Scale (SOAS) consists of five columns, each pertaining to specific aspects of aggressive behavior: the provocation, means used by the patient during the aggression, target of the aggression, consequences, and measures taken to stop aggressive behavior.[27] SOAS has been revised (SOAS-R) in order to develop a finer-grained severity scoring system.[28] The Modified Overt Aggression Scale (MOAS) collects the most serious incidents during the past week. It includes four dimensions: verbal and physical aggression, property damage, and self-inflicted harm.[29] The Social Dysfunction and Aggression Scale (SDAS) consists of nine items (SDAS-9) covering outward aggression and two items (SDAS-2) covering inward aggression.[30] All these scales intercorrelate highly.[31]

Some instruments have been developed to measure agitation. Positive and Negative Syndrome Scale-Excited Component (PANSS-EC) is a five-item subscale of the frequently used PANSS.[32] The Behavioral Activity Rating Scale (BARS) for acutely agitated psychotic patients scores behavioral activity from one (difficult or unable to arouse) to seven (violent).[33]

Etiology and Pathogenesis

Agitation is a common symptom of schizophrenia, bipolar disorder (manic and mixed episodes), and dementia. In particular, almost half of the patients with Alzheimer disease have agitation,[34] and behavioral disturbances are very common.[35] Agitation may also occur in catatonic states due to various causes and as an adverse effect of psychiatric medication.[36] The pathophysiology of agitation in these different states is not well understood.[11] In patients with psychosis, proposed mechanisms for agitation have included hyperdopaminergia in the basal ganglia, increased norepinephrine tone, and a reduction of inhibitory γ-aminobutyric acid influences.[37] Among patients with dementia, agitation is believed to be of multifactorial etiology.[38]

A number of theories have been developed to explain the reasons for inpatient aggression. These have been narrowed down to three models: the internal, the external, and the interactional models. The internal model sees mental illness as the cause of aggressive behavior. The external model is based on the assumption that environmental factors, like the type of regime on the ward or provision of privacy, contribute to the occurrence of aggressive incidents. The interactional model emphasizes the relationship between staff and patient. Patients perceive environmental conditions and poor communication to be a significant precursor of aggressive behavior. Nurses, in comparison, see the patients' mental illness to be the main reason for aggression. Although both groups are unsatisfied with the strategies used to control disruptive behavior, the suggestions for actions differ according to the assumed underlying cause. The use of medication and seclusion is supported by staff, but much less so by the patients, who prefer negotiation and de-escalation.[39]

Several studies have reported that the two most common types of patient assailants are the older male with a diagnosis of schizophrenia, past histories of violence toward others and substance use disorder, and the younger patient with personality disorder and past histories of violence toward others, personal victimization, and substance use disorder.[40,41] Other patient characteristics have also been associated with the threat of inpatient violence.[13,42–44] Little is known about the risk of aggression among those with affective psychoses. A study of patients with first-episode psychosis found those with a diagnosis of mania to be almost three times more likely to be aggressive at first contact than patients with schizophrenia.[19] From a clinical viewpoint it is useful to know that there are groups of repetitively violent patients who are responsible for a disproportionately large number of aggressive incidents.[45]

An interesting recent finding associated lifetime exposure to a life-threatening traumatic event with the use of seclusion or restraint during the hospital stay. The authors concluded that previous exposure to traumatic events enhances the risk of revictimization and retraumatization during inpatient treatment.[46] This view is often supported by the psychiatry survivor movement, that is, by patients who have experienced the existing mental health laws and practices as oppressive.

There is evidence that adverse incidents are more likely during and after weeks of high numbers of male admissions, during weeks when other incidents also occur, and during weeks of high regular staff absence through leave and vacancy.[47] Overcrowding[48] and boredom on wards[49] are associated with increased amount of violent incidents. Patients associate aggression on ward to negative and controlling staff attitudes.[50] There is some evidence that staff with poor clinical and interpersonal skills are at increased risk of violence.[51]

Many theories of inpatient violence see aggressive incidents as a result of complicated interactions between patient, staff, and environmental stressors. For instance, repeated inpatient aggression could be the result of a vicious circle: the patient's violent behavior increases the environmental and communicational stress on the patient and contributes to the risk of another violent outburst.[52]

Prediction of Aggressive Behavior

There are three types of risk factors: empiric, theoretic, and clinical. Predicting inpatient violence differs from predicting aggressive behavior in the community.[53] Purely theoretic predictors with high correlation with violence like poverty and segregation are useless from the clinical standpoint. Clinical approaches to violence prediction have been considered only slightly better than by chance,[54] but there are also reports of moderate accuracy.[55] Research in clinical violence prediction is difficult for several reasons. Assessment of the violence risk is judged to be one of the key competencies by many psychiatrists and is based on intuition and clinical experience, both hard to measure.[53] However, from the clinical viewpoint the true task of the clinician is to prevent violence, not to predict it. Predicted aggression leads to preventive actions, and therefore the prediction appears incorrect. Typical difficulties in clinical assessment of the risk of aggressive acts include vagueness of what is being assessed, relying on illusory correlations, failure to incorporate situational information, and ignoring statistical base-rate information.[56]

There has been some controversy over the usefulness of clinical versus actuarial prediction of aggression. In clinical judgment, the information about the probability of violence is processed inside the head of the decision maker, whereas in actuarial methods conclusions are drawn solely on the basis of established empirical knowledge.[55] On the basis of empirical findings, by far the best predictor of future violence is previous violent behavior.[53] The clinical approach involves expert clinical judgments of several factors in relation to the individual and the situation. Unaided clinical prediction of violent recidivism after hospital discharge does not function well, but clinical decision making can be accurate in estimating short-term aggression during psychiatric hospital care.[55] When making these clinical judgments, nurses rely on their personal knowledge of the patient, but also "tune in" on potentially violent situations as a whole and try to search causes for the violent behavior.[4] There is no difference in the accuracy of violence prediction between psychiatric nurses and psychiatrists.[57] Recently, a combination of clinical and actuarial approaches has been recommended. The emphasis is on developing evidence-based guidelines that promote systemization and consistency, but that are flexible enough to take account of specific cases and contexts.[56]

Some violence-related rating instruments to predict inpatient violence have proved to be useful, for example, the Bröset Violence Checklist (BVC).[45] The BVC assesses the presence of six observable patient behaviors, namely whether the patient is confused, irritable, boisterous, verbally threatening, and attacking objects. The sensitivity and specificity results indicate that BVC discriminates between the violent and nonviolent patients over the next 24-hour prediction period. It has shown to be 63% accurate in predicting that violence would occur within the next 24 hours and 92% accurate in predicting that violence would not occur.[58] BVC has been combined with the Visual Analog Scale (VAS) with good results.[59]

The Short-Term Assessment of Risk and Treatability (START)[60] is a new structured professional assessment aimed to guide assessment and management of diverse population of mentally disordered patients and to act as a clinical indicator of treatment progress.[61] START is specifically intended to be completed and used by an interdisciplinary team. It includes 20 dynamic risks and strength-related factors that give information concerning multiple risk domains relevant to everyday psychiatric clinical practice (e.g., risk to others, suicide, self-harm, self-neglect, substance abuse, unauthorized leave, and victimization). Preliminary findings have been promising.

Interventions

The evidence regarding interventions to treat violent or agitated behavior is limited.[62] It is also difficult to decide which interventions to use for which patients. Both agitation and aggression should be treated according to the underlying cause of the behavior when possible. For the present, treatment is usually identical for both agitation and aggression. Studies examining factors motivating inpatient aggression found that violent episodes can be categorized into three classes with different underlying causes.[63,64] The most common reason underlying an assault was disordered impulse control, often in situations that involved directing a patient to change his unwanted behavior and refusal of a patient request. Aggressive incidents due to organized assaults came second, and assaults motivated by psychosis were the least common.[64] Psychotically motivated assaults were due to positive psychotic symptoms, psychotic confusion, and disorganization.[63] All these should be treated differently and according to the cause. Psychosocial and pharmacological interventions for these states are discussed in the subsequent text and in Chapters 2 and 3, respectively.

POLICY LEVEL

As stated earlier, the use of different means to restrict the agitated and aggressive inpatient is determined not only by individual behavioral factors but also by cultural factors. Such factors arise from national policies for protection of human rights, cultural awareness of needs to protect human integrity, and staff attitudes formed during professional training.

Within psychiatry, awareness of and resistance to external influences is extremely important, as misuse of psychiatric inpatient treatment has been widely observed in totalitarian states. Psychiatric treatment practices are closely linked to the values of society, and international and national policies can have a decisive influence on clinical practice. The current international standards in the field of human rights were laid down by the Universal Declaration of Human Rights proclaimed by the General Assembly of the United Nations in 1948. The widely accepted principle of least restriction lays the ethical ground for treatment of the agitated and aggressive patient. This means that persons with mental disorders have the right to be cared for in the least restrictive environment and with the least restrictive or intrusive treatment, considering also the need to protect the safety of others. In practice, this means that de-escalation and behavioral techniques should always be preferred to seclusion, restraint, or forced medication.

Therefore, it is important that inpatients be informed about their rights as patients by easily available leaflets and access to an external competent person or body that can assist patients to understand and exercise their rights.

STIGMA

Stigma is a social construction that defines people in terms of some distinguishing characteristic or mark and devalues them as a consequence.[65] Stigma implies structural discrimination, and there are several examples of private and government policies that restrict the opportunities of the stigmatized groups.[66] When attitudes toward those with a mental illness are studied, schizophrenia is linked with chronicity and dangerousness. People with mental illness are seen as "different"—hard to talk with and unpredictable.[67] Stigma affects the interaction with people with mental illness. Mental health providers' beliefs do not differ from those of the population or are even more negative.[68] Professionals need to be sensitive to the ways their opinions affect their clinical behavior and judgments. Stigmatizing attitudes may lead to using exaggerated measures.

TRAINING OF HEALTH CARE AND ALLIED PROFESSIONALS

The power of habit is very enduring in clinical practice. This is well illustrated by the discussion of the use of "net beds" (beds surrounded by wire) or "cage beds" (beds surrounded by steel bars) in the Czech Republic. These methods of patient containment have long been condemned by human rights groups, yet some of the staff used to these methods consider them more humane than other restraint techniques like straps, isolation, or strong medication.[69]

Training courses in aggression management are widely offered to psychiatric staff. These often include knowledge-based elements about aggression and aggressive behavior, introducing different preventive measures and strategies, and acquiring practical "hands-on skills" such as breakaway techniques and holding methods. There is no evidence from controlled trials to prove the effectiveness of aggression management training courses.[62] There is one study showing a decrease in the use of coercive measures after training but not in the number of aggressive incidents.[70] Neither is there evidence that the courses affect nurses' perception of aggression.[71] One large study even showed an increase of violent incidents after training courses.[72] Training can make the staff feel safer,[73] although it has been shown that breakaway training does not result in the ability to use the techniques in real life. Assessing the effectiveness of the staff training programs is difficult. Most of them consist of training in different skills and it is difficult to differentiate among the effects of the training items.

HOSPITAL AND WARD LEVEL

The shortening of psychiatric hospital stays has changed the routines on hospital wards. In acute mental health care, clinical staff sometimes perceive that it is more important to care about safety, throughput, and cost than about the quality of clinical care.[74]

Patient satisfaction is a useful health care indicator and ward atmosphere is strongly correlated with it.[75] The staff's perceptions of the ward atmosphere do not directly reflect those of inpatients: the staff tends to consider the atmosphere more positive than patients do.[76] However, psychiatric inpatients are quite satisfied with their care in general, and most dissatisfaction is reported in the areas of information, restrictions, compulsory care, and ward atmosphere/physical milieu. A lack of meaningful activities on the ward and the necessity of sharing a room with other patients are evaluated especially negatively.[77] Because empty days are linked with disruptive incidents, the provision of meaningful activities to reduce boredom is thought to be important by both patients and staff.[49]

LEADERSHIP AND WARD MANAGEMENT

The success of implementing programs to reduce patient aggression on wards or limit the use of coercive treatment practices might depend on the organizational leadership.[78] Formal evaluations of systemic weaknesses contribute to the development of new interventions.[79] Psychiatric facilities commonly collect data on involuntary interventions. These data can be used for clinical, educational, managerial, and publicity purposes, and collection of data may in itself reduce the use of coercive practices.

PHYSICAL ENVIRONMENT

The occurrence of locked psychiatric wards differs between countries, and there is only a small correlation between the use of involuntary commitment and provision of treatment in a locked ward. The treatment of involuntarily committed patients in open wards is very common as is the treatment of voluntary patients in closed wards.[80] The most common reasons given for locked ward doors are preventing the patients from escaping, providing patients and others with safety and security, preventing import of drugs and other goods, preventing unwelcome visits, and staff's need for control.[81] Even high-security psychiatric wards can adopt therapeutic community principles by clarifying patient–staff communication, ward rules, and structure, and by improving environment and safety in order to increase staff satisfaction and decrease aggressive incidents.[82]

Environmental satisfaction with the ward is a significant predictor of overall satisfaction with hospital care, ranking below only perceived quality of nursing and clinical care. Studies show that the physical health care environment affects the well-being of patients. Positive effects have been found for sunlight, windows, odor, and seating arrangements, and inconsistent effects for sound, nature, spatial layout, television, and multiple stimuli interventions.[83] Recommendations for creating a therapeutic environment on a psychiatric ward include avoiding long corridors, incorporating spatial flexibility, reducing the institutional feeling, and incorporating a familiar tone. Safety considerations require shatterproof windows, tamperproof electrical outlets, and so on. Upholstered furniture is commendable, and furniture should not be easy to throw, yet one should be able to move it.[84] To avoid agitation, patients should be able to control their level of social contact: that means designing spaces where patients can retreat and have privacy.

Staffing

Several studies have examined the relationship between staff characteristics and inpatient aggression and agitation. The limited evidence suggests that some staff features are associated with increased occurrence of incidents of disturbed behavior: younger age, low level of experience, training and grade, male gender, and high level of limit-setting activities. However, there is little consistency across the studies. Considering the individual characteristics of a single staff member has not been customary, although they may have some importance. It has been observed that a small number of specific staff members are consistently self-delegated or delegated by coworkers to make the intervention decisions during crises. Consequently, a small number of "key decision makers" heavily influence the outcome of crisis situations or serve as crisis team leaders.[85] Also, differences in attitudes toward patient aggression may influence action in crisis situations. A nurse who has tolerance for agitated/aggressive behavior may remain calm during an interaction and may even employ a more low-intensity intervention (e.g., asking questions) and thereby successfully defuse a high-risk situation.[86] Patients defined as *difficult* by staff suggest the following qualities in good nursing: conveying respect, having normal conversations, receiving explanations from staff, and being able to achieve their aims by having enough control over their own treatment and goals.[87]

Psychological Management of Acutely and Chronically Violent Patients

Management of violent inpatients can be divided into short-term management of actual or anticipated aggression and longer-term treatment of the potential causes of aggressive behavior.[88]

SHORT-TERM MANAGEMENT OF ACTUAL OR ANTICIPATED AGGRESSION

Until recently, nonphysical conflict management and de-escalation have been rarely included in aggression management training programs or books on these topics in psychiatry.[89] Instead, physical techniques to manage aggressive and violent situations have been prevalent. However, the use of de-escalation techniques ("defusing," "talking-down"), including all verbal and nonverbal techniques

TABLE 12.1 BASIC PRINCIPLES OF CONFLICT MANAGEMENT

1. General attitude toward the patient should be emphatic, concerned, respectful, sincere, and fair with caring intention
2. The risk of each available option should be assessed realistically
3. The aim should be to gain control over the situation instead of the patient and, if possible, to find a satisfactory solution for both parties
4. De-escalation should be a one-on-one interaction, but risk assessment, decision making, responsibilities, and actions should be, if possible, based on teamwork
5. De-escalation is effective only as an early intervention but usually not appropriate in a high-risk and highly emotional situation
6. De-escalation is a way to gain time for considered decision and to reduce interpersonal tension
7. Sufficient physical distance is important for safety and to avoid anxious arousal and defensive actions in a patient
8. Applying de-escalation intervention requires apparent self-confidence without being provoking
9. Power plays and argumentation should be avoided with the patient
10. General safety issues of the ward should be clear to staff

used to defuse actual or anticipated violent situation,[90] is the initial step in the approach to the agitated or violent patient.[10,91]

The main goal of verbal de-escalation is try to regain the trust and confidence of the patient by active and emphatic listening.[89] Judgmental and critical comments, "why" questions, and closed questions should be avoided. Body language, facial expressions, and gestures, that is nonverbal communication is as important as verbal communication. Besides the knowledge of and training in different techniques, the use of de-escalation presumes stress management and self-awareness of the staff and the knowledge of basic principles of conflict management. Richter[89] has reviewed ten basic principles of conflict management (See Table 12.1).

LONGER-TERM TREATMENT OF THE POTENTIAL CAUSES OF AGGRESSIVE BEHAVIOR

Studies have shown the effectiveness of behavioral methods in reducing violent behavior in chronic institutionalized psychiatric patients,[88] and the authors recommend the use of behavioral methods in the treatment of severely affected neuropsychiatric and chronic psychotic patients who manifest violent behavior.[92] The goal is to modify both the stimuli and the consequences in order to reduce the frequency and intensity of the violent behavior in the long term. Applying these methods is preceded by a careful functional analysis attempting to identify individually the purpose of behavior by examining the events occurring before, during, and after the incident, and by assessing environmental, cognitive, psychological, and behavioral variables.[93]

Behavioral interventions can be divided into two principal classes, accelerative and decelerative techniques.[92] Accelerative techniques (e.g., token economy, aggression replacement, social skills training) strengthen behaviors that are incompatible with violent behavior or replace its function. The most well-known accelerative technique in psychiatric treatment is a token economy where patients receive tokens dependent on desirable behavior, and the tokens are later changeable to a meaningful object or privilege.[94] Aggression replacement encourages patients to find other activities to cope with aggression. Decelerative techniques (e.g., social or sensory extinction, time-out from reinforcement, seclusion, restraint) reduce violent behavior by producing neutral or negative consequences and for that reason they should be the last used. An example of the mildest form of decelerative techniques is social extinction by withdrawing attention. Seclusion and restraint should be a last resort.

Cognitive behavioral therapy-based anger management techniques (e.g., Stress Inoculation Training [SIT], cognitive restructuring, relaxation) are recommended for use among patients with mood, attentional, impulse control, and personality disorders,[92] but can also be used to support behavioral techniques among mentally disordered violent patients.[88] Research has focused on Novaco's (1975) application of Meichenbaum's SIT.[95] SIT is a three-phase intervention: cognitive preparation, skill acquisition, and application training. Many different techniques (e.g., cognitive reframing, relaxation training, imagery, modeling, and role-play) are applied to enhance patients' ability to cope with difficult situations. Linehan's[96] dialectical behavior therapy (DBT) is a comprehensive cognitive behavioral technique applied over the last decade to populations characterized by behavioral dyscontrol such as self-inflicted harm, violent behavior, and poor impulse control.[97,98] DBT enhances behavioral capabilities, improves motivation to change, assures that new capabilities generalize to the natural environment, structures the treatment environment, and enhances the capability and motivation of therapists. Four targeted skills are mindfulness, distress tolerance, emotion regulation, and interpersonal effectiveness.

Because acutely or chronically violent patients are not a homogeneous group, an individualized treatment plan[64] preceded by careful functional analysis[93] is an important tool to guide selection of suitable management strategies in individual cases.

CONSTANT OBSERVATION

Constant observation means an increased level of observation and supervision in which continuous, one-on-one monitoring techniques are utilized to assure the safety and well-being of an individual patient or others in the patient care environment.[99] Constant observation can mean intermittent checks on the patient and the most intrusive type of constant observation involves a health care professional being permanently with the patient. No evidence establishes the effectiveness of the procedure,[62] but it is widely used in mental health services.[100] Having a constant observation program can be both labor intensive and expensive for the hospital.[101] Nurses find close observation a stressful procedure. They report a feeling of being constantly observed themselves and a need to find ways of dealing with emotions caused by it. Lately, there have been successful projects to reduce formal observations and replace them with individual care interventions or structured group activities.[102]

BEHAVIORAL CONTRACTS AND THE USE OF EXPERT NURSES

Behavioral contracts are negotiated in mutual understanding by the patient and the health care team, which provides a clear delineation of the responsibilities of the patient and the health care professional with regard to the care delivered. Behavioral contracts may contain treatment plans that can be used if there is a threat of violent or disruptive behavior. Again, they are widely used, but there are no randomized controlled trials to prove their efficacy.[62]

In some psychiatric hospitals and emergency services there are response teams for behavioral emergencies.[103,104] They are specially trained staff members who are educated in different skills to defuse crises situations. There are also interesting experiences of placing expert nurses on the wards to assist the implementation of new techniques of conflict resolution.[105]

Pharmacotherapy

Pharmacotherapy is frequently used for aggressive patients.[106] In the pharmacologic management of aggression in repetitively aggressive adult patients only weak evidence of efficacy is found for antipsychotics, antidepressants, anticonvulsants, and β-adrenergic blocking drugs.[107] For rapid tranquilization several different drugs are used, and no medication has emerged as the gold standard.[108] Benzodiazepines and antipsychotics seem to be reasonably safe and effective. Again, there is a dearth of evidence base for the use of pro re nata (p.r.n.)—as needed—medication in the short-term management of aggressive behavior. This practice has no support from randomized trials but is based on clinical experience and habit.[109] These issues are discussed further in Chapter 3.

Seclusion and Restraint

Seclusion involves moving the patient alone to a locked room from which he or she is prevented from exiting freely.[110] Mechanical restraint includes different belts and handcuffs that partially or totally prevent the patient from moving. Physical restraint refers to the manual restriction of a patient by staff. No recommendations can be made on their effectiveness or benefits because of the absence of any controlled studies.[111] Seclusion and restraint can have substantial deleterious physical and more often psychological effects on both the patient and the staff.[79] Restraint is an intrinsically unsafe procedure, and both mechanical and physical restraints have been reported to be associated with deaths of patients.[112] In the last two decades new legislation, recommendations, professional guidelines, and some court cases have started to emerge to control the use of seclusion and restraint,[113] and successful programs to reduce the use of seclusion and restraint have started to emerge at the individual hospital level.[114] Apparently, the general opinion seems to be that because of the serious risks seclusion and restraint should be considered only as a last resort if nonpharmacologic (e.g., de-escalation) and pharmacologic interventions and strategies have failed. To achieve safe and effective implementation of seclusion and restraint, specific indications, authorization, initiation, duration, nature of the seclusion room or restraint, observation, care of the patient, release, and documentation should be addressed.[115]

Conclusions

Although violent behavior by people with mental disorders is far less common in the community setting than commonly perceived, agitation and aggression are common behavior in psychiatric ward settings. Evidence is limited, but the occurrence of agitated and aggressive behavior seems to be amendable by a range of interventions targeting patients, ward staff, and ward milieu. Restrictive measures, such as seclusion, restraint, or forced medication are the last resort, and should be used only if other measures have failed. More important are preventive measures aiming to improve ward environment and ambience as well as the use of behavioral techniques to reduce repeated violent behavior. In an acute situation, de-escalation techniques should be the initial approach. Measures that improve patient satisfaction with the environment and treatment and provide inpatients with meaningful activities contribute to reduction of inpatient agitation and aggression.

Evidence indicates that reduction of violence in psychiatric wards is most successful when employing complex interventions targeting several levels and different domains. Wards and hospital units with a high level of aggressive incidents need to develop long-term strategies for violence reduction including plans for improving staff–patient interactions, the physical environment, and treatment procedures. Clearly, the success of any such strategy needs to build on a shared set of values emphasizing human rights and integrity of psychiatric inpatients.

REFERENCES

1. Corrigan PW, Watson AC. Findings from the National comorbidity survey on the frequency of violent behavior in individuals with psychiatric disorders. *Psychiatry Res.* 2005;136(2-3): 153–162.

2. Fazel S, Grann M. The population impact of severe mental illness on violent crime. *Am J Psychiatry.* 2006;163(8):1397–1403.

3. White MC, Chafetz L, Collins-Bride G, et al. History of arrest, incarceration and victimization in community-based severely mentally ill. *J Community Health.* 2006;31(2):123–135.

4. Trenoweth S. Perceiving risk in dangerous situations: Risks of violence among mental health inpatients. *J Adv Nurs.* 2003;42(3):278–287.

5. Sells DJ, Rowe M, Fisk D, et al. Violent victimization of persons with co-occurring psychiatric and substance use disorders. *Psychiatr Serv.* 2003;54(9):1253–1257.

6. Noble P, Rodger S. Violence by psychiatric inpatients. *Br J Psychiatry.* 1989;155:384–390.

7. Needham I, Abderhalden C, Halfens RJ, et al. Non-somatic effects of patient aggression on nurses: A systematic review. *J Adv Nurs.* 2005;49(3):283–296.

8. Hunter M, Carmel H. The cost of staff injuries from inpatient violence. *Hosp Community Psychiatry.* 1992;43(6):586–588.

9. Appelbaum PS. Violence and mental disorders: Data and public policy. *Am J Psychiatry.* 2006; 163(8):1319–1321.

10. Marder SR. A review of agitation in mental illness: Treatment guidelines and current therapies. *J Clin Psychiatry.* 2006;67(Suppl 10):13–21.

11. Sachs GS. A review of agitation in mental illness: Burden of illness and underlying pathology. *J Clin Psychiatry.* 2006;67(Suppl 10):5–12.

12. Buckley PF, Noffsinger SG, Smith DA, et al. Treatment of the psychotic patient who is violent. *Psychiatr Clin North Am.* 2003;26(1): 231–272.

13. Ehmann TS, Smith GN, Yamamoto A, et al. Violence in treatment resistant psychotic inpatients. *J Nerv Ment Dis.* 2001;189(10):716–721.

14. Bowers L, Douzenis A, Galeazzi GM, et al. Disruptive and dangerous behaviour by patients

on acute psychiatric wards in three European centres. *Soc Psychiatry Psychiatr Epidemiol.* 2005;40(10):822–828.

15. Arango C, Calcedo Barba A, Gonzalez-Salvador T, et al. Violence in inpatients with schizophrenia: A prospective study. *Schizophr Bull.* 1999; 25(3):493–503.

16. Grassi L, Biancosino B, Marmai L, et al. Violence in psychiatric units: A 7-year Italian study of persistently assaultive patients. *Soc Psychiatry Psychiatr Epidemiol.* 2006;41(9):698–703.

17. Raja M, Azzoni A. Hostility and violence of acute psychiatric inpatients. *Clin Pract Epidemol Ment Health.* 2005;1:11.

18. Nijman HL, Palmstierna T, Almvik R, et al. Fifteen years of research with the Staff Observation Aggression Scale: A review. *Acta Psychiatr Neurol Scand.* 2005;111(1):12–21.

19. Dean K, Walsh E, Morgan C, et al. Aggressive behaviour at first contact with services: Findings from the AESOP First Episode Psychosis Study. *Psychol Assess.* 2007;37(4):547–557.

20. Foster C, Bowers L, Nijman H. Aggressive behaviour on acute psychiatric wards: Prevalence, severity and management. *J Adv Nurs.* 2007;58(2):140–149.

21. Maguire J, Ryan D. Aggression and violence in mental health services: Categorizing the experiences of Irish nurses. *J Psychiatr Ment Health Nurs.* 2007;14(2):120–127.

22. Kaltiala-Heino R, Tuohimäki C, Korkeila J, et al. Reasons for using seclusion and restraint in psychiatric inpatient care. *Int J Law Psychiatry.* 2003;26(2):139–149.

23. Bowers L, Simpson A, Alexander J. Patient-staff conflict: Results of a survey on acute psychiatric wards. *Soc Psychiatry Psychiatr Epidemiol.* 2003;38(7):402–408.

24. Marco CA, Vaughan J. Emergency management of agitation in schizophrenia. *Am J Emerg Med.* 2005;23(6):767–776.

25. Pulsford D, Duxbury J. Aggressive behaviour by people with dementia in residential care settings: A review. *J Psychiatr Ment Health Nurs.* 2006;13(5):611–618.

26. dosReis S, Barnett S, Love RC, et al. Maryland Youth Practice Improvement Committee. A guide for managing acute aggressive behavior of youths in residential and inpatient treatment facilities. *Psychiatr Serv.* 2003;54(10):1357–1363.

27. Palmstierna T, Wistedt B. Staff observation aggression scale, SOAS: Presentation and evaluation. *Acta Psychiatr Neurol Scand.* 1987;76(6):657–663.

28. Nijman H, Palmstierna T. Measuring aggression with the staff observation aggression scale – revised. *Acta Psychiatr Neurol Scand Suppl.* 2002;106(412):101–102.

29. Kay SR, Wolkenfeld F, Murrill LM. Profiles of aggression among psychiatric patients.

I. Nature and prevalence. *J Nerv Ment Dis.* 1988;176(9):539–546.

30. Wistedt B, Rasmussen A, Pedersen L, et al. The development of an observer-scale for measuring social dysfunction and aggression. *Pharmacopsychiatry.* 1990;23(6):249–252.

31. Steinert T, Wolfle M, Gebhardt RP. Measurement of violence during in-patient treatment and association with psychopathology. *Acta Psychiatr Neurol Scand.* 2000;102(2):107–112.

32. Battaglia J, Lindborg SR, Alaka K, et al. Calming versus sedative effects of intramuscular olanzapine in agitated patients. *Am J Emerg Med.* 2003;21(3):192–198.

33. Swift RH, Harrigan EP, Cappelleri JC, et al. Validation of the behavioral activity rating scale (BARS): A novel measure of activity in agitated patients. *J Psychiatr Res.* 2002;36(2):87–95.

34. Bartels SJ, Horn SD, Smout RJ, et al. Agitation and depression in frail nursing home elderly patients with dementia: Treatment characteristics and service use. *Am J Geriatr Psychiatry.* 2003;11(2):231–238.

35. Chen JC, Borson S, Scanlan JM. Stage-specific prevalence of behavioral symptoms in Alzheimer's disease in a multi-ethnic community sample. *Am J Geriatr Psychiatry.* 2000;8(2):123–133.

36. Davis JM, Chen N. Choice of maintenance medication for schizophrenia. *J Clin Psychiatry.* 2003;64(Suppl 16):24–33.

37. Lindenmayer JP. The pathophysiology of agitation. *J Clin Psychiatry.* 2000;61(Suppl 14): 5–10.

38. Madhusoodanan S. Introduction: Antipsychotic treatment of behavioral and psychological symptoms of dementia in geropsychiatric patients. *Am J Geriatr Psychiatry.* 2001;9(3):283–288.

39. Duxbury J, Whittington R. Causes and management of patient aggression and violence: Staff and patient perspectives. *J Adv Nurs.* 2005;50(5):469–478.

40. Flannery RB Jr. Characteristics of assaultive psychiatric inpatients: Updated review of findings, 1995–2000. *Am J Alzheimers Dis Other Demen.* 2001;16(3):153–156.

41. Flannery RB Jr, Juliano J, Cronin S, et al. Characteristics of assaultive psychiatric patients: fifteen-year analysis of the Assaulted Staff Action Program (ASAP). *Psychiatr Q.* 2006;77(3):239–249.

42. Calcedo-Barba AL, Calcedo-Ordonez A. Violence and paranoid schizophrenia. *Int J Law Psychiatry.* 1994;17(3):253–263.

43. Krakowski MI, Czobor P. Clinical symptoms, neurological impairment, and prediction of violence in psychiatric inpatients. *Hosp Community Psychiatry.* 1994;45(7):700–705.

44. James DV, Fineberg NA, Shah AK, et al. An increase in violence on an acute psychiatric

ward. A study of associated factors. *Br J Psychiatry*. 1990;156:846–852.

45. Björkdahl A, Olsson D, Palmstierna T. Nurses' short-term prediction of violence in acute psychiatric intensive care. *Acta Psychiatr Neurol Scand*. 2006;113(3):224–229.

46. Steinert T, Bergbauer G, Schmid P, et al. Seclusion and restraint in patients with schizophrenia: Clinical and biographical correlates. *J Nerv Ment Dis*. 2007;195(6):492–496.

47. Bowers L, Allan T, Simpson A, et al. Adverse incidents, patient flow and nursing workforce variables on acute psychiatric wards: The Tompkins Acute Ward Study. *Int J Soc Psychiatry*. 2007;53(1):75–84.

48. Nijman HL, Rector G. Crowding and aggression on inpatient psychiatric wards. *Psychiatr Serv*. 1999;50(6):830–831.

49. Meehan T, McCombes S, Hatzipetrou L, et al. Introduction of routine outcome measures: staff reactions and issues for consideration. *J Psychiatr Ment Health Nurs*. 2006;13(5):581–587.

50. Duxbury J. An evaluation of staff and patient views of and strategies employed to manage inpatient aggression and violence on one mental health unit: A pluralistic design. *J Psychiatr Ment Health Nurs*. 2002;9(3):325–337.

51. Spokes K, Bond K, Lowe T, et al. HOVIS – the Hertfordshire/Oxfordshire Violent Incident Study. *J Psychiatr Ment Health Nurs*. 2002;9(2):199–209.

52. Nijman HL, Campo JM, Ravelli DP, et al. A tentative model of aggression on inpatient psychiatric wards. *Psychiatr Serv*. 1999;50(6):832–834.

53. Steinert T. Prediction of inpatient violence. *Acta Psychiatr Neurol Scand Suppl*. 2002;106(412):133–141.

54. Lidz CW, Mulvey EP, Gardner W. The accuracy of predictions of violence to others. *JAMA*. 1993;269(8):1007–1011.

55. Nijman H, Merckelbach H, Evers C, et al. Prediction of aggression on a locked psychiatric admissions ward. *Acta Psychiatr Neurol Scand*. 2002;105(5):390–395.

56. Doyle M, Dolan M. Violence risk assessment: Combining actuarial and clinical information to structure clinical judgements for the formulation and management of risk. *J Psychiatr Ment Health Nurs*. 2002;9(6):649–657.

57. Haim R, Rabinowitz J, Lereya J, et al. Predictions made by psychiatrists and psychiatric nurses of violence by patients. *Psychiatr Serv*. 2002;53(5):622–624.

58. Almvik R, Woods P. Short-term risk prediction: The Broset Violence Checklist. *J Psychiatr Ment Health Nurs*. 2003;10(2):236–238.

59. Abderhalden C, Needham I, Dassen T, et al. Predicting inpatient violence using an extended version of the Broset-Violence-Checklist:

Instrument development and clinical application. *BMC Psychiatry*. 2006;6:17.

60. Webster CD, Nicholls TL, Martin ML, et al. Short-Term Assessment of Risk and Treatability (START): The case for a new structured professional judgment scheme. *Behav Sci Law*. 2006;24(6):747–766.

61. Nicholls TL, Brink J, Desmarais SL, et al. The Short-Term Assessment of Risk and Treatability (START): A prospective validation study in a forensic psychiatric sample. *Assessment*. 2006;13(3):313–327.

62. Muralidharan S, Fenton M. Containment strategies for people with serious mental illness. *Cochrane Database Syst Rev*. 2006;3:CD002084.

63. Nolan KA, Czobor P, Roy BB, et al. Characteristics of assaultive behavior among psychiatric inpatients. *Psychiatr Serv*. 2003;54(7):1012–1016.

64. Quanbeck CD, McDermott BE, Lam J, et al. Categorization of aggressive acts committed by chronically assaultive state hospital patients. *Psychiatr Serv*. 2007;58(4):521–528.

65. Dinos S, Stevens S, Serfaty M, et al. Stigma: The feelings and experiences of 46 people with mental illness. Qualitative study. *Br J Psychiatry*. 2004;184:176–181.

66. Corrigan PW, Watson AC, Heyrman ML, et al. Structural stigma in state legislation. *Psychiatr Serv*. 2005;56(5):557–563.

67. Gray AJ. Stigma in psychiatry. *J Assoc Adv Med Instrum*. 2002;95(2):72–76.

68. Schulze B. Stigma and mental health professionals: A review of the evidence on an intricate relationship. *Int Rev Psychiatry*. 2007;19(2):137–155.

69. Holt E. Rest and restraint. *Lancet*. 2004;364(9437):829–830.

70. Needham I, Abderhalden C, Meer R, et al. The effectiveness of two interventions in the management of patient violence in acute mental inpatient settings: Report on a pilot study. *J Psychiatr Ment Health Nurs*. 2004;11(5):595–601.

71. Needham I, Abderhalden C, Zeller A, et al. The effect of a training course on nursing students' attitudes toward, perceptions of, and confidence in managing patient aggression. *J Nurs Educ*. 2005;44(9):415–420.

72. Bowers L, Nijman H, Allan T, et al. Prevention and management of aggression training and violent incidents on U.K. Acute psychiatric wards. *Psychiatr Serv*. 2006;57(7):1022–1026.

73. Beech B, Leather P. Evaluating a management of aggression unit for student nurses. *J Adv Nurs*. 2003;44(6):603–612.

74. Quirk A, Lelliott P, Seale C. Service users' strategies for managing risk in the volatile environment of an acute psychiatric ward. *Soc Forces*. 2004;59(12):2573–2583.

75. Middelboe T, Schjodt T, Byrsting K, et al. Ward atmosphere in acute psychiatric inpatient care: Patients' perceptions, ideals and satisfaction. *Acta Psychiatr Neurol Scand.* 2001;103(3):212–219.

76. Rossberg JI, Friis S. Patients' and staff's perceptions of the psychiatric ward environment. *Psychiatr Serv.* 2004;55(7):798–803.

77. Kuosmanen L, Hatonen H, Jyrkinen AR, et al. Patient satisfaction with psychiatric inpatient care. *J Adv Nurs.* 2006;55(6):655–663.

78. Visalli H, McNasser G. Reducing seclusion and restraint: Meeting the organizational challenge. *J Nurs Care Qual.* 2000;14(4):35–44.

79. Fisher WA. Elements of successful restraint and seclusion reduction programs and their application in a large, urban, state psychiatric hospital. *J Psychiatr Pract.* 2003;9(1):7–15.

80. Rittmannsberger H, Sartorius N, Brad M, et al. Changing aspects of psychiatric inpatient treatment. A census investigation in five European countries. *Eur Psychiatry.* 2004;19(8):483–488.

81. Haglund K, van der Meiden E, von Knorring L, et al. Psychiatric care behind locked doors. A study regarding the frequency of and the reasons for locked psychiatric wards in Sweden. *J Psychiatr Ment Health Nurs.* 2007;14(1):49–54.

82. Mistral W, Hall A, McKee P. Using therapeutic community principles to improve the functioning of a high care psychiatric ward in the UK. *Int J Ment Health Nurs.* 2002;11(1):10–17.

83. Dijkstra K, Pieterse M, Pruyn A. Physical environmental stimuli that turn healthcare facilities into healing environments through psychologically mediated effects: Systematic review. *J Adv Nurs.* 2006;56(2):166–181.

84. Karlin BE, Zeiss RA. Best practices: Environmental and therapeutic issues in psychiatric hospital design: Toward best practices. *Psychiatr Serv.* 2006;57(10):1376–1378.

85. Schreiner GM, Crafton CG, Sevin JA. Decreasing the use of mechanical restraints and locked seclusion. *Adm Policy Ment Health.* 2004;31(6):449–463.

86. Whittington R, Higgins L. More than zero tolerance? Burnout and tolerance for patient aggression amongst mental health nurses in China and the UK. *Acta Psychiatr Neurol Scand Suppl.* 2002;106(412)37–40.

87. Breeze JA, Repper J. Struggling for control: The care experiences of 'difficult' patients in mental health services. *J Adv Nurs.* 1998;28(6):1301–1311.

88. Harris GT, Rice ME. Risk appraisal and management of violent behavior. *Psychiatr Serv.* 1997;48(9):1168–1176.

89. Richter D. Nonphysical conflict management and de-escalation. In: Richter D, Whittington R, eds. *Violence in mental health settings.* Causes, consequences, management LLC. Springer Science, Business Media; 2007.

90. Dix R. De-escalation techniques. In: Beer D, Pereira S, Paton C, eds. *Psychiatric intensive care.* London: Greenwich Medical Media; 2001.

91. Petit JR. Management of the acutely violent patient. *Psychiatr Clin North Am.* 2005;28(3):701–711

92. Alpert JE, Spillmann MK. Psychotherapeutic approaches to aggressive and violent patients. *Psychiatr Clin North Am.* 1997;20(2):453–472.

93. Daffern M, Howells K. Psychiatric inpatient aggression. *Aggress Violent Behav* 2002;7:477–497.

94. Wong SE, Woolsey JE, Innocent AJ, et al. Behavioral treatment of violent psychiatric patients. *Psychiatr Clin North Am.* 1988;11(4):569–580.

95. Beck R, Fernandez E. Cognitive-behavioral therapy in the treatment of anger: A meta-analysis. *Cognit Ther Res.* 1998;22:63–74.

96. Linehan M. Cognitive behavioral therapy of borderline personality disorder. New York: Guilford Press; 1993.

97. Evershed S, Tennant A, Boomer D, et al. Practice-based outcomes of dialectical behaviour therapy (DBT) targeting anger and violence, with male forensic patients: A pragmatic and non-contemporaneous comparison. *Crim Behav Ment Health.* 2003;13(3):198–213.

98. Berzins L, Trestman R. The development and implementation of dialectical behaviour therapy in forensic settings. *Int J For Ment Health* 2004;3(1):93–103.

99. Moore P, Berman K, Knight M, et al. Constant observation: Implications for nursing practice. *J Psychosoc Nurs Ment Health Serv.* 1995;33(3):46–50.

100. Fletcher RF. The process of constant observation: Perspectives of staff and suicidal patients. *J Psychiatr Ment Health Nurs.* 1999;6(1):9–14.

101. Blumenfield M, Milazzo J, Orlowski B. Constant observation in the general hospital. *Psychosomatics.* 2000;41(4):289–293.

102. Dodds P, Bowles N. Dismantling formal observation and refocusing nursing activity in acute inpatient psychiatry: A case study. *J Psychiatr Ment Health Nurs.* 2001;8(2):183–188.

103. Smith GM, Davis RH, Bixler EO, et al. Pennsylvania State Hospital system's seclusion and restraint reduction program. *Psychiatr Serv.* 2005;56(9):1115–1122.

104. D'Orio BM, Purselle D, Stevens D, et al. Reduction of episodes of seclusion and restraint in a psychiatric emergency service. *Psychiatr Serv.* 2004;55(5):581–583.

105. Brennan G, Flood C, Bowers L. Constraints and blocks to change and improvement on

acute psychiatric wards – lessons from the City Nurses project. *J Psychiatr Ment Health Nurs.* 2006;13(5):475–482.

106. Soliman AE, Reza H. Risk factors and correlates of violence among acutely ill adult psychiatric inpatients. *Psychiatr Serv.* 2001;52(1): 75–80.

107. Goedhard LE, Stolker JJ, Heerdink ER, et al. Pharmacotherapy for the treatment of aggressive behavior in general adult psychiatry: A systematic review. *J Clin Psychiatry.* 2006; 67(7):1013–1024.

108. NICE. *Clinical guideline 1. Schizophrenia. Core interventions in the treatment and management of schizophrenia in primary and secondary care.* 2002.

109. Whicher E, Morrison M, Douglas-Hall P. 'As required' medication regimens for seriously mentally ill people in hospital. *Cochrane Database Syst Rev* 2002;(2):CD003441.

110. Sailas E, Wahlbeck K. Restraint and seclusion in psychiatric inpatient wards. *Curr Opin Psychiatry.* 2005;18(5):555–559.

111. Sailas E, Fenton M. Seclusion and restraint for people with serious mental illnesses. *Cochrane Database Syst Rev.* 2000;(2):CD001163.

112. Mohr WK, Petti TA, Mohr BD. Adverse effects associated with physical restraint. *Can J Psychiatry.* 2003;48(5):330–337.

113. Keski-Valkama A, Sailas E, Eronen M, et al. A 15-year national follow-up: Legislation is not enough to reduce the use of seclusion and restraint. *Soc Psychiatry Psychiatr Epidemiol.* 2007;42(9):747–752.

114. Gaskin CJ, Elsom SJ, Happell B. Interventions for reducing the use of seclusion in psychiatric facilities: Review of the literature. *Br J Psychiatry.* 2007;191:298–303.

115. Fisher WA. Restraint and seclusion: A review of the literature. *Am J Psychiatry.* 1994;151(11):1584–1591.

Recurrently Readmitted Inpatient Psychiatric Patients: Characteristics and Care

WILLIAM H. SLEDGE AND CHRISTINE L. DUNN

Case Vignette

Pam is a 33-year-old mother of five children, divorced, with the diagnoses of mood disorder not otherwise specified (NOS), alcohol dependence, borderline personality disorder, and psychotic disorder NOS. She has had three hospitalizations in 3 months and has a history of cutting and impulsivity and chaotic personal relationships leading to the loss of custody of her children. The plan was to have involved her in a women's shelter program developing toward independent housing and in Alcoholics Anonymous (AA) and to organize her treatment at the local community mental health center. She was readmitted to the hospital approximately 6 weeks from the index hospital discharge for cutting and suicidal ideation but following discharge was lost to all efforts at follow-up.

"Recidivist," "frequent flyer," "revolving door," and "high user" are some of the not-so complimentary terms that have been used to refer to patients who are recurrently admitted to the hospital. This phenomenon is hard on everyone. There is no indication that patients find it a satisfactory way of engaging the mental health system (despite some older reports that these patients like to be in the hospital).[1,2] Patients' families and loved ones (when they are in the patients' lives) find it disruptive and alarming, and health care professionals frequently range from being annoyed to being substantially troubled. When employers of the patients are involved, they do not stay involved long. In general, it is not an effective way of getting mental health services to patients who need the services.

This pattern of use has been a preoccupation among health care professionals for some time, and that concern is represented in a robust literature that spans several eras of psychiatry in the last half of the 20th century. Geller,[3] one of the most creative and passionate investigators on the recurrent readmission (RR) phenomenon, provided a historical perspective in his account of a state hospital that spanned a 100 years during the last part of the 19th century and the first part of the 20th century. He suggests the RR phenomenon may be a nasty side effect of deinstitutionalization and the fragmented mental health care that resulted in many states.[3,4] (See also, Chpapter 1.)

This chapter will examine these and other perspectives as the authors review briefly some of the literature addressing the phenomenon of the recurrently admitted (to psychiatric hospitalization) patient. The authors will describe some of their work at the Yale-New Haven Psychiatric Hospital (YNHPH) in attempting to understand and intervene with this problem. The focus here will be on those patients who are recurrently admitted to the hospital. Although these patients may be a subset of those with persistent and severe mental illness, one of the repeated questions of the literature is to what degree the group of recurrently readmitted inpatient psychiatric patients (RRIPP) is coincident with the broader category of persistently and severely mentally ill and if there might be subcategories of RRIPP that are not typical of patients with severe and persistent mental illness.

Selected Review of the Literature

The RRIPP phenomenon has been explored and given different meanings over the years. Each era has imposed its particular issues on the phenomenon. The last 40 years have seen three substantial English language reviews[5–7] and one German review.[8] The authors will refer to these reviews and others as they develop a variety of themes and perspectives.

DEFINITION

What exactly is taken to constitute RR has varied in the literature, rendering comparisons among studies difficult and meta-analyses almost impossible. Not only have investigators used different rates of readmissions as the criterion, but also other measures have been suggested, such as days in hospital, time between hospitalizations, community tenure, and complex indices taking into consideration not only variables such as number of hospitalizations and rate, but also age at first hospitalization and associated costs. Byers and Cohen[9] reported the only study the authors of this chapter found that explored the relationships between some of these various outcomes. They found that readmission within 1 year correlated with number of days in the community at the 0.69 level and with the number of days to first readmission at 0.89, and that the number of days in the community correlated with number of days to first admission at the 0.71 level. These findings suggest that these different definitions are not too discordant from one another. Without a consensus for the definition of RR, naturally it will not be possible to get a consensus on who the RRIPP are. Nonetheless, a common picture does emerge when one puts together all the available evidence. The standard of using the rate of admission of three (or more) within 18 months has been more widely adopted than any other standard.

SALIENCE OF RECURRENT READMISSION

As the RR phenomenon emerged as a research focus in the 1970s, some authors asserted that these returnees were "failures" on the part of the hospital, either because the hospital could not effect appropriate psychological or situational change, or the hospital was unable to provide adequate aftercare.[5] More narrowly, DiScipio and Sommer[10] considered readmission within 30 days of a therapeutic failure, reflecting either an error in judgment or failure to provide proper aftercare. However, several authors questioned the use of the readmission rate as a measure of the quality of care, at least of the hospital. Voineskos and Denault,[11] Solomon and Doll,[12] and Erickson and Paige[13] all agreed that it is a fallacy to use the readmission rate as a measure of effectiveness of the hospital because the hospital did not control the actions of patients once they left, did not control the outpatient services, and did not have the ability to predict who might be vulnerable to return.

From 1955 to 2000, the population of state hospitals for the mentally ill went from 558,000 to 55,000,[4] varying, of course, by region and state. As this massive cutback of inpatient services was coming to a close, an emphasis emerged in the public sector on the organization and management of community-based treatments. This heralded a time of professional preoccupation with rehospitalization rates, the adequacy of community services, and the high cost of rehospitalization. Managed care or rather "managed cost" policies were prevalent in the practice of inpatient psychiatry. Some studies directly addressed the effects of managed care, such as the reduction of length of stay in the hospital. For example, Appleby et al.[14] examined whether patients who had a short length of stay were more likely to be readmitted. Length of stay was statistically significantly related to time to relapse after the effect of the number of previous admissions was taken into consideration. However, the small size of the effect raised questions about clinical significance. The authors argued that some patients need to stay in the hospital longer in order to recover sufficiently to remain out of the hospital because of the finding that the likelihood for readmission within 30 days was significantly higher in those with brief hospitalizations.

PREDICTION

Major themes of the literature have been the questions: Who are the RRIPPs? Can RR be predicted? And how did these patients end up using so much inpatient care? Many studies attempt to predict or show associations with RR even when the primary focus of the study is on some narrowly defined issue. Rather than discussing them individually and at length, the authors have summarized the results in Table 13.1 of studies that attempt to answer the questions in the preceding text. References in Table 13.1 are listed chronologically and include reports since 1970 that include a definition of RR and an inferential statistical approach to estimating the probability of variables' being associated with membership in the RR group. But because the definitions of RR differ widely, these results are not easily comparable. The authors' discussion in this section will take up measures of demographic variables, clinical features of symptoms and diagnoses, and attitudes toward clinical care and their illness. Later special issues and treatment and prevention approaches will be addressed.

Demographically, on first look the findings seem diverse and at times inconsistent among studies. Klinkenberg and Calsyn,[7] the review most oriented to research method, emphasized the shortcomings of the research designs and methods as a major cause of this variation through the use of underpowered studies and the failure to use multivariate statistics to control for multicollinearity. Nevertheless, summarizing from the table of 31 selected reviews spanning 33 years from 1973 to 2006, the authors find the following:

- No studies reported female gender more likely to be associated with RR; 4 reported male gender more likely to be associated with RR; and 30 found no difference or reported no gender findings.
- Race barely ever distinguished RRIPP from non-RRIPP.
- Youth was associated with RR status in nine studies, and no studies reported any other age-group more likely to be in the RR status.
- Being unmarried was associated with RR status in three studies, and being married was not associated with RR status in any study.
- Unemployment was positively associated with RR status in three studies.
- Educational level was not a factor in any study.

In general, taking the studies in Table 13.1 together, one could say that there was a trend for patients to be male, younger, unmarried, and unemployed. However, it is important to note that almost all these associations fell out when there was control for one or two other variables such as a history of recurrent hospitalizations. None of these demographic variables have the specificity and sensitivity to be considered predictors of the RR.

Patient attitudes toward care have received a fair amount of attention, especially compliance.[15–20] Of the authors' selected group of references, five reported a highly significant correlation between noncompliance with medication and frequent rehospitalization.

Diagnostically and clinically, psychosis is the more prevalent condition with nine references (four for schizophrenic diagnosis and five additional with psychotic symptoms). Yet other conditions were found in some studies, as follows: four for substance abuse and three for affective disorders. In addition to categoric diagnostic and symptom complex clinical characterizations, some studies reported correlations with RR through severe symptoms[2] or chronicity.[2] However, the main feature that was associated with RR status was former hospitalization: 13 studies reported an association and when multivariate statistics were used to control for multicollinearity, other associations usually dropped out of statistical significance.

Some, though, have found little difference between RRIPP and other patients. Lucas et al.[21] did a 6.5-year study of 193 inpatients who were heavy users of inpatient care and compared them with a control group of 400 inpatients. Heavy users were diagnostically and demographically similar to ordinary inpatients, despite the fact that they used services at roughly three times the rate of other inpatients in terms of health care costs.

Social issues have also been given strong consideration in the literature. Kent and Yellowlees[22] determined that social factors contributed to 39% of admissions. These social factors included relationship problems such as dysfunction and conflict in relationships, acute loneliness, social isolation, and lack of adequate continuous social supports, from either professionals or natural social networks. Another

TABLE 13.1 SUMMARY OF CITATIONS PREDICTING RECURRENT PSYCHIATRIC HOSPITALIZATION

Citation (First Author)	Date	Number of Subjects	RRIPP (%)	RRIPP Criteria	Study Design	Patient Qualities Associated with RRIPP		
						Demographic	Behavioral	Clinical
Buell	1973	78	100.0	≥2/6 mo	Rec rev, MV	None	Prev hsp	Length of last hospitalization
Fontana	1975	54	19/39	≥2/6, ≥2/12 mo	Prosp			Chronicity
Franklin	1975	107	33.6	≥2/12 mo	Random sample, prosp		Source of income, mar pblms	Sub ab (alcohol)
Voineskos	1978	572	13.6	≥5/24 mo	Rec rev	Male, unmarr, unempld	Prev hsp	
Byers	1979	129		≥2/12 mo	Rec rev, MV		Invl	
Joyce	1981	169	14.2	≥2/6 mo	Prosp and rec rev	Prev hsp		
Lambert	1983	22,062	25.0	≥2/69 mo	Rec rev, dis anlys	Age (−)	Lived in state, indigent	Psych syms
Abramowitz	1984	1,919	23.0	≥2/48 mo	Rec rev, MV		Invl	
Carpenter	1985	1,960	5.8	≥3/12 mo	Matched control		Noncmpy, prev hsp	Sub ab
Setz	1985	400	45.0	≥2/15 mo	Prosp, surv anlys	Age (−), ethnic (w)	Prev hsp	
Woogh	1986	1,722	7.0	≥3/72 mo	Rec rev	Males, age (−), unempld		Psychotic (47%)
Surber	1987	97		≥3/12 mo				
Green	1988	25		≥3/18 mo	Matched control, rec rev		Noncmpt	
Havassy	1989	300	32.0	≥2/12 mo	Rec rev, MV	Unempld	Prev hsp	Schz, affect dis, pers dis
Casper	1990	86			Rec rev	Unmarr	Noncmpt	Sub ab
Casper	1990	94	7.0		Rec rev, clus anlys			
Hadley	1990	11,399	5.0	≥rounded mean of costs		Age (−)		Schz and affect dis

Citation	Date	No. of subjects	% RRIPP	RRIPP criteria	Source/analysis	Predictor (demographic)	Predictor	Predictor
Appleby	1993	1,500	53.0	≥2/18 mo	Rec rev, surv anlys	Age (−)	Prev hsp	Psych syms
Casper	1993	416			Rec rev, clus anlys		Noncmpt	
Casper	1995	195	38.0	≥3/18 mo	Prosp, clus anlys		Homelessness, arrest	
Swett	1995	189	16.9	≥1/1 mo	—			Psych syms
Haywood	1995	135	89.0	Unclear	Prosp, MV		Noncmpt, prev hsp	Sub ab
Kent	1995	50		≥3/36 mo	Retrospective rev. with therapist and pts	Unmarr		Chronicity, sub ab
Postrado	1995	559		≥2/2 and ≥2/12 mo	Rec rev, MV		Prev hsp	Sev syms
Sanguineti	1996	1,755	17.9	>1/12 mo	Prosp	Age (−), male, AA		Schz
Lyons	1997	255	17.6	≥1/6 mo	Rec rev, MV			Sev sym
Perlick	1999	100	24/44	≥2/6, ≥2/15 mo	Prosp, surv anlys	Age (−)	Prev hsp	Neuroveg dep
Lucas	2001	193	10.0	Index	Matched control		Prev hsp	
Roick	2004	307	12.0	≥3/30 mo	Prosp, MV	Male, age (−)	Prev hsp	Psych syms
Bobo	2004	814	14.0	≥2/13 mo	Rec rev		Prev hsp	Hx child psych, psych aff dis
Rosca	2006	2,150		≥2/120 mo	Rec rev, MV	Age (−)	Invl	Schz

Citation, first author only; Date, of publication; Number of subjects, total population measured; % RRIPP, percent of total population that are recurrently admitted; RRIPP criteria, expressed in rate of admission per number of months; rec rev, archival source; prosp, prospective data; MV, multivariate analysis; surv anlys, survival analysis; pts, patients; RCD, random control design; dis anlys, discriminate analysis; clus anlys, cluster analysis; unmarr, unmarried; unempld, unemployed; AA, African American; prev hsp, previous hospitalization; psych, psychotic; syms, symptoms; schz, schizophrenic; noncmpt, noncompliant with treatment; invl, involuntary status; dx, diagnosis; dis, disorder; sub ab, substance abuse; mar pblms, martial problems. (Data from references 1,9,11,14–21,24,35–53.)

social issue of importance is the association of RR with homelessness in some studies.[23] Casper[24] found homelessness and a history of arrest to be important contributions to readmission.

Economic variables have been considered but not as much as one might hope or think. One economic issue, of course, is the extent and cost of RR. The 5% to 50% of patients who are RRIPP account for between 8% and approximately 40% of cost when it is measured. Weiden and Olfson[25] distinguished between noncompliance and loss of neuroleptic efficacy and estimated that the costs of neuroleptic efficacy accounted for 60% and noncompliance accounted for 40%.

TREATMENT AND MANAGEMENT APPROACHES

Several studies have been oriented toward efforts to control or reduce RR while providing appropriate care for the patients at risk. Dietzen and Bond[26] found that service intensity was not linearly related to client outcomes. They compared 14 programs and 155 clients and concluded that a minimum intensity of services is necessary to reduce hospital use for different clients with different needs. Dincin et al.[27] carried out a before and after test of implementation of an Assertive Community Treatment (ACT) team. The ACT team significantly reduced patient days and improved continuity of care. Net days were reduced by 28% compared to an increase of 15% in the hospital's other catchment areas. In the year after the program was implemented, the participants were hospitalized a mean of 27.7 days compared with a mean of 80 days in the year before.

Involuntary inpatient and outpatient treatment have not infrequently been used in the care of those who come back to the hospital repeatedly. Swartz et al.[28] did a randomized study to determine if involuntary outpatient commitment could reduce rehospitalization among individuals with severe mental illness. The control and outpatient commitments did not differ in hospital-based outcomes; however, in subjects who had sustained periods of outpatient commitment, there were 57% fewer readmissions and 20 fewer hospital days in the controls subjects. Sustained outpatient commitment was particularly effective for individuals with nonaffective psychotic disorders, reducing hospital readmissions in this group by 72%. They concluded that outpatient commitment can work to reduce hospital readmissions and total hospital days when court orders are sustained and combined with intensive treatment, especially for individuals with psychotic disorders.

Prince[29] examined the extent to which inpatient readmission among 264 patients with schizophrenia occurred within 3 months of discharge. Interventions in multiple domains were addressed, such as medication, education, symptom education, community service continuity, social skills, daily living, daily structures, and family issues. After accounting for demographic characteristics with logistic regression equations, they found that the interventions addressing symptom education, service continuity, and daily structure were most effective in preventing admission among individuals with four or more prior hospitalizations, but not among patients who had fewer than four previous inpatient stays.

The only randomized controlled study that prospectively identified RRIPP and attempted to treat them was the Swartz et al.,[28] cited in preceding text. Systems that employ assertive outreach and efforts at rehabilitation together with some kind of employment opportunity tend to do better in avoiding recurrent hospitalization with a general group of patients who are severely mentally ill. Again, the essential ingredients seem to be outreach, therapeutic relationship, and persistent engagement through a service such as case management.[29]

What emerges from the fog of time and multiple studies across cultures is a group of patients who tend to be difficult to engage with most institutions (mental health treatment programs, employment, and educational organizations) and people (family, friends, coworkers, etc.) for a variety of reasons (age, education, and psychopathology) and to whose needs organizations have trouble accommodating. What determines an RRIPP is dependent in part on the setting for delivery of mental health services. This includes how inpatient beds are managed, the level of oversight and application of specific criteria for admission, the goals of the inpatient care as well as the quality and goals of available outpatient and rehabilitative services, including nonclinical resources such as housing and integration into the community. Furthermore, how people with chronic illness, especially severe mental illnesses, are allowed to live in a particular culture will be important. Patient characteristics, of course, will be of major import. Anything that increases the opportunity for alienation and being cut off from the mainstream culture (youth, psychosis, lack of employment, and noncompliance with treatment) will foster this alienation as will personality characteristics that make social connections difficult.

Yale-New Haven Experience

Case Vignette

James was a 28-year-old unmarried, African American male who had the onset of a densely intractable psychotic condition at age 17 at which time he was admitted to a local psychiatric adolescent inpatient service with the delusions of being controlled by his family through the television. He had a long history of marijuana and alcohol use during adolescence and had been arrested for larceny and assault but was never sentenced. In the hospital, he was typically initially very difficult to engage and resorted to intimidation and threats to keep others at bay. But also typically, as he improved he would become quite interactive and revealed his great dependency on others, especially his mother, with whom he inevitably returned to live. Efforts to set up supported living separate from his mother were always undermined by his and her mixture of need and guilt. He had more than eight hospital admissions in a period of 2 years before he was found dead of an apparent arrhythmia secondary to cocaine use.

The authors' own clinical experience has not been different from others. Noticing what seemed to be an increasing rate of rehospitalization, the staff of YNHPH elected to implement a hospital-based approach to treatment planning attempting to ensure that patients who were at risk for recurrent hospitalization, based on their prior experience of being readmitted, would gain maximally from their stay in the hospital. For example, at the YNHPH, over the course of 12 months (March, 2003 to March, 2004) there were 56 patients (2.25% of annual discharges) who had inpatient psychiatric admissions more than three times a year. These 249 admission episodes entailed a total of 2,221 days of hospital care (~8.5% of total days and ~10% of total admission episodes) and amounted to approximately $1.7 million in total hospital costs.

The authors considered how a hospital with few associated outpatient programs might be effective in reducing the readmissions. In January 2005, they began organizing high-user treatment planning groups (HUTPGs) as suggested by one of their staff program leaders. These are structured, all-treater meetings held at the hospital and convened by hospital staff before the final plans were made for the patient's discharge. They asked for a HUTPG when patients were particularly problematic or had a history of recurrent hospitalizations. (Initially that term was not well defined. The authors eventually made it three or more hospitalizations within 12 months or one within 30 days of discharge from another hospitalization, but they modified that later to three or more within 18 months.) They asked the treaters who were expected to be part of the aftercare plan to join them in thinking through the details and putting in place elements that would have a chance of reducing hospitalization. Initially, the patients were not included but they quickly changed to include patients in some portion of the sessions. In the summer of 2005, the authors obtained a grant from Eli Lilly and Company that allowed them to do a pilot study of this intervention, as well as a chart review to characterize the patients who were recurrently being readmitted to their hospital. Consequently, they were able to get better agency buy-in to taking seriously the problem of recurrently readmitted patients and to systematize some of their work in addition to performing the studies noted in the subsequent text.

The Studies

CHART REVIEW

The goal of this study was to determine if the authors could identify distinctive characteristics of RRIPP. For the chart review they identified, over the period of slightly <9 months, 75 consecutive admissions of patients who were having a third (or more) psychiatric hospitalization within 18 months. These patients were then matched for comparison purposes with the next admitted patient who was not in the high-user category. After the close of the patient identification period, the recurrently admitted patients were compared with the nonrecurrently admitted patients. They discovered significant differences between these two groups. In regard to education, among the RRIPP only 51% had a high school degree or more, whereas among the comparison patients 71% had a high school degree or more. In regard to employment, 93% of recurrently were unemployed whereas 65% of the comparison group were unemployed. Diagnostically, RRIPP were much more likely to be schizophrenic (21% vs. 4%) or schizoaffective (31% vs. 7%), and these relationships were reversed when mood disorders were considered, such as 23% with depression in the comparison group versus 13% for the RRIPP. Taking all the psychotic diagnoses together, the RRIPP with a psychotic diagnosis had a period prevalence of 57%, whereas the comparison inpatients had a period prevalence of 30% with a psychotic diagnosis. The groups did not differ on age (both ~40 years old on average), on gender (both with slightly more females), or ethnicity (~59% white, 28% African American, 12% Hispanic).

The chart review helped the authors understand this group of patients in a general manner. It did not help them predict who will become RRIPP (as in other studies, these findings even when considered together are not sensitive or specific enough to be predictive). In that sense, the authors' work is like that of others.

PILOT STUDY OF THE HIGH-USER TREATMENT PLANNING GROUP

In addition to the chart review, the authors attempted a prospective pilot evaluation of the HUTPG approach. The design was to recruit patients as they came in who had a history or three or more admissions within the last 18 months and assign them to the HUTPG intervention that they designed; and to follow up patients for 6 months. The authors intended to compare patients' utilization experience before and after the HUTPG intervention in respect to the number of admissions and hospital days. They also planned to track how well patients were able to adhere to the conditions specified in their hospital-formulated HUTPG and to determine if particular features of the treatment plan were associated with outcome.

They were also able to do some community-based development work to maximize buy-in to the process and to document the ability of agencies to adhere to the requirement that all these patients have a hospital-based HUTPG. The agencies expecting to provide services agreed to send a senior member of their staff who was in a position to negotiate the allocation of resources on behalf of the patient. They held a half-day retreat with the appropriate agencies and used this occasion to review their understanding of these recurrently admitted patients and what was necessary to engage them in effective treatment. This turned out to be a very productive session that not only helped the authors develop a way of managing the HUTPG but also a way to think about a possible additional future intervention.

The HUTPG meetings were productive. A sensitive, concrete, and individualized treatment plan was formulated that included, at minimum, the following elements: (a) provision of safe and secure housing; (b) access to a clinical, sensitive treatment that included medication and psychological care; (c) case management services provided by the outpatient agency that would connect patients with critical resources, frequently provided by a visiting nurse group; and (d) plans for dealing with the sense of belonging in the community through social club participation, development of friendship patterns, development of social networks, and so on. A rating form was developed to capture the patient's adherence to the treatment plan once the patient left the hospital (see Table 13.2). The authors planned to follow up patients for 6 months after they were discharged, following treatment plan adherence, clinical condition, and rehospitalization experience.

Early on in the conduct of the research, the authors ran into a major difficulty. Although they found the number of recurrent admissions to be almost exactly what they expected; the recruitment rate

TABLE 13.2 FIDELITY RATINGS FORM

	Rating Date:				
Overall Ratings:	1	2	3	4	5
	No resemblance	Some elements in place	Half of essential elements in place	Some exceptions	Exactly as planned
Housing Plan Date:	**Rating Date:**			**Rating:**	
Housing Plan:	1	2	3	4	5
	Homeless	Unsuitable with family/friends	Shelter	Temporary but stable	Stable, consistent
Shelter Plan Date:	**Rating Date:**			**Rating:**	
Shelter Plan:	1	2	3	4	5
	No resemblance to plan	Some elements in place	Half of essential elements in place	Some exceptions	Exactly as planned
Food Plan Date:	**Rating Date:**			**Rating:**	
Food Plan:	1	2	3	4	5
	No provision	Inconsistent	Minimal	Variable but may be adaptable	Steady, consistent
Security Plan Date:	**Rating Date:**			**Rating:**	
Security Plan:	1	2	3	4	5
	Unsafe		Mostly stable, secure		Stable, secure

turned out to be a lowly 36% in contrast to the 75% rate that was planned. A variety of interventions were tried, including increasing the payment offered to patients for participation in follow-up interviews and reducing the amount of follow-up required, but none of these changes made a difference in the recruitment rate. They tried different interviewers including a team approach; but again, the patients showed an exquisite sensitivity to being followed, evaluated, and interviewed and seemed to share, in general, a feeling that they were better off by not being observed or followed in any way at all.

Although the initial participation of staff from the agencies was excellent, in studying the HUTPG, the authors found too much variation as time went on in how these groups were attended and conducted to provide a proper test of the intervention. Their efforts to have a consistent HUTPG intervention for all patients who qualified did not succeed. However, they were able to redefine a treatment review and planning process involving the major outpatient agency with whom they shared a bulk of the patients, a university-run community mental health center (the Connecticut Mental Health Center, [CMHC]) that serves the great majority of Department of Mental Health and Addiction Services (DMHAS) patients in the greater New Haven area, and for which YNHPH serves as the inpatient backup.

For the experimental project, 118 patients were deemed to be eligible for recruitment into the study during the 9-month recruitment time by virtue of their utilization experience. Of these, 91 were invited to participate in the study. Patients who were not invited to participate were either unable to give consent (because of the severity of their illness, their inability to read/speak English, or the presence of a developmental disability); or they were discharged before being approached by the recruiter. From these 91, 33 consented to being followed up after discharge from the hospital.

Of the 118 recidivists identified between September 2005 and May 2006, 53 (45%) patients had a HUTPG; 49 out of the 53 (92%) patients were present for and participated in their HUTPG; 33 of the 53 (62%) patients who participated in the HUTPG were rehospitalized within 6 months of the meeting was held. Of the 33 recidivists participating in the research follow-up study, 23 (70%) patients had a HUTPG before their discharge. Of the 33, 21 (64%) who were recruited to participate in the follow-up study were readmitted to YNHPH within 6 months of consenting to participate.

There was no difference in readmission between those for whom a HUTPG was held and those who did not have a HUTPG. However, the HUTPG assignment was not random, so that there may have been bias for sicker patients to have a HUTPG.

The authors did discover, however, that there were elements of the treatment planning process that predicted readmissions, some quite robustly. If they correlated elements of the treatment plan as it existed at discharge with subsequent readmission, they found that a variety of factors were associated with readmission. These included whether there was a good plan for food and housing, a clear plan for acquiring medication, the complexity of dosing regimens, whether case management was clearly available, how much the patient seemed to agree with the plan, and if the patient seemed motivated. These findings have been worked into a series of plans for change as noted in the subsequent text.

Case Vignette

Sonia is a 23-year-old African American, single female with multiple psychiatric admissions and various diagnoses, including borderline personality, schizoaffective disorder, and psychosis NOS. She also had set fires and was implicated in an ambiguous fire in her family's home 3 years before admission. As a teenager she had been bright and demonstrated promise, but she had become increasingly antisocial toward her family and uninvolved in school and had become involved with an antisocial, drug-using peer group.

Her treatment has been marked by multiple break-offs of therapeutic relationships and noncompliance with antipsychotic and mood-stabilizing medications. During her participation in the HUTPG she revealed that she had an interest in becoming a beautician, but had never had any formal training nor ever expressed this desire in a credible manner to others. She assumed that it was impossible to consider, given her circumstances. The treatment plan included a referral to a vocational rehabilitation agency that had the opportunity to provide her with beautician training. After a rocky discharge with some threatening and abusive behavior, she managed to settle down and attend the beautician training. She began to be minimally compliant with her medications as well.

At this writing, she has been out of the hospital for 24 months, longer than any time in the last 5 years, and seems to be participating effectively in becoming a beautician. She is on good terms with her family of origin.

Future

The future is well under way. Through the inspiration of the community-based meetings and the authors' experience with the treatment plan study patients, they have obtained funding to do a random allocation intervention study in which they train peer counselors to become "recovery guides"[30] and to use motivational interviewing as a technique to engage RRIPP while they are in the hospital and to follow up on them after hospitalization in an effort to assist them in becoming well connected to their service use. The recovery guide concept has been piloted in other settings in the Connecticut DMHAS for patients who have been hospitalized, but not particularly for RRIPP.[31] Furthermore, DMHAS has been successful in using motivational interviewing for training its peer counselors, so it is expected that this method will be possible to teach to people who are recovering from mental illness.

The recovery guides are patients who are in recovery and have the approval of their treatment teams to participate in a helping relationship with another patient. They receive 1 month of half-time training that emphasizes the role of a healing relationship from the provider's perspective. However, they do not have a formal clinical role and are not integrated into an ongoing clinical service. Their job is to try to connect with their mentees through at least twice-weekly, informal meetings, in order to provide a reassuring and inspirational presence as well as specific information about medication, services, and so on. They use motivational interviewing as a means to help the identified patients explore their ambivalence about psychiatric treatment, something that many of them are reluctant to do with mental health professionals.

In addition, the authors are making changes in their inpatient treatment approaches, centering upon the discharge and treatment planning processes. They have developed an approach that ensures that nursing staff and attending medical staff will review with patients their medication plan and all the elements as they approach discharge. Patients will be asked to demonstrate understanding and knowledge and will be invited to express any misgivings or reluctances. In addition, as a patient approaches discharge, medication administration is simplified as much as possible.

The authors continue to sponsor the HUTPG. Agencies providing services in the community will be encouraged to send their staff to the inpatient unit as referrals to their service approach discharge so that the patients will be familiar, at least in some manner, with those who are providing needed services. They believe that RRIPP are a group that justifies special efforts to engage them and bring them into the health care system on a collaborative basis. Not only is the expense of their recurrent hospitalizations wasteful, but also in a busy, oversubscribed system they can deny treatment to others through services being full or delay care to those who need it immediately through long waits in emergency rooms (ERs) and other places not set up to meet their needs.

LITERATURE ON TREATMENT

Geller[32] put forward the idea that for some frequently hospitalized patients, recidivism has become a way of life. Neither refractoriness to treatment nor noncompliance with medication explains their frequent admissions. His suggested treatment approach is still useful.

1. The patient's behavior is in response to some form of personal or interpersonal deficit.
2. The institution has some form of social meaning for the patient.
3. The problems and solutions are at the interface of the hospital and the community.
4. The patient's autonomy is not limitless.
5. The treatment plan must be comprehensive, consistent, and enforceable.
6. All treatment sites must endorse the treatment plan.
7. The patient must understand the treatment plan.
8. The providers and the patient should review the treatment plan at regularly scheduled intervals.
9. The treatment plan should be modified in response to patterns of behavior, not instances of behavior.
10. The long and short of it is that it is going to be long.

All systems of medical services that provide care for a broad range of patients have the experience that a few patients account for a disproportionate share of the resource use.[33] The hospitalizations of psychiatric patients is no exception. There will always be something of a mismatch between the needs of a small group of patients and the resources readily available for their care. The organization of health care systems does not allow for the routine responsiveness of individualized care to issues that are not relatively common or for which there are not clear solutions within the medical context. The American health care system is oriented toward responding to acute medical concerns, and psychiatric hospitalization is no exception to this approach. The rehabilitative and restorative functions that were served by some psychiatric hospitalization in the premanaged care era are no longer the function and goals of psychiatric hospitalization.

As Klinkenberg and Calsyn[7] noted in their literature review, a theoretic paradigm puts into perspective the various forces impinging on recidivism. This is summarized in Figure 13.1, adapted from

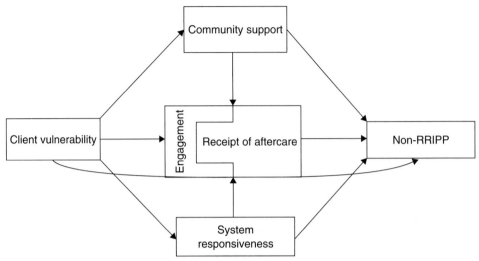

■ **Figure 13.1** Theoretic model of variables contributing to recurrent readmission and receipt of aftercare. RRIPP, recurrently readmitted inpatient psychiatric patients. (Modified from Klinkenberg WD, Calsyn RJ. Predictors of receipt of aftercare and recidivism among persons with severe mental illness: A review. *Psychiatr Serv.* 1996;47[5]:487–96.)

their review.[7] The literature has focused on the issues of client vulnerability, but system responsiveness and community support have not been emphasized in most studies. The authors' modification of this model would be to interpose capacity for engagement as an element of receipt of aftercare, as well as an important variable predicting RR. In many ways, the inability to collaborate and engage with others effectively is one of the substantial patient vulnerability or deficit issues that the RRIPP bring to their failures to stay out of the hospital. However, like any relationship concept, engagement, as a process issue, also belongs to the system responsiveness, community support, and client vulnerability domains. From the authors' literature review and their clinical experience, it is concluded that recurrent admission is associated with impairment in the ability to engage in treatment. This deficit derives from demographic and social factors, such as lack of education, lack of social support, youth, unemployment, and being unmarried; and also from factors intrinsic to a psychotic disorder. Consequently, special efforts should be made to provide alternative networks of advice and support upon which the patient may feel comfortable relying. Like the Klinkenberg and Calsyn model, this hypothesis is intended to be a heuristic device to focus efforts of future research as well as future program planning. The authors believe it is safe to say that recurrently admitted patients tend not to be so different on most measures from their less recurrently admitted peers.

The needs of RRIPP are not served by acute hospitalization except in a narrow sense of safety and relief of acute symptoms. Not infrequently, their needs are not met anywhere, in which case they may continue to bang on the door of whatever is available. Without appropriate services, they will inevitably default to a level of care that meets an essential experienced need but which has a level of intensity that is inappropriate overall, and consequently the costs are disproportionate to costs of needed services. In other words, the level of the care is frequently inappropriate. Such patients may be discharged before their nonmedical needs are met and, hence, get into trouble again. And their nonmedical needs can be overwhelming to most agencies that care for them.

Until some system of care has the managerial and programmatic resources to deal with these problematic patients effectively, there needs to be a way for those working in hospitals to cope with such clinical problems. What follows are some suggested elements to take into consideration. They are not particularly specific to RRIPP, for these patients are not a specific enough group to justify great specificity in treatment. Rather, these are intended to focus on what Geller[34] called the interface between the hospital and the community. These are sound practices for all treatment planning, only more so for dealing with the RR phenomenon.

1. *Treatment planning.* The authors' interest in this topic began with the idea that effective treatment planning was an approach that could help solve or modify this problem. They still believe this to be true. Treatment planning begins with the comprehensive understanding of the patient, historically and currently. For instance, it is essential to know the trend and pattern of the patient's illness and his or her attempts at adaptation to it. What have been the ups and downs? What has characterized the periods of stability as well as instability? What symptoms have been prominent in what circumstances? Also, what treatments have been tried and with what effect? And by treatments the authors mean the response not only to medication, but also to psychosocial treatments. Did the patient show an interest in activities that might lead to employment? Was the patient able to establish a friend or two outside the hospital? What was the drug, alcohol, and tobacco use? And, of course, the details of the patient's relationship to family, of origin as well as procreation, are extremely important.

2. *Communication.* It goes without saying that the process of treating complex, elusive patients is itself complex and involves many different disciplines: psychiatry, medicine, social work, nursing, psychology, and so on in many different roles. All members of the treatment team must communicate clearly and effectively with one another as well as with the patient and the patient's family. The individual roles of treatment team members must be clear to all concerned. Frequently, role is based on discipline such as physician, nurse, social worker, and so on. However, individuals are infinitely varied and some do some things better than others so that treatment teams almost always feature subtle differentiations of structure and function. This informal organization must be self-consciously understood, or there will be errors, failed assumptions, and miscommunications with resultant disappointments and resentments.

3. *Discharge process.* For RRIPP, it is wise to review everything in great detail, especially given our findings of the association of various elements of treatment planning and discharge before the patient leaves the hospital with their being subsequently readmitted. It is of major importance to make sure that the patient clearly understands and accepts all elements of the treatment plan. Ambivalences and uncertainties must be freely expressed and explored. A treatment plan must include having a place to live and eat, and all elements of clinical care, especially medications, must be clear, including not only dosage and administration but also how to acquire the medications. For patients on complex drug regimens, it makes sense to make the administration as simple as possible, opting for daily doses (rather than divided doses whenever possible), and making sure that the concrete elements of the treatment plan are clearly understood. Visual aids, calendars, diaries, and medications boxes can all make a difference. Someone on the team must ensure that these functions get covered.

4. *Effective collaborations.* For an acute inpatient service that takes care of seriously ill patients to function properly there must be collaborations with rehabilitative and outpatient services that can respond to treatment planning efforts and create an individualized treatment program that will be responsive to the patient's particular needs. There can be no taking for granted that patients are able to figure out what they need for the basics of independent or supported living outside the hospital. The treatment plan must provide adequate resources in the domains of food, shelter, clinical care, and case management as well as a rehabilitative program that includes socialization and as productive as possible a way of spending time.

5. *Program.* There needs to be a process that identifies patients at risk for RR and ensures that all that can be done on their behalf is accomplished. A tracking procedure at admissions should identify patients with previous recurrent admissions and bring their status to the attention of the treatment team so that resources can be put into place as soon as possible. The program should consist of special care of carrying out the principles noted in the preceding text.
   Of course there must be effective outpatient array of services that ensures basic food and shelter, as well as daily structure for a meaningful and appropriately stimulating community life. In this regard, there should be clear-cut arrangements with community services to make sure that the tried-and-true elements are in place: medication, psychosocial treatments, and meaningful community involvement combined with an active outreach and case management program.

6. *Review and evaluation.* As with any program, a process should monitor whether the desired processes and outcomes are being met. Although the procedures recommended in preceding text

are basically good care for all patients, their effectiveness depends on constant attention and rigorous administrative support. The only way to know for sure that they are being carried out is to have a continuous quality assessment and improvement plan.

Conclusion

The authors believe that there are solutions to the recurrently readmitted inpatient psychiatric (RRIP) phenomenon, despite the sometimes contradictory literature. High-quality treatment planning adhering to the standards noted in preceding text, with a particular emphasis on attention to engaging patients with their caretakers, has promise for breaking the "revolving door" in which some patients seem to be stuck. The care of those with severe mental illness is complex and seems at times to be open ended. Recurrently readmitted patients seem to be an exaggeration of all the disordered elements of patients' lives. The suffering of patients and families alone justifies the authors' greatest efforts at alleviation. They believe that creative, resourceful, and persistent treatment planning can be effective in relieving some of these problems.

REFERENCES

1. Franklin JL, Kittredge LD, Thrasher JH. A survey of factors related to mental hospital readmissions. *Hosp Community Psychiatry.* 1975;26(11):749–751.
2. Kinard EM. Discharged patients who desire to return to the hospital. *Hosp Community Psychiatry.* 1981;32(3):194–197.
3. Geller JL. A historical perspective on the role of state hospitals viewed from the era of the "Revolving Door". *Am J Psychiatry.* 1992;149(11): 1526–1533.
4. Grob GN. Deinstitutionalization of the mentally ill. Policy triumph or tragedy? *N J Med.* 2004; 101(12):19–30.
5. Rosenblatt A, Mayer JE. The recidivism of mental patients: A review of the past studies. *Am J Orthopsychiatry.* 1974;44(5): 697–706.
6. Kent S, Fogarty M, Yellowlees P. A review of studies of heavy users of psychiatric services. *Psychiatr Serv.* 1995;46(12):1247–1253.
7. Klinkenberg WD, Calsyn RJ. Predictors of receipt of aftercare and recidivism among persons with severe mental illness: A review. *Psychiatr Serv.* 1996;47(5):487–496.
8. Roick C, Gartner A, Heider D, et al. Heavy users of psychiatric care: A review of the state of research. *Psychiatr Prax.* 2002;29:334–342.
9. Byers ES, Cohen SH. Predicting patient outcome: The contribution of prehospital, inhospital, and posthospital factors. *Hosp Community Psychiatry.* 1979;30(5):327–331.
10. DiScipio WJ, Sommer G. Therapeutic failures: Patients who return within 30 days of hospital discharge. *Psychiatr Q.* 1973;47:371–376.
11. Voineskos G, Denault S. Recurrent psychiatric hospitalization. *CMAJ.* 1978;118:247–250.
12. Solomon P, Doll W. The varieties of readmission: The case against the use of recidivism rates as a measure of program effectiveness. *Am J Orthopsychiatry.* 1979;49(2):230–239.
13. Erickson RC, Paige AB. Fallacies in using lenth of stay and return rates as measures of success. *Hosp Community Psychiatry.* 1973;24(8):559–561.
14. Appleby L, Desai PN, Luchins DJ, et al. Length of stay and recidivism in schizophrenia: A study of public psychiatric hospital patients. *Am J Psychiatry.* 1993;150(1):72–76.
15. Carpenter MD, Mulligan JC, Bader SA, et al. Multiple admissions to an urban psychiatric center: A comparative study. *Hosp Community Psychiatry.* 1985;36(12):1305–1308.
16. Green JH. Frequent rehospitalization and noncompliance with treatment. *Hosp Community Psychiatry.* 1988;39(9):963–966.
17. Casper ES, Donaldson B. Subgroups in the population of frequent users of inpatient services. *Hosp Community Psychiatry.* 1990;41(2):189–191.
18. Casper ES, Egan JR. Reasons for admission among six profile subgroups of recidivists of inpatient services. *Can J Psychiatry.* 1993;38: 657–661.
19. Casper ES, Pastva G. Admission histories, patterns, and subgroups of the heavy users of a state psychiatric hospital. *Psychiatr Q.* 1990;61(2): 121–134.
20. Haywood TW, Kravitz HM, Grossman LS, et al. Predicting the "Revolving Door" phenomenon among patients with schizophrenic, schizoaffective, and affective disorders. *Am J Psychiatry.* 1995;152(6):856–861.
21. Lucas B, Harrison-Read P, Tyrer P, et al. Costs and characteristics of heavy inpatient service users in outer London. *Int J Soc Psychiatry.* 2001;47(1): 63–74.
22. Kent S, Yellowlees P. Psychiatric and social reasons for frequent rehospitalization. *Hosp Community Psychiatry.* 1994;45(4):347–350.
23. Appleby L, Desai PN. Documenting the relationship between homelessness and psychiatric hospitalization. *Hosp Community Psychiatry.* 1985;36:732–737.

24. Casper ES. Identifying multiple recidivists in a state hospital population. *Psychiatr Serv*. 1995; 46(10):1074–1075.

25. Weiden PJ, Olfson M. Cost of relapse in schizophrenia. *Schizophr Bull*. 1995;21(3):419–429.

26. Dietzen LL, Bond GR. Relationship between case manager contact and outcome for frequently hospitalized psychiatric clients. *Hosp Community Psychiatry*. 1993;44(9):839–843.

27. Dincin J, Wasmer D, Witheridge TF, et al. Impact of assertive community treatment on the use of state hospital inpatient bed days. *Hosp Community Psychiatry*. 1993;44(9):833–838.

28. Swartz MS, Swanson JW, Wagner HR, et al. Can involuntary outpatient commitment reduce hospital recidivism?: Findings from a randomized trial with severely mentally ill individuals. *Am J Psychiatry*. 1999;156(12):1968–1975.

29. Prince JD. Practices preventing rehospitalization of individuals with schizophrenia. *J Nerv Ment Dis*. 2006;194(6):397–403.

30. Davidson L, O'Connell M, Tondora J, et al. Recovery in serious mental illness: A new wine or just a new bottle? *Prof Psychol Res Pr*. 2005;36(5): 480–487.

31. Davidson L, Kirk T, Rockholz P, et al. Creating a recovery-oriented system of behavioral health care: Moving from concept to reality. *Psychiatr Rehabil J*. 2007;31(1):23–31.

32. Geller JL. In again, out again: Preliminary evaluation of a state hospital's worst recidivists. *Hosp Community Psychiatry*. 1986;37(4):386–390.

33. Mustard CA, Derksen S, Tataryn D. Intensive use of mental health care. *Can J Psychiatry*. 1996; 41:93–101.

34. Geller JL. Treating revolving-door patients who have "Hospitalphilia": Compassion, coercion, and common sense. *Hosp Community Psychiatry*. 1993;44(2):141–146.

35. Buell GJ, Anthony WA. Demographic characteristics as predictors of recidivism and posthospital employment. *J Couns Psychol*. 1973; 20(4):361–365.

36. Fontana AF, Dowds BN. Assessing treatment outcome II: The prediction of rehospitalization. *J Nerv Ment Dis*. 1975;161(4):231–238.

37. Joyce PR, Khan A, Jones AV. The revolving door patient. *Compr Psychiatry*. 1981;22(4): 397–403.

38. Lambert EW, Sherwood V, Fitzpatrick LJ. Predicting recidivism among first admissions at Tennessee's state psychiatric hospitals. *Hosp Community Psychiatry*. 1983;34(10): 951–953.

39. Abramowitz SI, Tupin JP, Berger A. Multivariate prediction of hospital readmission. *Compr Psychiatry*. 1984;25(1):71–76.

40. Setz PJ, Bond GR. Psychiatric recidivism in a psychosocial rehabilitation setting: A survival analysis. *Hosp Community Psychiatry*. 1985;36(5):521–524.

41. Woogh CM. A cohort through the revolving door. *Can J Psychiatry*. 1986;31:214–221.

42. Surber RW, Winkler EL, Monteleone M, et al. Characteristics of high users of acute psychiatric inpatient services. *Hosp Community Psychiatry*. 1987;38(10):1112–1114.

43. Havassy BE, Hopkin JT. Factors predicting utilization of acute psychiatric inpatient services by frequently hospitalized patients. *Hosp Community Psychiatry*. 1989;40(8):820–823.

44. Hadley TR, McGurrin MC, Pulice RT, et al. Using fiscal data to identify heavy service users. *Psychiatr Q*. 1990;61(1):41–48.

45. Swett C. Symptom severity and number of previous psychiatric admissions as predictors of readmission. *Psychiatr Serv*. 1995;46(5):482–485.

46. Kent S, Fogarty M, Yellowlees P. Heavy utilization of inpatient and outpatient services in a public mental health service. *Psychiatr Serv*. 1995;46(12):1254–1257.

47. Postrado LT, Lehman AF. Quality of life and clinical predictors of rehospitalization of persons with severe mental illness. *Psychiatr Serv*. 1995;46(11):1161–1165.

48. Sanguineti V, Samuel SE, Schwartz SL, et al. Retrospective study of 2,200 involuntary psychiatric admissions and readmissions. *Am J Psychiatry*. 1996;153(3):392–396.

49. Lyons JS, O'Mahoney MT, Miller SI, et al. Predicting readmission to the psychiatric hospital in a managed care environment: Implications for quality indicators. *Am J Psychiatry*. 1997; 154(3):337–340.

50. Perlick DA, Rosenheck RA, Clarkin JF, et al. Symptoms predicting inpatient service use among patients with bipolar affective disorder. *Psychiatr Serv*. 1999;50(6):806–812.

51. Roick C, Heider D, Kilian R, et al. Factors contributing to frequent use of psychiatric inpatient services by schizophrenia patients. *Soc Psychiatry Psychiatr Epidemiol*. 2004;39:744–751.

52. Bobo WV, Hoge CW, Messina MA, et al. Characteristics of repeat users of an inpatient psychiatry service at a large military tertiary care hospital. *Mil Med*. 2004;169:648–653.

53. Rosca P, Bauer A, Grinspoon A, et al. Rehospitalizations among psychiatric patients whose first admission was involuntary: A 10 year follow-up. *Isr J Psychiatry Relat Sci*. 2006;43(1):57–64.

CHAPTER 14

The Patient with Borderline Personality Disorder

ANTHONY W. BATEMAN

F ew areas of psychiatric investigation have seen such radical progress in the field of personality disorder (PD), particularly the understanding and treatment of borderline personality disorder (BPD). The advances in knowledge have been influenced and propelled by the discovery of relatively effective outpatient[1,2] and partial hospital[3] psychosocial treatments shown to accelerate improvement and the increasing recognition that the course of the disorder is not as chronic and malign as hitherto believed. Taken together, this emerging knowledge has resulted in a reappraisal of treatment contexts, organization of treatment, and focus of services for BPD. Until the 1990s, long-term inpatient treatment for BPD was considered desirable. Many hospitals offered inpatient treatment programmes lasting a year or more. This is now rare. The loss of long-term inpatient treatment for BPD, introduced for financial rather than clinical reasons, may inadvertently have led to significant improvement in the outcomes for the condition. In this chapter, the author will first explore this controversial suggestion. Second, he will consider the service changes in terms of an improving evidence base. Finally, he will discuss the current role of inpatient psychiatry in the treatment of BPD.

Borderline Personality Disorder

The key deficits, as opposed to descriptive characteristics, associated with BPD are normally thought to include impulsiveness, difficulty in managing emotions, and difficulties in relationships.[4] It has been suggested that these vulnerabilities in part arise out of problems with mentalization, that is a limited ability to perceive mental states in self and others accurately.[5] They may also be linked to problems with differentiating self and others and identity diffusion, which some authors see as central to BPD.[6-8] Certainly, difficulties with distinguishing self and others in BPD have been demonstrated in analog studies using film clips[9] and narratives of childhood experience.[10]

The development of mentalizing abilities has been discussed in detail elsewhere.[5,11] On the whole, the capacity to mentalize is a developmentally determined skill. Shutting down of mentalizing or inhibition of its development commonly occurs in response to attachment trauma. It is quite likely that high levels of arousal following traumatic experience contribute to suppressing the functioning of the frontal areas of the brain that normally underpin mentalization.[12,13] In effect, an interdependent process between environmental factors and neurobiologic development determines both an individual's baseline capacity to mentalize and the threshold at which their ability is lost during emotional states and in other stressful circumstances.

This developmental perspective is supported by family studies, a number of which have identified factors that may be important in the development of BPD. However, few of the studies point to the specific features of parenting that create a vulnerability for BPD. Physical, sexual, and emotional abuse all occur in a family context and high rates are reported in BPD.[14] Overall researchers have concluded that abuse alone is neither necessary nor sufficient for the development of BPD and that predisposing factors and contextual features of the parent–child relationship are likely to be mediating factors in its actual development. Parental responses play an important role in the pathogenetic effects of abuse with parental responsiveness (believing the reports, protecting, and not expressing high levels of anger) following reports of abuse promoting more rapid adjustment[15] and lack of emotional responsiveness as well as low support and inadequate validation possibly potentiating the effects. Therefore, caregiver response to the abuse may be more important than the abuse itself in long-term outcome.[16]

Taking all this into account, the mentalization approach to BPD predicts that it is not the fact of maltreatment but it is more the family environment that discourages coherent discourse concerning mental states and it is this that is likely to predispose the child to BPD—nonmentalizing processing leads to nonmentalizing responses. The mentalizing model suggests that individuals with BPD, while able to mentalize, are more likely to abandon the capacity under high emotional arousal, for example, in response to maltreatment, because mentalization was not well established during the first decade of life in part as a consequence of early maltreatment and its associated problems. The impact of trauma is most likely to be felt as part of a more general failure of consideration of the child's perspective through neglect, rejection, excessive control, unsupportive relationship, incoherence, and confusion. These can devastate the experiential world of the developing child and leave deep scars which are evident in their later social cognitive functioning and behavior.

This formulation converges with that advanced by Marsha Linehan[17] concerning the assumption of the invalidating family environments and developed further by Alan Fuzzetti et al.[18,19] These workers report that parental invalidation, in part defined as the undermining of self-perceptions of internal states, was not only associated with the young person's reports of family distress, their own distress, and psychological problems but also with aspects of social cognition, namely their ability to identify and label emotion. Along with other aspects contributing to the complex interaction described as invalidating, this amounts to a systematic undermining of a person's experience of their own mind by the replacement of their mind with another or a failure to encourage discrimination between their own feelings and experiences and those of the caregiver.

In BPD, inhibition of mentalization occurs specifically in the context of intimate attachment relationships. Although the deficit in mentalizing, characteristic of BPD, is partial, temporary, and relationship-specific, it is a core problem of the disorder. This is not a trivial point clinically because any treatment or any interactive context in which relationships are of significance, for example, psychotherapy or inpatient milieu will result in loss of mentalizing following stimulation of the attachment relationship. As a consequence, psychotherapies focusing on the relationship between patient and therapist and contexts intrinsically operating a high-pressure relational environment such as inpatient facilities might cause harm to borderline patients. There is some evidence for this.

LONG-TERM INPATIENT ADMISSION AND THE REALITY OF IATROGENIC HARM

Two carefully designed fully powered prospective studies have highlighted the inappropriateness of the attitudes that confined individuals with severe PD to the margins of even generous health care systems.[20] Most patients with BPD experience a substantial reduction in their symptoms far sooner than previously assumed.[21,22] This is in marked contrast to the evidence about the longitudinal course presented in the 1980s which suggested a chronic course leading to "burnt out borderlines." It transpires that after 6 years 75% of patients diagnosed with BPD achieve remission by standardized diagnostic criteria. Patients with BPD *can* undergo remission—a concept that had previously been solely used in the context of Axis I pathology. Approximately 50% remission rate has occurred by 4 years but the remission is steady (10% to 15% per year). Recurrences are rare, perhaps no more than 10% over 6 years. This contrasts with the natural course of many Axis I disorders, such as affective disorder, where improvement may be somewhat more rapid but recurrences are common. In the Collaborative Depression Study, 30% of the patients had not recovered at 1 year, 19% at 2 years, and 12% at 5 years.[23]

While improvements of BPD are substantial, it should be noted that it is symptoms such as impulsivity and associated self-mutilation and suicidality that show dramatic change and not affective symptoms or social and interpersonal functioning. The dramatic symptoms (self-mutilation, suicidality, quasi-psychotic thoughts often seen as requiring urgent hospitalization) recede but abandonment concerns, sense of emptiness, relationship problems, and vulnerability to depression are likely to remain present in at least half the patients. When dramatic improvements occur, they sometimes occur quickly, quite often associated with relief from severely stressful situations.[24]

It seems that certain comorbidities undermine the likelihood of improvement;[25] the persistence of substance use disorders decreases the likelihood of remission, suggesting that the latter must be treated.

But it also seems that treatment contexts can also subvert natural improvement. Negative findings to emerge from the literature in relation to intensive inpatient treatment concern the greater efficacy of briefer periods of hospitalization,[26] the general ineffectiveness of brief hospital admissions motivated by suicide threats,[27] and the uncertain value of combining short intensive inpatient admissions with structured psychotherapeutic interventions[28] in which only 48% of patients show clinically significant improvement (but see later). Chiesa et al. compared two models of psychosocial intervention for PD. People with PD were allocated (but not randomly) either to a one-stage treatment model (inpatient for 1 year with no specialist after care) or to a two-stage model (6-month inpatient admission followed by outreach treatment), and were prospectively compared. It was found that the subjects in the two-stage sample did significantly better on global assessment of mental health and in social adjustment at 12 months. Subjects with BPD allocated to the two-stage model improved significantly more than such patients in the one-stage model. The pattern was maintained in follow-up. Patients in shorter admission programme were found to self-mutilate, attempt suicide, and be readmitted significantly less at 24- and 36-month follow-up than patients in the longer-term inpatient group and these differences have now been shown to continue at 6-year follow-up.[29] In addition, patients admitted to the shorter programme were 5.5 times less likely to drop out early than those admitted to the more intensive admission.[30] Inevitably, the better outcome and less intensive intervention was more cost-effective.[31]

So what could be made of this evidence? Could the apparent improvement in the course of the disorder over the last decade be accounted for by harmful treatments, in this case prolonged inpatient treatment being less frequently offered? If correct, this is possibly more a consequence of the changing pattern of health care particularly in the United States[32] than recognition by clinicians of the possibility of iatrogenic deterioration and subsequent avoidance of damaging side effects. This suggestion is speculative but it requires further consideration although evidence from the recent longitudinal studies does not tell whether interventions that were delivered were effective or inappropriate.

Mechanism of Harm

If it is correct that borderline patients are more sensitive to protracted inpatient treatment than other groups of patients as suggested by the evidence, entering inpatient facilities is likely to be a highly stressful event. The very act of casting off everyday responsibilities to interact with a large group of patients is likely to stimulate the attachment system to a degree that easily overwhelms even the most robust individual. As previously mentioned, from a mentalizing perspective, the borderline patient is uniquely sensitive to stimulation of the attachment system and a rapid reduction in mentalizing capacity is inevitable when this occurs. Once mentalizing has been reduced, the mind goes "off line" and behavioral responses to stress are triggered.

The fact that starting treatment in an inpatient facility reduces mentalizing has been given more direct support from a study in Belgium. Vermote et al.[33] studied a group of patients with personality disorder admitted to a 1-year inpatient treatment programme. Defining three groups of patients—low, medium, and high symptom level—they identified different trajectories of treatment.

A small group of low-level patients presented few symptoms at the outset, had a high level of borderline personality organization, and were in crisis when admitted to the hospital. They recovered fast and did not need prolonged inpatient treatment for symptom amelioration.

The group with a high frequency of symptoms had a low-level borderline personality organization. *Post hoc* tests showed that they were considerably more paranoid, hostile, and vindictive than the other groups. The trajectory of this group is remarkable. They only improved in the last quarter of the treatment, an improvement that continued in the posttreatment phase.

The group with a moderate level of symptoms showed two distinct trajectories—one with a good outcome and the other with a poor outcome. This was not simply related to severity of borderline pathology and therefore, the authors investigated other characteristics finding that the good outcome group corresponded to those patients with dismissive avoidant attachment styles. The patients were characterized by avoidant, paranoid, schizoid, and narcissistic features. These features are similar to Blatt's categorization of an introjective group,[34,35] who are thought to do better with exploratory/interpretive therapy.[36] The poor outcome group showed all the features of BPD but with anaclitic features rather than controlling an introjective attitude. They reported more sexual abuse and other early traumas. Their poor outcome was considered to be related to the lack of support early in treatment. Vermote concludes that these patients were included too soon in a classic psychoanalytic interpretive group approach and were easily overwhelmed by the intensity of involvement on entering the inpatient facility.

During the first few weeks of admission all patients showed a reduction in mentalizing abilities as evidenced by the reflective function scale and the object relation inventory. Interestingly therapists rated this period as positive in contrast to the patients who only felt the considerable distress. This phenomenon of worsening of symptoms at the beginning of treatment has been considered as regression in the service of progression by therapists, but it is also the most likely cause of the high drop-out rate reported in studies of intensive treatments (36% in this study) as patients attempt to restabilize by leaving a toxic environment. This early reduction in mental capacity to manage emotional states should not be conflated with changes over the longer term. Gabbard et al.[37] observed little evidence of regression following prolonged inpatient treatment for PD. In a prospective study of 216 patients with severe PD treated at the Menninger Clinic for variable lengths of time in two psychoanalytically orientated inpatient units, they found positive change at discharge and 1-year follow-up, with no evidence of deleterious effects due to regression and dependency. But this finding applied to those patients who remained in the treatment programme and not to those who left in the first few weeks. So once the initial period of admission to inpatient treatment has been successfully negotiated borderline patients may do well.

Overall, the evidence suggests that loss in mentalizing triggered by a highly stimulating inpatient environment and treatment programme has to be managed if drop out is to be reduced and borderline patients are to be treated in inpatient programmes. Overall response of the patient to treatment and reaction to the early phase of inpatient treatment may also be determined by their personality characteristics. A high symptomatic group with anaclitic characteristics profits more from a supportive and structuring approach whereas an introjective group profits more by an explorative approach and may be able to manage the stimulation of inpatient treatment early on. Personality style is more important than severity of PD. Rather than blandly stating that long-term inpatient treatment is contraindicated for PD it seems that it may be a reasonable option for some patients depending on their personality style.

If long-term hospitalization for PD is to occur there are a number of practice points that need to be considered. Main's[38] classic paper should act as a reminder that regression and countertransference difficulties may pose considerable difficulties for teams treating patients intensively. Management structures need to be transparent, robust, and responsive so that decisions about admission, discharge, organization of the programme, and staff support can be taken rapidly. Leadership is important to instil appropriate attitudes and maintain a coherent therapeutic programme. Also it ensures that the staff feel empowered to work with patients who may be emotionally challenging and who may imperceptibly undermine carefully constructed boundaries. Supervision needs to be integrated into the work patterns of staff with consideration of countertransference responses toward patients. Unless a safe haven for discussion of countertransference is created destructive acting out may be the result.[39] Finally, the overall goals of the admission must be developed at the beginning of treatment with some agreement about the steps that are required to reach them. Development with the patient of ways to monitor progress is helpful to ensure that the focus on intermediate goals as stepping-stones to overall goals is maintained. This protects from admission interminable with the hope that the longer the patient continues in hospital the more likely he is to improve. This is not necessarily the case.

Team Work

Whenever borderline patients are admitted to hospital for acute or short- or long-term treatment good staff team work is essential. Developing a specialist team for borderline patients has been suggested as the best way forward.[40] Evidence from treatment trials suggests that specialist teams are important for successful outcomes and for reducing drop-out rates substantially. Even with a specialist team, good working relationships within the team and close collaboration are essential if treatment is to be consistent and implemented according to agreed protocols.

Reactions of even experienced staff to patients with BPD commonly subvert the task of treatment and lead to inappropriate actions on the part of staff.[41,42] Careful attention to countertransference in a good working team reduces the likelihood of unprofessional conduct. It is the lone practitioner who is at most risk of engaging in inappropriate behavior fuelled by unprocessed countertransference responses. Teams can protect each other by providing peer discussion and frequent clinical discussion.

Patients need to feel that those responsible for their care communicate frequently and effectively, resolve differences, and maintain clear boundaries of treatment. Integrating different perspectives is the very core of mentalizing. In order to understand different professional perspectives within a team of nurses, doctors, psychologists, and therapists some inpatient teams employ what has been called the *skill share model* of care[43] in which each member learns the skills of other members, at least at a basic level. The team is therefore never depleted of skills and team members can substitute for each other at times of absence. The skill share model may remove rivalry between professional disciplines but needs trust, good management, and leadership, especially if different members are paid different salaries.

Leadership is necessary to ensure that agreed interventions and protocols are implemented within a team and requires a willingness on the part of a team to assign the responsibility of leadership to a member of the team as well as that member being willing to undertake the leadership role. Underlying rivalries within a team will inevitably bring with them inconsistency as members of the team attempt to develop greater influence. For effective team work, the natural tendency of any one person to want to make an individual contribution has to become subdominant to the team itself. In order to achieve this, development of an iterative process is necessary in which the team moves toward a consensus that is then held by the team itself. New members of the team can then be educated by the team in the team perspective.

One of the reasons why those with PDs create so many problems in treatment is that they evoke inconsistency. From a psychodynamic perspective inconsistency arises when "splitting" occurs within teams. Splitting is regarded as arising for a number of reasons and, whenever it occurs, the most important point is to try to establish its meaning. Sometimes, externally manifested splitting may simply be a result of poor team communication whilst at other times it may be a representation of the internal processes of the patient. Yet at other times splitting within therapists or teams can result from their own unresolved transferences and have little to do with the patient. Different causes of splitting need different interventions. Splitting arising in the context of unresolved transferences needs team work rather than patient work but splitting emanating from projections of the patient may need clinical discussion within the team followed by dialogue with the patient. Gabbard[39] cautions against overzealous attempts to repair differences as they may be an important safety valve.

Restricting the people involved in care to those whose roles and tasks are clear reduces the chances of creating inconsistency. Consistency is likely to be improved by a specialist team approach as long as the team itself is cohesive which may necessitate good team support. Constancy and consistency of protocol implementation is necessary to avoid mirroring the fragmented mind of the patient with fragmented care. In order to do this, keeping the numbers of practitioners to a minimum level is helpful but the most important aspect is to avoid changes wherever possible. This is of particular relevance in the treatment of BPD in which changes in professionals may trigger experiences associated with loss, abandonment, and despair that are so common in their current and past relationships.[44] Senior figures who show few changes over time are clearly preferable and probably more so than in the management of other psychiatric disorders.

ANTISOCIAL PERSONALITY DISORDER

The iatrogenic effects of hospital admission may be worse for those patients who are comorbid for BPD and antisocial personality disorder (ASPD). This is probably a relatively common combination but most research studies on outcome of treatment often exclude such patients believing that their outcomes are poor. Paris[45] has argued that BPD and ASPD have common precursors but the expression of the underlying problem is influenced by gender with women being more likely to present with behaviors associated with BPD and men with those of ASPD. A further complication of this group is the presence of narcissistic problems which makes potential treatment extremely difficult. The admixture of borderline, antisocial, and narcissistic characteristics is a potent brew and may not be obvious at the time of presentation. Patients present more often with overt behavioral or emotional disturbance and so are more frequently considered to have BPD initially. It is only later that their disregard of others, their deceitfulness, and their irresponsibility become clearer. But by then it is too late and they already have a place in a treatment programme. Inpatient treatment may not only cause problems for the individual concerned but also the individual will create dissent within a harmonious group of patients, require excessive attention, subvert the system, and flout rules in a way that is difficult for staff to address. These patients often treat the hospital as an authoritarian institution and rapidly challenge obvious rules by returning to the ward drunk or bringing drugs on to the ward. This is done secretly but often staff is alerted to it by other patients or by obvious clinical signs. When they challenge the patient, they are themselves challenged to prove their "accusations" whilst the patient declares himself/herself misunderstood. In the end no one knows who is being truthful and the patient–staff relationship may deteriorate to one of accused/accuser. Overall, it may be necessary not to admit such a patient to an inpatient unit simply to protect the other patients from exploitation. Once admitted he may form relationships based on control and power often with a vulnerable dependent borderline patient. This is an area that requires thoughtful consideration.

Case Vignette

A 28-year-old male patient with ASPD was admitted to hospital following an overdose. He rapidly seemed to recover from his initial distress but then negotiated a longer admission to help him with his drug use and for advice about alcohol. This appeared to be a reasonable request and so a 4-week admission was planned. At the end of the first week, he was seen going out of the hospital with a 24-year-old female patient with depression and BPD. A few days later the staff, having seen them together on a number of occasions, asked them if they were having a relationship and informed them that the unit strongly recommended patients in the treatment programme did not have relationships. This was documented in the notes. Following this the two patients were not seen together by staff. But it turned out that they had continued to develop a relationship and when the male patient left hospital the female patient discharged herself to go to live with him. This was a surprise to staff who again cautioned strongly against it. Three months later the father of the borderline patient sued the hospital for not preventing his daughter being "used" by the male patient who had been physically abusive to her and imprisoned her in his flat to prevent her leaving him. The case was unsuccessful primarily because the staff had made clear notes of their recommendations to both patients and the patients themselves had actively prevented the staff from discovering their continuing relationship.

Despite these cautions, practitioners are in a difficult position with patients with ASPD. Their suicide rate is 3.7 times higher than comparable community subjects, 9 times greater if they are older than 30 years of age and they have a lifetime risk of at least 5%.[46] They are at considerable risk to themselves and perhaps not surprisingly their suicide attempts more often involve violent means.[47] However, it is unlikely that this risk to themselves is reduced by inpatient treatment and such patients are best managed as outpatients. Admission to hospital should be for the short-term only.

SHORT-TERM HOSPITALIZATION

The role of brief and short-term inpatient psychiatric treatment which have overtaken long-term specialist treatment as the commonest way of using hospital facilities in treatment of BPD will now be considered. There are distinct discernible uses of brief and short-term inpatient treatment. Brief admission of 3 to 10 days is used to stabilize a patient during a crisis. Short-term admission of approximately 3 months is used electively to treat specific symptoms and behaviors found to be unmanageable in the community. It is probably best to combine these to some extent so that any patient with BPD who is admitted to hospital for crisis management is also offered a full review of their treatment programme. If this cannot be done within a brief admission, the brief admission should develop in to a short-term admission if the treatment skills are available. If a crisis admission is a first presentation to services, inpatient admission should become part of the process of engaging the patient in treatment and organizing future treatment.

Brief Hospitalization for Crises

The lifetime risk of suicide in BPD is estimated to be approximately 9% and >70% of patients have a history of suicidal behavior.[48] Not surprisingly this worries clinicians who are likely to react to suicide threats with a recommendation of admission to hospital until the risk is reduced. Although admission to hospital may be a reasonable way to manage an acute risk, it is unlikely to make any difference to chronic risk. Admission cannot solely be based on a clinician's anxieties which may be related more to chronic risk than immediate risk and therefore, it is important to identify if a risk has changed and if so in what way before recommending admission to the patient.

Case Vignette

A patient presented to the emergency room complaining of suicidal impulses and requesting hospital admission. The psychiatrist asked about the patient's current suicidal thoughts and also about any specific plans the patient had to act on his thoughts. The patient reported that he had an image of himself falling from a balcony and that he had identified a specific shopping centre where he could jump over the balustrade. The psychiatrist decided that this merited hospital admission and did not explore other problems. On saying he would arrange admission, the patient changed his mind. In panic the psychiatrist said that he would compulsorily admit the patient at which point the patient became agitated and said that he was leaving and quickly left the clinic room. Persuaded to return by a nurse, the patient then talked about his suicidal plans further at which point it became apparent that they had been present over many years and their nature had shown no recent change. In fact, the request for admission was not specifically related to the complaint of suicide although this was the area that the psychiatrist had understandably explored. The initial demand to come into hospital was based on the patient's wish to get away from distressing home circumstances which themselves had not materially changed. He was presenting with a chronic risk masquerading as an acute risk.

An evidence-based approach to risk in PD offers a more objective way to make a decision. The goal of suicide assessment cannot be to predict suicide accurately because it is such a rare event that false positives abound. It is to place a person along a putative risk continuum, to appreciate the basis of the individual's suicidality, and to allow for a more informed intervention. A number of short-term factors increase the acute risk of borderline patients harming themselves especially when combined with long-term and unmodifiable factors such as being male and in an older age-group. Drug misuse and other psychiatric comorbidity increases the risk. Suicide attempters have more recent life events at home and with family, more difficulties financially, and have experienced more negative events (love, marriage, crime, legal) in the month preceding a suicide attempt.[49] Overall, high lethality status is predicted by low socioeconomic status, comorbid ASPD, extensive treatment histories, and greater intent to die.[50]

Once a decision to admit a patient during a crisis has been taken it is important for staff to know that there is an increased risk of suicide at discharge for BPD and this may be related to the terms they negotiate at the start of the admission. Yen et al.[49] reported that borderline patients were more likely to make suicide attempts if they were discharged after violating an inhospital contract when compared with a comparable group of borderline patients discharged from hospital with mutual agreement. This is significant because many borderline patients are placed on behavioral contracts when admitted in a crisis to an acute care inpatient ward in the belief that it will control their behavior although there is limited evidence for this. If contracts are used they must be achievable and linked to reward rather than discharge.

Frequent threats of suicide made by some borderline patients may inoculate staff's judgement of risk and prevent them taking threats seriously because they have "heard it all before." In addition, the problem of assessing the seriousness of previous multiple attempts, the evidence that patient's themselves underestimate the lethality of their acts and there is a dangerous mix of patient and staff factors that are likely to interfere with good risk assessment.

Staff

Borderline patients can be managed in acute care inpatient wards by generic nursing staff as long as they pay attention to the borderline patient's special needs. These include the careful assessment of risk taking into account the evidence mentioned earlier, providing appropriate structure, identifying and maintaining clear treatment goals, and having steady resolve to manage emotional crises and behavioral disturbance. Gunderson[7,51] suggests that if staff organize around the low-stimulus needs of long-term psychotic patients not only will they begin to resent the high-stimulus interactions of the borderline patients but also begin to believe that they have to set strict limits. When these are broken, as they inevitably will be, the limits may become increasingly punitive. This is a pathway to high-risk discharge. To this extent inpatient admission can increase rather than reduce risk.

Case Vignette

A borderline patient was admitted for a brief hospital admission because of self-harm. She had cut her neck and abdomen and sutures had been required. After admission, she cut herself again and therefore the staff placed her on individual observation. She was carefully monitored. When a nurse came to check whether the patient was alright when she was watching TV she swore at her and barricaded herself in her room. After considerable confusion the door was forcibly opened and the patient was given medication.

In this case the staff response to the self-harm led to overzealous monitoring which overstimulated the patient who then actively tried to prevent further intrusions by physical means because her mentalizing capacities were unable to process the persistent stimulation. Less monitoring and more structured verbal intervention might have been a better approach.

Ideally, staff within hospital programmes will show skills in developing personalized, structured, and achievable programmes with patients and show a capability to keep a focus on the patient's emotional state in relation to the aims of the inpatient admission. Borderline patients easily experience a sense of failure and shame at being unable to achieve what they believe is expected of them. Staff who anticipate this and organize a programme with small steps, sometimes on a daily basis, are more likely to succeed and to gain satisfaction in treating BPD.

Goals of Crisis Admission

Brief inpatient admission in a crisis is not only a way of reducing risk but also an opportunity to revisit treatment plans. Medication can be reviewed, daily living skills assessed, financial problems addressed, and physical evaluation completed if indicated.

Medication is an adjunct to psychotherapy in the treatment of BPD. It enhances the effectiveness of psychotherapy, improves symptoms, stabilizes mood, and may help patients attend psychotherapy sessions. Prescription needs to take into account transference and countertransference phenomena.

For example, medication may become the vehicle for enacting control and dependency transferences in which the clinician dominates the submissive patient. In addition, there is a tendency for anxious clinicians to overmedicate borderline patients, thereby potentially reducing rather than enhancing their ability to cope with everyday stressors. Many patients with BPD fail to take prescribed medication regularly, partly because of its relative inefficacy but in part due to their unstable lifestyle which militates against regularity and personal organization. Ashamed to tell the clinician about missing doses the patient builds up an increasingly large stock of medication which may then be taken impulsively in overdose during a crisis. Inpatient admission gives a chance for both patient and clinician to assess the effects of regular medication over a few weeks. Experience by the patient of beneficial effects is a more powerful driver of adherence to medication than exhortation from the clinician. In addition, the clinician himself can be clearer about the effects of medication and can feel justified in continuing a prescription. Finally, inpatient admission is an excellent time to rationalize medication. Zanarini found that at 2, 4, and 6 years after an index hospitalization 90% of her borderline sample were taking at least three medications at each time point and had been on medication longer than other patients.[52,53]

Many patients are reluctant to change their medication frightened that an alteration of dose will destabilize them. Conversely, some patients demand more and more medication leaving the hapless psychiatrist bewildered. It is best to set goals around medication use early during an admission and to plan any changes over time ensuring that discharge from hospital is not dependent on achieving the medication goals. Most changes of medication can be continued easily in outpatient treatment. Some patients may seek quick results, yet the effects of medication (e.g., antipsychotic and antidepressant drugs) may take some time to become apparent, therefore, it is necessary to warn patients of likely delay so that they do not give up after a few days. The best way forward during inpatient treatment is to arrange regular meetings to discuss changes in symptoms, side effects, and changes in dose. In general, patients should expect to take medication for a minimum of 2 weeks unless there are intolerable side effects and this "rule" is best agreed when medication is started. If the patient stops a drug unilaterally before the agreed time, no other drug is prescribed until the 2-week period is completed unless the cessation was due to intolerable side effects. This reduces the demand for drug after drug when no effect occurs within a few days and prevents "creeping" polypharmacy. Soloff et al.[54] have suggested that the exception to these type of rules is antipsychotic medication such as haloperidol and that the benefits may occur rapidly but wane within a few weeks. Many clinicians believe that borderline patients, whilst more prone to placebo responsiveness,[54] are also more sensitive to side effects and withdrawal effects of medication than other patients although there is little evidence that this is the case; nevertheless reducing medication slowly whilst implementing another is probably the best course.

It is important not to overestimate the borderline patient's capacities. Many patients present with apparent social and personal skills when in fact their ability to care for themselves is limited for long periods of time. Hospital rehabilitation programmes are a useful way of assessing everyday skills such as cooking, eating habits, financial management, and overall self-care. Focusing on these areas of competence may also guard against potential regression which, if induced, might prolong admission. To protect against loss of abilities during crisis and short-term elective admissions, staff are advised to follow some simple guidelines to ensure that they do not overprotect or overstimulate patients. First, it is important that patients feel understood and cared about —"I can see that things are really difficult at the moment and you don't know what to do. What can I do to help do you think?" Second, the staff and patient need to move to a collaborative relationship in which they both consider options to deal with manifest problems—"What sort of things do you think are the most important to address?" Third, a pathway to implementing the options needs to be defined—"What sort of ideas do you have to address them?" "Can we work out a way of going about that whilst you are here?" Finally, the intervention programme in the hospital needs to support the goals defined by the patient and staff. For example, problems with self-care could be addressed by therapeutic work on self-esteem and practical help in developing personal hygiene skills.

SHORT-TERM ELECTIVE ADMISSION

There remains a place for short-term elective admission to psychiatric inpatient facilities offering time limited but specialized treatment programmes. Although such facilities are relatively rare, hospitalization for a period of 2 to 3 months offers an opportunity to stabilize behavior not addressed in very brief admissions usually associated with a crisis. Lessons learned from these programmes can also be used to inform general management procedures in crisis admissions.

In general terms specific *short term inpatient programmes* are skills based with use of behavioral "ABCs," contingency management, and attempts to minimize positive reinforcement of maladaptive behaviors. Dialectical behavioral therapy (DBT) has been applied on an inpatient ward and early studies suggested promising results. Silk et al.[55] treated patients for 10 to 17 days as inpatients. Patients in the DBT programme when compared to patients assigned to a non-DBT discussion group perceived themselves as better able to manage difficult or emotional situations. In a more recent study[28] 31 patients who participated in a DBT inpatient program were compared with 19 patients who had been placed on a waiting list and received treatment as usual in the community. Posttesting was conducted 4 months after the initial assessment (i.e., 4 weeks after discharge for the DBT group). The waiting list group did not show any significant changes at the 4-month point. The DBT group improved significantly more than the participants on the waiting list on seven of the nine variables analyzed, including depression, anxiety, interpersonal functioning, social adjustment, global psychopathology, and self-mutilation. Analyses based on Jacobson's criteria for clinically relevant change indicated that 42% of those receiving DBT had clinically recovered on a general measure of psychopathology. The data suggest that 3 months of inpatient DBT treatment is significantly superior to nonspecific outpatient treatment but even so only 48% of patients showed improvement. This is in itself not surprising and the stability of recovery needs to be determined by long-term follow-up. More importantly for health care organizations it is the question of whether a time-limited inpatient treatment such as this one is better than a more specific intensive outpatient treatment which may be much cheaper. This remains unknown.

Conclusions

Long-term inpatient treatment for BPD is no longer a treatment of choice. For a subgroup of patients, this may have led to better outcomes over the long term either because they received more appropriate treatment or because they were able to take advantage of felicitous social and personal circumstances. Overly intensive treatments may induce deterioration in symptoms and behavior by overstimulating the attachment system which in turn "switches" off mentalization which is the very process that helps people manage difficult emotional states. But this danger is not specific to inpatient treatment and all treatment contexts need to balance the double jeopardy of understimulation and overstimulation. Whilst overstimulation may reduce mentalizing capacity and lead to a worsening of the symptoms of BPD, understimulation will prevent the patient working on maintaining mentalizing at the point at which it is in danger of being lost. This is the very essence of treatment for BPD. Despite these caveats, inpatient admission continues to have an important part to play in treatment of BPD particularly in acute crises and to stabilize otherwise intractable symptoms.

REFERENCES

1. Linehan MM, Armstrong H, Suarez A, et al. Cognitive-behavioural treatment of chronically parasuicidal borderline patients. *Arch Gen Psychiatry*. 1991;48:1060–1064.

2. Gieson-Bloo J, van Dyck R, Spinhoven P, et al. Outpatient psychotherapy for borderline personality disorder; randomized trial of schema-focused therapy versus transference focused therapy. *Arch Gen Psychiatry*. 2006; 63:649–658.

3. Bateman A, Fonagy P. The effectiveness of partial hospitalization in the treatment of borderline personality disorder – a randomised controlled trial. *Am J Psychiatry*. 1999;156: 1563–1569.

4. Sanislow CA, Grilo CM, Morey LC, et al. Confirmatory factor analysis of DSM-IV criteria for borderline personality disorder: Findings from the collaborative longitudinal personality disorders study. *Am J Psychiatry*. 2002;159:284–290.

5. Fonagy P, Bateman A. Mentalizing and borderline personality disorder. *J Ment Health*. 2007; 16:83–101.

6. Kernberg OF. Borderline personality disorder: A psychodynamic approach. *J Personal Disord*. 1987;1:344–346.

7. Gunderson JG. *Borderline personality disorder: a clinical guide*. Washington, DC: American Psychiatric Publishing; 2001.

8. Livesley WJ. *Practical management of personality disorder*. New York: Guilford Press; 2003.

9. Arntz A, Veen G. Evaluations of others by borderline patients. *J Nerv Ment Dis.* 2001; 189:513–521.

10. Fonagy P, Leigh T, Steele M, et al. The relation of attachment status, psychiatric classification, and response to psychotherapy. *J Consult Clin Psychol.* 1996;64(1):22–31.

11. Bateman A, Fonagy P. *Psychotherapy for borderline personality disorder: mentalisation based treatment.* Oxford: Oxford University Press; 2004.

12. Arnsten AF. The biology of being frazzled. *Science.* 1998;280(5370):1711–1712.

13. Phelps EA, LeDoux JE. Contributions of the amygdala to emotion provessing: from animal models to human behaviour. *Neuron.* 2005;48: 175–187.

14. Zanarini MC, Frankenburg FR, Reich DB, et al. Biparental failure in the childhood experiences of borderline patients. *J Personal Disord.* 2000; 14(3):264–273.

15. Everson MD, Hunter WM, Runyon DK, et al. Maternal support following disclosure of incest. *Am J Orthopsychiatry.* 1989;59:197–207.

16. Horwitz AV, Widom CS, McLaughlin J, et al. The impact of childhood abuse and neglect on adult mental health: A prospective study. *J Health Soc Behav.* 2001;42:184–201.

17. Linehan MM. *Cognitive-behavioral treatment of borderline personality disorder.* New York: Guilford Press; 1993.

18. Fruzzetti AE, Shenk C, Hoffman PD. Family interaction and the development of borderline personality disorder: A transactional model. *Dev Psychopathol.* 2005;17:1007–1030.

19. Fruzzetti AE, Shenk C, Lowry K, et al. Emotion regulation. In: O'Donohue WT, Fisher JE, Hayes SC, eds. *Cognitive behaviour therapy: applying empirically supported techniques in your practice.* New York: John Wiley and Sons; 2003: 152–159.

20. Zanarini MC, Frankenburg FR, Hennen J, et al. The longitudinal course of borderline psychopathology: 6-year prospective follow-up of the phenomenology of borderline personality disorder. *Am J Psychiatry.* 2003;160:274–283.

21. Zanarini MC, Frankenburg FR, Hennen J, et al. Prediction of the 10-year course of borderline personality disorder. *Am J Psychiatry.* 2006; 163(5):827–832.

22. Skodol AE, Gunderson JG, Shea MT, et al. The Collaborative Longitudinal Personality Disorders Study (CLPS): Overview and implications. *J Personal Disord.* 2005;19(5):487–504.

23. Keller MB, Lavori PW, Mueller TI, et al. Time to recovery, chronicity, and levels of psychopathology in major depression. A 5-year prospective follow-up of 431 subjects. *Arch Gen Psychiatry.* 1992;49(10):809–816.

24. Gunderson JG, Bender D, Sanislow C, et al. Plausibility and possible determinants of sudden "remissions" in borderline patients. *Psychiatry.* 2003;66(2):111–119.

25. Zanarini MC, Frankenburg FR, Hennen J, et al. Axis 1 comorbidity in patients with borderline personality disorder: 6-year follow-up and prediction of time to remission. *Am J Psychiatry.* 2004;161:2108–2114.

26. Chiesa M, Fonagy P, Holmes J, et al. Residential versus community treatment of personality disorders: A comparative study of three treatment programmes. *Am J Psychiatry.* 2004; 161:1463–1470.

27. Paris J. Is hospitalization useful for suicidal patients with borderline personality disorder? *J Personal Disord.* 2004;18:240–247.

28. Bohus M, Haaf B, Simms T, et al. Effectiveness of inpatient dialectical behavioral therapy for borderline personality disorder: A controlled trial. *Behav Res Ther.* 2004;42(5):487–499.

29. Chiesa M, Fonagy P, Holmes J. Six-year follow-up of three treatment programs to personality disorder. *J Personal Disord.* 2006;20(5):493–509.

30. Chiesa M, Drahorad C, Longo S. Early termination of treatment in personality disorder treated in a psychotherapy hospital: A quantitative and qualitative study. *Br J Psychiatry.* 2000;177:107–111.

31. Chiesa M, Bateman A, Wilberg T, et al. Patients' characteristics, outcome and cost-benefit of hospital-based treatment for patients with personality disorder: A comparison of three different programmes. *Psychol Psychother: Theory Res Pract.* 2002;75:381–392.

32. Lambert MJ, Bergin A, Garfield S. Introduction and historical overview. In: Lambert MJ, ed. *Bergin and Garfield's handbook of psychotherapy and behaviour change.* New York: John Wiley and Sons; 2004.

33. Vermote R, Vertommen H, Corveleyn J. *Touching inner change. Psychoanalytically informed hospitalisation-based treatment of personality disorders. A process-outcome study.* Doctoral Dissertation. Faculty of Psychology. Katholieke Universiteit, Leuven: 2005.

34. Blatt SJ, Blass R. Relatedness and self definition: a dialectic model of personality development. In: Noam GG, Fischer KW, eds. *Development and vulnerabilities in close relationships.* New York: Erlbaum; 1996:309–338.

35. Blatt SJ, Auerbach JS. Psychodynamic measures of therapeutic change. *Psychoanal Inq.* 2003;23:268–307.

36. Blatt SJ, Shahar G. Psychoanalysis: For what, with whom, and how: A comparison with psychotherapy. *J Am Psychoanal Assoc.* 2004;52:393–447.

37. Gabbard G, Coyne L, Allen J, et al. Evaluation of intensive in-patient treatment of patients with severe personality disorders. *Psychiatr Serv.* 2000;51:893–898.

38. Main T. The ailment. *Br J Med Psychol.* 1957;30: 129–145.
39. Gabbard GO. Splitting in hospital treatment. *Am J Psychiatry.* 1989;146:444–451.
40. Bateman A, Tyrer P. Services for personality disorder: Organisation for inclusion. *Adv Psychiatr Treat.* 2004;10:425–433.
41. Gabbard GO, Kay J. The fate of integrated treatment: Whatever happened to the biopsychosocial psychiatrist. *Am J Psychiatry.* 2001; 158:1956–1963.
42. Gabbard G. Psychodynamic psychotherapy of borderline personality disorder: A contemporary approach. *Bull Menninger Clin.* 2001;65: 41–57.
43. Tyrer P. The future of the community mental health team. *Int Rev Psychiatry.* 2000;12: 219–225.
44. Gunderson JG. The borderline patient's intolerance of aloneness: Insecure attachments and therapist availability. *Am J Psychiatry.* 1996;153(6): 752–758.
45. Paris J. Personality disorders over time: Precursors, course and outcome. *J Personal Disord.* 2003;17:479–496.
46. Laub JH, Vaillant GE. Delinquency and mortality: A 50-year follow-up study of 1,000 delinquent and non-delinquent boys. *Am J Psychiatry.* 2000;157(1):96–102.
47. Beautrais AL, Joyce PR, Mulder RT. Risk factors for serious suicide attempts among youths aged 13 through 24 years. *J Am Acad Child Adolesc Psychiatry.* 1996;35(9):1174–1182.
48. Paris J, Zweig-Frank H. A 27-year follow-up of patients with borderline personality disorder. *Compr Psychiatry.* 2001;42:482–487.
49. Yen S, Pagano ME, Shea MT, et al. Recent life events preceding suicide attempts in a personality disorder sample: Findings from the collaborative longitudinal personality disorders study. *J Consult Clin Psychol.* 2005;73(1):99–105.
50. Soloff P, Fabio A, Kelly TM, et al. High-lethality status in patients with borderline personality disorder. *J Personal Disord.* 2005;19:386–399.
51. Gunderson J, Gratz KL, Neuhaus EC, et al. Levels of care in treatment. In: Oldham J, Skodol AE, Bender D, eds. *Textbook of personality disorders.* Washington, DC: American Psychiatric Publishing; 2005.
52. Zanarini MC, Frankenburg FR, Khera GS, et al. Treatment histories of borderline patients. *Compr Psychiatry.* 2001;42:144–150.
53. Zanarini MC, Frankenburg FR, Hennen J, et al. Mental health service utilization by borderline personality disorder patients and axis II comparison subjects followed prospectively for 6 years. *J Clin Psychiatry.* 2004;65:28–36.
54. Soloff P, Cornelius J, George A. Efficacy of phenelzine and haloperidol in borderline personality disorder. *Arch Gen Psychiatry.* 1993;50:377–385.
55. Silk K, Eisner W, Allport C, et al. Focused time-limited in-patient treatment of borderline personality disorder. *J Personal Disord.* 1994;8:268–278.

CHAPTER 15

Evaluation and Management of Substance Use Disorders on the Inpatient Psychiatric Unit

CHRISTINE E. YUODELIS-FLORES, W. R. MURRAY BENNETT, JASON P. VEITENGRUBER, AND RICHARD K. RIES

T he need to evaluate, diagnose, and manage substance use disorders (SUDs) in patients admitted to a psychiatric unit has become increasingly common for the inpatient psychiatrist over the last decade. Frequently, the attending psychiatrist will find half or more of his or her inpatient service to have ongoing or past substance use issues that may profoundly impact diagnosis, treatment, and discharge planning. The complex challenges that patients with SUDs or co-occurring disorders present might engender feelings of apprehension, helplessness, or therapeutic nihilism on the part of a psychiatrist not experienced in treating addictive disorders. The clinician may be unclear about how to assess and treat addiction, a chronic disorder that severely affects the course and prognosis of mental illness. Clinicians unprepared to treat addictive disorders may feel the temptation to avoid treating the patient, referring the individual to another treatment program, or alternatively making treatment demands that the individual cannot achieve. By not having a clear understanding of addiction and minimizing its impact on mental illness, or by not knowing the impact of mental illness on the course of addiction, the psychiatrist risks treatment failure and recidivism. On the other hand, with practical clinical approaches better outcomes are possible and rewarding for both the patient and the clinician. In this chapter, after defining the problem and its prevalence, the authors will primarily focus on the practical management of substance use and co-occurring disorders. They will provide a framework to proceed in the complex task of evaluation and treatment, as well as delineate the role of medications, inpatient staff, group therapies, and self-help groups commonly used in co-occurring treatment units to assist the clinician in the daunting task at hand.

Epidemiology

PREVALENCE OF CO-OCCURRING DISORDERS IN GENERAL POPULATIONS

According to Diagnostic and Statistic Manual of Mental Disorders, Fourth Edition (DSM-IV), substance-related disorders are divided into two groups: SUDs (abuse and dependence) and substance-induced disorders. The co-occurrence of a SUD with another psychiatric disorder is often referred to as *dual diagnosis* or *co-occurring disorder*. The term may also refer to substance-induced psychiatric disorders that occur in the context of substance abuse or dependence.

Several epidemiologic surveys have been done in the general population, looking at lifetime and 12-month prevalence rates of comorbid disorders: the Epidemiologic Catchment Area (ECA) survey;[1] the National Comorbidity Survey (NCS);[2] and the National Epidemiological Survey on Alcohol and Related Conditions (NESARC).[3] Results from the ECA study found a lifetime prevalence rate of 29% for an addictive disorder in patients with mental disorders and a 61% lifetime prevalence rate for SUDs in those diagnosed with bipolar I. Conversely, those diagnosed with an alcohol disorder had a 37%

TABLE 15.1 TWELVE-MONTH PREVALENCE OF DIAGNOSTIC AND STATISTICAL MANUAL OF MENTAL DISORDERS (DSM-IV) INDEPENDENT MOOD AND ANXIETY DISORDERS AMONG RESPONDENTS WITH A 12-MONTH SUBSTANCE USE DISORDER (SUD)

Comorbid Disorder	Index Disorder: SUD					
	Any SUD (%)	Any Substance Dependence (%)	Any Alcohol Use Disorder (%)	Alcohol Dependence (%)	Any Drug Use Disorder (%)	Any drug Dependence (%)
Any mood disorder	19.67	29.19	18.85	27.55	31.80	55.02
Major depression	14.50	21.82	13.70	20.48	23.33	39.99
Any anxiety disorder	17.71	24.54	17.05	23.45	25.36	43.02

(Data from Grant BF, Stinson FS, Dawson DA, et al. Prevalence and co-occurrence of substance use disorders and independent mood and anxiety disorders: Results from the national epidemiologic survey on alcohol and related conditions. *Arch Gen Psychiatry*. 2004;61[8]:807–816. Copyright © [2004] American Medical Association.)

lifetime prevalence of mental disorders, and among those diagnosed with an addictive disorder other than alcoholism, 53% had a comorbid mental disorder. Among those diagnosed with schizophrenia there is a 34% prevalence rate of alcohol use disorders, and in those with bipolar disorder the prevalence rate is 46%. Of the individuals with affective disorder, the ECA study reported 32% also had a comorbid SUD.

According to results from the NESARC, the 12-month prevalence of SUD, alcohol use disorder, and drug use disorder in the general population is 9.35%, 8.46%, and 2.0%. The 12-month prevalence of SUD among those diagnosed with a mood disorder is 20%. Among those with anxiety disorders 15% have a SUD[4] (see Tables 15.1 and 15.2). The association of personality disorders and SUDs is also significant: the NESARC data report that among individuals with a personality disorder 16.4% reported a current alcohol use disorder and 6.5% had a drug use disorder. Conversely, among those with a current alcohol use disorder 28.6% had at least one personality disorder, and among those with a drug use disorder, 47.7% had a personality disorder.[5]

TABLE 15.2 TWELVE-MONTH PREVALENCE OF DIAGNOSTIC AND STATISTIC MANUAL (DSM-IV) SUBSTANCE USE DISORDERS AMONG RESPONDENTS WITH A 12-MONTH DSM-IV INDEPENDENT MOOD DISORDER

Comorbid Disorder	Index Disorder: Mood or Anxiety Disorder						
	Any Mood Disorder (%)	Major Depression (%)	Any Anxiety Disorder (%)	Panic Disorder with Agoraphobia (%)	Panic Disorder without Agoraphobia (%)	Social Phobia (%)	Generalized Anxiety Disorder (%)
Any substance use disorder	19.97	19.20	14.96	24.15	17.30	16.05	19.08
Any substance dependence	12.91	12.59	9.02	14.83	12.60	10.12	13.34
Any alcohol use disorder	17.30	16.40	13.02	18.81	15.29	13.05	14.82
Alcohol dependence	11.38	11.03	8.06	12.42	11.56	8.64	10.52
Any drug use disorder	6.90	6.61	4.58	10.58	6.32	5.52	8.06
Any drug dependence	3.74	3.54	2.43	5.94	4.16	2.94	5.24

(Grant BF, Stinson FS, Dawson DA, et al. Prevalence and co-occurrence of substance use disorders and independent mood and anxiety disorders: Results from the national epidemiologic survey on alcohol and related conditions. *Arch Gen Psychiatry*. 2004;61[8]:807–816. Copyright © [2004] American Medical Association.)

TABLE 15.3 PREVALENCE OF ACTIVE SUBSTANCE USE DISORDERS IN INPATIENT PSYCHIATRIC STUDIES

Dixon L, 1993	35%
Miller NS, 1994	30%
Lehman AF, 1994	56%
Lambert MT, 1996	58%
Dixon L, 1998	41%
Pages KP, 1998	42%
Averill PM, 2002	36%–66%

(Data from Dixon L, Dibietz E, Myers P, et al. Comparison of DSM-III-R diagnoses and a brief interview for substance use among state hospital patients. *Hosp Community Psychiatry* 1993;44[8]:748–752; Miller NS, Belkin BM, Gibbons R. Clinical diagnosis of substance use disorders in private psychiatric populations. *J Subst Abuse Treat* 1994;11[4]:387–392; Lehman AF, Myers CP, Corty E, et al. Prevalence and patterns of "dual diagnosis" among psychiatric inpatients. *ComprPsychiatry* 1994;35[2]:106–112; Lambert MT, Griffith JM, Hendrickse W. Characteristics of patients with substance abuse diagnoses on a general psychiatry unit in a VA Medical Center. *Psychiatr Serv* 1996;47[10]:1104–1107; Dixon L, McNary S, Lehman AF. Remission of substance use disorder among psychiatric inpatients with mental illness. *Am J Psychiatry* 1998;155[2]:239–243; Pages KP, Russo JE, Wingerson DK, et al. Predictors and outcome of discharge against medical advice from the psychiatric units of a general hospital. *Psychiatr Serv* 1998;49[9]:1187–1192; Averill PM, Veazey C, Shack A, et al. Acute mental illness and comorbid substance abuse: Physician-patient agreement on comorbid diagnosis and treatment implications. *Addict Disord Treat* 2002;1:119–125.)

PREVALENCE OF POLYSUBSTANCE DEPENDENCE

Results from the NESARC show an overwhelmingly positive correlation between alcohol use and drug use disorders. Persons with alcohol dependence have a 13%, 12-month prevalence of any drug use disorder. Those with cocaine dependence have an 89% prevalence of alcohol use disorder, and among those with opioid dependence the prevalence of alcohol use disorder is 74%. Among individuals with cannabis dependence and amphetamine dependence, the prevalence of alcohol use disorder is 68% and 78%, respectively.[6]

PREVALENCE OF SUBSTANCE USE DISORDERS IN INPATIENT PSYCHIATRIC POPULATIONS

Substance use worsens the course and complicates the treatment of mental illness. In patients with severe mental illness, substance use is associated with higher rates of medication noncompliance and increased relapse and readmission rates.[7,8] It is linked to self-harm and suicide,[9] poor health and self-care,[10] increased episodes of violence and victimization,[11,12] incarceration,[13] and homelessness.[14] Substance use can both cause and exacerbate mental illness, and it is associated with impulsivity and poor judgment.

For the reasons mentioned in the preceding text, it is no surprise that various inpatient psychiatric populations have a higher rate of concurrent SUDs than outpatient populations reported in surveys. Various studies report that 30% to 66% of psychiatric inpatients have an active SUD (see Table 15.3).

Diagnostic Considerations

The relationship between psychiatric illness and substance use is complex. Psychoactive drugs and alcohol both produce and exacerbate psychiatric symptoms through several pharmacologic mechanisms. Symptoms associated with acute and chronic intoxication and withdrawal may overlap with symptoms of psychiatric and cognitive disorders. Substance use also exacerbates coexisting psychiatric disorders, often being the primary reason for decompensation as well as causing psychosocial consequences that contribute to the worsening of the psychiatric illness. Substance-induced psychiatric disorders may be misdiagnosed as primary depression, anxiety disorders, psychosis, and personality disorders. In diagnosing a co-occurring psychiatric disorder in a person with an active SUD, the physicians must often assign a provisional diagnosis and delay a more definitive diagnosis until a period of abstinence has been obtained. This is increasingly difficult to do in an inpatient setting as inpatient stays are becoming less frequent and of shorter duration. The length of abstinence necessary for diagnosis depends on the substance of abuse and the psychiatric diagnosis being assessed. To diagnose a substance-induced psychiatric disorder, DSM-IV criteria specify that the psychiatric symptoms arise within 1 month of substance intoxication or withdrawal. A co-occurring disorder rather than a substance-induced disorder is probable if the symptoms have been present during abstinence, if they are persistent despite the cessation of acute withdrawal or intoxication, or if symptoms are substantially in excess of what would be expected, given the amount and type of substance used.

Despite the high rates of dual diagnosis in the psychiatric inpatient populations, SUDs are frequently underdiagnosed.[15,16] Treatment of addictive disorders may be ignored or mismanaged, in part because of the patients' underreporting of substance use and denial or minimization, clinicians' inexperience with dual diagnosis, low rates of reimbursement by insurance companies for treatment of substance-induced disorders, or the program's lack of resources for appropriate treatment.

Clinical Model for Treatment

In the following section, division of the clinical model for treatment into acute and subacute phases is designed to assist the clinician develop a practical approach to initial and subsequent steps in assessment, diagnosis, and treatment of dual disorders. This approach also serves to underscore the therapeutic process of developing a treatment alliance with dual diagnosis patients, beginning with the initial interview and building on that foundation in subsequent interviews through motivational techniques and behavioral interventions designed to facilitate a patient's understanding and acceptance of the complex association of addiction and mental illness.

ACUTE PHASE MEDICAL STABILIZATION: DAYS 1 TO 2 OF HOSPITALIZATION

At this initial point, questions the clinician should be asking him/herself include: Is the patient intoxicated and/or in danger of acute, possibly life-threatening substance withdrawal? Is this condition medically or psychiatrically substance-related? Are there emergent conditions such as head injury, toxic encephalopathy, overdose, infections, cardiac, hepatic or renal failure, and thiamine deficiency that will necessitate acute medical stabilization?

Given the high degree of substance-associated psychiatric illness in the acute care setting, it is important during the initial psychiatric evaluation to also focus on a substance use history by asking direct and detailed questions in a respectful and nonjudgmental manner regarding the patient's substance use. Several screening instruments, such as the CAGE questionnaire,[17] Alcohol Use Disorders Identification Test (AUDIT),[18] the TWEAK questions,[19] and the Brief Michigan Alcoholism Screening Test (Brief MAST),[20] are available to assess SUDs. In the authors' experience, however, it is preferable to conduct a detailed substance use history, as the clinician can utilize this interview process to engage the client, develop rapport, and underscore the importance of evaluating and treating SUDs during inpatient psychiatric evaluation and treatment.

The clinician should ascertain specific information such as doses and types of substances used, duration and frequency of use, time of last use, and a history of withdrawal symptoms and previous substance abuse treatment. This detailed questioning is important to determine the need for acute medical stabilization and detoxification as well as to determine if the psychiatric disorder is substance related. Of course, minimization, evasion, or denial may be present to some degree, and indeed is common not only in those with primary SUDs, but also in those with psychiatric disorders uncomplicated by substance use. The authors' experience in an acute psychiatric inpatient service of an urban public hospital is that patients will often initially underreport or avoid discussions of addictive disorders, but they estimate that perhaps only 5% or 10% of psychiatric

CAGE Questionnaire

Have you ever:

1. Felt you should **C**ut down on your drinking?
2. Felt **A**nnoyed by criticism of your drinking?
3. Felt bad or **G**uilty about your drinking?
4. Taken a drink in the morning (**E**ye-opener) to steady your nerves or get rid of a hangover?

(Reprinted with permission from Ewing JA. Detecting alcoholism. The CAGE questionnaire. *JAMA* 1984;252[14]:1905–1907. Copyright ©1984, American Medical Association. All rights reserved.)

"Dual CAGE" Questions

Have you ever:

1. **C**ut down (or stopped) Because mental symptoms worsened? Because mental health doctor or therapist suggested?
2. Felt **A**nnoyed when your drug/alcohol use was discussed? Felt **A**nnoyed, anxious or angry, or had fights when using? Been **A**dmitted to emergency room (ER) or hospital for psychiatric problems, when using or not? ADHD as a child?
3. Felt **G**uilty about use? Felt **G**uilty, depressed, suicidal when using or not? Ever made a suicide attempt when using or not?
4. Taken an *eye-opener* drink or drug in the morning to feel better? Taken a drink or drug to blot out symptoms? Taken drink or drug with psychiatric medications? Not taken medications because of using drug/alcohol (forgot, avoid mixing, etc.)?

   What are 2 or 3 reasons you use alcohol/drugs?
   What are 2 or 3 reasons you might want to stop or cut down?

patients with addictive disorders will deny their existence and refuse to participate in dual diagnosis treatment.

Case Vignette

Ms. S was admitted to the psychiatric unit for symptoms of depression and suicide attempt. She denied a drug or alcohol use disorder; however, she admitted that she had been drinking the night of her suicide attempt. The clinician provided education about depression and added information about the disinhibiting effects of alcohol and the dangers of drinking when depressed or suicidal. She asked Ms. S to attend the dual diagnosis therapy group to explore this issue, and although initially reluctant Ms. S agreed to do so.

Most patients become willing and even enthusiastic participants in dual diagnosis treatment if the addictive disorder in importance is elevated to the level of the psychiatric disorder in the authors'

TABLE 15.4 PATIENT ADMITTED FOR DEPRESSION AND SUICIDAL BEHAVIOR: CAGE STYLE INTERVIEW

Psychiatrist:	"Do you use any drugs or alcohol?"
Patient:	"I don't use drugs but I drink now and then."
Psychiatrist:	"Now and then?"
Patient:	"Yes, mostly on weekends."
Psychiatrist:	"Do you ever feel the need to drink in order to cope with stress or depression?"
Patient:	"Yes, maybe I've been drinking more since I've been feeling so bad."
Psychiatrist:	"How much is "more"?"
Patient:	"Oh … up to a six-pack of beer."
Psychiatrist:	"How often?"
Patient:	"Maybe 3 or 4 times a week … not every day."
Psychiatrist:	"When was the last time you drank?"
Patient:	"Last night before I came in."
Psychiatrist:	"Do you ever get out of control when you drink a lot?"
Patient:	"I can handle my liquor pretty well."
Psychiatrist:	"How much does it take for you to feel "tipsy"?"
Patient:	"Maybe 5 or more beers."
Psychiatrist:	"Have you ever had to drink to control shakiness?"
Patient:	"No"
Psychiatrist:	"Do you ever think you might be drinking too much?"
Patient:	"No … it's not a problem."
Psychiatrist:	"Has any one else ever worried about your drinking?"
Patient:	"Well … I guess my ex-wife didn't like it very much."
Psychiatrist:	"Did you ever think you might have a drinking problem?"
Patient:	"I used to drink a lot when I was in college, but I stopped that because it was getting out of hand."
Psychiatrist:	"Out of hand?"
Patient:	"Yea … those days were pretty wild and crazy."
Psychiatrist:	"Did it get you in trouble?"
Patient:	"That's why I had to cool it … a cop stopped me after leaving a party and it was either that or jail."

subsequent discussions with the patient. To minimize denial, it is helpful to utilize an empathetic, respectful, and nonjudgmental style to engage the client, such as is demonstrated in the dialogue in Table 15.4.

A medical history and physical examination, as well as a review of symptoms, should be done, focusing on possible substance-related medical conditions such as recent falls or injuries; neurologic problems such as visual and balance difficulties, blackouts, seizures, and memory difficulties; infections and skin wounds or tracks; cardiac diseases such as cardiomyopathy, hypertension, or endocarditis; and liver and gastrointestinal problems such as hepatitis, ulcers, or pancreatitis. Laboratory tests include a urine toxicology screen, blood alcohol level, liver function tests, complete blood count (CBC), and comprehensive chemistry panel. If neuropsychological symptoms are present, a head computed tomography (CT) should be performed. As a rule, if alcohol abuse or dependence is suspected, patients should receive thiamine 50 mg IM or PO immediately and orally for the subsequent 3 days in addition to multivitamins as alcoholics are at risk for thiamine deficiency, which may lead to Wernicke disease and the Wernicke-Korsakoff syndrome.

Acute Phase: Detoxification

Management of polydrug detoxification is a common problem, and this potential should be determined during the initial evaluation of SUDs. Particularly difficult is a combined sedative-hypnotic, alcohol, and opioid withdrawal. In these cases, the substance that could potentially cause the most medically severe withdrawal sequelae (alcohol or sedative-hypnotic) should take precedence, and the clinician should focus primarily on managing that withdrawal rather than withdrawal from opiates.

Case Vignette

Mr. T was admitted for suicidal ideation in the context of heroin dependence and difficulty tolerating the symptoms of withdrawal. When questioned about the amount and types of substances used, he admitted to frequent heavy alcohol, cocaine, and benzodiazepine use to enhance his opiate "highs" and mitigate withdrawal effects. Because of concerns about alcohol and benzodiazepine withdrawal, the clinician decided against using buprenorphine for opiate detoxification and instead initiated an alcohol/benzodiazepine withdrawal protocol using chlordiazepoxide with a clonidine withdrawal protocol added when signs of opiate withdrawal emerged. After inpatient day 3, the patient was tolerating detoxification, but was still using an average of 300 mg of chlordiazepoxide daily and 0.2 mg of clonidine t.i.d. At this point it was decided to discontinue the protocols and begin a 3-day taper of chlordiazepoxide and continue the clonidine at 0.2 mg t.i.d. for an additional 2 days before tapering by 0.2 mg per day. On day 7, after discontinuing chlordiazepoxide, the patient endorsed worsening anxiety, restlessness, and insomnia as well as muscle twitching. Symptoms were managed by addition of gabapentin 300 mg t.i.d. and trazodone 50 mg at bedtime. By discharge on day 10, Mr. T denied withdrawal symptoms and was preparing to enter a residential addiction treatment program. He was instructed to continue gabapentin for an additional 2 weeks before tapering over a third week and to continue the trazodone as needed for insomnia over the subsequent month.

Alcohol

Alcohol withdrawal may occur after a heavy drinker stops or reduces the amount of alcohol intake. Symptoms of alcohol withdrawal include signs of autonomic hyperactivity such as tachycardia, hypertension, fever, and sweating. Other signs are anxiety, insomnia, psychomotor agitation, nausea or vomiting, and tremor. Rarely, transient visual, tactile, or auditory hallucinations can occur as well as withdrawal-associated seizures. Symptoms of withdrawal usually peak around the second day and improve after day 5, although prolonged subclinical withdrawal syndromes may take months to resolve. Approximately 5% of alcohol-dependent patients will develop severe withdrawal consisting of seizures or alcohol-induced delirium, commonly known as *delirium tremens*.[21] Alcohol detoxification is done on the psychiatric unit using protocols for alcohol withdrawal, which include administering the Clinical Institute Withdrawal Assessment for Alcohol Scale-Revised (CIWA-Ar)[22] every 2 hours while awake and giving chlordiazepoxide 50 to 100 mg or lorazepam 1 to 2 mg for scores >8–9. Chlordiazepoxide is less reinforcing than lorazepam and longer acting; however, lorazepam is preferred for patients with significant liver dysfunction. For patients at risk for withdrawal seizures, anticonvulsants such as divalproex sodium, carbamazepine, or gabapentin can be used as adjunctive agents. Gabapentin can also be used in place of benzodiazepines for withdrawal, starting at 300 mg three times a day and increasing if necessary to up to 600 mg every 6 hours.[23–25]

Opiates

Clinical manifestations of acute opioid withdrawal are due to noradrenergic hyperactivity and rebound effects and include tachycardia, hypertension, fever, mydriasis, lacrimation, rhinorrhea, piloerection, perspiration, nausea, vomiting, diarrhea, abdominal cramping, myalgia, muscle spasms, restlessness, irritability, insomnia, craving, and yawning. Onset of withdrawal symptoms depends on the half-life of the substance: as short as 4 to 6 hours for heroin and up to 36 hours for methadone. Severity of withdrawal varies with dose and duration of use. Duration of the withdrawal syndrome is shortest with short-acting agents: heroin withdrawal generally peaks at 36 to 72 hours and lasts 7 to 14 days, while methadone withdrawal syndromes last approximately 4 to 8 weeks. Protracted withdrawal syndromes persisting for up to 6 months have been reported. Management of opioid detoxification depends on underlying medical conditions such as hepatitis C, hepatic disease, and pregnancy. Opioid withdrawal during pregnancy can lead to fetal distress and premature labor, so methadone maintenance during pregnancy is the treatment of choice, and pregnant women should be referred to a local methadone maintenance program.

It can be extraordinarily difficult to manage opiate withdrawal in patients hospitalized with co-occurring psychiatric illness, and patients may abruptly leave the inpatient unit against medical advice if the withdrawal syndrome is not managed appropriately. The most common pharmacologic therapies used to manage opiate withdrawal include opioid agonist substitution with taper and clonidine detoxification. In patients who are withdrawing from alcohol or sedative-hypnotics as well as opiates, caution must be taken to avoid adverse drug interactions such as excessive respiratory suppression due to combining protocols using opioid agonists and benzodiazepines. In these cases, the clinician must primarily focus on the alcohol or sedative-hypnotic withdrawal (which can be far more medically serious than opioid withdrawal) and avoid or limit opioid doses used. Clonidine detoxification would be preferred over an opioid detoxification to avoid respiratory suppression.

Opiate Agonist Substitution with Taper

The most common opioids used for detoxification include methadone and buprenorphine. To use buprenorphine in detoxification, physicians must complete an 8-hour training, or be certified in Addiction Medicine, or boarded in Addiction Psychiatry and apply to the Drug Enforcement Administration (DEA) through a Notification of Intent (NOI) to use buprenorphine for the treatment of opioid treatment or detoxification.

Methadone detoxification. Inpatient methadone substitution and taper with patients who illicitly use drugs can be difficult, as knowledge of the exact dosage of heroin or other narcotic is not usually available. Patients may over- or underestimate their use, and the purity of street drugs is notoriously variable. The physician must guess at the initial methadone dosage. As little as 40 mg of methadone could be fatal to someone who is nontolerant to opiates. To ensure safety, it is important to start with a methadone dose of 10 to 20 mg, and closely observe the patient to assess the effects of the dose. If the initial dose does not suppress withdrawal symptoms within 1 hour, an additional dose of 5 to 10 mg methadone can be given. No greater than 30 mg of methadone should be given within the first 24 hours of detoxification unless there is documented evidence that the patient uses >40 mg of methadone equivalents per day. On day 2 of detoxification, the initial dosage used to stabilize a patient in withdrawal should be repeated. Subsequently, the dosage can be adjusted by 5 mg every 2 days if the patient is having continued symptoms of withdrawal. Blood levels will continue to rise on the same daily dose of methadone for the next 4 days. Once the patient is stabilized, the methadone dosage can be decreased by 5 mg per day until a zero dosage is achieved. This method of methadone tapering can take anywhere from 5 to 10 days.

Buprenorphine detoxification. Buprenorphine is a partial μ-receptor agonist and antagonist approved by the U.S. Food and Drug Administration (FDA) in 2002 for detoxification and maintenance treatment of opioid dependence. Sublingual tablets are available both with and without naloxone added (Suboxone and Subutex). The addition of naloxone, a powerful opioid antagonist which is very poorly absorbed sublingually, is to reduce risks of buprenorphine abuse. Snorting or dissolving and injecting a crushed tablet containing naloxone will precipitate acute opiate withdrawal. In patients who are dependent on shorter-acting opioids, buprenorphine detoxification is effective, better tolerated, and safer than methadone detoxification on an inpatient unit.[26] Because of the long half-life of methadone, however, it is much more difficult to use buprenorphine to detoxify methadone-dependent patients, and the authors do not recommend it for this purpose. Because of the partial agonist–antagonist effects, a precipitated opiate withdrawal syndrome can occur if buprenorphine is given to the patient before he or she is in clear opiate withdrawal. Therefore, the key to successful buprenorphine detoxification lies in waiting a sufficient time until mild to moderate symptoms of opiate withdrawal are documented (usually 12 to 24 hours after the last dose of heroin). At that time, an initial 4 mg dose of buprenorphine is administered sublingually. If the patient is still in opiate withdrawal 2 hours after the buprenorphine is given, an additional 4 mg of sublingual buprenorphine can be administered. The following days the patient can be given 4 mg, 8 mg, or 12 mg sublingually to relieve withdrawal symptoms, and then on subsequent days the dose can be reduced by 2 to 4 mg per day until zero dosage is achieved. A buprenorphine detoxification taper usually takes from 3 to 7 days. The use of benzodiazepines is a relative contraindication in those being detoxified from opiates with buprenorphine, as there have been several reports of adverse events such as accidental overdose in those on this combination.[27,28]

Clonidine detoxification. An α_2 agonist and antihypertensive agent, clonidine ameliorates adrenergic-mediated symptoms by blocking activation of the locus ceruleus that shows increased activity during opioid withdrawal. It decreases opioid withdrawal symptoms; however, myalgias, craving, insomnia, and restlessness may still persist. The use of clonidine is limited by the hypotensive effects and it should be used with caution in patients with hypotension or on antihypertensive agents. Many inpatient psychiatric units have an opiate withdrawal protocol using clonidine. Inpatient detoxification can be accomplished with a 6- to 8-day scheduled clonidine taper, using 0.1 to 0.2 mg every 4 to 6 hours up to 1.0 mg total the first day and increasing as tolerated up to a maximum of 1.2 mg total in divided doses on days 2 to 4. For withdrawal from shorter-acting opiates, by day 5 clonidine can be tapered by 0.2 mg per day, to avoid hypertensive rebound, until zero dosage. For detoxification from longer-acting opiates such as methadone, clonidine should be maintained at a dose sufficient to ameliorate withdrawal symptoms for up to 5 additional days before a 0.2 mg per day taper. During detoxification, vital signs should be monitored before each dosing, and clonidine should be held for systolic blood pressures <100 mm Hg and diastolic readings <50 mm Hg.

Adjunct medications used in opioid detoxification. Often, patients undergoing opioid detoxification have severe anxiety, insomnia, muscle/joint pain, gastrointestinal distress, or restlessness not ameliorated by clonidine. Acetaminophen, ibuprofen, or a muscle relaxant such as methocarbamol can be added during the acute withdrawal period. On the basis of the authors' clinical experience, low-dose hydroxyzine or lorazepam can be used during the first few days of a clonidine detoxification to manage excessive anxiety, insomnia, or restlessness, and then tapered at the end of detoxification. Gastrointestinal distress, manifested by nausea, vomiting, or diarrhea, can be managed with adjunct medications such as promethazine for nausea and vomiting and loperamide for diarrhea.

Sedative-Hypnotics

Drugs in this class are among the most widely used prescription medications in the United States. If used over a period of time, these agents can cause psychological and physical dependence and withdrawal. Psychiatric diagnoses associated with benzodiazepine or sedative-hypnotic use disorders are primarily anxiety disorders, sleep disorders, and depression. Patients with underlying anxiety disorders, who are physiologically dependent, and are withdrawn from these agents will experience rebound anxiety or recurrence of their anxiety disorder. Ideally, they should be withdrawn in an outpatient setting, gradually, over an extended period of time, unless their use of the agent is unsafe or abusive. Agents commonly associated with severe withdrawal states include methaqualone ("Quaalude," Sopor), glutethimide (Doriden), chloral hydrate, and benzodiazepines such as alprazolam and triazolam. Drugs associated with less severe clinical withdrawal states include meprobamate (Miltown, Equanil), diazepam, chlordiazepoxide, clonazepam, and lorazepam.[29] Clinical manifestations of sedative-hypnotic withdrawal are similar to alcohol withdrawal and include tachycardia, hypertension, fever, tinnitus, agitation, anxiety, restlessness, delirium, hallucinations, insomnia, irritability, nightmares, sensory or perceptual disturbances, tremor, muscle tension, anorexia, diarrhea, and nausea. Signs of a severe withdrawal syndrome include seizures, delirium, and severe autonomic instability that could result in death. Time course and severity of the withdrawal syndrome depend on the dose, duration of use, and duration of drug action. Cessation of short-acting benzodiazepines will produce onset of withdrawal within 24 hours with peak severity in 1 to 5 days. Onset of withdrawal from long-acting benzodiazepines occurs within 5 days with peak severity occurring at 1 to 9 days. Duration of the withdrawal syndrome is shorter for the short-acting benzodiazepines but could last up to 3 weeks, whereas duration of withdrawal syndromes for long-acting benzodiazepines last 10 to 28 days. Prolonged withdrawal syndromes lasting several months are possible in patients with long-term benzodiazepine use.

Management of sedative-hypnotic withdrawal. Gradual dose reduction of the agent, or substitution with phenobarbital or a long-acting benzodiazepine such as clonazepam or chlordiazepoxide (Librium), with gradual dose reduction, are the preferred methods of managing withdrawal. Dose reduction on an outpatient basis should be only 10% per 1 to 2 weeks for patients who have been on benzodiazepines for more than 1 year; however, based on the authors' experience and a controlled trial by Ries et al.,[30] this tapering schedule can be significantly accelerated to 3 to 10 days on an inpatient unit with the addition of carbamazepine 200 mg t.i.d., which effectively attenuates the benzodiazepine withdrawal syndrome. Carbamazepine should be continued for at least 2 to 3 weeks after the taper is completed. Case reports of divalproex sodium or gabapentin used in assisting benzodiazepine withdrawal syndromes are also reported in the literature. Management of rebound anxiety is best accomplished with behavioral interventions such as cognitive behavioral therapy or relaxation therapy and, in the authors' experience, pharmacologic interventions using nonaddictive medications such as antidepressants that are effective for anxiety disorders: buspirone, gabapentin, or hydroxyzine.

Stimulants: Cocaine, Methamphetamine, Amphetamines, Methylenedioxymethamphetamine

Cocaine. Cocaine is the second most widely used illicit drug in the United States, and it is highly associated with legal substance use (alcohol and tobacco). Symptoms associated with cocaine withdrawal include depression, hypersomnia, fatigue, anxiety, irritability, poor concentration, increased appetite, paranoia, and drug craving. Medical complications associated with cocaine withdrawal include hypertension and stroke as well as cardiac abnormalities such as prolonged QTc interval and a potential for arrhythmia and myocardial infarction. Seizures and hyperthermia may also be a complication of cocaine intoxication and may occur during withdrawal. Rhabdomyolysis is a common complication of cocaine binging and should be ruled out by checking a plasma creatine kinase (CK) level. There are no specific pharmacologic interventions for treatment of cocaine withdrawal unless medical complications are present. Patients are encouraged to sleep, eat, and remain well hydrated. During acute withdrawal, it can be difficult to encourage patients to attend groups or interact with staff because of hypersomnia and irritability. This should resolve by day 2 or 3 of hospitalization. Psychiatric symptoms during cocaine withdrawal can include psychosis, severe depression, and suicidal behavior.

Methamphetamine and amphetamines. Use of methamphetamine has had devastating effects on society, health care, and the environment as well as the legal system. It is a stimulant with longer half-life and longer duration of euphoric effects than cocaine. Symptoms of stimulant withdrawal are remarkably similar for methamphetamine, amphetamines, and cocaine. However, acute methamphetamine withdrawal tends to be of longer duration. Those who have been using intravenous methamphetamine or smoke "crank," also known as *glass* or *ice*, usually have more severe withdrawal symptoms. The first 2 weeks of abstinence are colloquially described as "the crash," consisting of hypersomnia, anergia, irritability, hyperphagia, anhedonia, and sadness. Supportive measures are advised including adequate hydration, nutrition, and time for restorative sleep. The crash period is followed by an intermediate withdrawal phase characterized by fatigue, loss of energy, and anhedonia. During the late withdrawal phase, patients experience intense craving. If severe symptoms such as psychosis or suicidality emerge, it is advisable to consider psychiatric hospitalization for safety and to start treatment with appropriate antipsychotic or antidepressant medications. Similarly to cocaine, medical complications can arise including rhabdomyolysis, seizures, cardiac arrhythmias, and stroke. Long-term methamphetamine use is associated with psychosis, which can take months or years to resolve. Methamphetamine-related psychosis can be indistinguishable from schizophrenia, and patients may experience paranoid ideation, auditory and visual hallucinations, bizarre delusions, and delusions of reference. Patients with schizophrenia and other psychotic disorders can develop acute exacerbation of psychosis with even a small amount of methamphetamine.

Methylenedioxymethamphetamine. Methylenedioxymethamphetamine (MDMA), a designer drug commonly known as *Ecstasy*, is a popular stimulant used in the "rave scene." Ingestion of MDMA increases the release of serotonin, dopamine, and norepinephrine from presynaptic neurons as well as inhibiting monamine oxidase, which slows the metabolism of these neurotransmitters. Effects of intoxication include stimulant and hallucinogenic properties similar to methamphetamine and empathogenic action enhancing empathy, sociability, and feeling of well-being. Adverse effects of intoxication include bruxism, agitation, anxiety, delirium, tachycardia, hypertension, arrhythmias, hyperthermia, rhabdomyolysis, and serotonin syndrome. Long-term exposure produces long-term memory and learning impairment secondary to serotonergic neuronal damage. Psychosis similar to methamphetamine psychosis can also be seen in chronic users of MDMA.[31] Depression, hypersomnia, poor concentration, and fatigue are the most common withdrawal effects. Depression or dysphoria can be present for weeks to months after discontinuing use. Memory deficits may also persist for long periods of time. Psychopharmacologic management of withdrawal symptoms is not usually necessary and patients are managed similarly to cocaine withdrawal. However, for agitation or psychosis, patients should be treated with benzodiazepines or atypical antipsychotics.

γ-Hydroxy butyrate. Abuse of this novel agent is found amongst urban nightclub attendees, participants in the "rave scene," and bodybuilders. γ-hHydroxy butyrate (GHB) is a metabolite of the inhibitory neurotransmitter γ-aminobutyric acid (GABA) and has the effects of relaxation, euphoria, sedation, and disinhibition at lower doses. Higher doses will cause respiratory and central nervous system (CNS) depression. It has a remarkably narrow dose range, is not detected by urine toxicology screens, and has risk of significant drug-to-drug interactions. Accidental overdoses associated with CNS depression are common, leading to emergency department visits safely managed with supportive measures, protected airway, and expectant management. Dependence on GHB is rare as it has a short half-life of just a few hours. In chronic users of GHB, symptoms of withdrawal mimic alcohol or sedative-hypnotic withdrawal and include anxiety, tremor, and insomnia which can last for weeks after stopping the drug.[32] Severe withdrawal is dangerous and difficult to manage, marked by seizures, psychosis, bizarre behavior, delirium, and agitation. Current best medical practice is to follow a sedative-hypnotic withdrawal protocol using tapered benzodiazepines in an inpatient setting.[33] However, "benzodiazepine-resistant" cases requiring >1,100 mg lorazepam over 4 days have been discussed widely in case reports. Consequently, there has been some discussion in the literature about the adjunct use of low-dose, second-generation antipsychotic agents such as risperidone or olanzapine. The authors advise vigilant use of the sedative-hypnotic withdrawal protocol with strong consideration for the addition of a low-dose atypical antipsychotic agent.

Cannabis. Cannabis is the most commonly used illicit drug in the United States. Dependence, occurring in approximately 10% of individuals, is associated with a gradual increase in use and tolerance to the effects. Intoxication is associated with short-term memory loss and difficulties in concentration. Acute marijuana withdrawal is reported by approximately half of those seeking treatment for marijuana dependence.[34] Symptoms of withdrawal, usually mild and self-limited, include anxiety, irritability, restlessness, anorexia, and insomnia. Marijuana usually does not cause psychiatric disorders; however, several studies have linked its use with an increased risk of psychosis and psychotic relapse.[35,36] Owing to anxiolytic properties, cannabis use is common in those with comorbid anxiety disorders, and its use will behaviorally interfere with long-term treatment strategies employed to treat the anxiety disorder.

Tobacco. Tobacco use is extremely common among patients with psychiatric disorders and is responsible for higher morbidity and mortality than all of the other substances of abuse combined. However, the psychoactive effects of tobacco rarely contribute to other axis I disorders, and so the authors will not focus on tobacco dependence in this chapter, except to mention management of tobacco withdrawal. As inpatient units are generally nonsmoking, and patients are often detained involuntarily and need to be supervised closely, the privileges of smoking may be withheld from patients until their security and stability is assured. Management of tobacco withdrawal is easily accomplished with the use of a daily nicotine patch, or nicotine gum on an as-needed basis, for those patients in discomfort from abstention.

Acute Phase Diagnostic Considerations: Acute Psychiatric and Substance Use Diagnoses

Often the initial admitting diagnoses are mood disorder Not Otherwise Specified (NOS) or psychosis NOS in addition to a SUD because of the difficulty of diagnosing a primary psychiatric disorder in the presence of intoxication or withdrawal. During the first couple of days of psychiatric hospitalization, the task is to sort out and refine the psychiatric and substance use diagnoses as well as determine their overlay. The best way to differentiate between substance-induced psychiatric syndromes and psychiatric disorders complicated by substance use is to observe the psychiatric symptoms during a prolonged period of abstinence. This may be impossible when evaluating patients on an acute inpatient psychiatric unit where the average length of stay can be only 5 to 7 days. Determining whether the psychiatric disorder is entirely due to substance use or only coincident with or exacerbated by substance use can be elucidated by obtaining a history of use in relation to the psychiatric symptoms. Is the patient's psychiatric syndrome present during prolonged periods of abstinence? Which disorder appeared first in the patient's chronologic history? Of course, people can be notoriously poor historians when asked to recall psychiatric and substance use history over a long period of time, and additional information from laboratory examination and outside sources such as family, past clinicians, or previous hospitalizations should be obtained. In general, a greater length and severity of substance dependence, as measured by the history of use and present severity of intoxication or withdrawal symptoms, will predict a greater likelihood of a substance-induced psychiatric disorder, but does not rule out the possibility of a co-occurring psychiatric disorder. Having a family history of the psychiatric disorder, a history of mental disorders during a prolonged period of abstinence, or a history of previous psychiatric illness before substance dependence will suggest a co-occurring disorder. In many cases, it will not be possible to establish a definitive psychiatric diagnosis until the patient has at least 1 month of abstinence.

Acute Phase Psychiatric Stabilization: Acute Pharmacologic and Behavioral Management

Despite the uncertainty of a definitive psychiatric diagnosis at this stage, acute symptoms of agitation, severe anxiety, mania, and psychosis need to be treated emergently and pharmacologic management is indicated. If alcohol or sedative-hypnotic withdrawal is occurring, the agitation, anxiety, and psychosis may represent a withdrawal delirium that could be life threatening. Reassessing the doses and frequency of administration of the agent used for withdrawal (usually a benzodiazepine) is important, and if autonomic hyperactivity is not prominent and dosing appears adequate, additional medication for acute anxiety and agitation should be limited to nonbenzodiazepines (on an as-needed basis) such as hydroxyzine, gabapentin, or low doses of quetiapine, which have been effective based on the authors' clinical experience. During alcohol or sedative-hypnotic withdrawal, psychotic symptoms in the absence of a clouded sensorium can be treated with low doses of an atypical antipsychotic, in conjunction with benzodiazepines administered according to the withdrawal protocol. Insomnia is common and difficult to treat during this stage and preferably should be managed with reassurance, behavioral and sleep hygiene techniques, and non-habit-forming sleep aids such as trazodone or diphenhydramine.

Anxiety and agitation due to acute opiate withdrawal might not respond to a clonidine detoxification and low doses of a benzodiazepine such as lorazepam during the first few days of detoxification may be necessary along with sleep aids. Alternatively, the clinician may need to switch from a clonidine withdrawal protocol to a buprenorphine withdrawal, which is usually better tolerated.[37] Psychotic symptoms during opiate withdrawal are uncommon, unless there is an underlying psychotic disorder, and should be treated with atypical antipsychotic medications, which could also help with insomnia, agitation, or anxiety.

Psychotic symptoms, especially paranoia, during cocaine or stimulant withdrawal are particularly common and often severe or problematic. Psychosis in stimulant withdrawal should be managed with an atypical antipsychotic. Psychosis remits within 3 to 5 days of intoxication and withdrawal from cocaine. With methamphetamine-induced psychosis, the psychotic symptoms usually remain much longer after acute detoxification, especially if the duration or severity of use is long or great. In this case, antipsychotic treatment is necessary for several months or longer, until the psychotic symptoms resolve and the patient's methamphetamine dependence is in remission.

SUBACUTE PHASE: DAYS 2 TO 5+ OF HOSPITALIZATION

Diagnostic Considerations

After acute withdrawal symptoms have attenuated, patients should be reassessed for severity of psychiatric symptoms and suicidality. At this point, if the psychiatric syndrome is substance-induced, signs of remission may be present. For example, in cocaine-induced mood disorder, the authors find that sleep, energy, mood, and appetite disturbances often remit in the first few days of detoxification. During the subacute stage, gathering information from prior hospitalizations, outpatient clinicians, and family members also assists in diagnostic assessment and treatment planning.

Case Vignette

Mr. Q presented with acute suicidal and paranoid ideation as well as cocaine dependence. On inpatient day 1, he could barely be aroused for the psychiatric evaluation, but endorsed irritability, suspiciousness, sleeplessness before admission, low energy and motivation, hopelessness, poor concentration, weight loss, and feelings of guilt/shame. On day 2, Mr. Q endorsed a good appetite and although he continued to express low energy, depressed mood, and hypersomnia, he was able to attend most of his group therapies and denied psychotic symptoms. He progressively improved over the next 3 days and denied symptoms of depression or psychosis by discharge on day 5.

Psychosocial and Behavioral Interventions

Daily Rounds: Keep the Focus on Chemical Dependency Issues

In treatment of co-occurring disorders, both problems, although they may not be equally severe, are considered equally important and should be addressed concurrently. This means that during daily rounds, the psychiatrist may need to focus on the SUD as much as the psychiatric disorder. Usually, additional information about the addictive disorder not obtained during the first interview is needed to determine treatment planning and includes obtaining a history of legal, social, and medical problems associated with the substance use; a family history of SUDs; and a history of previous chemical dependency treatment and the successes/failures in treatment. It is appropriate to assess the patient's awareness of the SUD and its relation to the psychiatric illness as well as the degree of motivation for treatment. Exploring the connections between the SUD and the course of psychiatric illness, periods of abstinence and treatment episodes, and probing for negative consequences of substance use can be done gradually on a daily basis. Throughout this evaluative process, it is helpful to maintain an attitude of nonjudgmentally exploring the patient's ambivalence to improve rapport and set the stage for change.

Evaluation of Motivation and Treatment Readiness

Successful treatment for chemical dependency depends to a large degree on an individual's commitment to change and belief that he or she can be successful in changing a behavior. Therefore, it is critical to assess a person's motivation to address the SUD. The degree of motivation will vary and is influenced by an individual's insight into the role of substance use in creating his or her problems. Motivation is also affected by the individual's desire to change, the belief that change is possible, the balance between reasons to change versus reasons to stay the course, and the perceived difficulties associated with change. As described by Prochaska and DiClemente,[38] change is a process that proceeds through five identifiable stages: precontemplation, contemplation, preparation, action, and maintenance. During the stage of precontemplation, the patient considers his or her substance use as enjoyable and not causing any problems. In the contemplation stage, the patient is aware that substance use is a problem,

Core Principles of Motivational Interviewing

1. **Express empathy:** communicate respect for the client through reflective listening
2. **Develop discrepancy:** enhance client's perception of discrepancy between where they are and where they want to be with regard to drug use
3. **Avoid argumentation:** avoid direct argumentation or confrontation which evokes resistance
4. **Roll with resistance:** new ways of thinking about the problem are invited but not imposed
5. **Support self-efficacy:** client will not move toward change unless there is hope for success

considers the advantages and disadvantages of the behavior, and contemplates change. Patients are in the preparation stage when they have decided that change is important, and they begin to actively prepare for changing the behavior. The action stage begins when a patient stops the behavior. The final stage, of maintenance, occurs when the patient has made the change and actively avoids relapse into the old behavior.

Success in changing behavior can be predicted by determining the stage at which an individual is and promoted by facilitating progression to the next stage. A patient in the stage of precontemplation is unlikely to consider his substance abuse a problem and would not be likely to consider changing his or her behavior. Those in a precontemplative or contemplative stage are less likely to have success in an addiction treatment program until they have reached the preparation stage. Therefore, the clinician's task at hand is to facilitate progression from one stage to the next.

Motivational Interviewing

Motivational interviewing (MI), a counseling style developed by Miller and Rollnick,[39] is designed to elicit behavior change by helping a person explore and resolve ambivalence. Motivational Enhancement Therapy (MET) is a brief directive therapy focusing on interventions designed to enhance motivation for change and facilitate transition from one stage to the next. There are five core principles of MI as described by Miller and Rollnick[40] and listed in the box.

Miller and Rollnick emphasize four core techniques which go by the acronym of open-ended questions; affirmations; reflective listening; summaries (OARS) (see Table 15.5). According to MET, specific interventions should be matched with stages of change. For an individual in the stage of precontemplation, clinicians should work on engaging the client and raising awareness of risky and problematic drug or alcohol-related behavior. Educating the patient about the role of substance use in sustaining or worsening the symptoms is helpful at this stage. Once patients become aware of the need for change, they are in the contemplative stage. At this stage, they have ambivalence regarding changing the behavior, and their task would be to facilitate exploring the pros and cons of behavior change through a decision balance analysis and heightening the discrepancy between the individual's goals or

TABLE 15.5 MOTIVATIONAL INTERVIEW USING OPEN-ENDED QUESTIONS, AFFIRMATIONS; REFLECTIVE LISTENING; SUMMARIES (OARS) TO ELICITE SELF-MOTIVATIONAL BEHAVIOR

OARS:	
Open-ended questions:	"What was going on that led to your seeking help?" "What do you think about all of this?" and "So what makes you feel it might be time for a change?"
Affirmation:	"That must have been hard to handle," "So even though you think it will be hard, you're still not ready to give up," "It is difficult to commit to such a drastic change."
Reflection (focusing on change talk):	"So it sounds like you are saying . . . ," "It sounds like you haven't made up your mind that this is really a problem," "Maybe you have mixed feelings about this . . . on the one hand/on the other hand . . . "
Summarizing:	"Let me see if I've got this straight . . . "

TABLE 15.6 EXAMPLE OF MOTIVATIONAL INTERVIEWING

Psychiatrist:	"Yesterday when we met, we had a discussion about some problems you had with alcohol in the past."
Patient:	"Yes that was in the past."
Psychiatrist:	"All that was a long time ago and it doesn't concern you now."
Patient:	"Not really, I am a responsible drinker now."
Psychiatrist:	"That is good to hear … Responsible. Tell me what that means to you."
Patient:	"Well, I would never drink and drive now … too much to lose."
Psychiatrist:	"Yes, that would be foolish and dangerous. What other things mean "responsible drinking" to you?"
Patient:	"I wouldn't let my drinking interfere with my work."
Psychiatrist:	"So you don't want your alcohol use to cause dangerous or risky situations. And you don't want to end up in jail or out of a job. How about other problems?"
Patient:	"Like what?"
Psychiatrist:	"Well, how about problems with physical or emotional health?"
Patient:	"I don't think alcohol hurts me."
Psychiatrist:	"Do you think it can hurt you?"
Patient:	"Yes, if you drink too much."
Psychiatrist:	"Tell me what you would consider too much."
Patient:	"Like so much that you get brain damage or liver problems."
Psychiatrist:	"So you might consider your drinking a problem if you had brain or liver damage."
Patient:	"Yes. That would be a definite sign that it has become a problem."
Psychiatrist:	"Do you know if you have those problems?"
Patient:	"Me? Of course not!"
Psychiatrist:	"How would you know if you had health problems or emotional problems because of alcohol?"
Patient:	"I don't know … maybe ask my doctor."
Psychiatrist:	"Would you like to know how a doctor would determine that?"
Patient:	"Yes."
Psychiatrist:	"So you would like to have more information about this so you can determine if you drink too much or if alcohol is causing health and emotional problems for you."
Patient:	"Yes."
Psychiatrist:	"That sounds like a wise and responsible thing to do. Maybe we can help you find information on that."

values and his or her substance use. It can be helpful to create a timeline of illness, substance use, and adverse consequences to underscore connections between the behavior and the current problems. Other motivational techniques include exploring with the patient what led to prior relapses, exploring alternatives and options, and helping the patient problem solve around barriers to success. The problem of demoralization may arise. Often patients have unsuccessfully tried many times to deal with their addiction and become demoralized with successive treatment failures. A clinician should question this perspective by empathizing, affirming the individual's strengths, and offering an alternative perspective. It is valuable to point out discrepancies in self-defeating statements and maintain that successful change is always possible. Frustration with relapses can be reframed as increased motivation for what must change. When a patient is preparing for action, or in the action stage, the clinician should encourage self-efficacy and provide assistance in creating an effective plan that is acceptable for the patient (see Table 15.6).

Dealing with Resistance

Often patients with co-occurring disorders are in denial and/or resistant to interventions. This is particularly common in those with severe mental illness and co-occurring substance abuse because they tend to have heightened sensitivity to the effects of psychoactive substances[41] and may use much lower amounts of substances than addicted individuals in the general population. Perhaps they are not convinced that their drug or alcohol use influences their psychiatric condition, or else they are not prepared to face the hardship of giving up a habit that they enjoy or feel they need to practice in order to avoid discomfort.

Case Vignette

Mr. U, admitted for acute exacerbation of schizophrenia, relates chronic heavy alcohol use and does not see a problem with this as he has never undergone symptoms of withdrawal. He was referred to the dual diagnosis therapy group and developed acquaintances with other group members with similar problems. Over the course of his hospitalization, he and his clinician explored issues with adherence, analyzed precipitating factors in past psychotic episodes, discussed ways to develop new supportive relationships, and how to prevent future hospitalizations. By discharge, Mr. U has made plans to attend an outpatient dual diagnosis group at his community mental health center along with another patient whom he knew was having similar problems.

Possibly, family members or friends may also have addictive disorders, and the patient may feel dependent on the relationships and unwilling to give up substance use, which may jeopardize these relationships.

Case Vignette

Mr. R, age 20, was admitted with psychotic symptoms and marijuana abuse. After a brief intervention and a trial on antipsychotic medications, his symptoms resolved. He endorsed a desire to stop marijuana use; however, he was concerned that he would be socially isolated from friends, should he refrain from smoking pot.

Often, they may have found outpatient clinicians willing to prescribe medicines with abuse potential and are unwilling to consider contradicting recommendations. The clinician can impact the patient's perspective by keeping the focus on the addictive disorder, using a motivational style to reframe statements, and validate reasons for resisting change. Once validated, the patient becomes less defensive, and at that point the clinician will find that eliciting patient goals and highlighting discrepancies will lead to more prochange talk, preparing the patient for progression to the next stage of change (see Tables 15.7 and 15.8).

Dual Diagnosis Group Therapy

Group therapy for co-occurring disorders is vital for any psychiatric inpatient program. Many of the concepts associated with addiction treatment are also used in the treatment of psychiatric patients

TABLE 15.7 DEALING WITH RESISTANCE-I

Dr:	"Tell me about your experience with AA."
Patient:	"AA doesn't work for me."
Dr:	"You haven't found AA to be helpful in the past."
Patient:	"Yes, I just hear the same old stories. I leave feeling like I want a drink."
Dr:	"So going to AA triggers cravings for you."
Patient:	"Yes."
Dr:	"I can see how you wouldn't want that. It sounds like you haven't found the right group yet. Have you tried other meetings?"

TABLE 15.8 DEALING WITH RESISTANCE-II

Patient:	"AA never worked for me."
Dr:	"What was it that bothered you about it?"
Patient:	"I am not a religious person."
Dr:	"So you have trouble relating to the religious aspect of AA."
Pt:	"Yes, all that God talk makes me uncomfortable."
Dr:	"I've heard that before. It seems many people feel uncomfortable with it. Do you think AA could be different for you if it wasn't for that?"
Pt:	"Yes."
Dr:	"Maybe you could explore alternatives to the traditional AA. For example, Did you know that there are also agnostic/atheist AA groups or Secular Organization for Sobriety groups available around town?"

either in group or individual therapy. Topics in common include the acceptance of and recovery from chronic illness, the importance of asking for help, the problem of demoralization, overcoming denial and shame, analysis of coping skills, and how to actively use treatment. Group topics in co-occurring disorder groups also focus on education and the functional analysis of SUDs, dual diagnosis and influences of substance use on psychiatric disorders, the role of psychiatric disorders in addiction relapse, the importance of adherence to medication and treatment, and the role of social support and self-help groups such as Alcoholics Anonymous (AA). Co-occurring disorder groups also teach relapse prevention skills, such as recognizing and coping with craving, problem-solving skills, and how to evaluate past and future high-risk situations. Not only actively using individuals can benefit from these dual diagnosis groups: Patients who have achieved abstinence and those with family members who have addictive disorders can also benefit from the group and provide valuable perspectives (see Table 15.9).

Dual Diagnosis 12-Step Meetings

The importance of 12-step attendance and peer support in establishing and maintaining long-term sobriety has been established in several outcome studies of AA attendees.[42–46] Support and assistance from AA group members and sponsors has been shown to be the best predictor of success in recovery.[47] Dual diagnosis AA groups, commonly known as *dual recovery anonymous*, or *double trouble groups*, are also very helpful in promoting both medication adherence and maintenance of sobriety.[48] These groups are particularly helpful to an inpatient psychiatric program with patients with co-occurring disorder. Although privacy concerns prohibit AA groups on the psychiatric inpatient unit, stable patients can attend groups off the unit but on or near the hospital grounds. Adjunct AA groups serve as an important introduction to self-help resources, provide a form of no-cost aftercare, and often are of key importance to an individual continuing both psychiatric treatment and maintenance of sobriety after discharge from an acute inpatient unit. Official AA literature advocates the seeing of psychiatrists for mental disorders and the taking of appropriate psychiatric medications.[49]

TABLE 15.9 EXAMPLE OF DUAL DIAGNOSIS UNIT ACTIVITIES

- Screening for co-occurring disorders
- Daily psychiatric rounds that focus on chemical dependency (CD) as well as psychiatric issues
- Meeting with addiction counselor for individualized assessment and treatment planning
- Daily dual diagnosis group therapy, women's dual diagnosis group
- Alcoholics Anonymous (AA) meetings, especially dual diagnosis meetings close to unit (on hospital grounds) at least three times a week
- Evening videos on addiction topics twice a week
- Family conference to discuss dual diagnosis and treatment
- Discharge planning with social worker and addiction counselor that focuses on follow-up treatment for dual diagnosis, sober housing, and support groups; planning should include active referral: setting up appointments with addiction program or sober housing, providing options, AA group schedules

Integrated Therapeutic Model of Treatment for Dual Disorders

The roles of nursing staff, therapists, social workers, and chemical dependency counselors are crucial in promoting and developing an integration of addiction and mental health treatment for the patient with co-occurring disorder. Staff members' interpersonal skills, therapeutic efficacy, and knowledge of addictive disorders and treatment can vary widely. Therapeutic nihilism and demoralization of staff in providing care to CD patients is a common problem. When treating people with dual disorders, it is important to maintain a realistic longitudinal perspective of addiction and relapse. Focusing on a motivational method of treatment serves to combat not only patient demoralization but also clinicians' therapeutic nihilism, which can become problematic.

Psychosocial interventions coordinated by staff should include scheduling a family conference to promote family participation in focusing on addiction as well as psychiatric treatment. Discharge planning should include assessment of the patient's living environment and the need for clean and sober housing. The chemical dependency counselor should provide an introduction to AA and outpatient addiction treatment programs. Active referrals to outpatient treatment programs and assisting patients in scheduling intake appointments, rather than simply providing a list of resources, can be very important to facilitate follow-up care. Even if non-MD staff are the chief therapeutic managers of the addictions part of the patient's condition, it is crucial that MD staff inquire about addictions issues and support therapeutic interventions, including 12-step referrals, during daily rounds.

Principles of Pharmacotherapy for Co-occurring Disorders

Consensus recommendations in improving the psychiatric care of individuals with severe and persistent mental illness and SUDs[50] discuss the following key principles of pharmacotherapy for patients with dual diagnosis:

1. **Avoid treating nonspecific complaints.** Medications should be limited to treating symptom clusters related to an axis I disorder in order to avoid reinforcing self-medication behavior. Anxiolytic p.r.n. medication should be assessed behaviorally as one coping strategy with pros and cons and discussed as such with patients.
2. **Consider safety and side effect profiles and be aware of potential interactions between medications and drugs of abuse.** Clinicians should be aware of the synergistic effects that drugs of abuse combined with psychiatric medications may have on the CNS. Medications that increase sedation, lower seizure thresholds, cause liver toxicity or cardiac effects, and cause delirium, including those with strong anticholinergic or orthostatic side effects may adversely affect the individual who relapses on drugs or alcohol while prescribed those medications. Suicide risk may increase during relapse or acute intoxication, and therefore medications with a lower risk in overdose are recommended. Discharge recommendations to outpatient clinicians may include limiting or monitoring the amounts of prescribed medications.
3. **Avoid medications with abuse liability or addiction potential.**
4. **Choose strategies that promote medication adherence.** Providing education on the proper use of medication and simplifying medication regimens will enhance adherence. Staff should teach patients about filling "medisets" and strategies for remembering times of dosing.

Pharmacologic Treatment of Schizophrenia Spectrum Disorders in Individuals with Co-occurring Addiction

Even small amounts of drugs of abuse increase psychotic symptoms in patients with primary psychotic disorders. Psychotic symptoms can be present during intoxication and withdrawal of alcohol, sedatives, stimulants, MDMA, cannabis, hallucinogens, opioids, and phencyclidine. Substance-induced psychotic disorder is common in chronic cocaine, methamphetamine, and other stimulant dependence.[51,52] Cocaine-induced psychosis usually persists for a few days after cessation of use. Methamphetamine-induced psychosis may present as a protracted psychotic illness similar to schizophrenia lasting for more than 6 months.[53] Atypical antipsychotics are effective in treating psychosis complicated by substance use, and recent research suggests that clozapine[54] and quetiapine in particular[55,56] may be effective in reducing substance craving and relapse as well as the psychosis.

Pharmacologic Treatment of Bipolar Disorder in Individuals with Addictive Disorders

Bipolar disorder and SUDs commonly co-occur, and the presence of substance misuse will worsen the clinical course of bipolar disorder. Compared with nonsubstance abusers, bipolar patients with SUDs have more frequent hospitalizations, earlier onset of the affective disorder, and a higher incidence of rapid cycling and mixed mania.[57,58] A few studies have evaluated the effects of valproate and lithium in treating substance-abusing patients with bipolar disorder, but much further research is needed. Geller et al.[59] reported lithium to be effective in adolescents with bipolar disorder and substance abuse, but Bowden[60] found substance abuse to be a predictor of a poor response to lithium. It has also been reported that lithium is not as effective as valproate in individuals with rapid cycling and dysphoric mania, conditions that are more common in substance abusers. Brady et al.[61] concluded that valproate is effective and relatively safe in mixed manic bipolar patients with substance dependence, and Albanese and Clodfelter[62] also found valproate to be effective for substance-abusing bipolar patients. Salloum et al.,[63] in a double-blind placebo-controlled study, evaluated valproate in alcoholic bipolar patients and reported significant improvement in alcohol use and stabilization of mood. Goldberg et al.[64] reported a higher remission rate for mania in hospitalized patients with SUDs treated with valproate compared to lithium. Salloum et al.[65] reported on the outcomes of treatment of cocaine-abusing bipolar I patients in a pilot study, and the results revealed significant improvement in cocaine abuse as well as in symptoms of mania, depression, and sleep symptoms. One concern, however, about the use of valproate in bipolar patients with SUDs is the possibility of worsening hepatic dysfunction in patients with liver disease, so liver function tests should be routinely monitored.

Treatment of Anxiety Disorders in Individuals with Addictive Disorders

Managing symptom recurrence in addicted patients with co-occurring anxiety disorders can be problematic. The patient should be reassured that anxiety and sleep disturbance are common in early abstinence and may take months to resolve in protracted withdrawal syndromes. Benzodiazepines should be avoided in these individuals. Selective serotonin reuptake inhibitors (SSRIs) are considered to be first-line treatment for anxiety disorders in addicted patients. Adjunct treatment with buspirone[66,67] and gabapentin[68] may be considered in those with generalized anxiety disorder, social phobia, and panic disorder. For protracted insomnia, trazodone can be used.[69]

Treatment of Co-occurring Depression in Individuals with Addictive Disorders

Results from controlled medication trials in co-occurring alcohol use and depressive disorders modestly support the use of antidepressants, and in particular the SSRIs, in treating depressive symptoms in this patient population; however, antidepressants have little impact on reducing alcohol or other drug abuse.[70–72] Newer approaches emphasize the addition of pharmacotherapy specifically targeting the alcohol dependence. In patients with co-occurring drug use disorders and depression, there have been no placebo-controlled studies on antidepressant effectiveness.

Pharmacologic Interventions for Substance Use Disorders

Alcohol Dependence

Two types of medication are used for treatment of alcoholism: aversive medication that deters the patient from drinking and anticraving medication that reduces the patient's desire to drink. Disulfiram has been used for aversive medication treatment of alcoholism since the late 1940s. Anticraving medications approved by the FDA include naltrexone and acamprosate. Medications given for treatment of alcohol dependence should be given in conjunction with addiction counseling.

Disulfiram. Disulfiram (Antabuse) is an alcohol-sensitizing agent, which causes alcohol ingestion to be toxic by inhibiting aldehyde dehydrogenase that catalyzes the oxidation of aldehyde to acetic acid. The disulfiram–ethanol reaction is caused by a buildup of acetaldehyde in the blood. In cases of a small amount of alcohol ingestion, symptoms include flushing of the skin, increased heart rate, and lowered blood pressure. Other symptoms include nausea, vomiting, shortness of breath, sweating, anxiety, dizziness, and blurred vision. In a more severe reaction, symptoms can include confusion, marked tachycardia, hypotension, bradycardia, and even cardiovascular collapse and death. Severe reactions are associated with higher doses of disulfiram and >2 oz of alcohol. It is not recommended that patients with hepatic or cardiac disease be started on disulfiram. Psychosis can also be exacerbated by disulfiram because it inhibits the enzyme dopamine β-hydroxylase, causing a rise in dopamine levels. Disulfiram inhibits a wide variety of liver enzymes and therefore it will reduce clearance rates of drugs including chlordiazepoxide, diazepam, desipramine, imipramine, phenytoin, and warfarin (Coumadin). Serious adverse effects such as optic neuritis, peripheral neuropathy, and hepatotoxicity are rare.

It is recommended to start disulfiram at a daily dose of 250 mg. Efficacy of disulfiram depends on patient compliance. Administration of disulfiram should be avoided in those who are noncompliant or who have difficulty in understanding or following instructions on avoidance of not only alcohol ingestion but also ingestion of substances containing alcohol. These include foods and over-the-counter medications such as mouthwash, cold medications, or cosmetics with alcohol as an ingredient. Educating the patient about disulfiram and providing written information about interactions are important.

Naltrexone. The opioid antagonist naltrexone is an anticraving medication for alcohol dependence that acts by blocking endogenous opioids which induce the euphoria and relaxation effects of alcohol. It is well tolerated and results in significantly less alcohol craving, fewer drinking days, and less drinks per occasion.[73-75] Provided the patient is not on opiates, naltrexone is given as 25 mg for a starting dose and increased to 50 mg PO daily and is well tolerated; side effects include nausea. Hepatotoxicity is a potential adverse effect, and liver function tests should be monitored during naltrexone treatment. A sustained-release (depot) preparation has recently been FDA approved for monthly use, eliminating the problem of patient noncompliance.

Acamprosate. Acamprosate, FDA approved for the treatment of alcohol dependence, acts on the N-methyl-D-aspartate (NMDA) receptor to modulate glutamate release. It has been shown to decrease desire to drink and enhances treatment retention and maintenance of abstinence in several European trials.[76-79] However in more recent American[80,81] and Australian trials,[82] results are mixed and it may not be as effective as naltrexone.

Pharmacotherapy for Opioid Dependence

Methadone maintenance. Methadone maintenance therapy for opiate addicts is a proven and effective treatment for heroin addiction. Good treatment retention, improved psychosocial adjustment, and reduced criminal activity are other reported benefits.

Buprenorphine maintenance. Outpatient buprenorphine maintenance treatment using the sublingual combination tablet containing buprenorphine and naloxone (Suboxone) is also a safe and effective treatment for opiate dependence. Buprenorphine treatment is available at specialized addiction treatment programs as well as through private physicians who are trained and DEA approved to prescribe it. A list of physicians who are licensed to prescribe buprenorphine in various regions is available through the Substance Abuse and Mental Health Services Administration (SAMHSA) website (www.buprenorphine.samhsa.gov).

Naltrexone therapy. This long-acting opioid antagonist provides complete blockade of opioid receptors when taken at a dosage of 50 mg a day. Naltrexone treatment retention rates are very low, only approximately 20% to 30% over 6 months.[83] Those who have external incentives to comply with treatment (e.g., health care professionals, business executives, people on probation) are good candidates for naltrexone treatment of opioid dependence. The new long-acting depot preparation of naltrexone, mentioned earlier, should improve compliance rates.

Naltrexone is started at 25 mg PO on the first day after withdrawal from opiates is completed. There should be at least a 5- to 7-day period free from short-acting opioids and a 7- to 10-day period for long-acting opioids in order to avoid precipitated withdrawal syndromes. If naltrexone is tolerated, the subsequent doses can be administered at 50 mg every day or 100 mg q.o.d. Nausea and vomiting are common side effects, and there is a potential for liver toxicity.

Pharmacotherapy for Sedative-Hypnotic Dependence

There is no FDA-approved pharmacotherapy for treatment of sedative-hypnotic dependence. As discussed earlier, detoxification from benzodiazepines and sedative-hypnotics using long-acting benzodiazepines or phenobarbital is necessary to avoid life-threatening withdrawal syndromes. After detoxification is complete, rebound anxiety and other symptom reemergence is common and may be managed with antidepressants and cognitive-behavioral therapies. Other approaches used include augmentation with carbamazepine, gabapentin, tricyclics, or buspirone, and the use of sedating antidepressants and nonaddictive sleep aids such as mirtazapine, trazodone, or ramelteon.

Cocaine/Stimulant Dependence

Cocaine and stimulant abuse and dependence are associated with several psychiatric illnesses: depression, bipolar disorder, anxiety disorders, personality disorders, psychosis, and suicidal behavior.[51,65,84–87] The FDA has not approved any medication for the indication of treatment of cocaine addiction, and there is little consensus on effective pharmacotherapy for cocaine dependence. Medication treatment should target psychiatric symptoms associated with cocaine and stimulant dependence, such as psychosis and depression that does not remit during the acute withdrawal phase.

Conclusions

In most psychiatric residency programs, specific training in the treatment of addictive disorders consists of a 2- or 3-month rotation. This is proving to be inadequate for the inpatient clinician, given the prevalence of addictive disorders in psychiatric inpatients. Several organizations have websites that include excellent resources and publications available to the practitioner. The National Institute on Alcohol Abuse and Alcoholism (NIAAA) website (www.niaaa.nih.gov) publishes the quarterly peer-reviewed journal *Alcohol Research and Health* as well as monographs and publications on treatment of co-occurring disorders. The National Institute on Drug Abuse (NIDA) website (www.nida.nih.gov) features publications for treatment clinicians, and the peer-reviewed journal *NIDA Science and Practice Perspectives*. The SAMHSA website also has a publication site and includes the Center for Substance Abuse Treatment (CSAT) (www.csat.samhsa.gov) page, where Treatment Improvement Protocols (TIPs) publications can be ordered at no cost. The authors highly recommend the TIP publications which are evidence-based best practice guidelines providing a wealth of information from consensus panels of nationally known substance use experts and professionals in related areas of mental health, primary care, and social services.

REFERENCES

1. Regier DA, Farmer ME, Rae DS, et al. Comorbidity of mental disorders with alcohol and other drug abuse: Results from the epidemiologic catchment area (ECA) study. *JAMA.* 1990; 264:2511–2518.
2. Kessler RC, McGonagle KA, Zhao S, et al. Lifetime and 12-month prevalence of DSM-III-R psychiatric disorders in the united states. Results from the national comorbidity survey. *Arch Gen Psychiatry.* 1994;51(1):8–19.
3. Grant BF, Stinson FS, Dawson DA, et al. Co-occurrence of 12-month alcohol and drug use disorders and personality disorders in the united states: Results from the national epidemiologic survey on alcohol and related conditions. *Arch Gen Psychiatry.* 2004;61(4):361–368.
4. Grant BF, Stinson FS, Dawson DA, et al. Prevalence and co-occurrence of substance use disorders and independent mood and anxiety disorders: Results from the national epidemiologic survey on alcohol and related conditions. *Arch Gen Psychiatry.* 2004;61(8):807–816.
5. Grant BF, Stinson FS, Dawson DA, et al. Co-occurrence of DSM-IV personality disorders in the united states: Results from the national epidemiologic survey on alcohol and related conditions. *Compr Psychiatry.* 2005;46(1):1–5.
6. Stinson FS, Grant BF, Dawson DA, et al. Comorbidity between DSM-IV alcohol and specific drug use disorders in the united states: Results from the national epidemiologic survey on alcohol and related conditions. *Drug Alcohol Depend.* 2005;80(1):105–116.
7. Drake RE, Brunette MF. Complications of severe mental illness related to alcohol and drug use disorders. *Recent Dev Alcohol.* 1998;14:285–299.

8. Haywood TW, Kravitz HM, Grossman LS, et al. Predicting the "Revolving door" Phenomenon among patients with schizophrenic, schizoaffective, and affective disorders. *Am J Psychiatry.* 1995;152(6): 856–861.

9. Comtois KA, Russo JE, Roy-Byrne P, et al. Clinicians' assessments of bipolar disorder and substance abuse as predictors of suicidal behavior in acutely hospitalized psychiatric inpatients. *Biol Psychiatry.* 2004;56(10):757–763.

10. Rosenberg SD, Goodman LA, Osher FC, et al. Prevalence of HIV, Hepatitis B, and Hepatitis C in people with severe mental illness. *Am J Public Health.* 2001;91(1):31–37.

11. Goodman LA, Rosenberg SD, Mueser KT, et al. Physical and sexual assault history in women with serious mental illness: Prevalence, correlates, treatment, and future research directions. *Schizophr Bull.* 1997;23(4):685–696.

12. Swartz MS, Swanson JW, Hiday VA, et al. Violence and severe mental illness: The effects of substance abuse and nonadherence to medication. *Am J Psychiatry.* 1998;155(2): 226–231.

13. Abram KM, Teplin LA. Co-occurring disorders among mentally ill jail detainees. Implications for public policy. *Am Psychol.* 1991;46(10): 1036–1045.

14. Hurlburt MS, Hough RL, Wood PA. Effects of substance abuse on housing stability of homeless mentally ill persons in supported housing. *Psychiatr Serv.* 1996;47(7):731–736.

15. Appleby L, Dyson V, Luchins DJ, et al. The impact of substance use screening on a public psychiatric inpatient population. *Psychiatr Serv.* 1997;48(10):1311–1316.

16. Averill P, Veazey C, Shack A, et al. Acute mental illness and comorbid substance abuse: Physician-patient agreement on comorbid diagnosis and treatment implications. *Addict Disord Treat.* 2002; 1:119–125.

17. Ewing JA. Detecting alcoholism. The cage questionnaire. *JAMA.* 1984;252(14):1905–1907.

18. Babor TF, de la Fuente J, Saunders J, et al. *Audit – the alcohol use disorders identification test: guidelines for use in primary health care.* Geneva, Switzerland: World Health Organization; 1992.

19. Russell M, Martier SS, Sokol RJ, et al. Screening for pregnancy risk-drinking. *Alcohol Clin Exp Res.* 1994;18(5):1156–1161.

20. Pokorny AD, Miller BA, Kaplan HB. The brief mast: A shortened version of the michigan alcoholism screening test. *Am J Psychiatry.* 1972; 129(3):342–345.

21. Schuckit MA, Tipp JE, Reich T, et al. The histories of withdrawal convulsions and delirium tremens in 1648 alcohol dependent subjects. *Addiction.* 1995;90(10):1335–1347.

22. Sullivan JT, Sykora K, Schneiderman J, et al. Assessment of alcohol withdrawal: The revised clinical institute withdrawal assessment for alcohol scale (CIWA-Ar). *Br J Addict.* 1989;84(11):1353–1357.

23. Bonnet U, Specka M, Leweke FM, et al. Gabapentin's acute effect on mood profile – a controlled study on patients with alcohol withdrawal. *Prog Neuropsychopharmacol Biol Psychiatry.* 2007;31(2):434–438.

24. Malcolm R, Myrick LH, Veatch LM, et al. Self-reported sleep, sleepiness, and repeated alcohol withdrawals: A randomized, double blind, controlled comparison of lorazepam versus gabapentin. *J Clin Sleep Med.* 2007;3(1):24–32.

25. Mariani JJ, Rosenthal RN, Tross S, et al. A randomized, open-label, controlled trial of gabapentin and phenobarbital in the treatment of alcohol withdrawal. *Am J Addict.* 2006;15(1): 76–84.

26. Reed LJ, Glasper A, de Wet CJ, et al. Comparison of buprenorphine and methadone in the treatment of opiate withdrawal: Possible advantages of buprenorphine for the treatment of opiate-benzodiazepine codependent patients? *J Clin Psychopharmacol.* 2007;27(2):188–192.

27. Lai SH, Yao YJ, Lo DS. A survey of buprenorphine related deaths in singapore. *Forensic Sci Int.* 2006;162(1-3):80–86.

28. Reynaud M, Petit G, Potard D, et al. Six deaths linked to concomitant use of buprenorphine and benzodiazepines. *Addiction.* 1998;93(9): 1385–1392.

29. Dickenson W, Mayo-Smith M, Eickelberg S. Management of sedative-hypnotic intoxication and withdrawal. In: Graham A, Schultz T, Mayo-Smith M, eds. *Principles of addiction medicine,* 3rd ed. Chevy Chase: American Society of Addiction Medicine; 2003:633–649.

30. Ries R, Cullison S, Horn R, et al. Benzodiazepine withdrawal: Clinicians' ratings of carbamazepine treatment versus traditional taper methods. *J Psychoactive Drugs.* 1991;23(1):73–76.

31. Landabaso MA, Iraurgi I, Jimenez-Lerma JM, et al. Ecstasy-induced psychotic disorder: Six-month follow-up study. *Eur Addict Res.* 2002; 8(3):133–140.

32. Galloway GP, Frederick SL, Staggers FE Jr, et al. Gamma-hydroxybutyrate: An emerging drug of abuse that causes physical dependence. *Addiction.* 1997;92(1):89–96.

33. McDonough M, Kennedy N, Glasper A, et al. Clinical features and management of gamma-hydroxybutyrate (GHB) withdrawal: A review. *Drug Alcohol Depend.* 2004;75(1):3–9.

34. Budney AJ, Novy PL, Hughes JR. Marijuana withdrawal among adults seeking treatment for marijuana dependence. *Addiction.* 1999; 94(9):1311–1322.

35. Semple DM, McIntosh AM, Lawrie SM. Cannabis as a risk factor for psychosis: Systematic review. *J Psychopharmacol.* 2005;19(2):187–194.

36. van Os J, Bak M, Hanssen M, et al. Cannabis use and psychosis: A longitudinal population-based study. *Am J Epidemiol.* 2002;156(4): 319–327.

37. Nigam AK, Ray R, Tripathi BM. Buprenorphine in opiate withdrawal: A comparison with clonidine. *J Subst Abuse Treat.* 1993;10(4):391–394.

38. Prochaska JO, DiClemente CC, Norcross JC. In search of how people change. Applications to addictive behaviors. *Am Psychol.* 1992;47(9): 1102–1114.

39. Rollnick S, Miller W. What is motivational interviewing? *Behav Cogn Psychother.* 1995;23: 325–334.

40. Miller WR, Rollnick S. *Motivational interviewing: preparing people for change.* 2nd ed. New York: Guilford Press; 2002.

41. Drake RE, Mueser KT. Psychosocial approaches to dual diagnosis. *Schizophr Bull.* 2000;26(1): 105–118.

42. Emrick C, Tonigan J, Montgomery H, et al. Alcoholics anonymous: what is currently known? In: McCrady B, Miller W, eds. *Research on alcoholics anonymous: opportunities and alternatives.* New Brunswick: Rutgers Center of Alcohol Studies; 1993:41–76.

43. Humphreys K, Moos RH, Cohen C. Social and community resources and long-term recovery from treated and untreated alcoholism. *J Stud Alcohol.* 1997;58(3):231–238.

44. Kaskutas LA, Ammon L, Delucchi K, et al. Alcoholics anonymous careers: Patterns of AA involvement five years after treatment entry. *Alcohol Clin Exp Res.* 2005;29(11):1983–1990.

45. Timko C, Moos RH, Finney JW, et al. Long-term outcomes of alcohol use disorders: Comparing untreated individuals with those in alcoholics anonymous and formal treatment. *J Stud Alcohol.* 2000;61(4):529–540.

46. Tonigan JS, Toscova R, Miller WR. Meta-analysis of the literature on alcoholics anonymous: Sample and study characteristics moderate findings. *J Stud Alcohol.* 1996;57(1):65–72.

47. Kaskutas LA, Bond J, Humphreys K. Social networks as mediators of the effect of alcoholics anonymous. *Addiction.* 2002;97(7):891–900.

48. Laudet AB, Magura S, Cleland CM, et al. The effect of 12-step based fellowship participation on abstinence among dually diagnosed persons: A two-year longitudinal study. *J Psychoactive Drugs.* 2004;36(2):207–216.

49. Alcoholics Anonymous World Services. *The AA member-medications & other drugs.* Available from: http://www.alcoholics-anonymous.org/en_services_for_members.cfm?PageID=189, 1984.

50. Ziedonis DM, Smelson D, Rosenthal RN, et al. Improving the care of individuals with schizophrenia and substance use disorders: Consensus recommendations. *J Psychiatr Pract.* 2005;11(5):315–339.

51. Brady KT, Lydiard RB, Malcolm R, et al. Cocaine-induced psychosis. *J Clin Psychiatry.* 1991; 52(12):509–512.

52. Srisurapanont M, Ali M, Marsden J, et al. Psychotic symptoms in methamphetamine psychotic inpatients. *Int J Neuropsychopharmacol.* 2003;6:347–352.

53. Sato M. A lasting vulnerability to psychosis in patients with previous methamphetamine psychosis. *Ann N Y Acad Sci.* 1990;654:160–170.

54. Green AI. Pharmacotherapy for schizophrenia and co-occurring substance use disorders. *Neurotox Res.* 2007;11(1):33–40.

55. Potvin S, Stip E, Lipp O, et al. Quetiapine in patients with comorbid schizophrenia-spectrum and substance use disorders: An open-label trial. *Curr Med Res Opin.* 2006;22(7):1277–1285.

56. Sattar SP, Bhatia SC, Petty F. Potential benefits of quetiapine in the treatment of substance dependence disorders. *J Psychiatry Neurosci.* 2004; 29(6):452–457.

57. Sonne SC, Brady KT. Substance abuse and bipolar comorbidity. *Psychiatr Clin North Am* 1999; 22(3):609–627, ix

58. Sonne SC, Brady KT, Morton WA. Substance abuse and bipolar affective disorder. *J Nerv Ment Dis.* 1994;182(6):349–352.

59. Geller B, Cooper TB, Sun K, et al. Double-blind and placebo-controlled study of lithium for adolescent bipolar disorders with secondary substance dependency. *J Am Acad Child Adolesc Psychiatry.* 1998;37(2):171–178.

60. Bowden CL. Predictors of response to divalproex and lithium. *J Clin Psychiatry.* 1995;56(Suppl 3): 25–30.

61. Brady KT, Sonne SC, Anton R, et al. Valproate in the treatment of acute bipolar affective episodes complicated by substance abuse: A pilot study. *J Clin Psychiatry.* 1995;56(3):118–121.

62. Albanese MJ, Clodfelter RC Jr, Khantzian EJ. Divalproex sodium in substance abusers with mood disorder. *J Clin Psychiatry.* 2000; 61(12):916–921.

63. Salloum IM, Cornelius JR, Daley DC, et al. Efficacy of valproate maintenance in patients with bipolar disorder and alcoholism: A double-blind placebo-controlled study. *Arch Gen Psychiatry.* 2005;62(1):37–45.

64. Goldberg JF, Garno JL, Leon AC, et al. A history of substance abuse complicates remission from acute mania in bipolar disorder. *J Clin Psychiatry.* 1999;60(11):733–740.

65. Salloum IM, Douaihy A, Cornelius JR, et al. Divalproex utility in bipolar disorder with co-occurring cocaine dependence: A pilot study. *Addict Behav.* 2007;32(2):410–415.

66. Kranzler HR, Burleson JA, Del Boca FK, et al. Buspirone treatment of anxious alcoholics.

A placebo-controlled trial. *Arch Gen Psychiatry.* 1994;51(9):720–731.

67. McRae AL, Sonne SC, Brady KT, et al. A randomized, placebo-controlled trial of buspirone for the treatment of anxiety in opioid-dependent individuals. *Am J Addict.* 2004;13(1):53–63.

68. Pande AC, Davidson JR, Jefferson JW, et al. Treatment of social phobia with gabapentin: A placebo-controlled study. *J Clin Psychopharmacol.* 1999;19(4):341–348.

69. Le Bon O, Murphy JR, Staner L, et al. Double-blind, placebo-controlled study of the efficacy of trazodone in alcohol post-withdrawal syndrome: Polysomnographic and clinical evaluations. *J Clin Psychopharmacol.* 2003;23(4):377–383.

70. Nunes EV, Levin FR. Treatment of depression in patients with alcohol or other drug dependence: A meta-analysis. *JAMA.* 2004;291(15):1887–1896.

71. Pettinati HM. Antidepressant treatment of co-occurring depression and alcohol dependence. *Biol Psychiatry.* 2004;56(10):785–792.

72. Sullivan LE, Fiellin DA, O'Connor PG. The prevalence and impact of alcohol problems in major depression: A systematic review. *Am J Med.* 2005;118(4):330–341.

73. Chick J, Anton R, Checinski K, et al. A multicentre, randomized, double-blind, placebo-controlled trial of naltrexone in the treatment of alcohol dependence or abuse. *Alcohol Alcohol.* 2000;35(6):587–593.

74. Oslin D, Liberto JG, O'Brien J, et al. Naltrexone as an adjunctive treatment for older patients with alcohol dependence. *Am J Geriatr Psychiatry.* 1997;5(4):324–332.

75. Volpicelli JR, Alterman AI, Hayashida M, et al. Naltrexone in the treatment of alcohol dependence. *Arch Gen Psychiatry.* 1992;49(11):876–880.

76. Paille FM, Guelfi JD, Perkins AC, et al. Double-blind randomized multicentre trial of acamprosate in maintaining abstinence from alcohol. *Alcohol Alcohol.* 1995;30(2):239–247.

77. Sass H, Soyka M, Mann K, et al. Relapse prevention by acamprosate. Results from a placebo-controlled study on alcohol dependence. *Arch Gen Psychiatry.* 1996;53(8):673–680.

78. Tempesta E, Janiri L, Bignamini A, et al. Acamprosate and relapse prevention in the treatment of alcohol dependence: A placebo-controlled study. *Alcohol.* 2000;35(2):202–209.

79. Whitworth AB, Fischer F, Lesch OM, et al. Comparison of acamprosate and placebo in long-term treatment of alcohol dependence. *Lancet.* 1996; 347(9013):1438–1442.

80. Anton RF, O'Malley SS, Ciraulo DA, et al. Combined pharmacotherapies and behavioral interventions for alcohol dependence: The combine study: A randomized controlled trial. *JAMA.* 2006;295(17):2003–2017.

81. Mason BJ, Goodman AM, Chabac S, et al. Effect of oral acamprosate on abstinence in patients with alcohol dependence in a double-blind, placebo-controlled trial: The role of patient motivation. *J Psychiatr Res.* 2006; 40(5):383–393.

82. Morley KC, Teesson M, Reid SC, et al. Naltrexone versus acamprosate in the treatment of alcohol dependence: A multi-centre, randomized, double-blind, placebo-controlled trial. *Addiction.* 2006;101(10):1451–1462.

83. Kleber HD, Topazian M, Gaspari J, et al. Clonidine and naltrexone in the outpatient treatment of heroin withdrawal. *Am J Drug Alcohol Abuse.* 1987;13(1-2):1–17.

84. Cassidy F, Ahearn EP, Carroll BJ. Substance abuse in bipolar disorder. *Bipolar Disord.* 2001; 3(4):181–188.

85. Kranzler HR, Satel S, Apter A. Personality disorders and associated features in cocaine-dependent inpatients. *Compr Psychiatry.* 1994; 35(5):335–340.

86. O'Brien MS, Wu LT, Anthony JC. Cocaine use and the occurrence of panic attacks in the community: A case-crossover approach. *Subst Use Misuse.* 2005;40(3):285–297.

87. Rounsaville BJ. Treatment of cocaine dependence and depression. *Biol Psychiatry.* 2004; 56(10):803–809.

CHAPTER 16

The Elderly Psychiatric Inpatient

VASSILIOS LATOUSSAKIS, SIBEL A. KLIMSTRA, DIMITRIS N. KIOSSES, BALKRISHNA KALAYAM, AND GEORGE S. ALEXOPOULOS

Aging is associated with physiological and psychological changes that may alter the manifestation, course, and treatment response of both general medical and psychiatric disorders. With advancing age, mental health problems develop ever more frequently in the context of medical and neurologic illness. Adopting a "geriatric-friendly" approach means to be attuned to those age-associated changes and to the complex interactions of mental and physical factors in the elderly population.

Beginning in the early 1980s, many recognized the benefits of treating medically ill elderly patients in specialized geriatric units as opposed to mixed-age medical units.[1,2] Similarly, elderly patients (i.e., those older than 64 years) in need of acute inpatient psychiatric care may benefit more from an admission into a specialized geropsychiatric unit as opposed to a mixed-aged unit. Over the last 25 years, an increasing number of geropsychiatric units have been established in general hospitals in recognition of the uniqueness of this age-group and the importance of integrating psychiatric and medical care in this population.

On a specialized geropsychiatric unit, elders are more likely to receive comprehensive medical and cognitive assessments, monitoring of psychopharmacologic side effects and blood levels, and aging-sensitive aftercare referral.[3]

Within a geropsychiatric unit, multidisciplinary teamwork and the use of mental health assessment protocols have been found clinically important.[4] In a study of 31 inpatient psychiatry units across the country, geriatric professionals were surveyed to understand what practices were adopted for optimal care. Physical modifications included handrails, tub lifts, specialized furniture such as moveable geri-chairs, recliners, lowered and/or electric beds and hospital beds, wheelchair accessibility, specialized flooring, and increased walking areas. Safety emphasis included restraint reduction, fall prevention plans with protocols and screening, and monitoring of physical signs and symptoms such as pain, dysphagia, and oral intake. Increased family contact was encouraged. More than 75% of all specialized geriatric units provided reminiscence groups, family and patient education, exercise and music groups, and recreational/leisure activities. Fifty-five percent of the units used nurse-led groups. Challenges to care included nursing staffing shortages, lack of staff training in geriatric psychiatry, patient medical acuity, balancing restraint/seclusion regulations with fall prevention, and discharge placement difficulties. Excellence in multidisciplinary care (67% of respondents) was the factor most commonly identified for a successful unit. Additional factors included availability of geriatric medicine physicians and on-unit services.[5] Readily available on-unit geriatric medicine and neurology consultation services are optimal, given the high degree of medical comorbidity.

The adaptation of successful geriatric psychiatry inpatient care within existing mixed-age frameworks is an alternative milieu model to an independent geropsychiatry unit that, while perhaps ideal, may not be feasible for administrative or financial reasons. Faced with these limitations, one study describes an inpatient "geropsychiatric unit without walls." A senior team program for geropsychiatric inpatients was created within an existing adult inpatient unit of a general hospital. Geriatric patients were clustered together, physical modifications were made including a senior team lounge near the nursing station, and staff received geriatric care training. Remarkably, over the first 14 months of the program, the elderly "fall" rate was reduced and no geriatric patient required restraints.[6] Additional geriatric milieu management requires awareness that cognitive impairment may limit psychotherapy; the use of "behavior as communication" becomes critical. Tolerance of wandering behaviors, while monitoring safety, is encouraged.[7]

The most common primary diagnosis among elderly psychiatric inpatients is depression, which accounts for 33% to 73% of cases. Dementia complicated by psychosis or behavioral disturbances is the second most common primary diagnosis, followed by psychotic disorders (10%), bipolar disorder (8% to 10%), substance-related disorders (6% to 7%), and delirium (4% to 5%).[8–11]

Despite the general trend toward shortened inpatient length of stay,[12] certain factors predict protracted stays among psychogeriatric patients:[8] higher Brief Psychiatric Rating Scale positive symptoms scores, electroconvulsive therapy (ECT), falls, pharmacologic complications, history of multiple psychiatric hospitalizations, legal proceedings for continued inpatient treatment, delays in consultations, and lack of ECT on weekends.

The chapter is organized along the lines of the customary phases of inpatient work: admission, evaluation, management, and discharge. This is done more for convenience of organization than to suggest that there are clear demarcating lines between those phases.

Admission

Psychiatry patients who are older than 64 years are almost twice as likely to be treated as inpatients, compared with younger adults.[13] They can be admitted from a variety of settings—medical inpatient units, assisted living or skilled nursing facilities, or the community.

Two clinical problems are especially relevant in the elderly and frequently trigger a psychiatric inpatient admission: suicidality and inability to care for oneself.

Case Vignette

The 81-year-old white retired accountant took his own life by shooting himself in the head. His daughter had returned unexpectedly to pick up something she needed for an errand and was horrified to discover him lying on the floor of his bedroom. On the bed, he had left a note directing her on financial matters. She had known that he was having a rough time lately. A few years ago, his wife had passed away after a long battle with colon cancer. Since then, he had seemed more sullen, but things had taken a turn for the worse several months previously when his oldest son and his family moved away to another state. Usually keeping to himself, the only things he had enjoyed were spending time with his grandchildren and taking care of the garden. After they left, he had grown more silent and made frequent cynical and pessimistic remarks about himself and the world in general all the while denying feeling depressed. He had stopped attending to his garden and did not leave the house for days. His heart was failing him too. Three weeks before his death, he had visited his primary care doctor who had made some changes in his regimen for congestive heart failure and prescribed clonazepam for anxiety. More recently, his sleep had deteriorated; he paced for hours in the middle of the night and, on a couple of occasions, his daughter had heard him talking to himself or somebody else with harsh words. He had refused to seek psychiatric help throughout this period and had gotten increasingly upset when she urged him to talk to someone about the way he felt.

Suicidality affects the elderly disproportionately. Although they represent 13% of the population, they account for 18% of completed suicides.[14] Elderly white males are mostly responsible for the increased suicide rate, which, for those older than 75 years, is almost double that of the general population.[15] Elderly persons attempt suicide less frequently than younger adults, but when they do they use more violent means of suicide and are more likely to succeed in taking their own lives.[16] Firearms, which account for 70% of suicides among those 70 years and older, independently increase the risk for suicide.[17]

As the vignette illustrates, elderly with depression are less likely to report depressed mood or suicidal ideation compared with younger people.[18],[19] Indeed, most of the elderly who commit suicide have never made a previous attempt and have never received psychiatric treatment. The single most significant risk factor for suicide in the elderly is a depression diagnosis. Both major and nonmajor depression increase the risk for suicide,[20] although depression severity is highly correlated with suicide risk in the elderly.[21] Psychotic depression, active or remitted alcohol and substance use disorders, impaired functional level, and bereavement or recent loss also increase the risk of suicide in the elderly.[22],[23] Psychotic depression often requires inpatient treatment because of the increased suicide risk, and the likely need for combination pharmacotherapy or ECT warranting close monitoring, especially in the frail elderly with medical comorbidities.[24]

Case Vignette

Mrs. R, now almost 75, always preferred to have lunch at the local senior citizen center. Her chronic bronchitis, congestive heart failure, and marked obesity restricted her agility and it took her almost 45 minutes each way to walk the three blocks from her first-floor walk-up apartment to the center. The social workers greeted her with warmth everyday. These short exchanges were, on most days, the only meaningful interaction for Mrs. R, who had been estranged from her two adult children and lived alone for as long as anybody remembered. Every few years or so, she would draw attention upon herself by accusing a staff member or one of her senior peers of something sinister, usually stealing, eavesdropping, or plotting something against her. Her accusations were never substantiated. In the wake of such an incident, she would stop dropping in for lunch for a few days but then she would reappear. After one such incident though, she was not seen at the center for more than a month. The senior social worker alerted the adult protection services and a field worker paid a visit to Mrs. R. With the help of the building's superintendent, they entered her apartment only to discover Mrs. R lying on the floor, unable to get up, mumbling something about "strange odors coming from the people upstairs." She was malodorous, had not eaten or taken her medications for days, but kept insisting they leave her alone.

Cognitive impairment and medical comorbidities frequently coexist in elderly psychiatric inpatients. Elders with dementia are often admitted for severe behavioral disturbances or uncontrolled aggression. As in the case just described, when a community-dwelling older person becomes incapable of self-care, an admission is warranted. Such patients may be dehydrated, malnourished, and unable to adhere to their medication regimens. Because of their physical frailty, cognitive deficits, or medical comorbidities, it may be unsafe to evaluate and treat their psychiatric problems as outpatients.[25] When medically ill or medically high-risk patients require inpatient psychiatric treatment, a combined medical/psychiatric geriatric unit offering integrated monitoring and treatment[26] or a psychiatric unit within a general medical hospital are preferred treatment settings.

Diagnostic Evaluation

Evaluation should systematically attend to elderly specific factors such as the frequent coexistence of general medical and neurologic illnesses. Elderly psychiatric inpatients, like elderly general medical inpatients, have on average five to six active medical problems.[10] The inpatient psychiatrist needs to collect historical information about psychiatric, general medical, and neurologic issues including all medical conditions and medicines. Inquiry about any cognitive decline or deterioration in function or nutritional status is essential. Other sources of information such as family members, caregivers, and previous treaters should be sought because psychiatric illness as well as cognitive impairment may impair recollection or insight in the elderly.

Alcohol and over-the-counter and prescription medicines such as opiate analgesics and benzodiazepines are more commonly abused than illicit substances in the elderly[27] and warrant specific inquiry. Such substances may cause mood and/or cognitive disorders and lead to withdrawal syndromes.

Past psychiatric history should attempt to differentiate between early-onset and late-onset disorders such as depression, mania, or schizophrenia because they may be associated with distinct clinical and treatment–response characteristics. Family history should include episodes of mood or cognitive illness in blood relatives, attempted or completed suicides, as well as any medical or neurologic illness giving rise to a psychiatric syndrome. An elderly-specific social history should focus on social support or isolation, including whether involved family members live locally, financial and retirement status, and any recent losses leading to bereavement. The ability to perform basic and instrumental activities of daily living is also included here.

Mental status assessment is not complete without a cognitive assessment. A brief, widely used, global standardized instrument is the Mini Mental State Examination (MMSE). It assesses domains of orientation, memory, concentration, language, and constructional ability. It is not sensitive in assessing executive function, a domain that may be impaired in dementias and geriatric depression. The clock drawing test, also a brief and standardized instrument, can reveal executive dysfunction in the depressed elderly[28] and in elderly patients with a normal MMSE.[29] Another brief and effective tool for dementia detection is the Mini-Cog,[30] which combines a three-item recall question and the clock drawing test, and performs at least as well as the MMSE in culturally diverse elderly populations.[31]

A targeted but systematic physical, including neurologic, examination is necessary. Normal neurologic changes found in aged populations—such as head or neck tremors, muscle atrophy of the hands, restricted conjugate upward gaze, reduced vibration sense, and nonspecific gait disturbance—should not be confused with neurologic disease. On admission, the nutritional and functional status should be routinely assessed, including gait assessment and fall risk. Risk factors for falls in the inpatient geropsychiatric setting include cardiac arrhythmias, degenerative neurologic disorders (Parkinson disease, dementias), and use of mood stabilizers or ECT.[32] Postural hypotension also predisposes to falls[33] and sitting/standing vital signs should be a routine part of vital sign assessment.

Laboratory tests may assist in differential diagnosis, especially when medical factors are thought to contribute to or cause psychiatric signs and symptoms, and are routinely used to assess the safety of initiating a medication trial (e.g., lithium) or ECT. Upon admission, laboratory screening may include electrolytes, blood urea nitrogen/creatinine, fasting blood glucose, liver function tests, thyroid function tests, lipid profile, complete blood count, urinalysis, urine toxicology, and possibly blood alcohol level. Drug levels for nortiptyline, desipramine, lithium, valproic acid and digoxin, and prothrombin time/international normalized ratio (if warfarin is prescribed) should be ordered. Chest x-ray is usually part of the pre-ECT and delirium workups. Electrocardiogram (ECG) is often ordered.[34] For dementia workup, routine laboratory orders include serum chemistries, renal, liver and thyroid function tests, vitamin B_{12}, and complete blood count. Syphilis serology, urinalysis, erythrocyte sedimentation rate, heavy metal and toxicology screening, human immunodeficiency virus (HIV) testing, chest x-ray, electroencephalogram (EEG), ECG, and lumbar puncture may be ordered based on clinical suspicion.[35] Initial dementia evaluations generally include a structural neuroimaging study such as magnetic resonance imaging (MRI) or noncontrast computed tomography (CT), especially in those younger than 65, in the presence of vascular risk factors, and when focal neurologic lesions are suspected. Functional neuroimaging studies are currently limited to special circumstances. In particular, Medicare will cover a positron emission tomography (PET) study as part of the differential diagnosis of patients with clinical symptoms of frontotemporal dementia.

Management

The main goal of inpatient psychiatric treatment is to initiate safe and effective acute-phase therapies while managing medical comorbidities, maintaining the patient in a supportive environment, and providing appropriate aftercare referral and treatment recommendations.

For ease of presentation, this section will examine medication and psychosocial approaches separately. The treatment of delirium and dementia with behavioral disturbances will be discussed first, followed by schizophrenia, geriatric depression, and geriatric bipolar disorder. Emphasis will be placed on the treatment of the two most common geropsychiatric syndromes in the inpatient setting, severe depression and dementia with behavioral disturbances.

PSYCHOPHARMACOLOGIC APPROACHES

Guiding Principles of Inpatient Geriatric Psychopharmacology

1. Starting dose and titration speed should be individualized. Although side effects often appear at lower dosages in the elderly compared to younger adults, chronologic age is only one factor to be considered. Equally important is the knowledge of general physical health status and co-occurring general medical and psychiatric disorders. In light of this, "start low and go slow" may apply differently to different elderly patients.
2. Usual target doses depend on diagnosis and class of medication used. Selective serotonin reuptake inhibitors (SSRIs) and serotonin-norepinephrine reuptake inhibitors (SNRIs) have similar target doses in the elderly as in younger adults, whereas the target dose for neuroleptics in the elderly is diagnosis-dependent. Compared with younger adults, the elderly require lower target doses for schizophrenia and lower doses still for dementia-related psychosis and behavioral disturbances.[36,37] Because adequate target dose is critical, the "start low and go slow" principle may have to be revised to "start low, go slow, but get there."
3. The list of coadministered medicines should be scrutinized to uncover potential drug–drug or disease–drug interactions A number of on-line drug information databases[38] as well as software programs for handheld devices[39] can be used to assist in the detection of drug–drug interactions. Their routine use by clinicians, on admission and when adding a new medicine, should be considered.
4. Caution is advised when psychotropic medicines are used on an as-needed (p.r.n.) basis. Such use may cloud the clinical picture and result in knee-jerk reactions in response to fleeting symptoms rather than a targeted treatment plan. It is crucial to review the use of p.r.n. medication regularly to prevent drug accumulation.

Delirium

The increased prevalence of dementia, multiple medical and neurologic comorbidities, and polypharmacy in the elderly make that age-group particularly susceptible to delirium. Differential diagnosis from common psychiatric syndromes such as dementia, depression, hypomanic and manic states, schizophrenia, and substance use disorders is not an easy task. Especially in patients who are not hyperactive or agitated, and therefore do not present an acute behavioral problem in the inpatient setting, delirium is frequently missed.[40,41] Delirium should be viewed as a medical emergency that, unless treated, may lead to significantly worsened outcomes including greater mortality and morbidity, prolonged hospital stays, and increased rates of institutionalization. Therefore, when in doubt, it is prudent to assume the diagnosis of delirium. Key clinical features of delirium include the acute or subacute development of disturbances in attention and orientation, sleep–wake cycle, and psychomotor functions.

Psychomotor disturbances in delirium may give rise to hyperactive, mixed, or hypoactive clinical subtypes. The latter two subtypes are more common than the hypoactive and less likely to be recognized despite being associated with a more severe illness.[40,42] A systematic workup must then proceed while attending to the safety of the delirious patient. A careful history and physical and neurologic examination may guide the selection of more tailored workups.

In the search for possible etiologies of delirium, it is helpful to remember that (a) delirium is often multifactorial;[43] (b) risk factors already identified during the admission assessment could guide further workup; and (c) delirium is frequently caused by non–CNS-related conditions such as infections (e.g., urinary tract infection), dehydration, and polypharmacy.[44]

While basic workup (complete blood count, electrolytes, liver and renal function tests, glucose, ECG, urinalysis, chest x-ray, and erythrocyte sedimentation rate) is being completed, medical or neurologic consultation may be sought. Further patient-specific tests may be warranted. Management should proceed hand in hand with diagnostic assessment. Environmental measures are an integral part of management and should always be considered. The main goals of environmental manipulations are (a) to correct or optimize any sensory deficits (use of glasses, hearing aids and dentures, adequate lighting, noise reduction, etc.), (b) to promote familiarity or orientation to surroundings (a visible clock and calendar, presence of a relative or family photos, frequent reality orientations, etc.), and (c) to ensure a reassuring and clear communication style by staff and family members.

Antipsychotic medications are the mainstay of pharmacologic management of delirium. Benzodiazepines should be avoided, except in alcohol or benzodiazepine withdrawal. Haloperidol, administered orally or intramuscularly, is helpful in most agitated patients. More recently, atypical antipsychotics have emerged as alternative options but further study is warranted before advocating their use.[44]

Dementia with Neuropsychiatric and Behavioral Disturbances

Neuropsychiatric and behavioral disturbances associated with dementia include psychosis and a spectrum of agitated behaviors, such as aggressive, physically nonaggressive, and verbal/vocal agitated behaviors. When such behavioral disturbances present a danger to self or others or cause a significant decline in functioning, an inpatient psychiatric admission is warranted for the elderly demented patient. During the inpatient geropsychiatric stay, specific targeted treatment symptoms should be identified and tracked. Because the etiology of behavioral disturbances in dementia is often multifactorial, a comprehensive assessment is warranted. Common causes of agitation in patients with dementia include delirium (superimposed on dementia), depression, and psychosis. Other important causes include dyspnea, dysuria, abdominal discomfort from constipation, and pruritus.[36,45] Finally, a number of patients present with "idiopathic" agitation syndromes, that is, behavioral disturbances in the context of a dementing disorder with no other identifiable cause(s).

NONPHARMACOLOGIC APPROACHES

Common and perhaps easily reversible causes of problematic behaviors in the demented elderly patient include space restriction, environmental over- or understimulation, a sudden decline in a patient's ability to communicate, and problems in the approach or style of the caregiver toward the patient.[36,46] Environmental manipulations, although frequently overlooked, may be beneficial and include optimizing hearing and vision, reduction of overstimulation, speaking in a soft and supportive tone, improving communication through nonverbal means, or attending to the patient during calm periods as well.

PHARMACOLOGIC APPROACHES

First, delirium should be ruled in or out and, if necessary, treated appropriately. In the presence of agitated depressive symptoms, an SSRI trial is indicated. When delusions are present, antipsychotics are recommended by expert consensus. Antipsychotics are favored by experts even in nondelusional patients, although they may not be as efficacious as when delusions are present.[36]

However, more recently, antipsychotic use in the elderly has come under increased scrutiny. The U.S. Food and Drug Administration (FDA), in April of 2005, issued a public health advisory, which required all manufacturers of atypical antipsychotics to add a Boxed Warning to their labeling describing a 1.6- to 1.7-fold mortality increase, primarily due to cardiac-related events or infections, in elderly patients with dementia and behavioral disturbances (FDA, 2005). An independent meta-analysis of randomized controlled studies of atypical antipsychotics found death occurring slightly more frequently with atypical antipsychotics versus placebo (3.5% vs. 2.3%).[47] Another large retrospective mixed diagnosis study found that elderly patients on antipsychotic medication for 180 days or less had a higher risk of death with conventional compared to atypical antipsychotics (relative risk = 1.37).[48] More recently, the National Institutes of Mental Health–sponsored Clinical Antipsychotic Trial of Intervention Effectiveness-Alzheimer disease (CATIE-AD) conducted a double-blind, placebo-controlled study of ambulatory outpatients with Alzheimer dementia and behavioral problems such as psychosis, agitation, or aggression. Patients were randomized to treatment with olanzapine, quetiapine, risperidone, or placebo and followed up for up to 36 weeks. Time to treatment discontinuation for any reason did not differ significantly among the medication and placebo groups. Median time to discontinuation due to lack of efficacy was significantly longer with olanzapine (22.1 weeks) or risperidone (26.7 weeks) than with quetiapine (9.1 weeks) or placebo (9.0 weeks). Discontinuation rates due to intolerance, adverse effects, or death were 24% with olanzapine, 18% with risperidone, 16% with quetiapine, and 5% with placebo. However, findings from this ambulatory study may not directly apply to the demented elderly inpatient with likely more severe behavioral problems.

Therefore, it is prudent to exercise judgment in the use of all antipsychotics—atypical or conventional—for severe behavioral disturbances in dementia. The inpatient clinician initiating an antipsychotic trial should keep in mind that antipsychotic response times differ depending on diagnosis. Whereas dementia-related behavioral response may take several weeks, antimanic response may be seen in 2 to 4 days and antipsychotic response in schizophrenia within 1 week. For that reason, clinicians are in danger of generalizing their experiences, which may lead to overdosing and serious side effects. A useful inpatient strategy is to initiate and maintain atypical antipsychotics at low dosages, using, for a time-limited period, low-dose standing benzodiazepines (with heightened fall precautions) to treat dementia-related agitation symptomatically until the therapeutic effect of antipsychotics is established. Agitated and aggressive behaviors in AD have responded to risperidone at a dosage of 1 mg per day or olanzapine a dosage of 5 to 10 mg per day.[48,49] The clinician should discuss with the family the risks with antipsychotic use, including the risk of metabolic syndrome, cerebrovascular accidents (CVAs), or even death. Clinicians should document (a) their rationale for using an antipsychotic, including a discussion of the risk/benefit ratio, (b) other approaches considered or attempted first, and (c) the risk of withholding antipsychotic treatment.

Cognitive enhancers such as cholinesterase inhibitors or memantine, although not useful in the acute control of behavioral disturbances in demented inpatients, may be helpful in the long term because they have shown to improve not only cognitive, but also behavioral, emotional, and psychotic symptoms.[50–54] Similarly, SSRIs, although likely more useful in preventing future episodes than treating the current one, may be considered for dementia-related behavioral disturbances.

Schizophrenia

Early- versus late-onset schizophrenia

Diagnostic and Statistical Manual of Mental Disorders, Fourth Edition, Text Revision (DSM-IV-TR) does not distinguish between late-onset and early-onset schizophrenia. Part of the reason may be that even the age after which the term *late onset* applies is unclear, with some requiring onset after age 40, others at 45 or even 60.[55] Nevertheless, there are clinical, neuropsychological, and genetic differences. Although delusions and hallucinations are common to both groups, symptoms tend to be milder in late-onset schizophrenia, with negative symptoms, thought disturbances, and first-rank Schneiderian symptoms being less prominent. Neurocognitive deficits exist in both chronic and late-onset schizophrenia. There is disagreement as to whether patterns of cognitive impairment are similar or markedly different with cognitive decline and dementia occurring earlier (within 5 years) in the late-onset schizophrenic group.[56] First-degree relatives of patients with late-onset schizophrenia have lower prevalence of the disease compared to first-degree relatives of patients with early-onset schizophrenia.[57]

Schizophrenia inpatient treatment

Clinicians should first rule out other causes of late-onset psychotic symptoms such as dementia and mood or delusional disorders. The mainstay of treatment for geriatric schizophrenia is antipsychotic pharmacotherapy. In the elderly, such treatment has been associated with an increased risk of cerebrovascular adverse events and even death. Most, if not all, of those risks were observed in demented patients with behavioral disturbances and it is unclear whether they pertain to other elderly clinical samples. In a recent mixed-age study, there was similar effectiveness (a measure of efficacy and tolerability) between atypical and typical antipsychotics.[58] Required antipsychotic doses for elderly patients with schizophrenia are intermediate to those for younger patients with schizophrenia and patients with dementia (see Table 16.1).[36]

TABLE 16.1 ANTIPSYCHOTIC DOSING FOR THREE DIFFERENT SYNDROMES

Drug	Dementia with Behavioral Disturbances	Schizophrenia in Late Life	Schizophrenia in Young and Middle Adulthood
Olanzapine	5.0–7.5 mg/d	7.5–15 mg/d	10–30 mg/d
Quetapine	50–150 mg/d	100–300 mg/d	300–800 mg/d
Risperidone	0.5–2.0 mg/d	1.25–3.5 mg/d	2–8 mg/d

(Data from Alexopoulos GS, et al. Expert Consensus Panel for Using Antipsychotic Drugs in Older Patients: Using antipsychotic agents in older patients. *J Clin Psychiatry*. 2004;65[Suppl 2]:5–102; Weiden P, et al. Translating the psychopharmacology of antipsychotics to individualized treatment for severe mental illness: A Roadmap. *J Clin Psychiatry*. 2007;68[Suppl 7]:1–48; Lehmann AF, et al. Practice guideline for the treatment of patients with schizophrenia, second edition. *Am J Psychiatry*. 2004;161[Suppl 2]:1–56.)

Bipolar Disorder

Elderly patients with bipolar disorder are approximately four times more likely to have had an inpatient psychiatric admission in the preceding 6 months compared with the elderly with unipolar depression.[59] Length of inpatient psychiatric hospitalization for older patients with bipolar disorder is twice that of their younger bipolar counterparts, perhaps due to slower symptom resolution or greater medical comorbidity.[60]

Case Vignette

Mrs. A was a 61-year-old woman who was admitted to the hospital voluntarily. She was accompanied by her husband who reported that, for the last 3 weeks, she attempted to spend all their retirement savings on a vacation home. She became irritable with him when he prevented her from purchasing anything but had not been at all violent. She was overly energetic and stayed up at night incessantly making phone calls. She also seemed confused and had not been caring for herself well, including not bathing or eating as much. She had no prior history of mood disorder, no family history of bipolar disorder, and no history of alcohol or substance use disorders, including prescription drugs. Her medical history was significant for hypertension, atrial fibrillation, and diabetes mellitus.

Compared with younger patients with bipolar disorder, elderly patients with bipolar disorder suffer less from comorbid substance use disorders; however, they experience greater impairment in functioning[60] and more disorientation and confusion.[61] This patient presents with late-onset manic symptoms and the distinction between early- versus late-onset illness is important clinically. Compared with early-onset elderly patients, those with late-onset illness are less likely to require emergency petition or to manifest aggression or threatening behaviors before inpatient psychiatric admission. They are also less likely to be medication nonadherent.[62] This patient has vascular disease, which is a risk factor for late-onset bipolar disorder. Specifically, hypertension, stroke, coronary artery disease, atrial fibrillation, diabetes mellitus, hypercholesterolemia, and hyperlipidemia are present more frequently in age-matched patients with late-onset versus early-onset bipolar disorders.[63] Also, neurologic disease and, to a lesser extent, decreased family history, are more strongly associated with late-onset illness.[11]

Differential diagnosis

Differential diagnosis should first exclude secondary mania in elderly patients with new-onset symptomatology. There are many causes of secondary mania and most can occur in the elderly. Because late-onset mania is associated with vascular disease, the clinician needs to be diligent in pursuing workup and treatment of these conditions, such as diabetes, hypertension, stroke, and cardiovascular disease.[64] Additional disorders particularly pertinent to the elderly include right-hemispheric and thalamic stroke, central nervous system [CNS] tumors, fall-related traumatic brain injury, hyperkinetic movement disorders, temporal lobe epilepsy, multiple sclerosis, and tertiary syphilis. Common medicines associated with mania include antidepressants, corticosteroids, dopaminergic drugs used to treat Parkinson disease, sympathomimetics, and benzodiazepines.[65]

Treatment

Patients with bipolar disorder who are older than 65 have twice the psychiatric inpatient length of stay of younger patients with bipolar disorder, which may be due to the increased rates of medical or psychiatric comorbidities.[11] The American Psychiatric Association's Practice Guideline for the Treatment of Patients with Bipolar Disorder[66] provides some guidance in the treatment approach. An evidence-based review of pharmacologic treatment in late-life bipolar disorder noted that lithium and divalproex are the two most common antimanic agents studied, and uncontrolled studies suggest that they are efficacious. However, there is little evidence on therapeutic concentration ranges or adequate duration for acute treatment with antimanic agents in the elderly. There is a paucity of systematic drug treatment studies in geriatric bipolar depression. Likewise, there are no studies comparing ECT and pharmacotherapy.[67] A retrospective study found no difference among lithium, valproic acid, and carbamazepine treatment in length of geriatric inpatient stay or improvement in global assessment of functioning scores.[68] A multicenter, randomized, double-blind, prospective National Institutes of Mental Health (NIMH)-funded trial is under way to assess the acute treatment efficacy of lithium versus divalproex in geriatric mania. Until more data are available, the strategies listed in the subsequent text may be useful for the inpatient treatment of geriatric bipolar disorder.[67]

1. For geriatric mania, the treatment of choice is monotherapy with a mood stabilizer. A dosage of lithium producing serum lithium levels of 0.4 to 0.8 mEq per L is reasonable as an initial target, but patients may require doses producing levels in the range of 0.8 to 1.0 mEq per L. Divalproex sodium may be given with target serum concentrations used for younger adults. Carbamazepine should be considered a second-line treatment. For partial responders to monotherapy with a mood stabilizer, adding an atypical antipsychotic or a second mood stabilizer may be useful.
2. For geriatric bipolar depression, monotherapy with lithium may be given. Lamotrigine should be considered using the same dosing strategies as for younger adults. If necessary, an antidepressant may be added.
3. ECT may be considered in either phase of geriatric bipolar disorder. Its use is indicated in the severely ill elderly patient where rapid response is critical, when medication trials present more risks than ECT, in medication refractory illness, and when medication side effects are intolerable,[69] as is often seen in the frail, medically compromised elderly. Management with ECT is discussed further in Chapter 10.

Geriatric Depression

DSM-IV criteria for major depressive disorder[70] are the same for young, midlife, and elderly adults, although depressive symptom expression may vary between age-groups. For example, major depression in the elderly may not be accurately diagnosed because geriatric patients often deny the subjective feeling of depressed mood and endorse instead an inability to derive pleasure from activities or focus on somatic or cognitive symptoms such as poor sleep, low energy, or memory difficulties.[71] In some cases, those physical or cognitive complaints may be incorrectly attributed to comorbid medical or dementing disorders, whereas in others physical and cognitive symptoms are indeed caused by such comorbid disorders with the depressive illness intensifying the clinical picture. Sad mood, frequent tearfulness, and recurrent thoughts of suicide and death are more reliable in diagnosing major depression in the elderly with the symptoms of anhedonia, social isolation, hopelessness, helplessness, worthlessness, nondelusional guilt, psychomotor activation or retardation, and impairment in decision making and daily planning of activities further assisting in establishing the diagnosis.

Major depression is often associated with neuropsychological deficits, such as concentration difficulties, slowed mental processing, and executive dysfunction.[72] Those deficits may persist, albeit ameliorated, after depressive symptoms remit.[73]

According to DSM-IV criteria,[70] psychotic depression is recognized only as a severe form of major depressive disorder, and the diagnosis can be made if delusions or hallucinations are present in the context of a major depressive episode. Approximately 40% of all depressed elderly inpatients manifest psychotic features.[74] Nevertheless, delusions—most frequently of guilt, nihilism, hypochondriasis, persecution, or jealousy[75]—and hallucinations are frequently not elicited or recognized as such by clinicians.[76] Across all age ranges, approximately 25% of inpatient psychotic depression is misdiagnosed, most frequently due to lack of recognition of psychosis.[77]

Several syndromes of late-life depression have been described, which may have clinical significance for treatment or prognosis.

Depression with Reversible Dementia

Dementia presenting during depressive episodes in old age at times subsides after remission of depression. This is particularly likely to occur in elderly patients with late-onset major depression. In many cases, some cognitive deficits persist, albeit in an ameliorated form, after depressive remission. In 40% of cases an irreversible dementia develops within 3 years of follow-up.[78] Therefore, reversible dementia may herald a permanent dementing syndrome, which needs to be identified and treated as early as possible.

Vascular Depression

Depressive syndromes in old age frequently coexist with cerebrovascular lesions and risk factors and often develop in the wake of strokes.[79] These observations formed the basis of the vascular depression hypothesis according to which cerebrovascular disease may predispose to, precipitate, or perpetuate some geriatric depressive syndromes.[80,81] The elderly with vascular depression have more apathy, retardation, and lack of insight and less agitation, and guilt than those with nonvascular depression.[81,82] Verbal fluency and naming are the most impaired cognitive functions in vascular depression. Finally, patients with this form of depression have greater disability compared to those who are depressed but have no vascular stigmata.[82]

The vascular depression hypothesis has clinical ramifications. Ameliorating cerebrovascular risk factors (e.g., hypertension or hypercholesterolemia) or employing agents promoting vascular integrity (e.g., antiplatelet agents, calcium channel blockers, or antioxidants) might reduce the risk of vascular depression. A study using the calcium channel blocker nimodipine as an augmenting agent led to improved antidepressant treatment outcomes compared to antidepressant monotherapy among patients with vascular depression.[83] Furthermore, the choice of antidepressant treatment might be guided by the presumptive knowledge of the underlying vascular etiology. Catecholaminergic agents promote functional recovery from ischemic brain lesions in contrast to serotoninergic agents or antidepressants with α-blocking action.[80]

Depression-Executive Dysfunction Syndrome

Clinical, structural and functional neuroimaging, and neuropathology studies point to frontostriatal limbic dysfunction as the biological substrate predisposing to at least some late-life depressive syndromes. The depression-executive dysfunction syndrome has been conceptualized as an entity with pronounced frontostriatal limbic dysfunction. Clinically, it is characterized by reduced interest in activities, psychomotor retardation, impaired instrumental activities of daily living, suspiciousness, impaired insight, and limited vegetative signs.[84] This syndrome has also been shown to have a poor, slow, and unstable response to antidepressant medications[85–87] and may respond better to problem-solving therapy (PST).[88]

Late-Onset Illness

Elderly patients who present with their first major depressive episode later in life, generally after age 50 to 60, have distinct characteristics compared with those with an earlier onset. These include a higher prevalence and a greater risk of developing dementia on follow-up,[89] more pronounced neuropsychological impairment as well as structural neuroimaging abnormalities (ventriculomegaly, white matter hyperintensities),[90] more sensorineural hearing loss,[91] less frequent family history of mood disorders, and less psychiatric comorbidity.[92]

However, use of age of onset as a distinguishing characteristic of geriatric depression introduces methodological and conceptual problems.[75] Methodologically, it is difficult to ascertain the time of onset of depressive symptoms, especially when those symptoms are mild.[93] Conceptually, brain abnormalities may contribute to a depressive episode occurring after age 50, regardless of whether the patient experienced other episodes earlier in life. Furthermore, depressive episodes earlier in life may predispose to brain abnormalities and thereby increase the risk of late-life depression.

Acute-phase inpatient treatment of late-life depression

Severe unipolar major depressive disorder without psychotic features. Combination pharmacotherapy and psychotherapy is the treatment of choice. Another first-line option is pharmacotherapy alone. Treatment should consist of single antidepressant trials, dosed adequately and given for an adequate duration. If there is no response, monotherapy with another antidepressant should follow. If there is partial response, augmentation strategies should be initiated.

SSRIs are the antidepressants of choice because they are as efficacious as the older tricyclic antidepressants (TCAs) and safer in overdose. However, SSRI use in the elderly may carry certain risks. A large population-based study of older adults (age older than 50 years) found that daily SSRI use increased the risk of falls and doubled the risk of fragility fractures.[94] Other studies associate SSRI use with an increased risk of suicide. Compared with other antidepressants, one study reported almost a fivefold increase in the risk of elderly suicide, but only during the first month after SSRI initiation and not at later time points. The absolute suicide risk was low (1 in 3,353 SSRI-treated patients), and many of these deaths were likely due to depressive illness, not to medication. SSRI treatment benefits appear to outweigh this small risk.[95] Clinicians should monitor suicidality throughout the course of treatment, and especially during the first month after antidepressant initiation.

SNRIs are another first-line option. Although uncommon, elevation of supine diastolic blood pressure is a potential side effect with these agents.[96,97] Other options include buproprion, mirtazine, and finally, in patients without cardiac conduction defects, TCAs. Among TCAs, nortriptyline and desipramine are preferred due to a better side effect profile. Doxepin, imipramine, amitriptyline, and trazodone should be avoided.

ECT may also be offered to severely depressed elderly inpatients. ECT has been shown to be effective in the elderly[98] and safe in patients with comorbid general medical conditions.[75] Indications for ECT use include failure of two adequate trials of antidepressants, acute suicide risk, and medical comorbidity complicating antidepressant medication treatment.

Unipolar major depressive disorder with psychotic features. According to expert consensus guidelines, psychotic depression in the elderly should be treated either with a combination of an antidepressant and an atypical antipsychotic or with ECT.[99] SSRIs and SNRIs are the preferred antidepressants, although direct empirical testing in the elderly is lacking. However, in the first randomized efficacy study in elderly delusional depression, combination nortriptyline and perphenazine, although well tolerated, did not separate from nortriptyline alone in efficacy.[100] Results from the Study of the Pharmacotherapy of Psychotic Depression (STOP-PD), a 12-week randomized, controlled, multicenter trial comparing olanzapine plus sertraline with olanzapine plus placebo, are awaited.

PSYCHOSOCIAL APPROACHES

Psychotherapies

Traditional psychotherapy models have not been adequately tested in the acute geropsychiatric inpatient setting. However, clinicians need to be aware of basic psychotherapeutic principles relevant to the elderly psychiatric patient to guide discharge recommendations. The best-studied psychotherapy application is for the treatment of late-life major depression. The optimal acute treatment strategy for geriatric depression is combination psychotherapy and psychopharmacology.[101] Cognitive behavioral therapy (CBT), interpersonal therapy (IPT), and PST are the three therapies best shown to have efficacy in geriatric major depression.

Additional therapies have encouraging results. Brief dynamic therapy can be effective and achieve similar outcome improvement to that of CBT and behavioral therapy.[101,102] Reminiscence therapy (RT), developed specifically for the older adult, is Eriksonian in theory and employs life review and reminiscence to resolve the integrity versus despair conflict.[103] Although literature supports the efficacy of RT in geriatric depression, PST has shown superiority over RT.[104] Finally, group dialectical behavior therapy (DBT), as an adjunct to antidepressant medication, was found more effective than antidepressant medication alone.[105]

Geriatric depression is frequently complicated by cognitive deficits (Alexopoulos et al.[84]), and approaches addressing this comorbidity offer distinct advantages. PST has shown efficacy in depressed elders with mild executive dysfunction.[106] Both IPT and PST have been modified for depressed elders with moderate cognitive impairment and may be useful discharge treatment recommendations for this population and their caregivers.

Psychotherapeutic approaches have been found effective in reducing depression and institutionalization in demented patients.[107] Caregivers' training in behavioral and problem-solving techniques was effective in reducing depression in patients with Alzheimer disease and had a sustained effect at 6-month follow-up.[108] Exercise training combined with teaching caregivers behavioral management techniques can improve depression and physical health in patients with Alzheimer disease.[109,110] Psychological support for caregivers as well as psychoeducation and problem solving has been found effective in reducing institutionalization and time to nursing home placement.[110,111] Other strategies indicated for demented patients involve behavior-oriented techniques based on identification of factors triggering behavioral disturbance with subsequent environmental modifications. Supportive psychotherapy may be helpful for patients with early dementia in dealing with the issue of loss.

Psychosocial Assessment and Education

Psychoeducational efforts are best conducted after a thorough assessment of the status of the patient–caregiver dyad. Even before admission, an assessment of the patients' living circumstances, the availability of caregivers, and the expectations of patients and family members regarding discharge arrangements can guide education efforts. The geriatric social worker ideally establishes family contact within the first 24 hours of admission. Psychosocial assessment should cover at minimum the following areas: (a) safety of current living arrangements, including the ability to function independently (e.g., is the patient still driving, can he or she be safely left alone, etc.); (b) evidence of abuse toward either the patient or the caregiver; (c) the caregiver's physical and mental ability to function in his/her role including any cognitive, emotional, or skill impediments; and (d) the degree of social support available to the dyad of patient–caregiver.[112]

An important and frequently overlooked focus of the assessment is the caregiver, with emphasis on caregiver abilities and depression. Approximately one third of caregivers for patients with moderate to advanced dementia in the community experience significant depressive symptoms. Caregiver characteristics associated with an increased risk of caregiver depression include wife designation, increased time spent caregiving, and impairment in physical functioning. Younger age, lower education, white or Hispanic ethnicity, increased dependency for activities of daily living, and behavioral disturbance are patient characteristics associated with increased caregiver depression.[113]

Family member roles can range from support to surrogate decision making, depending on the patient's physical and cognitive state. Inpatient psychoeducation should emphasize increased caregiving skills and resource awareness. Family involvement during a geropsychiatric hospitalization is related to the complexity and awareness of the patient's needs and to the altered caregiver role on discharge.[114]

Helping families and caregivers through transitions is another task for the inpatient social worker. Patients admitted from a nursing home frequently have severe behavioral disturbances complicated by medical problems and transfers can happen quickly. The patient and family have little time to process this change and are often in a state of shock and anger. Social workers can help family members recognize and process those emotions as well as educate them on disease processes, including cognitive, mood, and behavioral changes.

Social workers can help caregivers identify successful patient-specific behavioral strategies. Along with the rest of the treatment team, they search for environmental triggers and behavioral strategies for the management of agitated or aggressive states. For example, noise-related sleep deprivation is a common environmental cause of agitation in the nursing home and relatively easy to modify. Social workers are also integrally involved in discharge plans. Patients who are treated on specialized psychogeriatric inpatient units receive more appropriate age-specific aftercare referrals.[3]

Occupational and Recreational Therapies

Activity programs can benefit psychogeriatric patients in multiple domains: physical, cognitive, emotional, spiritual, and social. A blend of physical and mental tasks is offered and patients are encouraged to perform as independently as possible. The book *Activities for the Elderly: A Guide to Quality Programming*[115] describes specific activities. Recreational group activities need to adapt to the physically impaired elderly, including the nonambulatory and sensory impaired. Geriatric occupational therapy (OT) uses rehabilitation models of functional status and emphasizes physical skills such as strengthening and positioning.[7] OT groups may emphasize skills in activities of daily living with the dual purpose of social activity and individual skill assessment and intervention. To accommodate most levels of physical skill, group activity can be modified to include either seated or standing exercise.

Groups reviewing current events can enhance memory and orientation. Higher functioning patients can profit from wellness groups, which focus on health-related behaviors such as exercise and nutrition, social activity, stress, and anger management. Cognitive stimulation techniques should take into consideration the level of cognitive impairment to prevent frustration and catastrophic reactions.[25]

Geropsychiatric inpatients may profit from music therapy, an intervention found to improve agitation and aggressive behaviors in patients with dementia in long-term care settings.[116] Pet therapy may reduce ECT-associated fear[117] and dementia-related irritability[120] and can also be used in inpatient geriatric units.

Management of Suicide and Aggression

Almost half of elderly suicides among patients admitted to psychiatric inpatient units occur during the first week after admission or the first week after discharge, an observation highlighting the impact of transitions and the importance of rigorous vigilance during those times.[119] The elderly inpatient should be assessed for suicidal risk and risk of harming others immediately on admission and throughout the inpatient stay. An appropriate observational status should be ordered. Geriatric inpatient suicide risk assessment parallels adult risk assessment and includes such factors as history of attempts, active suicidal ideation with lethal plan, and psychosis. However, general elderly suicide risk factors cannot adequately predict individual suicide risk. A study of mixed-age psychiatric inpatients who completed suicide highlighted the importance of 1:1 observation of the high-risk patient (as opposed to 15-minute checks) and targeting severe anxiety/agitation as a means of improving suicide risk assessment and intervention.[120] The use of lithium for patients with bipolar disorder and clozapine for patients with schizophrenia or schizoaffective disorder has been shown to decrease suicidality in mixed-age or young adult outpatient populations[121–123] and may be a reasonable strategy for reducing chronic suicide risk.

Management of Aggressive Behaviors

Up to 30% of all elderly psychiatric inpatients manifest violent or assaultive behavior over a 3-day period, and these events significantly prolong hospital stay.[124] The presence of "organic mental disorders" predicts violence. Aggressive behaviors in this diagnostic group are also more likely to persist. Compared with younger psychiatric inpatients, fellow patients, as opposed to professional staff, are the more common assault victims.[125–127] Evaluation and treatment algorithms for this diagnostic group have been described previously under Neuropsychiatric and Behavioral Disturbances Associated with Dementia. The clinician should search for an underlying pattern to the aggressive outbursts (e.g., occurring at times of care or only with a specific staff member). Environmental interventions should always be tried first. If there is a specific syndrome present (psychosis, depression, or mania), appropriate medication trials should be initiated. Acute management of an assaultive geriatric patient may require treatment with atypical antipsychotics or benzodiazepines. In the elderly, dementia-related aggressive behaviors frequently respond to lower doses of antipsychotics than violence associated with primary psychotic and mood disorders. Benzodiazepines are associated with a risk of falls and increased confusion. Agents, such as lorazepam, that lack primary hepatic metabolites are preferred.

Seclusion and Restraints

In an inpatient geropsychiatric unit, seclusion rooms should be used in preference to physical restraints given the physical frailty of many elderly. Restraints can be used either for behavioral health management or to support medical/surgical care management. The monitoring and documentation requirements differ in these two situations. When physical restraints (e.g., mittens, helmets, tabletops, siderails, vest restraints, two- or four-point extremity restraints) are used, it is important to document the situation that necessitated their use according to institutional and/or state policies. Reduction of stimulation and use of behavioral techniques (e.g., distraction) frequently lead to de-escalation of acute problematic behaviors in demented elderly and should always be considered first. Fall prevention monitoring devices, such as chair and bed alarms, are not restraints. They alert staff when patients at increased risk of falls attempt to transfer independently.

Discharge

Elderly psychiatric inpatients have more discharge needs than simple outpatient referral. Level of disability, social support, and degree of medical and psychiatric care needs should be evaluated on the first admission day. Caregivers too have various needs: educational, psychiatric, medical, psychosocial, and financial. The inpatient team should assess families' strengths and weaknesses and help them cope while respecting their preferences and autonomy. Bolstering their strengths has the potential to improve quality of life for both patients and caregivers and delay of institutionalization for the elderly patient.[128] The psychiatric team needs to assess the patient's level of functioning and then link the patient and caregiver dyad to the appropriate services. Following an inpatient geropsychiatric stay, patients may benefit from a partial hospitalization program as an intermediate level of care to ensure further improvement or continued stabilization and prevent rehospitalization.[129,130] Alternatively, patients may return home with the appropriate home-based services or, at the other end of the spectrum, be admitted or returned to a long-term care facility. Cost coverage restrictions imposed by Medicare or other programs as well as changing eligibility criteria are ever-present barriers to access to services. The community service network for seniors becomes increasingly complex and inpatient practitioners must acquire basic information to educate patients, families, and other health professionals about the support services available in each specific community. Cultivating ongoing collaborations between the inpatient psychiatric team and facilities and community programs is crucial to ensure continuity of care and effective transitions.

REFERENCES

1. Rubenstein LZ, Josephson KR, Wieland GD, et al. Effectiveness of a geriatric evaluation unit. A randomized clinical trial. *N Engl J Med.* 1984; 311(26):1664–1670.

2. Collard AF, Bachman SS, Beatrice DF. Acute care delivery for the geriatric patient: An innovative approach. *QRB Qual Rev Bull.* 1985;11(6): 180–185.

3. Yazgan IC, Greenwald BS, Kremen NJ, et al. Geriatric psychiatry versus general psychiatry inpatient treatment of the elderly. *Am J Psychiatry.* 2004;161(2):352–355.

4. Ngoh CT, Lewis ID, Connolly PM. Outcomes of inpatient geropsychiatric treatment: The value of assessment protocols. *J Gerontol Nurs.* 2005; 31(4):12–18.

5. Smith M, Specht J, Buckwalter KC. Geropsychiatric inpatient care: What is state of the art? *Issues Ment Health Nurs.* 2005;26(1):11–22.

6. Nadler-Moodie M, Gold J. A geropsychiatric unit without walls. *Issues Ment Health Nurs.* 2005; 26(1):101–114.

7. Inventor BR, Henricks J, Rodman L, et al. The impact of medical issues in inpatient geriatric psychiatry. *Issues Ment Health Nurs.* 2005;26(1):23–46.

8. Blank K, Hixon L, Gruman C, et al. Determinants of geropsychiatric inpatient length of stay. *Psychiatr Q.* 2005;76(2):195–212.

9. Blixen CE, McDougall GJ, Suen LJ. Dual diagnosis in elders discharged from a psychiatric hospital. *Int J Geriatr Psychiatry.* 1997;12(3): 307–313.

10. Zubenko GS, Marino LJ, Jr., Sweet RA, et al. Medical comorbidity in elderly psychiatric inpatients. *Biol Psychiatry.* 1997; 41(6):724–736.

11. Depp CA, Jeste DV. Bipolar disorder in older adults: A critical review. *Bipolar Disord.* 2004; 6(5):343–367.

12. Weintraub D, Mazour I. Clinical and demographic changes over ten years on a psychogeriatric inpatient unit. *Ann Clin Psychiatry.* 2000;12(4):227–231.

13. Colenda CC, Mickus MA, Marcus SC, et al. Comparison of adult and geriatric psychiatric practice patterns: Findings from the American Psychiatric Association's Practice Research Network. *Am J Geriatr Psychiatry.* 2002;10(5):609–617.

14. Arias E, Anderson RN, Kung HC, et al. Deaths: Final data for 2001. *Natl Vital Stat Rep.* 2003;52(3):1–115.

15. Kochanek KD, Murphy SL, Anderson RN, et al. Deaths: Final Data for 2002. *Natl Vital Stat Rep.* 2004;53(5):1–116.

16. Conwell Y, Duberstein PR, Caine ED. Risk factors for suicide in later life. *Biol Psychiatry.* 2002;52(3):193–204.

17. Conwell Y, Duberstein PR, Connor K, et al. Access to firearms and risk for suicide in middle-aged and older adults. *Am J Geriatr Psychiatry.* 2002;10(4):407–416.

18. Lyness JM, Cox C, Curry J, et al. Older age and the underreporting of depressive symptoms. *J Am Geriatr Soc.* 1995;43(3):216–221.

19. Duberstein PR, Conwell Y, Seidlitz L, et al. Age and suicidal ideation in older depressed inpatients. *Am J Geriatr Psychiatry.* 1999;7(4):289–296.

20. Waern M, Runeson BS, Allebeck P, et al. Mental disorder in elderly suicides: a case-control study. *Am J Psychiatry.* 2002;159(3):450–455.

21. Alexopoulos GS, Bruce ML, Hull J, et al. Clinical determinants of suicidal ideation and behavior in geriatric depression. *Arch Gen Psychiatry.* 1999;56(11):1048–1053.

22. Alexopoulos GS, Katz IR, Reynolds CF, et al. Pharmacotherapy of depression in older patients: A summary of the expert consensus guidelines. *J Psychiatr Pract.* 2001;7(6):361–376.

23. Waern M. Alcohol dependence and misuse in elderly suicides. *Alcohol.* 2003;38(3): 249–254.

24. Meyers BS, Chester JG. Acute management of late-life depression. In: Copeland JRM, Abou-Saleh MT, Blazer DG, eds. *Principles and practice of geriatric psychiatry.* New York: John Wiley & Sons; 1994:563–567.

25. Rabins PV, Blacker D, Rovner BW, et al. American Psychiatric Association practice guideline for the treatment of patients with Alzheimer's disease and other dementias. Second edition. *Am J Psychiatry.* 2007;164(Suppl 12):5–56.

26. Folks DG, Kinney FC. The medical psychiatry inpatient unit. In: Copeland JRM, Abou-Saleh MT, Blazer DG, eds. *Principles and practice of geriatric psychiatry*, 2nd ed. John Wiley & Sons; 2002:709–712.

27. Bartels SJ, et al. Substance abuse and mental health among older americans: the state of the knowledge and future directions. Rockville: Older American Substance Abuse and Mental Health Technical Assistance Center; 2005.

28. Woo BK, Rice VA, Legendre SA, et al. The clock drawing test as a measure of executive dysfunction in elderly depressed patients. *J Geriatr Psychiatry Neurol.* 2004;17(4):190–194.

29. Juby A, Tench S, Baker V. The value of clock drawing in identifying executive cognitive dysfunction in people with a normal mini-mental state examination score. *Can Med Assoc J.* 2002; 167(8):859–864.

30. Borson S, Scanlan JM, Chen P, et al. The Mini-Cog as a screen for dementia: Validation in a population-based sample. *J Am Geriatr Soc.* 2003;51(10):1451–1454.

31. Borson S, Scanlan JM, Watanabe J, et al. Simplifying detection of cognitive impairment: Comparison of the Mini-Cog and mini-mental state examination in a multiethnic sample. *J Am Geriatr Soc.* 2005;53(5):871–874.

32. de Carle AJ, Kohn R. Risk factors for falling in a psychogeriatric unit. *Int J Geriatr Psychiatry.* 2001;16(8):762–767.

33. Tinetti ME, Gordon C, Sogolow E, et al. Fall-risk evaluation and management: Challenges in adopting geriatric care practices. *Gerontologist.* 2006;46(6):717–725.

34. Vergare MJ, Binder RL, Cook IA, et al. Practice guideline for the psychiatric evaluation of adults. In: *Practice guidelines for the treatment of psychiatric disorders.* Arlington: American Psychiatric Association; 2006:1–64.

35. Boyle LL, Ismail MS, Porsteinsson AP. The dementia workup. In: Agronin ME, Maletta GJ, eds. *Principles and practice of geriatric psychiatry.* Philadelphia: Lippincott Williams & Wilkins; 2006:137–152.

36. Alexopoulos GS, et al. Expert consensus panel for using antipsychotic drugs in older patients: Using antipsychotic agents in older patients. *J Clin Psychiatry.* 2004;65(Suppl 2):5–102.

37. Madhusoodanan S, Shah P, Brenner R, et al. Pharmacological treatment of the psychosis of Alzheimer's disease: What is the best approach? *CNS Drugs.* 2007;21(2):101–115.

38. Clauson KA, Marsh WA, Polen HH, et al. Clinical decision support tools: Analysis of online drug information databases. *BMC Med Inform Decis Mak.* 2007;7:7.

39. Mattana J, Charitou M, Mills L, et al. Personal digital assistants: A review of their application in graduate medical education. *Am J Med Qual.* 2005;20(5):262–267.

40. Armstrong SC, Cozza KL, Watanabe KS. The misdiagnosis of delirium. *Psychosomatics.* 1997;38(5):433–439.

41. Johnson JC, Kerse NM, Gottlieb G, et al. Prospective versus retrospective methods of identifying patients with delirium. *J Am Geriatr Soc.* 1992;40(4):316–319.

42. Young J, Inouye SK. Delirium in older people. *Br Med J.* 2007;334(7598):842–846.

43. Meagher DJ, Norton JW, Trzepacz PT. Delirium in the Elderly. In: Agronin ME, Maletta GJ, eds. *Principles and practice of geriatric psychiatry.* Philadelphia: Lippincott Williams & Wlikins; 2006:332–348.

44. Inouye SK. Delirium in older persons. *N Engl J Med.* 2006;354(11):1157–1165.

45. Alexopoulos GS, Jeste DV, Chung H, et al. The expert consensus guideline series. Treatment of dementia and its behavioral disturbances. Introduction: Methods, commentary, and summary. *Postgrad Med.* 2005:6–22.

46. Cohen-Mansfield JJ. Nonpharmacologic interventions for inappropriate behaviors in dementia: A review, summary, and critique. *Am J Geriatr Psychiatry.* 2001;9(4):361–381.

47. Schneider LS, Dagerman KS, Insel P. Risk of death with atypical antipsychotic drug treatment for dementia: Meta-analysis of randomized placebo-controlled trials. *JAMA.* 2005;294(15):1934–1943.

48. Wang PS, Schneeweiss S, Avorn J, et al. Risk of death in elderly users of conventional versus atypical antipsychotic medications. *N Engl J Med.* 2005;353(22):2335–2341.

49. Sink KM, Holden KF, Yaffe K. Pharmacological treatment of neuropsychiatric symptoms of dementia: A review of the evidence. *JAMA.* 2005;293(5):596–608.

50. Tariot PN, Farlow MR, Grossberg GT, et al. Memantine treatment in patients with moderate to severe Alzheimer disease already receiving donepezil: A randomized controlled trial. *JAMA.* 2004;291(3):317–324.

51. Trinh NH, Hoblyn J, Mohanty S, et al. Efficacy of cholinesterase inhibitors in the treatment of neuropsychiatric symptoms and functional impairment in Alzheimer's disease: A meta-analysis. *JAMA.* 2003;289(2):210–216.

52. Cummings JL, Schneider L, Tariot PN, et al. Reduction of behavioral disturbances and caregiver distress by galantamine in patients with Alzheimer's disease. *Am J Psychiatry.* 2004;161(3):532–538.

53. Beier MT. Treatment strategies for the behavioral symptoms of Alzheimer's disease: Focus on early pharmacologic intervention. *Pharmacotherapy.* 2007;27(3):399–411.

54. Cummings JL, Donohue JA, Brooks RL. The relationship between donepezil and behavioral disturbances in patients with Alzheimer's disease. *Am J Geriatr Psychiatry.* 2000;8(2):134–140.

55. Andreasen NC. I don't believe in late-onset schizophrenia. In: Howard R, Rabins PV, Castle DJ, eds. *Late onset schizophrenia.* Stroud: Wrightson Biomedical Publishing Ltd; 1999:111–123.

56. Almeida OP, Fenner S. Bipolar disorder: Similarities and differences between patients with illness onset before and after 65 years of age. *Int Psychogeriatr.* 2005;14(03):311–322.

57. Castle DG, Howard R. What do we know about the aetiology of late-onset schizophrenia? *Eur Psychiatry.* 1992(7):99–108.

58. Schneider LS, Tariot PN, Dagerman KS, et al. Effectiveness of atypical antipsychotic drugs in patients with Alzheimer's disease. *N Engl J Med.* 2006;355(15):1525–1538.

59. Bartels SJ, Forester B, Miles KM, et al. Mental health service use by elderly patients with bipolar disorder and unipolar major depression. *Am J Geriatr Psychiatry.* 2000;8(2):160–166.

60. Depp CA, Lindamer LA, Folsom DP, et al. Differences in clinical features and mental health service use in bipolar disorder across the lifespan. *Am J Geriatr Psychiatry.* 2005;13(4):290–298.

61. McDonald WM. Epidemiology, etiology, and treatment of geriatric mania. *J Clin Psychiatry.* 2000;61(Suppl 13):3–11.

62. Lehmann SW, Rabins PV. Factors related to hospitalization in elderly manic patients with early and late-onset bipolar disorder. *Int J Geriatr Psychiatry.* 2006;21(11):1060–1064.

63. Cassidy F, Carroll BJ. Vascular risk factors in late onset mania. *Psychol Med.* 2002;32(02):359–362.
64. Sajatovic M, Madhusoodanan S, Coconcea N. Managing bipolar disorder in the elderly: Defining the role of the newer agents. *Drugs Aging.* 2005;22(1):39–54.
65. Van Gerpen MW, Johnson JE, Winstead DK. Mania in the geriatric patient population: A review of the literature. *Am J Geriatr Psychiatry.* 1999;7(3):188–202.
66. RM Hirshfeld, et al., eds. American Psychiatric Association. *Practice guideline for the treatment of patients with bipolar disorder.* Washington, DC: American Psychiatric Publishing; 2002:851–932.
67. Young RC, Gyulai L, Mulsant BH, et al. Pharmacotherapy of bipolar disorder in old age: Review and recommendations. *Am J Geriatr Psychiatry.* 2004;12(4):342–357.
68. Sanderson DR. Practical geriatrics: Use of mood stabilizers by hospitalized geriatric patients with bipolar disorder. 1998;49:1145–1147.
69. Weiner RD, Coffey CE. The practice of electroconvulsive therapy: recommendations for treatment, training, and privileging: a task force report of the American Psychiatric Association. American Psychiatric Publishing; 2001.
70. American Psychiatric Association. *Diagnostic and statistical manual of mental disorders* 4th ed, text revision. Washington, DC: American Psychiatric Press; 2000.
71. Gallo JJ, Rabins PV. Depression without sadness: Alternative presentations of depression in late life. *Am Fam Physician.* 1999;60(3):820–826.
72. Elderkin-Thompson V, Mintz J, Haroon E, et al. Executive dysfunction and memory in older patients with major and minor depression. *Arch Clin Neuropsychol.* 2006;21(7):669–676.
73. Murphy CF, Alexopoulos GS. Longitudinal association of initiation/perseveration and severity of geriatric depression. *Am J Geriatr Psychiatry.* 2004;12(1):50–56.
74. Meyers BS. Late-life delusional depression: Acute and long-term treatment. *Int Psychogeriatr.* 1995;7(Suppl):113–124.
75. Alexopoulos GS. Late-Life Mood Disorders. In: Sadavoy J, et al., eds. *Comprehensive textbook of geriatric psychiatry.* New York: W. W. Norton & Company; p. 2004:609–653.
76. Rothschild AJ, Mulsant BH, Meyers BS, et al. Challenges in differentiating and diagnosing psychotic depression. *Psychiatr Ann.* 2006;36(1):40–46.
77. Rothschild AJ, et al. Misdiagnosis of psychotic depression at 4 academic medical centers. *Am J Psychiatry.* (in press).
78. Alexopoulos GS, Meyers BS, Young RC, et al. The course of geriatric depression with "reversible dementia": A controlled study. *Am J Psychiatry.* 1993;150(11):1693–1699.
79. Robinson RG. Vascular depression and post-stroke depression: Where do we go from here? *Am J Geriatr Psychiatry.* 2005;13(2):85–87.
80. Alexopoulos GS, Meyers BS, Young RC, et al. 'Vascular depression' hypothesis. *Arch Gen Psychiatry.* 1997;54(10):915–922.
81. Krishnan KR, Hays JC, Blazer DG. MRI-defined vascular depression. *Am J Psychiatry.* 1997;154(4):497–501.
82. Alexopoulos GS, Meyers BS, Young RC, et al. Clinically defined vascular depression. *Am J Psychiatry.* 1997;154(4):562–565.
83. Taragano FE, Bagnatti P, Allegri RF. A double-blind, randomized clinical trial to assess the augmentation with nimodipine of antidepressant therapy in the treatment of "vascular depression". *Int Psychogeriatr.* 2005;17(3):487–498.
84. Alexopoulos GS, Kiosses DN, Klimstra S, et al. Clinical presentation of the "depression-executive dysfunction syndrome" of late life. *Am J Geriatr Psychiatry.* 2002;10(1):98–106.
85. Kalayam B, Alexopoulos G. Prefrontal dysfunction and treatment response in geriatric depression. *Arch Gen Psychiatry.* 1999;56(8):p713–p718.
86. Alexopoulos GS, Meyers BS, Young RC, et al. Executive dysfunction and long-term outcomes of geriatric depression. *Arch Gen Psychiatry.* 2000;57(3):285–290.
87. Alexopoulos GS, Kiosses DN, Heo M, et al. Executive dysfunction and the course of geriatric depression. *Biol Psychiatry.* 2005;58(3):204–210.
88. Alexopoulos GS, Raue P, Arean P. Problem-solving therapy versus supportive therapy in geriatric major depression with executive dysfunction. *Am J Geriatr Psychiatry.* 2003;11(1):46–52.
89. Alexopoulos GS, Young RC, Meyers BS. Geriatric depression: Age of onset and dementia. *Biol Psychiatry.* 1993;34(3):141–145.
90. Alexopoulos GS, Young RC, Shindledecker RD. Brain computed tomography findings in geriatric depression and primary degenerative dementia. *Biol Psychiatry.* 1992;31(6):591–599.
91. Kalayam B, Meyers BS, Kakuma T, et al. Age at onset of geriatric depression and sensorineural hearing deficits. *Biol Psychiatry.* 1995;38(10):649–658.
92. Lyness JM, Conwell Y, King DA, et al. Age of onset and medical illness in older depressed inpatients. *Int Psychogeriatr.* 1995;7(1):63–73.
93. Wiener P, Alexopoulos GS, Kakuma T, et al. The limits of history-taking in geriatric depression. *Am J Geriatr Psychiatry.* 1997;5(2):116–125.

94. Richards JB, Papaioannou A, Adachi JD, et al. Effect of selective serotonin reuptake inhibitors on the risk of fracture. *Arch Intern Med.* 2007;167(2):188–194.

95. Juurlink DN, Mamdani MM, Kopp A, et al. The risk of suicide with selective serotonin reuptake inhibitors in the elderly. *Am J Psychiatry.* 2006;163(5):813–821.

96. Thase ME. Effects of venlafaxine on blood pressure: A meta-analysis of original data from 3744 depressed patients. *J Clin Psychiatry.* 1998; 59(10):502–508.

97. Staab JP, Evans DL. Efficacy of venlafaxine in geriatric depression. *Depress Anxiety.* 2000; 12(Suppl 1):63–68.

98. Tew JD Jr., Mulsant BH, Haskett RF, et al. Acute efficacy of ECT in the treatment of major depression in the old-old. *Am J Psychiatry.* 1999; 156(12):1865–1870.

99. Alexopoulos GS, Katz IR, Reynolds CF, et al. *Pharmacotherapy of depressive disorders in older patients – the expert consensus guideline series.* Postgraduate Medicine Special Report, 2001:1–86.

100. Mulsant BH, Sweet RA, Rosen J, et al. A double-blind randomized comparison of nortriptyline plus perphenazine versus nortriptyline plus placebo in the treatment of psychotic depression in late life. *J Clin Psychiatry.* 2001;62(8):597–604.

101. Arean PA, Cook BL. Psychotherapy and combined psychotherapy/pharmacotherapy for late life depression. *Biol Psychiatry.* 2002; 52(3):293–303.

102. Thompson LW, Gallagher D, Breckenridge JS. Comparative effectiveness of psychotherapies for depressed elders. *J Consult Clin Psychol.* 1987;55(3):385–390.

103. Bohlmeijer E, Roemer M, Cuijpers P, et al. The effects of reminiscence on psychological well-being in older adults: A meta-analysis. *Aging Ment Health.* 2007;11(3):291–300.

104. Arean PA, Perri MG, Nezu AM, et al. Comparative effectiveness of social problem-solving therapy and reminiscence therapy as treatments for depression in older adults. *J Consult Clin Psychol.* 1993;61(6):1003–1010.

105. Lynch TR, Morse JQ, Mendelson T, et al. Dialectical behavior therapy for depressed older adults: A randomized pilot study. *Am J Geriatr Psychiatry.* 2003;11(1):33–45.

106. Alexopoulos GS, Raue P, Areán P. Problem-solving therapy versus supportive therapy in geriatric major depression with executive dysfunction. *Am J Geriatr Psychiatry.* 2003;11(1):46–52.

107. Livingston GG, Johnston K, Katona C, et al. Systematic review of psychological approaches to the management of neuropsychiatric symptoms of dementia. *Am J Psychiatry.* 2005; 162(11):1996–2021.

108. Teri L, Logsdon RG, Uomoto J, et al. Behavioral treatment of depression in dementia patients: A controlled clinical trial. *J Gerontol B Psychol Sci Soc Sci.* 1997;52(4):66.

109. Teri L, Gibbons LE, McCurry SM, et al. Exercise plus behavioral management in patients with Alzheimer disease: A randomized controlled trial. *JAMA.* 2003;290(15):2015–2022.

110. Eloniemi-Sulkava U, Notkola IL, Hentinen M, et al. Effects of supporting community-living demented patients and their caregivers: A randomized trial. *J Am Geriatr Soc.* 2001; 49(10):1282–1287.

111. Mittelman MS, Ferris SH, Shulman E, et al. A family intervention to delay nursing home placement of patients with Alzheimer disease. A randomized controlled trial. *JAMA.* 1996; 276(21):1725–1731.

112. Thompson LW, et al. The geriatric caregiver. In: Agronin ME, Maletta GJ, eds. *Principles and practice of geriatric psychiatry.* Philadelphia: Lippincott Williams & Wilkins; 2006:37–49.

113. Covinsky KE, Newcomer R, Fox P, et al. Patient and caregiver characteristics associated with depression in caregivers of patients with dementia. *J Gen Intern Med.* 2003; 18(12):1006–1014.

114. Owens SJ, Qualls SH. Family involvement during a geropsychiatric hospitalization. *J Clin Geropsychol.* 2002;8(2):87–99.

115. Parker SD, Will C, Burke CL. *Activities for the elderly: a guide to quality programming*, Vol. 1. Ravensdale: Idyll Arbor Inc; 1999.

116. Gerdner LA. Music, art, and recreational therapies in the treatment of behavioral and psychological symptoms of dementia. *Int Psychogeriatr.* 2005;12(S1):359–366.

117. Barker SB, Pandurangi AK, Best AM. Effects of animal-assisted therapy on patients' anxiety, fear, and depression before ECT. *J ECT.* 2003;19(1):38–44.

118. Zisselman MH, Rovner BW, Shmuely Y, et al. A pet therapy intervention with geriatric psychiatry inpatients. *Am J Occup Ther.* 1996; 50(1):47–51.

119. Erlangsen A, Zarit SH, Tu X, et al. Suicide among older psychiatric inpatients: An evidence-based study of a high-risk group. *Am J Geriatr Psychiatry.* 2006;14(9):734–741.

120. Busch KA, Fawcett JJ, Jacobs DG. Clinical correlates of inpatient suicide. *J Clin Psychiatry.* 2003;64(1):14–19.

121. Tondo L, Hennen J, Baldessarini RJ. Lower suicide risk with long-term lithium treatment in major affective illness: A meta-analysis. *Acta Psychiatr Scand.* 2001;104(3):163–172.

122. Meltzer HY, Alphs L, Green AI, et al. Clozapine treatment for suicidality in schizophrenia: International Suicide Prevention Trial (InterSePT). *Arch Gen Psychiatry.* 2003;60(1):82–91.

123. Meltzer HY, Baldessarini RJ. Reducing the risk for suicide in schizophrenia and affective disorders. *J Clin Exp Psychopathol Q Rev Psychiatry Neurol.* 2003;64(9):1122–1129.

124. Patel V, Hope RA. Aggressive behaviour in elderly psychiatric inpatients. *Acta Psychiatr Scand.* 1992;85(2):131–135.

125. Miller RRJ, Zadolinnyj KK, Hafner RRJ. Profiles and predictors of assaultiveness for different psychiatric ward populations. *Am J Psychiatry.* 1993;150(9):1368–1373.

126. Cooper AJ, Mendonca JD. A prospective study of patient assaults on nurses in a provincial psychiatric hospital in Canada. *Acta Psychiatr Scand.* 1991;84(2):163–166.

127. Wystanski MM. Assaultive behaviour in psychiatrically hospitalized elderly: A response to psychosocial stimulation and changes in pharmacotherapy. *Int J Geriatr Psychiatry.* 2000;15(7):582–585.

128. Schulz R, Martire LM, Klinger JN. Evidence-based caregiver interventions in geriatric psychiatry. *Psychiatr Clin North Am.* 2005;28(4):1007–1038.

129. Hoe J, Ashaye K, Orrell M. Don't seize the day hospital! Recent research on the effectiveness of day hospitals for older people with mental health problems. *Int J Geriatr Psychiatry.* 2005;20(7):694–698.

130. Boyle DP. The effect of geriatric day treatment on a measure of depression. *Clin Gerontol.* 1997;18(2):43–63.

CHAPTER 17

The Brain-Injured or Developmentally Disabled Psychiatric Inpatient

DAVID B. ARCINIEGAS AND C. ALAN ANDERSON

T he neuropsychiatric consequences of acquired brain injury (ABI) and developmental disabilities (DD) are many and varied and include problems such as depression, mania, affective lability, anxiety, apathy, psychosis, aggression, agitation, and self-injurious behavior. Neuropsychiatric disorders may arise in this population as a direct physiologic consequence of ABI or DD, an independent comorbid psychiatric condition, a manifestation of environmental or psychosocial problems, or a combination of these factors. When neuropsychiatric problems develop in a person with ABI or DD, they may be difficult to identify correctly because of the cognitive and communication problems often experienced by these individuals.[1] This difficulty is often compounded by the sometimes atypical presentations of neuropsychiatric conditions in this population, which frequently cross conventional psychiatric diagnostic boundaries or occur only in partial forms.[2] Consequently, the task of evaluating and treating neuropsychiatric problems in persons with ABI and DD is necessarily complex. Unfortunately, most psychiatrists are afforded little experience in care of persons with ABI and DD during medical school or residency training.[3–5] Despite suggestions that psychiatric training should require experience in the management of persons with DD,[6,7] the availability of supervised clinical experience in this area during residency remains highly variable and is in many cases optional.[3] Calls for similar experience in the neuropsychiatric management of persons with ABI and DD are either embedded in the suggested curriculum for psychosomatic medicine rotations[8] or instead incorporated specifically into fellowship-level curricula.[9,10]

Nonetheless, the high prevalence of ABI and DD, which collectively affect >5% of the US population,[11,12] and the high rates of severe neuropsychiatric disorders associated with these conditions[13–19] all but ensure that inpatient psychiatrists will be called upon to participate in the care of persons with DD and ABI.

A complete review of the ABI and DD and their neuropsychiatric features is beyond the scope of this chapter, which may be supplemented by information presented elsewhere.[20–22] Because the goal is to offer inpatient psychiatrists practical guidance on the management of neuropsychiatric problems in persons with ABI and DD, the authors discuss the etiology and pathogenesis of ABI and DD only in general terms except where a more detailed understanding of these matters informs their treatments.

Definitions of Acquired Brain Injury and Developmental Disability

ACQUIRED BRAIN INJURY

ABI is a broad category that refers to any noncongenital, nondegenerative injury to the brain. The causes of ABI are numerous and include trauma, hypoxia, vascular disruption, infections, inflammatory or demyelinating conditions, cerebral neoplasms (primary or metastatic), metabolic and nutritional disorders, endocrine disturbances, toxic exposures, substance abuse or dependence, some chemotherapies, and electrical injuries. From a practical standpoint, ABI implies the development of a static or potentially reversible neurologic condition that results in cognition, emotional, behavioral, and/or physical impairments which interfere with the ability to function independently in the absence of special services, support, or other forms of assistance.

Neurodegenerative conditions are generally excluded from the category of ABI based on their progressive, rather than static or potentially reversible, nature. Similarly, some clinicians might exclude inflammatory disorders (e.g., multiple sclerosis [MS], progressive multifocal leukoencephalopathy), infectious diseases (e.g., human immunodeficiency virus [HIV]), cerebral neoplasms (e.g., primary or metastatic), some cerebrovascular diseases (e.g., Binswanger disease, cerebral autosomal dominant arteriopathy with subcortical infarcts and leukoencephalopathy [CADASIL]), and other progressive neurologic conditions from the category of ABI.

Notwithstanding arguments regarding the boundaries of this category, the authors suggest that an inclusive formulation of ABI is often the most practical one by which to help patients, their families, and other health care providers understand the role of structural and/or functional brain disturbances on the development and treatment of neuropsychiatric problems. Traumatic brain injuries (TBIs) and hypoxic-ischemic (anoxic) brain injuries, however, are the most common intended referents of ABI in the medical literature. Most studies of treatments for the neuropsychiatric consequences of ABI are conducted in these contexts, and particularly in the setting of TBI. In the authors' experience, the principles of evaluation and treatment of persons with neuropsychiatric problems following TBI generalize reasonably well to the broader category of ABI. Treatment recommendations offered in this chapter therefore draw heavily upon this literature.

Obviously, some patients require condition-specific treatments (e.g., immunomodulatory therapies in demyelinating disorders, antiviral therapies in HIV, chemo- or radiotherapies in cerebral neoplasms, antispasticity therapies, etc.) that influence the selection or dosing of psychopharmacologic agents. In the less common context of recurrent or long-term inpatient psychiatric hospitalizations, or when presented with the opportunity to establish realistic long-term management strategies with the patient and his or her care providers, the treating psychiatrist also may be able to offer treatment recommendations that anticipate needs entailed by the natural course of a specific ABI.

Persons of any age may develop a condition that merits the designation ABI. However, when one or more of these conditions develop before the age of 22, they are most often discussed under the rubric of DD.

DEVELOPMENTAL DISABILITY

The U.S. Department of Health and Human Services-Administration for Children and Families (USDHHS-ACF)[23] defines DD as a severe chronic disability attributable to a mental and/or physical impairment acquired before 22 years that results in substantial functional limitations in three or more areas of major life activity. These areas include self-care, receptive and expressive language, learning, mobility, self-direction, capacity for independent living, and economic self-sufficiency. This formulation of DD also requires that such limitations reflect the need for services, individualized supports, or other forms of assistance that are of lifelong or extended duration and that require individual planning and coordination. The category of DD also includes individuals from birth to 9 years of age with substantial developmental delays or specific congenital or acquired conditions who, while not presently suffering substantial functional limitations in three or more of the above-mentioned areas, have a high probability of developing such limitations later in life.

Many administrative formulations of DD require an impairment of intellectual function resulting in a full-scale intelligence quotient (IQ) of 70 (two standard deviations below age-adjusted performance expectations) or less. While such formulations may assist with the allocation of publicly funded services, the neuropsychiatric treatment needs of patients with milder intellectual impairments or substantial impairments in adaptive behavior resulting from communicative disorders, behavioral disturbances, or physical (including sensory) impairments may benefit from a diagnostic and treatment approach that defines DD more broadly.

The causes of DD include chromosomal abnormalities, other genetic factors, prenatal and perinatal neurodevelopmental insults, childhood ABIs, environmental exposures, and sociocultural factors.[24] These and other factors contribute to the broad array of clinical diagnoses that are grouped under the heading of DD. The most common of these clinical diagnoses are mental retardation, cerebral palsy, epilepsy, autism, sensory (vision, hearing) or communicative disorders, and other childhood-onset neurologic conditions that result in impairment of general intellectual functioning or adaptive behavior.

When the specific cause of DD in an individual patient is known, the treatment of the acute neuropsychiatric problems with which that patient presents may require modification tailored to concurrently administered medical or neurologic treatments (e.g., anticonvulsants in epilepsy, endocrine or metabolic therapies, etc.). In many cases, despite a thorough evaluation, the etiology of the patient's DD will either be unclear (cryptogenic) or presumed to be multifactorial. Accordingly, the neuroanatomy and putative neurochemistry of both the DD and its neuropsychiatric sequelae often remain a source of uncertainty, particularly as regards their implications for psychopharmacologic interventions. A general approach to the evaluation and treatment of the neuropsychiatric manifestations of DD, similar to that offered for the psychiatric management of persons with ABI, is therefore often the most practical strategy available to the inpatient psychiatrists providing care to patients with DD.

General Principles of Evaluation and Treatment

NEUROPSYCHIATRIC EVALUATION

Before initiating any treatment of the patient with ABI or DD, obtaining a thorough developmental, neurologic, psychiatric (including substance), social, family, and treatment history is essential. In general, the initial inpatient evaluation of persons with ABI and DD is similar to that of patients with primary psychiatric illnesses. However, Silka and Hauser[24] offer several additional recommendations with which to adjust this evaluation for the needs of this population.

The evaluation should be conducted promptly to avoid escalating behavioral disturbances due to the unfamiliar and often intense milieu, of the inpatient psychiatric setting. The evaluation is best conducted in as safe, private, and quiet environment as is feasible. If the patient is accompanied by caregivers or professional staff that the patient usually finds comforting, inviting them into the interview may be useful. Conversely, if the initial evaluation suggests that the presence of such individuals is distressing or disruptive to the patient, excusing them from the interview of the patient may be necessary.

As with any patient, the presenting problem should be identified as clearly as possible. In this population, defining clearly the presenting problem is sometimes more challenging than among patients with primary psychiatric illnesses. Patients with ABI and DD and their caregivers may be biased to under- or overreport psychiatric symptoms.[1,26,27] Limited awareness regarding the pathological nature of some behaviors, fear of stigmatization associated with psychiatric diagnoses, attempts to avoid impugning the efforts of other care providers, and pessimism regarding the effectiveness or tolerability of treatment may result in caregivers' minimizing or withholding potentially important historical details. Conversely, frustration over or intolerance of challenging behaviors may result in magnification of the reported severity of such symptoms and requests for prescription of psychiatric medications that are in fact unnecessary.[25]

The initial evaluation should also seek not only neuropsychiatric symptoms but also potential causes or contributors, including medical, neurologic, psychiatric, substance, and environmental factors, as well as current treatments (discussed further in the subsequent text) and the individuals providing them. With regard to this latter issue, clinicians should be mindful that a change in residence, the residents or caregivers in that residence, disruptions of daily routines, or other similar events may produce acute emotional and/or behavioral disturbances among persons with ABI and DD. Clinicians also should be vigilant for signs of abuse or maltreatment of patients with ABI and DD, particularly among those who are able to communicate their distress only by their behavior and among those whose unwanted behaviors may engender further abuse.[28–30] Although pharmacologic treatment may be required to address the emotional or behavioral consequences of environmental problems, sometimes the most appropriate recommendation will be to use no medicines at all if a change in the environment or the provision of nonpharmacologic interventions (e.g., supportive psychotherapy, staff retraining, change in caregivers, etc.) will suffice.

Finally, observations made of the patient at the time of admission must be regarded as preliminary; placed suddenly in the unfamiliar emergency or inpatient psychiatric ward, patients may behave quite differently (better or worse) from how they behave in their usual environment. Additionally, the frequently severe cognitive, behavioral, and communication impairments experienced by persons with ABI or DD, as well as the often limited availability of collateral history from reliable informants and medical records, may make it difficult to arrive at a well-informed diagnosis, and therefore a rational treatment plan, at the time of admission to a psychiatric unit. With this in mind, remaining circumspect with respect to diagnosis and treatment until the presenting problem and the context in which it occurs are characterized fully is prudent.

CHARACTERIZING NEUROPSYCHIATRIC SYMPTOMS

For many of the reasons noted earlier, characterizing neuropsychiatric symptoms requiring treatment among persons with ABI and DD presents substantial challenges to the inpatient psychiatrist. These challenges may, at least in part, be overcome by the use of objective rating scales of neuropsychiatric status. In addition to facilitating the timely identification of neuropsychiatric symptoms requiring clinical intervention, use of such scales provides a means by which to develop a common frame of reference for discussion of neuropsychiatric symptoms between the inpatient psychiatrist, the patient, and other parties involved in the patient's care. They also serve as a reference to measure the response to pharmacologic and behavioral interventions.

When the patient with ABI or DD is cognitively and linguistically capable of participating in a structured clinical interview of neuropsychiatric functioning, the Neurobehavioral Rating Scale-Revised (NRS-R)[31] is particularly well suited to this task. Derived from the Brief Psychiatric Rating Scale,[32] a widely used psychiatric research assessment, the NRS-R includes 29 items that assess five domains of neuropsychiatric function: cognition, positive symptoms, negative symptoms, mood and affect, and oral/motor function. Completing the interview portion of the NRS-R typically requires only 15 to 20 minutes. During the interview, structured clinical observations are made and then supplemented by collateral data gathered from reliable informants on the patient's day-to-day functioning. This relatively brief assessment thereby provides the clinician with a useful method of initial symptom identification, diagnostic formulation, and serial assessment, as well as a means by which to resolve discrepancies between the history provided by the patient and his or her caregivers. Although the NRS-R was originally developed for use among persons with TBI specifically, in the authors' experience this assessment is similarly useful among persons with ABI and DD more generally.

When patients are not able to participate directly in the provision of history, the initial assessment may be limited to observation of the patient supplemented by review of records and interview of a reliable informant on the patient's neuropsychiatric status. In the authors' experience, the Neuropsychiatric Inventory (NPI)[33] is a useful means by which to obtain neuropsychiatric symptom assessment in such circumstances. Originally developed for use among persons with dementias, the NPI assesses ten domains of psychopathology (i.e., delusions, hallucinations, agitation/aggression, dysphoria, anxiety, euphoria, apathy, disinhibition, irritability/lability, and aberrant motor behavior) commonly experienced by patients with many types of neurobehavioral disorders. A screening question for each domain is asked of the informant; this approach allows the clinician to identify potential areas of neuropsychiatric disturbance and to avoid potentially unrewarding avenues of inquiry. The NPI generally requires 10 to 20 minutes to complete, although interviews of caregivers unfamiliar with the distinctions between certain domains of neuropsychiatric dysfunction (i.e., depression vs. apathy, agitation/aggression vs. irritability/lability) may require explanations of these distinctions, thereby necessitating a longer initial interview. Educating caregivers provides them with a framework to monitor the patient's behavior and improve future reporting.

After the initial administration, a questionnaire form of this instrument, the Neuropsychiatric Inventory-Questionnaire (NPI-Q),[34] may be completed by the informant alone. A version of the NPI for use in institutional settings, the Neuropsychiatric Inventory-Nursing Home (NPI-NH),[35] is also available; this version is predicated on clinician interview of staff members familiar with the patient's neuropsychiatric functioning and adds two additional domains, nighttime behaviors and appetitive disturbances, to the assessment. Like the NRS-R, the NPI, in its several forms, provides the clinician with a useful method of initial symptom identification, diagnostic formulation, and serial assessment among patients with severe cognitive, behavioral, or communication impairments.

On the basis of data yielded by the NRS-R or the NPI, clinicians may further characterize the patient's presenting problem with one or more symptom-specific scales (e.g., Hamilton Depression Rating Scale,[36] Young Mania Rating Scale,[37] Overt Aggression Scale,[38] and Apathy Evaluation Scale,[39] etc.). Because neuropsychiatric disturbances in persons with ABI and DD often cross conventional diagnostic boundaries or present in only partial forms,[2,40] identifying symptoms requiring therapeutic intervention, rather than adhering strictly to a Diagnostic and Statistical Manual of Mental Disorders, Fourth Edition, Text Revision (DSM-IV-TR)-based[41] categorical diagnoses, is often the most productive clinical approach.

Although not included in either the NRS-R or the NPI, screening for "spells" is also necessary. Epilepsy, particularly of the complex partial (with or without secondary generalization) type, is a common comorbidity among persons with DD[42,43] and ABI[44] and may be a cause of behavioral disturbances during or after seizures. Additionally, nonepileptic events, including pseudoseizures, are not uncommon in these populations.[45,46] When the history identifies paroxysmal behavioral events, characterizing those events with respect to the presence or absence of other manifestations of seizures, and particularly the presence or absence of alteration in consciousness during or after the event, as well as event precipitants, potential behavioral reinforcers, and the effects of interventions (e.g., antiepileptic medications) is essential. Because many patients are unable to accurately report the character of their spells and subsequent behaviors, direct observation of their typical spells, sometimes using video-electroencephalographic monitoring, and obtaining descriptions from reliable informants is recommended before offering a diagnosis of either seizure or nonepileptic seizures. Identification of seizure-related behavioral disturbances will direct treatment toward epilepsy rather than its behavioral manifestations, thereby avoiding unnecessary psychopharmacologic interventions. Conversely, identification of nonepileptic events may permit the discontinuation of anticonvulsant medications and refocus treatment on the psychological and/or environmental precipitants as well as reinforcers of those events.

As a corollary to defining target symptoms, identifying not only what but also who requires treatment is essential. Although the medical convention is to regard the patient as the focus of treatment, the evaluation of neuropsychiatric problems among persons with ABI and DD cannot be decontextualized. The emotional or behavioral problems of the patient are better understood as a problem in the interaction between the patient and his environment.

Case Vignette

A 29-year-old, right-handed man with a remote severe TBI was referred by his insurance case manager for inpatient evaluation and pharmacologic treatment of "intractable aggression." The preadmission history suggested daily, unpredictable aggressive behavior toward his wife and young children. Admission evaluation was remarkable for severe cognitive impairments, but agitation was noted only when the ward staff observed the patient's wife speaking to him in a rapid, loud, and impatient manner and at a level of complexity inconsistent with his verbal communication skills. The raucous behavior of the patient's young children increased his agitation. Staff intervention directed toward calming the wife and children, or escorting them out of the patient's room, allowed resolution of the patient's agitation.

These observations prompted education of the patient's wife regarding the nature of his condition and the relationship between the family's interactions with him and the patient's unwanted behaviors. Despite extensive training of the patient's wife, she was unable to modify her own behavior and her supervision of their children to meet the patient's needs. He was discharged to a residential living center for persons with ABI where he had minimal agitation and staff there perceived no need for pharmacologic intervention.

This case is an example of a severe behavioral problem arising from the interaction between the patient and his environment. The evaluation yielded a clearer understanding of the antecedents of his agitation/aggression, allowed discharge to a setting in which the safety of the patient and his family was maintained, and obviated the need for pharmacotherapy of his agitated/aggressive behaviors. This example serves as a reminder to clinicians that proper treatment of the patient with ABI or DD necessitates assessment of both the patient and the context in which his or her neuropsychiatric disturbances arise.

REVIEW OF PRIOR INTERVENTIONS

In addition to the types of history taking and symptom identification described in the preceding text, pretreatment assessment of the patient with ABI or DD requires review of past and current treatments. A comprehensive assessment of pharmacologic, nonpharmacologic, prescribed, and self-administered treatments is encouraged, and should focus on three key issues: (a) the indications for such treatments; (b) the effects (positive, neutral, or negative) of those treatments; and (c) whether current symptoms reflect side effects of those treatments.

Consultation with other treating clinicians may be required to decide whether a current medicine is necessary or whether a new medicine might be helpful. When reviewing the indications for current treatments, avoiding the artificial distinction between "psychiatric" and "nonpsychiatric" medicines is recommended. By definition, patients with ABI and DD have an underlying neurologic condition. These neurologic conditions often require treatment in their own right (e.g., antiviral, anti-inflammatory, immunomodulatory, or antineoplastic agents) or produce other nonbehavioral problems (e.g., hemiparesis, spasticity, incontinence, etc.) that require treatment. Unfortunately, some agents used for these purposes may produce a wide range of problematic neuropsychiatric symptoms,[47–52] including mood disorders, other affective disturbances, psychotic symptoms, and agitation, among others. Sometimes such treatments have not been properly applied, are predicated on misdiagnosis of the problem, or are the result of poor communication among treating professionals regarding the problem in question. Conversely, some medicines initiated for other conditions may have neuropsychiatric benefits and can play a role in the treatment plan. Examples include β-blockers started for hypertension that can reduce aggression and anticonvulsants given for seizures that can stabilize mood. Accordingly, identifying relationships between neuropsychiatric disturbances and treatments prescribed for the neurologic or medical conditions of persons with ABI and DD is an essential element of the pretreatment assessment.

Similarly, review of treatments directed at reduction of neuropsychiatric symptoms and unwanted behaviors is also required before undertaking additional therapeutic interventions of any kind. Although many medicines may alleviate neuropsychiatric disturbances among patients with ABI and DD, some agents may produce such problems. For example, paradoxical agitation, although an uncommon problem, may develop in response to treatment with benzodiazepines,[53] valproate,[54] or more rarely with cholinesterase inhibitors.[55] Depression, psychosis, and other behavioral disturbances occur with some anticonvulsants.[50,52,56] Lingering effects of previously prescribed treatments, and particularly antipsychotic-induced extrapyramidal syndromes such as tardive akathisia[57–59] are also potential causes of behavioral disturbances among persons with ABI and DD. Where possible, eliminating or reducing potentially problematic medicines—particularly when a temporal relationship between treatment with such agents and problematic behaviors or psychiatric symptoms can be established—may alleviate such symptoms and thereby avoid prescription of additional agents.

In some cases, a potentially effective medicine or nonpharmacologic intervention has not been beneficial because it has been offered in a dose that is inadequate or for a period of time that is too brief. In such circumstances, undertaking an empiric trial of an intervention that was previously deemed "unhelpful" may be very useful. If a previous treatment was maximally employed but affected only a partial improvement in the symptom for which it was used, reinstituting that treatment and augmenting it with another, whether pharmacologic or behavioral/environmental, with a complementary mechanism of action may be helpful. This strategy may also help the clinician avoid serial empiric trials of several individually ineffective, or only partially effective, treatments.

COGNITIVE EXAMINATION

Cognitive impairments and related functional disabilities should be identified in persons with ABI and DD admitted to an inpatient psychiatric unit. However, such information is often more usefully gathered from history than by formal assessment at the time of inpatient psychiatric admission.

As noted earlier, most administrative formulations of DD require intellectual impairment. The severity of impairment graded by age-appropriate full-scale IQ: 50 to 70 = mild, 35 to 50 = moderate, 20 to 35 = severe, and <20 = profound. Among patients admitted to an inpatient psychiatric unit with a history of DD, information regarding the severity of intellectual disability will have been acquired at some point in the past. Obtaining that information may be a useful guide with which to formulate a treatment plan that is adjusted to the patient's cognitive abilities and disabilities and that is communicated to the patient in a manner sensitive to his or her ability to understand it.

Among persons with ABI, cognitive impairments also are an expected part of the clinical presentation. The types and severities of impairments vary with the types and severities of ABI, although the correspondence between initial injury severity and long-term cognitive impairment is not strict.[2] By the time a person with an ABI is admitted to an inpatient psychiatric setting, an assessment of post-ABI cognitive impairments and related functional disabilities often has been performed. When available, that information should be obtained before treatment initiation. Among patients with ABI, and particularly TBI, without prior assessments clinicians are advised to maintain a high level of suspicion for cognitive impairments of possible clinical significance and to undertake at least a preliminary cognitive assessment.

Psychiatric conditions of severity sufficient to necessitate inpatient hospitalization tend to impair performance on tests of cognitive ability. Accordingly, performing such assessments at the time of admission may overestimate the severity of cognitive impairments. When not understood in the context of, and perhaps at least in part as a product of, the psychiatric condition for which the patient was admitted, such testing may foster erroneous negative assumptions about the patient's ability to participate in treatment planning, behavioral and other nonpharmacologic treatments, and disposition determinations.

This assessment should include evaluation of level of arousal, with vigilance for signs of either hypo- or hyperarousal; attention, including at least the ability to select and sustain focus to relevant environmental targets and freedom from attention to hallucinatory stimuli; speed of information processing; language, and particularly impairments in the ability to communicate suggestive of aphasia; memory, including the ability to retrieve previously learned information, the ability to learn and recall new information, and the ability to learn new procedures; praxis (the ability to perform previously learned skilled purposeful movements on command), including single-step and multistep sequences; recognition (gnosis) in visual, auditory, and tactile domains; visuospatial function, with particular vigilance for signs of hemi-inattention or neglect; and executive function (retrieval, sequencing and organization of information, conceptualization/abstraction, judgment, and insight).

For most patients, bedside cognitive "screening" measures, such as the Mini Mental State Examination,[60] one of the various versions of the clock drawing test, the Frontal Assessment Battery[61] and related executive function measures are usually sufficient for the purpose of identifying major domains of cognitive impairment that may affect the patient's ability to participate in the development and execution of a treatment plan. When the patient is not able to participate in a structured cognitive assessment, an observational cognitive assessment anchored to the domains described in the preceding text should be performed.

When cognitive impairments are identified, it is essential that the clinician discuss these findings with reliable informants and/or review of medical records to confirm that such impairments are a known part of the patient's preadmission history. If they appear to be new, then the clinician must determine whether they reflect the effects of the psychiatric illness on cognition (e.g., impaired attention due to hallucinations, memory and executive impairments due to depression, disorganized thought and behavior due to severe psychosis) or instead suggest a nonpsychiatric cause of cognitive impairment. Among the nonpsychiatric problems of greatest concern are medical conditions or intoxication/withdrawal states causing delirium and also acute neurologic processes producing focal neurobehavioral syndromes (i.e., stroke-causing aphasia and apraxia, fall-producing bifrontal subdural hematomas and executive dysfunction, etc.). In either case, reevaluating apparent "psychiatric" symptoms as possible manifestations of an acute or subacute medical, substance-related, or neurologic condition and undertaking timely medical and neurologic evaluations (discussed in the subsequent text) is necessary.

If the cognitive impairments observed are felt to reflect the effects of the patient's psychiatric illness or are stable sequelae of the patient's ABI or DD, further evaluation of cognitive function specifically may not be necessary. Understanding the nature and severity of the patient's cognitive impairment allows staff to adjust communication and behavioral expectations to the patient's strengths and limitations. This information is also used to develop behavioral interventions for the neuropsychiatric problems that prompted psychiatric hospitalization.

PHYSICAL AND NEUROLOGIC EXAMINATIONS

Performing a thorough physical and neurologic examination before initiating treatment among persons with ABI or DD is highly recommended.[62] Patients with ABI and DD may require more frequent explanation and reassurance about interview and examination procedures than might ordinarily be offered to patients with primary psychiatric disorders. Such explanations should be stated simply and succinctly and offered as frequently as needed to maintain the patient's attention to the task at hand.

These examinations should include evaluation for signs of systemic disease (e.g., hypothyroidism and other endocrine disturbances, infectious or inflammatory disorders), substance abuse (e.g., physical hallmarks of alcohol or drug use), and impairments in elementary neurologic function. Identification of untreated physical or neurologic problems that, although not causes of neuropsychiatric problems *per se*, are potentially important comorbidities may alter treatment recommendations. For example, patients with neuropsychiatric disturbances after TBI frequently experience headaches and other types of pain (e.g., due to spasticity, traumatic neuropathies), which may exacerbate depression, anxiety, or agitation/aggression. If these comorbidities are left untreated, the response of the neuropsychiatric problem of concern to pharmacotherapies and other treatments may be limited. Additionally, untreated sensory (e.g., hearing, vision) problems may limit the effectiveness of psychotherapy and other behavioral interventions requiring verbal or written communication.

Similarly, although alcoholism and other substance use disorders appear to be less common among persons with DD than in the general population[63] their identification is essential before instituting an inpatient psychiatric treatment plan. Such problems are more common among persons with many forms of ABI, and particularly TBI, and they adversely affect medical, neuropsychiatric, and psychosocial functioning.[64] Given the potential for limited self-report of such problems among persons with DD and ABI, examination for the physical signs of alcohol and drug abuse may identify both important contributors to neuropsychiatric disturbances[64,65] as well as comorbidities requiring specific intervention.

In some cases it may be necessary to initiate preliminary treatment of severely disruptive or aggressive behaviors in order to examine the patient.[24] Among the initial treatment of greatest concern is the use of seclusion or restraint. Except under circumstances of imminent harm to the patient or staff, seclusion and restraint should be avoided if at all possible. Cognitively impaired patients often have difficulty understanding the rationale for the use of such measures and may escalate behaviorally when they are employed, thereby delaying further the interview and examinations needed to inform treatment.

LABORATORY ASSESSMENTS

Routine screening for laboratory abnormalities among persons hospitalized for psychiatric disturbances only rarely identifies previously unrecognized medical problems requiring intervention.[66] Testing patients with ABI or DD may be more productive.[62,66,67] In particular, assessment of serum glucose, creatinine and blood urea nitrogen, vitamin B_{12}, folate and thyroid-stimulating hormone levels, urinalysis and urine toxicology, and, when appropriate, pregnancy testing and serum drug levels (e.g., anticonvulsants, tricyclic antidepressants [TCAs], and/or some antipsychotic medications) may be clinically informative. The selection of such laboratory assessments is best guided by identification of historical and/or physical examination findings that suggests a reason for their performance. However, in the ABI and DD populations clinical suspicion for occult medical problems (e.g., urinary tract infection) should be high and the threshold for undertaking laboratory assessments low, especially when the ability to perform a thorough history or physical examination is limited.

ELECTROENCEPHALOGRAPHY

Routine, or screening, electroencephalography (EEG) is not recommended. However, if the history suggests the possibility of previously unrecognized epilepsy or encephalopathy then EEG may be useful. Although a "negative" EEG does not exclude the possibility of epilepsy, interictal epileptiform discharges, severe diffuse or focal slowing, or other markedly abnormal EEG findings (e.g., periodic lateralized discharges, periodic sharp waves, triphasic waves, etc.) may indicate a need for additional evaluation of medical or neurologic problems requiring specific intervention.

NEUROIMAGING

When available, review of previously performed structural neuroimaging studies (computed tomography [CT] or magnetic resonance imaging [MRI]) may be informative. If such imaging is not available or has not previously been performed, it may be useful to obtain and review anatomic brain studies before instituting a definitive psychiatric treatment plan. In addition to offering information regarding the possible anatomic bases of the patient's cognitive, emotional, or behavioral symptoms, the type of neuroimaging findings may inform the treatment approach.

Among persons with severe TBI, damage to the anterior and orbital frontal cortices as well as anterior temporal cortices is relatively common. Given the behaviorally inhibitory functions served by these areas, loss of cortex in these areas is commonly associated with disinhibited and/or aggressive behavior. In addition to suggesting a need for environmental interventions that decrease antecedents to such behaviors, neuroimaging findings of this sort suggest that pharmacologic interventions directed toward decreasing the limbic drive toward disinhibited or aggressive behavior (e.g., selective serotonin reuptake inhibitors [SSRIs], anticonvulsants, or atypical antipsychotics) may be more useful than those intended to augment the function of residual ventral anterior frontal and temporal cortices (e.g., psychostimulants, cholinesterase inhibitors).

Similarly, severe injury to dominant hemisphere lateral temporal and/or parietal cortex is associated with impairments in language comprehension (e.g., Wernicke or transcortical sensory aphasias) and, more occasionally, paranoid interpretation of the actions of others.[68] Among patients with deficits in language comprehension, therapeutic interventions predicated on verbal reassurance, redirection, and/or limit setting are unlikely to succeed, and pharmacologic interventions intended to improve language function are similarly unlikely to be successful. Armed with knowledge of the anatomy and severity of the brain injury underlying the patient's failure to respond to verbal cueing and to aphasia-targeted pharmacotherapy, the clinician will be better equipped to educate staff and caregivers about the nature of the patient's condition and the need for nonverbal interventions.

By contrast, neuroimaging that demonstrates injury restricted to cerebral white matter with axonal sparing, or even no overt evidence of brain damage, suggests a higher likelihood of improving neurobehavioral function through pharmacologic and/or environmental interventions. In such circumstances, instituting treatments directed toward augmentation of cortical areas required to effect neurobehavioral improvement may be useful—particularly when the treatment suggested seems counterintuitive to other staff members (e.g., stimulants or other catecholaminergically active agents in the hyperactive and impulsive brain-injured patient[69]).

Case Vignette

A 55-year-old, right-handed man was admitted to a long-term inpatient psychiatric unit at a state hospital from a nursing home for intractable psychotic and aggressive symptoms.

(continued)

The available history suggested onset of such problems approximately 30 years earlier, necessitating a series of unsuccessful inpatient psychiatric and nursing home placements spanning decades. The patient was unable (or "unwilling" according to staff members) to provide any historical information and was widely disliked by staff because of his apparent uncooperativeness with treatment (and particularly verbal redirection and limit setting). His verbal output, spontaneously or with prompting, was severely limited, generally consisting of single-word and frequently unintelligible utterances. The patient appeared to be responding to internal auditory stimuli, prompting a paranoid and aggressive behavior directed at anyone near him.

A neuropsychiatric evaluation identified a comment in a record from a prior hospitalization suggesting that the patient had been in a motorcycle accident approximately 30 years previously. Neurologic examination identified bilateral *mitgehen*-type paratonia, a mild spastic catch on extension of the right upper extremity, right-sided hyperreflexia, Babinski and Hoffman signs, and multiple primitive reflexes. In light of a history suggesting a possible remote TBI and an abnormal neurologic examination, MRI of the brain was recommended.

The MRI of the brain (see Fig. 17.1) identified a bilateral (left greater than right) anterior temporal porencephalic cysts, bilateral anterior frontal porencephalic cysts, bifrontal cortical atrophy, and severe bifrontal (left greater than right) white matter injury, consistent with a remote, severe TBI. This study suggested neuroanatomic bases for his impaired language function (left frontal and temporal damage), disinhibited and aggressive behavior (bilateral anterior and ventral frontal damage), and schizophreniform psychosis (severe left frontotemporal damage with bifrontal and bitemporal involvement[70]).

Communication of these findings to nursing staff allowed them to reframe his "unwillingness" to communicate verbally as an inability to do so because of nonfluent aphasia, to view his behaviors as products of his TBI rather than as intentional "uncooperativeness," and to understand his psychosis as reflective of very severe TBI. Environmental interventions designed to eliminate the antecedents to his unwanted behaviors and to enhance nonverbal communication were then able to be implemented more successfully. Additionally, staff members had more reasonable expectations regarding the likelihood of response to treatment of his aggression and psychosis with anticonvulsants and antipsychotic medications.

Although functional imaging (single photon emission computed tomography [SPECT], positron emission tomography [PET], and functional magnetic resonance imaging [fMRI]) is increasingly available, its use in the inpatient psychiatric evaluation and treatment of persons with ABI and DD does not often add therapeutically useful information to the evaluation of such patients. Accordingly, the use of functional imaging is not recommended in this context.

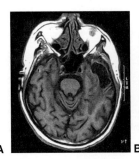 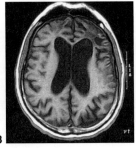 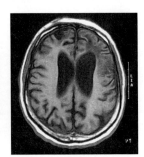

A   **B**   **C**

■ **Figure 17.1** T1-weighted coronal images of the brain.

Treatment of Neuropsychiatric Disturbances in Acquired Brain Injury and Developmental Disabilities

PSYCHOLOGICAL INTERVENTIONS

Psychological, behavioral, and environmental assessment and management is the cornerstone of treatment of patients with ABI and DD.[71,72] In all cases, supportive counseling—even if directed only toward engagement in treatment[73]—is recommended. When patients are cognitively and linguistically capable of engaging in other forms of psychotherapy, including cognitive-behavioral therapy, dialectical behavioral therapy, interpersonal therapy, and group (including family) therapy, such therapies should be offered.[74–78] Use of such interventions, particularly cognitive-behavioral therapies, improves coping skills among persons with ABI and DD.[74,75] Cognitive-behavioral therapies also appear particularly useful for the treatment of depressive, anxious, and anger symptoms in these populations.[79–81]

Hurley offered several principles that guide the performance of psychotherapeutic interventions for persons with ABI or DD.[82] As suggested in the preceding text, the technique employed should be adapted to meet the patient's cognitive abilities. Rather than assuming a neutral or passive approach, therapies are most useful when offered in a more directive manner. However, remaining flexible, rather than prescriptive, in the manner in which therapy is offered is prudent. Rather than performing psychotherapy with the patient alone, engaging significant others in the therapeutic (and particularly educational and problem-solving) process is generally necessary. Patients with ABI and DD, including those with severe cognitive impairments, should be expected to develop transferences to the treating clinician and the setting in which treatment is offered. Countertransferences involving both the patient and their families/caregivers arise during the provision of any such treatment and require careful management. Finally, addressing directly the issues of diagnosis (ABI and DD), disability, and the psychological consequences attendant to these problems is recommended.

BEHAVIORAL ANALYSIS AND INTERVENTION

Developing a treatment plan for the inpatient with ABI or DD and neuropsychiatric disturbances begins with nonpharmacologic interventions. As illustrated by the case vignettes offered earlier, an analysis of behaviors using an A-B-C (antecedents, behaviors, and consequences) approach is useful,[83] particularly when aggressive, violent, or other disinhibited behaviors are the focus of treatment.[83–86]

Antecedents to problematic behaviors or neuropsychiatric symptoms are many and varied, but are frequently identifiable with careful attention to the history. Common causes of problematic behaviors include previously unrecognized or undertreated medical, neurologic, psychiatric (and especially mood), or substance use disorders; communication difficulties between patient and caregivers; and environmental factors (e.g., poor fit between patient and residence, including persons with whom the patient resides or interacts). Suspicion for the latter of these antecedents should be particularly high when, following admission, the patient fails to demonstrate the neuropsychiatric problems that necessitated hospitalization. Once identified, the treatment plan includes patient and caregiver education and/or training aimed at eliminating or modifying antecedents to problematic behaviors. Although such interventions may not obviate the need for pharmacologic treatment of neurobehavioral disturbances, particularly among patients with more severe cognitive impairments,[71] pharmacotherapy is less likely to succeed when undertaken without addressing the triggers of problematic behaviors.

In addition to characterizing the type and severity of behaviors requiring treatment in the manner described earlier, the possible meanings of those behaviors also require consideration before developing a treatment plan.[87] Although neuropsychiatric problems (e.g., psychosis, depression, mania, anxiety, aggression, and apathy) may arise directly as a result of brain dysfunction attributable to ABI or DD, some problematic behaviors may represent attempts (even if maladaptive one) to communicate physical symptoms and/or emotional reactions to depression, anxiety, losses, conflicts, or other social/psychological stressors.[88,89] With this in mind, data derived from the types of history taking described earlier in this chapter should be followed by an attempt to understand the patient's neuropsychiatric symptoms in neurobiological, psychological, and environmental terms. While such formulations will often remain speculative, they nonetheless serve as the bases for hypotheses that are subsequently tested through empiric trials of nonpharmacologic and pharmacologic interventions.

Finally, attempts should be made to identify the consequences of the patient's behaviors. In some cases, caregivers—including inpatient staff—may misunderstand the reasons for a patient's behavior. That misunderstanding may lead them to fail to provide the consequences needed to ameliorate it or, worse, to provide consequences that inadvertently reinforce it. For example, agitation may represent an attempt to communicate pain, fatigue, hunger, the need to urinate or defecate, or environmental overstimulation. When responded to only with limit setting or redirection (an inappropriate response to behavior generated by these factors), remission of the behavior should not be expected. Conversely, if the patient is attended to only when he or she becomes agitated, that behavior is reinforced and therefore should be expected to recur and likely increase.

Although the paradigm of operant conditioning (i.e., behavior X is followed by consequence Y, thereby reinforcing [positively or negatively] behavior X) may seem simplistic, it remains a powerful method by which to analyze complex clinical situations and reduce unwanted (maladaptive) behaviors and encourage wanted (adaptive) ones among persons with ABI and DD.[84,90,91]

PHARMACOLOGIC TREATMENTS

General Principles

Few controlled clinical trials have assessed the effects of medication in persons with ABI or DD, and no medicine has received approval for the treatment of any neuropsychiatric sequelae of these conditions. Accordingly, all pharmacologic treatments offered to persons with neuropsychiatric problems due to ABI or DD are "off-label." Given the dearth of information regarding the benefits, risks, and side effects of psychopharmacologic agents in these populations, approaching the use of medication is best undertaken with caution and after obtaining informed consent from the patient or his legally authorized proxy medical decision makers.

The decision regarding which medicine (if any) to prescribe may be informed by published treatment studies, where these are available. Absent such studies, medication selection is guided by (a) current knowledge of the efficacy of the medicine in other psychiatric disorders, (b) side effect profiles of the medicine, (c) consideration of the potential for increased sensitivity to side effects, (d) analogies made between brain injury–related symptoms and those that occur in idiopathic psychiatric syndromes (e.g., amotivational syndrome after TBI may be analogous to the deficit syndrome in schizophrenia), and (e) hypotheses, when such can be developed, regarding the neuroanatomic and neurochemical disturbances produced by a specific type of ABI or DD and the mechanisms of action of the medicine selected.

When selecting a pharmacotherapy, define the target symptoms of each medicine prescribed. Monotherapy is preferable to polypharmacy; because many medicines may treat several neuropsychiatric symptoms effectively (e.g., atypical antipsychotics for psychosis, aggression, and insomnia; anticonvulsants for mania, aggression, insomnia, and seizures), selecting an agent with the broadest possible benefits and the fewest possible adverse effects (e.g., avoiding typical antipsychotics, benzodiazepines, and agents with potent anticholinergic properties) is encouraged. Nonetheless, clinicians should remain open to the possible use of multiple medicines when a single agent will not suffice or proves ineffective for one or more target symptoms. When possible, it is prudent to initiate each treatment sequentially rather than concurrently to understand as clearly as possible both the beneficial and adverse effects of each medicine prescribed. Also define "successful outcome" (even if only an improvement sufficient enough to permit transition to a less restrictive treatment setting) and the duration of treatment expected to achieve that outcome as clearly as possible, recognizing that both may require modification as treatment proceeds. Communicate these definitions to the patient, his or her significant others, and the staff of the psychiatric unit to establish a shared set of expectations regarding the purpose and duration of pharmacotherapy. Anticipating potential adverse responses (e.g., paradoxical agitation with benzodiazepines) allows for contingency planning. Finally, if possible, initiate new treatments when the patient's environment is stable. In the authors' experience, starting new treatments over weekends, holidays, or periods with significant staff turnover is less effective.

Once treatment is initiated, a "start low and go slow" approach to dosing is recommended. Although it is important to alleviate the suffering of patients as quickly as possible, many psychotropic medicines (e.g., antidepressants, antiaggressive agents, etc.) must be titrated slowly and used for several weeks before the effects become fully apparent. Toward that end, it is prudent to expect that standard (or higher) doses of some medicines, even if arrived slowly, may be required to achieve optimal effects.

Reassess the target symptom(s) at a predefined interval (e.g., daily, twice weekly, weekly) and adhere to the proposed treatment plan as much as possible. The present authors encourage the use of the same standardized scales used to identify the symptom(s) rather than depending on subjective reports from the patient and staff. The recurrence of an unwanted behavior—however disruptive and distressing that behavior may be—does not necessarily demonstrate that the current treatment is ineffective. Instead, it may simply indicate the need for additional time or increased dosing of the medicine prescribed. Bear in mind that general medical (e.g., urinary tract infection, metabolic disturbances) and neurologic (e.g., seizure) comorbidities may produce a recurrence of unwanted behaviors and exacerbation of psychiatric symptoms as well. Evaluating the patient for such problems when unwanted behaviors arise should also be considered.

Remain vigilant for adverse effects and drug–drug interactions; when such develop, lower the dose of the most recently prescribed (or increased) medicine before discontinuing that treatment entirely. When such reductions result in recurrence of the target symptom, consider augmenting the first medicine with a second agent. The selection of a supplementary (or augmenting) medicine should be based on consideration of the possible complementary or contrary mechanisms of action of such agents, the individual and combined side effect profiles of the initial and secondary agents, and their potential pharmacokinetic and pharmacodynamic interactions. If the augmentation strategy is successful, attempt to discontinue the first medicine in the service of determining whether monotherapy with the "augmentation" agent is sufficient to treat the target symptom; if it is not, continue treatment with the lowest possible effective dose of both agents.

Depression

Depression is a common problem among persons with ABI and DD and is amenable to pharmacologic intervention.[92–94] Treatment of depression may alleviate not only the mood disturbance but also reduce other neurobehavioral disturbances such as impulsivity, aggression, and self-injurious behaviors.[95] Although many factors (e.g., sleep disturbance, fatigue [anergia], difficulty concentrating, and anhedonia [apathy]) may produce or contribute to apparent depressive symptoms, when there are sufficient symptoms (or behavioral equivalents) to merit a diagnosis of depression an antidepressant treatment should be initiated. Apathy can be misinterpreted as depression and should be considered in the case formulation (see subsequent text).

Somatic therapies for depression among persons with ABI and DD include SSRIs, serotonin-norepinephrine reuptake inhibitors (SNRIs), tricyclic and tetracyclic agents (TCAs), novel antidepressants (e.g., trazodone, mirtazapine, venlafaxine, bupropion), monoamine oxidase inhibitors (MAOIs), and psychostimulants. Given the relatively favorable profile of the selective SSRIs, these agents are suggested as the first-line treatment for depression among persons with ABI and DD.

Although there is no evidence to suggest that any SSRI is clearly superior to the others for the treatment of depression (with or without other behavioral disturbances) in these populations, the physicians generally recommend using agents with relatively short half-lives, limited CYP-450 inhibition, and no anticholinergic effects. With these considerations in mind, sertraline, citalopram, and escitalopram are considered first-line treatments. When cost considerations, treatment intolerance, or patient/caregiver preference preclude use of these agents, fluoxetine and paroxetine are reasonable to consider and would, in general, be expected to be similarly effective. However, their use may require more careful consideration of possible drug–drug interactions (mediated through their effects on CYP-450 drug metabolism) and, in the case of paroxetine, on cognition (through its anticholinergic effects).

The TCAs are used less commonly for the treatment of depression in general as well as for depression among persons with ABI or DD, and the authors regard them as second-line treatments for this purpose. The possibility of increased side effects associated with these agents, reports of more limited effectiveness of these agents among persons with TBI,[96,97] waning familiarity with the use of these agents on the part of recently trained clinicians, or some combination of these factors may explain the declining use of these agents. Nonetheless, these agents may be helpful for some patients and merit consideration among those unable to tolerate or unwilling to take SSRIs. When a TCA is used, nortriptyline and desipramine are recommended due to their more favorable side effect profiles.

Common clinical experience[98] suggests that the novel antidepressants may be useful in the treatment of depression among persons with ABI and DD, but their use must be undertaken cautiously given the very limited data describing the benefits and risks attendant to their use in these populations. Bupropion is of particular concern because of its dose-related incidence of seizures, which appear to be more common among persons with underlying neurologic conditions.[99,100]

MAOIs are infrequently used to treat depression in persons with ABI and DD. Their limited use reflects the high likelihood of difficulties with patient adherence to the complex dietary restrictions required during use of these medications, particularly among persons with cognitive impairments. Additionally, the literature offers little support for the effectiveness of these medicines in these populations.[96,97]

Psychostimulants, and particularly methylphenidate and dextroamphetamine, may improve depression and other behavioral disturbances among persons with ABI.[101–104] When a rapid response to depression is required, these agents may be particularly useful. In such circumstances, these agents are generally used as an initial intervention, which is then followed with a standard antidepressant (usually an SSRI) for long-term treatment. In some cases, these agents may be used long term. As suggested earlier in this chapter, the decision to employ a psychostimulant may be informed by a review of neuroimaging; among patients with severe ventral frontal cortical injury or frank disconnection due to destructive white matter lesions interrupting frontal–subcortical circuits, these agents may worsen impulsive/aggressive behavior, whereas they tend to improve depression and behavior among patients with relatively preserved frontolimbic anatomy.

In addition to the psychostimulants, augmentation with lithium, triiodothyronine (T3), and/or pindolol[98,105] may be considered on the basis of the beneficial effects of these agents as augmentation strategies for depressive disorders in otherwise neurologically healthy persons.[105] However, their use for this purpose among persons with ABI and DD has not been systematically evaluated and must therefore be undertaken with caution and with careful monitoring for adverse effects.

Mania

Mania and bipolar disorder may develop among persons with ABI and DD, although this appears to be more common among persons with DD[71] than among persons with ABI.[106,107] Treatment of acute manic states may include any of several pharmacologic approaches, including use of anticonvulsants, atypical antipsychotics, typical antipsychotics, and/or benzodiazepines. Prophylaxis against manic episodes is typically undertaken with lithium carbonate, carbamazepine, or valproate. There are very few reports regarding the treatment of mania following ABI, whether that treatment is for acute manic states or for long-term prophylaxis against recurrent mania. However, studies performed to date suggest that treatment with lithium carbonate, carbamazepine, and valproate may be useful in this population as well. Neurologic comorbidities including seizures, migraine, and other pain syndromes may guide the selection of a specific medicine.

Absent evidence demonstrating the clear superiority of one of these agents over the others, the authors generally recommend valproate as a first-line treatment given its effectiveness for acute mania, rapid-cycling bipolar disorder, and antimanic prophylaxis as well as its reasonable tolerability in persons with ABI and DD. Although valproate may exacerbate cognitive impairments,[108] it appears less likely to do so than either carbamazepine or lithium. Nonetheless, its use should include careful and ongoing assessment of cognition as well as typical treatment-related side effects such as tremor, weight gain, diarrhea, blood dyscrasias, hepatotoxicity, and hair loss.

Lithium carbonate may be useful for the treatment of mania in persons with ABI and DD, although partial response, relapse of symptoms, or need for a second mood-stabilizing medicine are common.[109–113] Lithium appears more likely to produce nausea, tremor, ataxia, and lethargy in persons with neurologic disorders than in the general psychiatric population, and lithium may lower seizure threshold.[114] These observations emphasize the need for vigilance for adverse effects when using this agent in persons with ABI or DD and to titrate cautiously to beneficial effect or medication intolerance. Manic episodes occurring after TBI may also respond to carbamazepine. Because carbamazepine may produce or exacerbate cognitive and motor impairments among persons with TBI,[108] monitoring carefully for adverse effects when using this agent in patients ABI or DD is recommended.

Although there is emerging enthusiasm in general psychiatry for the use of other antimanic agents, including several of the newer anticonvulsants (e.g., lamotrigine, oxcarbazepine) and the atypical antipsychotics (risperidone, olanzapine, quetiapine, ziprasidone, and aripiprazole), reports describing the use of these agents in persons with ABI and DD are few. Clinicians interested in using these agents for the treatment of ABI and DD patients with mania are advised to undertake such treatments cautiously; in particular, use of the atypical antipsychotics for this purpose should entail careful monitoring for adverse cognitive, motor, cardiac, and metabolic side effects.

Pathologic Laughing and Crying

In contrast to mood disorders, conditions in which the baseline emotional state is pervasively disturbed over a relatively long period of time (i.e., weeks), disorders of affect denote conditions in which the more moment-to-moment variation and regulation of emotion is disturbed. The classic disorder of affect dysregulation is pathological laughing and/or crying (PLC), also known as *emotional incontinence* or *pseudobulbar affect*.[115] Patients with this condition experience involuntary and uncontrollable episodes of involuntary crying and/or laughing that may occur many times per day, are provoked by trivial (i.e., often not sentimental) stimuli, are quite stereotyped in their presentation, may be of a valence contradictory to the context in which they occur (i.e., crying when laughing would be expected and vice versa), and do not produce a persistent change in the prevailing mood.

The prevalence of PLC among persons with ABI and DD is not clear, but may be as high as 11% among persons with TBI,[116] 34% among persons with stroke,[117] and 10% among persons with MS.[118] Although this condition is an uncommon reason for admission to an inpatient psychiatric setting, its lack of inclusion in the DSM-based diagnostic system may foster misdiagnosis and hence a perceived need for hospitalization. Patients presenting with paroxysms of crying are often diagnosed as "depressed" and patients with paroxysms of crying and laughing are often misdiagnosed as "bipolar" despite the absence of pervasive and sustained disturbances of mood, psychological, and neurovegetative symptoms required for these diagnoses. The misdiagnosis of PLC as bipolar disorder, and especially of the rapid cyling or ultrarapid cycling types, is particularly concerning given the dissimilarity of treatments between these conditions.

The treatment literature overwhelmingly supports the use and effectiveness of relatively low doses (often well below typical antidepressant doses) of serotonergically and noradrenergically active antidepressants.[119-122] Collectively, these reports suggest that the SSRIs are effective treatments for affective lability and PLC following TBI, and the present authors recommend them as first-line agents for this purpose. Given that the use of these agents in the absence of a mood stabilizer of some sort would not be prudent in patients with bipolar disorder, as well as the apparently limited benefit of mood-stabilizing medications on most forms of PLC, the importance of diagnostic accuracy in this context cannot be overstated.

As for the treatment of depression, no SSRI is clearly superior for treatment of PLC. However, using agents with relatively short half-lives, limited drug–drug and CYP-450 interactions, and favorable side effect profiles is recommended. TCAs may also be effective for PLC, with nortriptyline being the most favorable of these agents. Although psychostimulants and other medications that enhance dopamine and/or norepinephrine neurotransmission are used most often for the treatment of cognitive impairments and/or diminished motivation following ABI, they may also concurrently afford relief from PLC. Among patients in whom PLC is accompanied by irritability/anger, aggressive, or self-destructive behaviors, treatment with anticonvulsants or lithium may be of some benefit.

Anxiety Disorders and Post-traumatic Stress Disorder

Anxiety disorders, including generalized anxiety disorder, panic disorder, phobias, obsessive compulsive disorder, and/or post-traumatic stress disorder, may develop among persons with ABI and DD, and may be a source of substantial morbidity for persons with these problems and their families. When any of these conditions are present, clinicians should carefully assess patients for comorbid conditions (medical, psychiatric, substance related, etc.) and environmental factors that may be driving the anxiety symptoms and, when possible, treat such conditions before specifically targeting anxiety symptoms.

The authors generally prefer to treat complaints of anxiety in these patients with supportive psychotherapy and social interventions most appropriate to the specific anxiety disorder with which the patient presents before adding an anxiolytic medication. However, when anxiety symptoms are so severe that they require pharmacological intervention, treatment with SSRIs, benzodiazepines, or buspirone may be needed. Among these medications, SSRIs are preferred for the treatment of anxiety disorders following TBI given their considerable benefits on a host of anxiety disorders in the general psychiatric population and also their relatively favorable side effect profiles.

When SSRIs fail to produce adequate and sustained relief of anxiety, it may be necessary to consider treatment with a benzodiazepine or buspirone. Although benzodiazepines offer the benefit of rapid anxiolysis, their use among persons with ABI and DD is concerning given their tendency to produce a variety of potentially problematic side effects, including memory and motor impairments. This constellation of adverse effects makes the use of benzodiazepines for the treatment of anxiety in patients with ABI, in particular, undesirable. Their use as first-line treatments for anxiety in this context is not encouraged. When these agents are used, agents with moderate half-lives (lorazepam, oxazepam) are preferable to those with very short half-lives (which are highly reinforcing and may produce rebound anxiety between doses) or very long half-lives (which may result in cumulative adverse effects with repeated administrations).

Buspirone appears to carry less risk of worsening cognitive functioning in patients with ABI than benzodiazepines, and use of buspirone is not associated with dependency. Unfortunately, therapeutic effects of buspirone appear to require several weeks to develop and not all patients respond to this agent. The prolonged latency of action sometimes necessitates short-term treatment with another anxiolytic, usually one of the benzodiazepines, and/or more intensive psychotherapy to keep the patient engaged in the use of this medicine.

Apathy

States of diminished motivation, or apathy, are relatively common consequences of many types of ABI.[123] In this context, apathy denotes a clinically significant decrease in goal-directed cognition, emotion, and/or behavior. Each of these manifestations of the apathy syndrome may be present in varying degrees in individual patients; however, when present to any degree they may interfere with rehabilitation efforts and functioning in everyday life.

Apathetic states occur on a continuum of severity, with states of mildly diminished motivation at one end of that continuum and akinetic mutism at the other end. Although apathy may be a feature of depression, it often arises independent of this condition. Clinicians unfamiliar with the syndrome of apathy as a distinct sequela of ABI may be misled diagnostically by the apathetic patient's presentation. When patients present with diminished affective responsivity ("flat affect"), they are frequently described by caregivers as "depressed." However, patients with depression suffer from a state of persistent and excessive distress—by self-report, observation, or both—whereas patients with apathy are more correctly described as suffering from an absence of emotion. Making this distinction is imperative as first-line treatments for depression (e.g., SSRIs, TCAs) often fail to improve or worsen apathy.

Psychostimulants (e.g., methylphenidate, dextroamphetamine) and other dopaminergically active medications (e.g., amantadine, bromocriptine, carbidopa/L-dopa) are the principal pharmacotherapies.[124] Among patients in whom motivational deficits and memory impairments co-occur, cholinesterase inhibitors (donepezil, rivastigmine, and galantamine) may be of benefit for both symptoms.[125] Protriptyline, a secondary amine tricyclic agent, has been suggested to have sufficient stimulant properties to permit its use for anergia and diminished motivation in some patients with ABI.[126,127] Amitriptyline and desipramine also may improve arousal and initiation,[128] possibly as a result of their pronoradrenergic effects of these agents. Despite these case reports, however, the authors suggest that TCAs are best regarded as treatments of last resort for apathy in light of their potential for exacerbating cognitive impairments and less favorable side effect profiles.

Complicating the treatment of apathy is its not uncommon co-occurrence with behavioral dyscontrol (disinhibition, impulsivity, and aggression). This seemingly odd combination of behavioral problems occurs in the setting of injury to both the anterior cingulate-subcortical circuits (resulting in apathy) and lateral orbitofrontal-subcortical circuits (resulting in a behavioral dyscontrol syndrome). Patients with comorbid apathy and behavioral dyscontrol usually appear apathetic at baseline but demonstrate episodic behavioral dyscontrol when an environmental or somatic stimulus is sufficiently potent to produce aggressive and/or appetitive behaviors. Those automatic behaviors may be understood, somewhat simplistically, as reflecting an automatic response to environmental or somatic stimuli sufficient to activate limbic-subcortical circuits involved in appetitive or aggressive behaviors despite a lack of activity in those circuits to sustain motivation more generally. The combination of apathy and behavioral dyscontrol presents a substantial therapeutic challenge, as the therapies used to improve apathy may worsen behavioral dyscontrol and the therapies for behavioral dyscontrol may worsen apathy. Patients and their caregivers are often better able to tolerate and manage apathy than behavior dyscontrol, and some may elect to intervene pharmacologically on the latter even knowing that it may exacerbate the former. When both symptoms require intervention, it is best to maximize nonpharmacologic approaches, use the lowest possible dose of pharmacologic treatments sufficient to permit management of these behaviors, and anticipate the possibility of using one of the previously mentioned agents to improve apathy concurrent to the use of another to limit the frequency and severity of behavioral excesses (described in the subsequent text).

Psychosis

Among persons with ABI and DD, schizophreniform, schizoaffective, and delusional disorders[70,71,129] occur with a frequency higher than that observed in the general population and their treatment may require inpatient hospitalization.[130] Identification of psychotic symptoms may be particularly challenging among patients with severe cognitive and communicative impairments. In these patients, behavioral disturbances may be the more obvious problem, but careful evaluations using the methods described previously may facilitate the identification of psychosis as the prompt for those behaviors.

Although typical antipsychotic medications are sometimes used to treat psychosis and attendant behavioral disturbances (e.g., agitation, aggression, impulsivity) among persons with ABI and DD, these agents are used less often since the advent of the second-generation, or atypical, antipsychotics. However, there is at present a dearth of reports to guide selection among the atypical antipsychotic agents in these populations. Clozapine, the prototype of this class, may be useful in the treatment of psychosis and aggressive behavior among persons with ABI and DD.[127,131,132] Unfortunately, this treatment carries a relatively high risk of adverse effects including seizures and agranulocytosis. Additionally, the laboratory-monitoring protocol required during its use is for many clinicians and patients too cumbersome to be practical. Nonetheless, it may be a useful therapy for patients who do not respond to or are unable to tolerate treatment with another atypical antipsychotic.[133]

With these concerns in mind, risperidone, olanzapine, quetiapine, ziprasidone, and aripiprazole are generally used for the treatment of psychosis and related behavioral disturbances among persons with ABI and DD.[70,129,134] Each of these medicines may be of benefit in this population, but specific benefits and side effect profiles attendant to their use among persons with ABI and DD are not characterized fully at this time. On the basis of the literature[129,135,136] and the authors' clinical experience in this area, risperidone, olanzapine, or quetiapine is recommended as first line for the treatment of psychosis following TBI.

In general, starting doses of these agents are generally one third to one half of those used among persons with primary psychotic disorders. However, gradual titration to doses similar to those used in other contexts may be required to effect improvement in psychosis and related behavior disturbances. Baseline assessment of and periodic monitoring for cardiac problems (i.e., prolonged QTc) and also metabolic syndrome during treatment with any atypical antipsychotic medication are recommended. Additionally, vigilance for the development of treatment-emergent movement disorders such as dystonias, dyskinesias, and akathisia,[137] neuroleptic malignant syndrome, and seizures is particularly important in these patients, who may be susceptible to such problems.

Aggression, Agitation, and Self-Injurious Behaviors

Aggressive, agitated, and self-injurious behaviors are common reasons for inpatient psychiatric admission among persons with ABI and DD.[130] A multimodal, multidisciplinary, collaborative approach to treatment is essential, and the nonpharmacologic treatments described in the preceding section of this chapter should be regarded as first-line interventions. As highlighted there, diagnosis must precede treatment: determining the mental status of the patient before the agitated or aggressive events occurs (including co-occurring medical, neurologic, psychiatric, and substance use disorders), carefully characterizing the behaviors and the contexts in which they develop, identifying possible reinforcers of these behaviors, and implementing nonpharmacologic treatments are prerequisites to pharmacotherapy. When medication is used, treatment of comorbid neuropsychiatric conditions (depression, psychosis, insomnia, anxiety, and delirium), when present, takes precedence and should be undertaken before initiating treatment specifically for agitation or aggression.

When a pharmacotherapy for aggression or agitation is required, using agents that may improve both these problems and also the comorbid neuropsychiatric conditions driving them is recommended. Additionally, employing agents with a specific neurochemical target in mind may help avoid redundancy when serial medication trials are required to effect reduction in aggression and/or agitation. Hypotheses regarding the selection of pharmacotherapies for the treatment of aggression and agitation include inhibition of excessive activity in temporolimbic areas with anticonvulsants, reduction of "hyperactive" limbic monoaminergic neurotransmission with β-adrenergic receptor antagonists (e.g., propranolol) or dopamine-receptor antagonists (e.g., haloperidol), augmentation of orbitofrontal and/or dorsolateral prefrontal cortical activity with monoaminergic agonists (e.g., amantadine, methylphenidate, and perhaps buspirone), or modulation of limbic and frontal activity through augmentation of serotonergic activity (e.g., SSRIs).[138] However, the neurochemistry of aggression in this or any other clinical context is not understood completely, and these hypotheses must be regarded as preliminary at best. Consequently, the pharmacologic treatment of these problems often entails a trial-and-error approach to find a medicine that is both effective and tolerable. Finally, clinicians should bear in mind that patients may not respond to just one medicine, but may require combination treatment, similar to the pharmacotherapeutic treatment for refractory posttraumatic depression.

When employing a pharmacotherapy for aggression, agitation, and self-injurious behavior, it may be helpful to consider the treatment of acute and chronic problems of these sorts separately. Antipsychotics and benzodiazepines are the most commonly used medicines in the treatment of acute aggressive, agitated, and self-injurious behaviors among persons with ABI and DD.[139] When an antipsychotic agent is used, atypical antipsychotics (e.g., risperidone, olanzapine, quetiapine) are best regarded as first-line treatments,[136,137,140] and are most effective among patients in whom such behaviors are psychosis related. As with their use in the treatment of psychosis among persons with ABI and DD, starting dose of antipsychotic agents should be low and repeated at frequent intervals until control of the target behavior is achieved. If after several administrations of these agents the patient's behavior does not abate, the dose may be increased until sedation is achieved. Subsequently, the daily dose is decreased gradually (e.g., by $\sim$25% per day) to determine the minimally effective dose for continued control of the problematic behavior(s). Chronic treatment with the agents may be required in some cases, and particularly among those with comorbid psychotic symptoms.

Although these agents are appropriate and may be particularly effective when such behaviors arise as a result of psychosis, their use should not be undertaken lightly due to the potential for serious treatment-related adverse events including movement disorders, seizures, and neuroleptic malignant syndrome. In the absence of psychosis, the sedative side effects of antipsychotics are most likely the mechanisms by which treatment (or, more accurately, masking) of these behaviors is effected. Unfortunately, tolerance to the sedative effects of these agents is not uncommon, thereby necessitating increasing doses and incurring greater risk for other adverse effects. Of particular concern, even with the atypical antipsychotics, is the development of akathisia. When this problem develops, agitation, restlessness, and self-injurious behaviors may increase and be misunderstood as an indication for dose escalation, thereby setting in motion a cycle of increasing antipsychotics doses and worsening akathisia. With this in mind, increasing behaviors of these sorts in response to treatment with an antipsychotic agent should prompt consideration of the use of a different class of medication.

The sedative properties of benzodiazepines may be helpful in the management of acute agitation and aggression.[139] However, benzodiazepines predictably impair memory, motor function, coordination and balance, all of which are common problems among persons with ABI and DD. Although a rare adverse effect of benzodiazepine treatment, paradoxical agitation, aggression, and self-injurious behavior are also problems of concern in these populations. For these reasons, benzodiazepines are generally avoided whenever possible for these behaviors in this context. However, when a benzodiazepine is required for the treatment of acute aggression, agitation, or self-injurious behaviors, those with moderate half-lives, relatively few drug–drug interactions, and no active metabolites (e.g., lorazepam, oxazepam) are recommended.

When a patient exhibits chronic aggression, agitation, and/or self-injurious behaviors, chronic pharmacotherapy (framed as prophylaxis in some cases) may be required. As noted in the preceding text, selection of pharmacotherapy is guided by identification of comorbid neuropsychiatric symptoms or syndromes (e.g., depression, mania, anxiety) the treatment of which necessitates use of a medicine relatively specific to that comorbidity. When these behaviors are not clearly related to another neuropsychiatric symptom or syndrome or are sufficiently severe to require their own treatment, there is no consensus on their optimal management. The present authors' approach is to begin treatment with the least potentially problematic medications and undertake serial empiric trials of medications from different pharmacologic classes in pursuit of the most effective and well-tolerated medication for each patient.

Serotonergically active antidepressants may improve aggressive, agitated, and self-injurious behaviors and tend to do so with relatively few adverse effects.[95,139,141–144] Among these agents, the SSRIs are the first-line agents and are used in dosages similar to those for depression. Although there is no *a priori* expectation of differences between the SSRIs on these behaviors, some patients may respond favorably to one SSRI but not another. Additionally, some patients respond better to trazodone or to a TCA. Clinicians may wish to consider serial empiric trials within the general class of serotonergically active antidepressants before proceeding to the next medication class in the authors' approach, anticonvulsants.

Agitation, aggression, and self-injurious behavior may respond to treatment with anticonvulsants such as carbamazepine[145–147] and valproate.[148–152] Between these agents, valproate is generally recommended as a first-line treatment given its effectiveness, tolerability, and more limited set of drug–drug interactions. Although newer anticonvulsants such as oxcarbazepine, gabapentin, lamotrigine, and levetiracetam are tempting to employ as treatments for these behaviors,[153–155] their use in these populations is less well studied than either carbamazepine or valproate. The clinical experience with oxcarbazepine as an alternative to carbamazepine is encouraging, but useful only as anecdote. Several reports describe worsening of agitation and aggression among persons with ABI and DD during treatment with gabapentin,[156–158] lamotrigine,[159] and levetiracetam.[160] Accordingly, their use is best undertaken after valproate and carbamazepine prove ineffective or intolerable, and then with caution and with careful monitoring for treatment-related worsening of such behaviors.

When treatment with serotonergically active antidepressants and/or anticonvulsants does not improve aggressive, agitated, or self-injurious behaviors, the next step in treatment is addition of an atypical antipsychotic. As suggested for the acute management of these behaviors, risperidone, olanzapine, and quetiapine are suggested as first-line agents.[136,137,140] If the addition of such a medicine meets with behavior improvement, an empiric trial of monotherapy with it will suffice as treatment for the behavioral disturbance. There is also evidence suggesting clozapine as a treatment for these behavioral problems among persons with ABI and DD;[127,131,161] it is regarded as an antipsychotic treatment of last resort given the cumbersome administration and monitoring requirements, its tendency to lower seizure threshold, and risk for potentially life-threatening blood dyscrasias. When any of the atypical antipsychotics are used long-term either as monotherapy or an augmentation agent, baseline and serial reassessment for cardiac, metabolic, and other antipsychotic-induced adverse effects (as discussed previously) is recommended.

Lithium,[139,162,163] β-adrenergic receptor antagonists,[139,147,164–167] buspirone,[168–171] long-acting benzodiazepines such as clonazepam,[172] and, among persons with preserved ventral frontal-subcortical systems, even catecholamine-augmenting agents such as methylphenidate[173] and amantadine[174,175] may reduce aggression, agitation, and self-injurious behaviors among persons with ABI and DD. Among these, lithium and β-adrenergic receptor antagonists are generally regarded as the most effective agents,[139] but their use is often complicated by adverse systemic and neurologic side effects in these populations. Nonetheless, these agents merit consideration—particularly as augmentation strategies—when serotonergically active antidepressants, anticonvulsants, and/or atypical antipsychotics have proved ineffective, only partially effective, or intolerable at doses required to effect behavioral improvements.

Electroconvulsive Therapy

Electroconvulsive therapy (ECT) remains a highly effective and underutilized treatment in general, and the same is true in persons with ABI and DD.[176–179] Similar to its beneficial effects on a variety of primary psychiatric disorders, ECT appears to be an effective and safe treatment of chronic, severe neuropsychiatric disorders due to ABI and DD.[178–188] The literature suggests that ECT improves refractory depression, mania, and psychosis in these populations with similar speed and comparable rates of side effects to those observed among persons with primary psychiatric disorders who receive ECT.

When ECT is considered, the principal issue of concern will be consent to treatment. Given the effectiveness and safety of ECT, a cogent ethical justification for the use of ECT can be offered when other behavioral and pharmacologic treatments have failed. Discussing the benefits and risks, and acknowledging that neither of these issues is understood completely, with the patient and his or her legally authorized proxy medical decision maker is imperative.

In the service of minimizing treatment-emergent delirium, hypomania, and cognitive impairment, the authors recommend treatment with the lowest possible energy levels that will generate a seizure of adequate duration (>20 seconds), using pulsatile currents, increased spacing of treatments (2 to 5 days between treatments), and fewer treatments in an entire course (4 to 6). In general, nondominant unilateral ECT is the preferred technique.

Conclusions

In this chapter, the authors reviewed the evaluation and treatment of psychiatric disturbances among patients with ABI and DD most relevant to care provided in the inpatient psychiatric setting. Despite the limited training in the care of persons with ABI and DD provided to psychiatrists during medical school and residency, those working in inpatient settings will be called upon to provide psychiatric services to individuals with these conditions. Treatment planning in this population requires a more extensive pretreatment evaluation than is often required by patients with primary psychiatric illnesses, the general principles of which were reviewed herein. The authors suggested that the pretreatment evaluation focus on the review of collateral information provided by reliable informants and medical records; use of standardized measures of neuropsychiatric symptoms to define potential targets of treatment; detailed review of environmental issues and prior treatments, including medical, neurologic, and psychiatric interventions both pharmacologic and nonpharmacologic; thorough cognitive, physical, and neurologic examinations; problem-focused laboratory and electroencephalographic assessments; and review of neuroimaging findings.

Psychological, behavioral, and environmental management is the cornerstone of treatment of neuropsychiatric disturbances in patients with ABI and DD. When specific neuropsychiatric symptoms require pharmacologic treatment as well, using medicines that are broadly effective (i.e., able to treat multiple target symptoms concurrently) in the lowest effective dose and with careful monitoring for adverse effects is recommended. Specific treatments were described for the neuropsychiatric problems that most often result in inpatient psychiatric hospitalization, including depression, mania, PLC, anxiety disorders, apathy, psychosis, and agitated, aggressive, and self-injurious behaviors. The treatment literature is encouraging of the potential for these problems to respond to a combination of psychological, behavioral, environmental, and pharmacotherapies. Among patients in whom pharmacotherapy is not effective or tolerated, ECT remains a reasonable, effective, and generally safe treatment of severe and refractory neuropsychiatric disturbances among patients with ABI and DD.

REFERENCES

1. Costello H, Bouras N. Assessment of mental health problems in people with intellectual disabilities. *Isr J Psychiatry Relat Sci.* 2006;43(4): 241–251.

2. McAllister TW, Arciniegas D. Evaluation and treatment of postconcussive symptoms. *Neurorehabilitation.* 2002;17(4):265–283.

3. Lunsky Y, Bradley E. Developmental disability training in Canadian psychiatry residency programs. *Can J Psychiatry.* 2001;46(2): 138–143.

4. Lennox N, Chaplin R. The psychiatric care of people with intellectual disabilities: The perceptions of trainee psychiatrists and

psychiatric medical officers. *Aust N Z J Psychiatry.* 1995;29(4):632–637.

5. Menolascino FJ, Fleisher MH. Training psychiatric residents in the diagnosis and treatment of mental illness in mentally retarded persons. *Hosp Community Psychiatry.* 1992;43(5):500–503.

6. Reinblatt SP, Rifkin A, Castellanos FX, et al. General psychiatry residents' perceptions of specialized training in the field of mental retardation. *Psychiatr Serv.* 2004;55(3):312–314.

7. Trestman RL, Sevarino KA, Kelly M. Management of psychiatric issues in patients with intellectual disability. *Conn Med.* 2004;68(8):495–498.

8. Gitlin DF, Schindler BA, Stern TA, et al. Recommended guidelines for consultation-liaison psychiatric training in psychiatry residency programs. A report from the Academy of Psychosomatic Medicine Task Force on Psychiatric Resident Training in Consultation-Liaison Psychiatry. *Psychosomatics.* 1996;37(1):3–11.

9. Arciniegas DB, Kaufer DI. Core curriculum for training in behavioral neurology and neuropsychiatry. *J Neuropsychiatry Clin Neurosci.* 2006;18(1):6–13.

10. Palmer FB, Percy AK, Tivnan P, et al. Certification in neurodevelopmental disabilities: The development of a new subspecialty and results of the initial examinations. *Ment Retard Dev Disabil Res Rev.* 2003;9(2):128–131.

11. Hirtz D, Thurman DJ, Gwinn-Hardy K, et al. How common are the "common" neurologic disorders? *Neurology.* 2007;68(5):326–337.

12. NIH Consensus Development Panel. Consensus conference. Rehabilitation of persons with traumatic brain injury. NIH Consensus Development Panel on rehabilitation of persons with traumatic brain injury. *JAMA.* 1999;282(10):974–983.

13. Max JE, Sharma A, Qurashi MI. Traumatic brain injury in a child psychiatry inpatient population: A controlled study. *J Am Acad Child Adolesc Psychiatry.* 1997;36(11):1595–1601.

14. Deb S. Almost half of people suffering traumatic brain injury may later be diagnosed with axis I disorders. *Evid Based Ment Health.* 2003;6(2):59.

15. Hibbard MR, Uysal S, Kepler K, et al. Axis I psychopathology in individuals with traumatic brain injury. *J Head Trauma Rehabil.* 1998;13(4):24–39.

16. Koponen S, Taiminen T, Portin R, et al. Axis I and II psychiatric disorders after traumatic brain injury: A 30-year follow-up study. *Am J Psychiatry.* 2002;159(8):1315–1321.

17. Linaker OM, Nitter R. Psychopathology in institutionalised mentally retarded adults. *Br J Psychiatry.* 1990;156:522–525.

18. Mandell DS, Cao J, Ittenbach R, et al. Medicaid expenditures for children with autistic spectrum disorders: 1994 to 1999. *J Autism Dev Disord.* 2006;36(4):475–485.

19. Sevin JA, Bowers-Stephens C, Crafton CG. Psychiatric disorders in adolescents with developmental disabilities: longitudinal data on diagnostic disagreement in 150 clients. *Child Psychiatry Hum Dev.* 2003;34(2):147–163.

20. Silver JM, McAllister TW, Yudofsky SC. *Textbook of traumatic brain injury.* Washington, DC: American Psychiatric Publishing; 2004.

21. Zasler ND, Katz DI, Zafonte RD. *Brain injury medicine: principles and practice.* New York: Demos Medical Publishing; 2007.

22. Brown I, Percy M. *A comprehensive guide to intellectual and developmental disabilities.* Baltimore: Brookes Publishing; 2007.

23. Administration on Developmental Disabilities (ADD). U.S. Department of Health & Human Services Administration for Children & Families, http://www.acf.hhs.gov/programs/add/ddact/DDA.html. 7-29-2005, 6-16-2007.

24. Silka VR, Hauser M. Psychiatric assessment of the person with mental retardation. *Psychiatr Ann.* 1997;27(3):162–169.

25. Stolker JJ, Koedoot PJ, Heerdink ER, et al. Psychotropic drug use in intellectually disabled group-home residents with behavioural problems. *Pharmacopsychiatry.* 2002;35(1):19–23.

26. Des Noyers HA. Psychiatric disorders in children and adolescents with mental retardation and developmental disabilities. *Curr Opin Pediatr.* 1996;8(4):361–365.

27. Baker BL, Heller TL, Blacher J, et al. Staff attitudes toward family involvement in residential treatment centers for children. *Psychiatr Serv.* 1995;46(1):60–65.

28. Strand M, Benzein E, Saveman BI. Violence in the care of adult persons with intellectual disabilities. *J Clin Nurs.* 2004;13(4):506–514.

29. McCartney JR, Campbell VA. Confirmed abuse cases in public residential facilities for persons with mental retardation: A multi-state study. *Ment Retard.* 1998;36(6):465–473.

30. Marchetti AG, McCartney JR. Abuse of persons with mental retardation: Characteristics of the abused, the abusers, and the informers. *Ment Retard.* 1990;28(6):367–371.

31. McCauley SR, Levin HS, Vanier M, et al. The neurobehavioural rating scale-revised: Sensitivity and validity in closed head injury assessment. *J Neurol Neurosurg Psychiatry.* 2001;71(5):643–651.

32. Overall JE, Gorham DR. The brief psychiatric rating scale. *Psychol Rep.* 1962;10:799–812.

33. Cummings JL, Mega M, Gray K, et al. The Neuropsychiatric Inventory: Comprehensive assessment of psychopathology in dementia. *Neurology.* 1994;44(12):2308–2314.

34. Kaufer DI, Cummings JL, Ketchel P, et al. Validation of the NPI-Q, a brief clinical form of the Neuropsychiatric Inventory. *J Neuropsychiatry Clin Neurosci.* 2000;12(2):233–239.

35. Wood S, Cummings JL, Hsu MA, et al. The use of the neuropsychiatric inventory in nursing home residents. Characterization and measurement. *Am J Geriatr Psychiatry*. 2000;8(1):75–83.

36. Hamilton M. Development of a rating scale for primary depressive illness. *Br J Soc Clin Psychol*. 1967;6:278–296.

37. Young RC, Biggs JT, Ziegler VE, et al. A rating scale for mania: Reliability, validity and sensitivity. *Br J Psychiatry*. 1978;133:429–435.

38. Silver JM, Yudofsky SC. The Overt Aggression Scale: Overview and guiding principles. *J Neuropsychiatry Clin Neurosci*. 1991;3(2):S22–S29.

39. Marin RS, Biedrzycki RC, Firinciogullari S. Reliability and validity of the Apathy Evaluation Scale. *Psychiatry Res*. 1991;38:143–162.

40. Arciniegas DB, Topkoff J, Silver JM. Neuropsychiatric aspects of traumatic brain injury. *Curr Treat Options Neurol*. 2000;2(2):167–186.

41. American Psychiatric Association. *Diagnostic and statistical manual of mental disorders*, 4th ed, Text revision. Washington, DC: American Psychiatric Association; 2000.

42. Huber B, Seidel M. Update on treatment of epilepsy in people with intellectual disabilities. *Curr Opin Psychiatry*. 2006;19(5):492–496.

43. Mayville EA, Matson JL. Assessment of seizures and related symptomatology in persons with mental retardation. *Behav Modif*. 2004;28(5):678–693.

44. Frey LC. Epidemiology of posttraumatic epilepsy: A critical review. *Epilepsia*. 2003;10(Suppl 44):11–17.

45. Paolicchi JM. The spectrum of nonepileptic events in children. *Epilepsia*. 2002;3(Suppl 43):60–64.

46. Hudak AM, Trivedi K, Harper CR, et al. Evaluation of seizure-like episodes in survivors of moderate and severe traumatic brain injury. *J Head Trauma Rehabil*. 2004;19(4):290–295.

47. Sleijfer S, Bannink M, Van Gool AR, et al. Side effects of interferon-alpha therapy. *Pharm World Sci*. 2005;27(6):423–431.

48. Onder G, Pellicciotti F, Gambassi G, et al. NSAID-related psychiatric adverse events: Who is at risk? *Drugs*. 2004;64(23):2619–2627.

49. Warrington TP, Bostwick JM. Psychiatric adverse effects of corticosteroids. *Mayo Clin Proc*. 2006;81(10):1361–1367.

50. Besag FM. Behavioural effects of the newer antiepileptic drugs: An update. *Expert Opin Drug Saf*. 2004;3(1):1–8.

51. Ketter TA, Post RM, Theodore WH. Positive and negative psychiatric effects of antiepileptic drugs in patients with seizure disorders. *Neurology*. 1999;53(2 Suppl 5):S53–S67.

52. Trimble MR. Anticonvulsant-induced psychiatric disorders. The role of forced normalisation. *Drug Saf*. 1996;15(3):159–166.

53. Smith VM. Paradoxical reactions to diazepam. *Gastrointest Endosc*. 1995;41(2):182–183.

54. Sobhan T, Munoz C, Ryan W. Agitation as a paradoxical effect of divalproex sodium: A case report. *J Neuropsychiatry Clin Neurosci*. 2001;13(4):528–530.

55. Dunn NR, Pearce GL, Shakir SA. Adverse effects associated with the use of donepezil in general practice in England. *J Psychopharmacol*. 2000;14(4):406–408.

56. Mendez MF, Doss RC, Taylor JL, et al. Depression in epilepsy. Relationship to seizures and anticonvulsant therapy. *J Nerv Ment Dis*. 1993;181(7):444–447.

57. Sachdev P. Drug-induced movement disorders in institutionalised adults with mental retardation: Clinical characteristics and risk factors. *Aust N Z J Psychiatry*. 1992;26(2):242–248.

58. Brasic JR, Barnett JY, Kowalik S, et al. Neurobehavioral assessment of children and adolescents attending a developmental disabilities clinic. *Psychol Rep*. 2004;95(3 Pt 2):1079–1086.

59. Ganesh S, Murti Rao JM, Cowie VA. Akathisia in neuroleptic medicated mentally handicapped subjects. *J Ment Defic Res*. 1989;33(Pt 4):323–329.

60. Folstein MF, Folstein SE, McHugh PR. Mini-mental state: a practical method for grading the cognitive state of patients for the clinician. *J Psychiatr Res*. 1975;12:189–198.

61. Dubois B, Slachevsky A, Litvan I, et al. The FAB: A frontal assessment battery at bedside. *Neurology*. 2000;55:1621–1626.

62. Battaglia A, Bianchini E, Carey JC. Diagnostic yield of the comprehensive assessment of developmental delay/mental retardation in an institute of child neuropsychiatry. *Am J Med Genet*. 1999;82(1):60–66.

63. McGillicuddy NB. A review of substance use research among those with mental retardation. *Ment Retard Dev Disabil Res Rev*. 2006;12(1):41–47.

64. Jorge RE, Starkstein SE, Arndt S, et al. Alcohol misuse and mood disorders following traumatic brain injury. *Arch Gen Psychiatry*. 2005;62(7):742–749.

65. Taggart L, McLaughlin D, Quinn B, et al. An exploration of substance misuse in people with intellectual disabilities. *J Intellect Disabil Res*. 2006;50(Pt 8):588–597.

66. Anfinson TJ, Kathol RG. Screening laboratory evaluation in psychiatric patients: A review. *Gen Hosp Psychiatry*. 1992;14:248–257.

67. Catalano G, Catalano MC, O'Dell KJ, et al. The utility of laboratory screening in medically ill patients with psychiatric symptoms. *Ann Clin Psychiatry*. 2001;13(3):135–140.

68. Fuchs T. Delusion syndromes in sensory impediment – overview and model presentation. *Fortschr Neurol Psychiatr*. 1993;61(8):257–266.

69. Jin C, Schachar R. Methylphenidate treatment of attention-deficit/hyperactivity disorder secondary to traumatic brain injury: A critical appraisal of treatment studies. *CNS Spectr.* 2004; 9(3):217–226.

70. Arciniegas DB, Harris SN, Brousseau KM. Psychosis following traumatic brain injury. *Int Rev Psychiatry.* 2003;15(4):328–340.

71. Ferrell RB, Wolinsky EJ, Kauffman CI, et al. Neuropsychiatric syndromes in adults with intellectual disability: Issues in assessment and treatment. *Curr Psychiatry Rep.* 2004;6(5): 380–390.

72. Borgaro S, Caples H, Prigatano GP. Non-pharmacological management of psychiatric disturbances after traumatic brain injury. *Int Rev Psychiatry.* 2003;15(4):371–379.

73. Judd D, Wilson SL. Psychotherapy with brain injury survivors: An investigation of the challenges encountered by clinicians and their modifications to therapeutic practice. *Brain Inj.* 2005;19(6):437–449.

74. Coetzer R. Psychotherapy following traumatic brain injury: Integrating theory and practice. *J Head Trauma Rehabil.* 2007;22(1):39–47.

75. Delmonico RL, Hanley-Petersen P, Englander J. Group psychotherapy for persons with traumatic brain injury: Management of frustration and substance abuse. *J Head Trauma Rehabil.* 1998; 13(6):10–22.

76. Prout HT, Nowak-Drabik KM. Psychotherapy with persons who have mental retardation: An evaluation of effectiveness. *Am J Ment Retard.* 2003;108(2):82–93.

77. Beail N. Psychoanalytic psychotherapy with men with intellectual disabilities: A preliminary outcome study. *Br J Med Psychol.* 1998; 71(Pt 1):1–11.

78. Pfadt A. Group psychotherapy with mentally retarded adults: Issues related to design, implementation, and evaluation. *Res Dev Disabil.* 1991;12(3):261–285.

79. Tiersky LA, Anselmi V, Johnston MV, et al. A trial of neuropsychologic rehabilitation in mild-spectrum traumatic brain injury. *Arch Phys Med Rehabil.* 2005;86(8):1565–1574.

80. Burg JS, Williams R, Burright RG, et al. Psychiatric treatment outcome following traumatic brain injury. *Brain Inj.* 2000;14(6): 513–533.

81. Lindsay WR, Howells L, Pitcaithly D. Cognitive therapy for depression with individuals with intellectual disabilities. *Br J Med Psychol.* 1993;66(Pt 2):135–141.

82. Hurley AD. Individual psychotherapy with mentally retarded individuals: A review and call for research. *Res Dev Disabil.* 1989;10(3): 261–275.

83. Alpert JE, Spillmann MK. Psychotherapeutic approaches to aggressive and violent patients. *Psychiatr Clin North Am.* 1997;20(2): 453–472.

84. Uomoto JM, Brockway JA. Anger management training for brain injured patients and their family members. *Arch Phys Med Rehabil.* 1992;73(7):674–679.

85. Rao V, Handel S, Vaishnavi S, et al. Psychiatric sequelae of traumatic brain injury: A case report. *Am J Psychiatry.* 2007;164(5):728–735.

86. Willner P, Brace N, Phillips J. Assessment of anger coping skills in individuals with intellectual disabilities. *J Intellect Disabil Res.* 2005; 49(Pt 5):329–339.

87. Leftoff S. Psychopathology in the light of brain injury: A case study. *J Clin Neuropsychol.* 1983;5(1):51–63.

88. Persinger MA. Personality changes following brain injury as a grief response to the loss of sense of self: Phenomenological themes as indices of local lability and neurocognitive structuring as psychotherapy. *Psychol Rep.* 1993; 72(3 Pt 2):1059–1068.

89. Block SH. Psychotherapy of the individual with brain injury. *Brain Inj.* 1987;1(2):203–206.

90. Roane HS, Lerman DC, Vorndran CM. Assessing reinforcers under progressive schedule requirements. *J Appl Behav Anal.* 2001;34(2):145–166.

91. Vollmer TR, Progar PR, Lalli JS, et al. Fixed-time schedules attenuate extinction-induced phenomena in the treatment of severe aberrant behavior. *J Appl Behav Anal.* 1998;31(4):529–542.

92. Alderfer BS, Arciniegas DB, Silver JM. Treatment of depression following traumatic brain injury. *J Head Trauma Rehabil.* 2005;20(6): 544–562.

93. Janowsky DS, Davis JM. Diagnosis and treatment of depression in patients with mental retardation. *Curr Psychiatry Rep.* 2005;7(6):421–428.

94. Verhoeven WM, Veendrik-Meekes MJ, Jacobs GA, et al. Citalopram in mentally retarded patients with depression: A long-term clinical investigation. *Eur Psychiatry.* 2001; 16(2):104–108.

95. Janowsky DS, Shetty M, Barnhill J, et al. Serotonergic antidepressant effects on aggressive, self-injurious and destructive/disruptive behaviours in intellectually disabled adults: A retrospective, open-label, naturalistic trial. *Int J Neuropsychopharmacol.* 2005;8(1):37–48.

96. Saran AS. Depression after minor closed head injury: Role of dexamethasone suppression test and antidepressants. *J Clin Exp Psychopathol Q Rev Psychiatry Neurol.* 1985;46(8):335–338.

97. Dinan TG, Mobayed M. Treatment resistance of depression after head injury: A preliminary study of amitriptyline response. *Acta Psychiatr Scand.* 1992;85(4):292–294.

98. Patel NC, Crismon ML, Rush AJ, et al. Practitioner versus medication-expert opinion on psychiatric pharmacotherapy of mentally retarded

patients with mental disorders. *Am J Health Syst Pharm*. 2001;58(19):1824–1829.

99. Davidson J. Seizures and bupropion: A review. *J Clin Psychiatry*. 1989;50(7):256–261.

100. Johnston JA, Lineberry CG, Ascher JA, et al. A 102-center prospective study of seizure in association with bupropion. *J Clin Psychiatry*. 1991;52(11):450–456.

101. Gualtieri CT, Evans RW. Stimulant treatment for the neurobehavioral sequelae of traumatic brain injury. *Brain Inj*. 1988;2(4):273–290.

102. Lee H, Kim SW, Kim JM, et al. Comparing effects of methylphenidate, sertraline and placebo on neuropsychiatric sequelae in patients with traumatic brain injury. *Hum Psychopharmacol*. 2005;20(2):97–104.

103. Masand P, Murray GB, Pickett P. Psychostimulants in post-stroke depression. *J Neuropsychiatry Clin Neurosci*. 1991;3(1):23–27.

104. Woods SW, Tesar GE, Murray GB, et al. Psychostimulant treatment of depressive disorders secondary to medical illness. *J Clin Psychiatry*. 1986;47(1):12–15.

105. Schweitzer I, Tuckwell V, Johnson G. A review of the use of augmentation therapy for the treatment of resistant depression: Implications for the clinician. *Aust N Z J Psychiatry*. 1997; 31(3):340–352.

106. Jorge RE, Robinson RG, Starkstein SE, et al. Secondary mania following traumatic brain injury. *Am J Psychiatry*. 1993;150(6):916–921.

107. Starkstein SE, Pearlson GD, Boston J, et al. Mania after brain injury. A controlled study of causative factors. *Arch Neurol*. 1987;44(10): 1069–1073.

108. Massagli TL. Neurobehavioral effects of phenytoin, carbamazepine, and valproic acid: Implications for use in traumatic brain injury. *Arch Phys Med Rehabil*. 1991;72(3):219–226.

109. Parmelee DX, O'Shanick GJ. Carbamazepine-lithium toxicity in brain-damaged adolescents. *Brain Inj*. 1988;2(4):305–308.

110. Stewart JT, Hemsath RH. Bipolar illness following traumatic brain injury: Treatment with lithium and carbamazepine. *J Clin Exp Psychopathol Q Rev Psychiatry Neurol*. 1988;49(2):74–75.

111. Starkstein SE, Mayberg HS, Berthier ML, et al. Mania after brain injury: Neuroradiological and metabolic findings. *Ann Neurol*. 1990;27(6): 652–659.

112. Bamrah JS, Johson J. Bipolar affective disorder following head injury. *Br J Psychiatry Suppl*. 1991;158:117–119.

113. Zwil AS, McAllister TW, Cohen I, et al. Ultra-rapid cycling bipolar affective disorder following a closed-head injury. *Brain Inj*. 1993;7(2):147–152.

114. Massey EW, Folger WN. Seizures activated by therapeutic levels of lithium carbonate. *South Med J*. 1984;77(9):1173–1175.

115. Arciniegas DB, Topkoff J. The neuropsychiatry of pathologic affect: An approach to evaluation and treatment. *Semin Clin Neuropsychiatry*. 2000;5(4):290–306.

116. Tateno A, Jorge RE, Robinson RG. Pathological laughing and crying following traumatic brain injury. *J Neuropsychiatry Clin Neurosci*. 2004;16(4):426–434.

117. Kim JS, Choi-Kwon S. Poststroke depression and emotional incontinence: Correlation with lesion location. *Neurology*. 2000;54(9):1805–1810.

118. Feinstein A, Feinstein K, Gray T, et al. Prevalence and neurobehavioral correlates of pathological laughing and crying in Multiple Sclerosis. *Arch Neurol*. 1997;54:1116–1121.

119. Wortzel HS, Anderson CA, Arciniegas DB. Treatment of pathologic laughing and crying. *Curr Treat Options Neurol*. 2007;9(5):371–380.

120. Schiffer RB, Herndon RM, Rudick RA. Treatment of pathological laughing and weeping with amitriptyline. *N Engl J Med*. 1985;312:1480–1482.

121. Andersen G, Vestergaard K, Riis JO. Citalopram for post-stroke pathological crying. *J Lancet*. 1993;342:837–839.

122. Robinson RG, Parikh RM, Lipsey JR, et al. Pathological laughing and crying following stroke: Validation of a measurement scale and a double-blind treatment study. *Am J Med Genet B Neuropsychiatr Genet*. 1993;150:286–293.

123. Marin RS, Fogel BS, Hawkins J, et al. Apathy: A treatable syndrome. *J Neuropsychiatry Clin Neurosci*. 1995;7(1):23–30.

124. McAllister TW. Apathy. *Semin Clin Neuropsychiatry*. 2000;5(4):275–282.

125. Cummings JL. Cholinesterase inhibitors: A new class of psychotropic compounds. *Am J Psychiatry*. 2000;157(1):4–15.

126. Wroblewski B, Glenn MB, Cornblatt R, et al. Protriptyline as an alternative stimulant medication in patients with brain injury: A series of case reports. *Brain Inj*. 1993;7(4):353–362.

127. Antonacci DJ, de Groot CM. Clozapine treatment in a population of adults with mental retardation. *J Clin Psychiatry*. 2000;61(1):22–25.

128. Reinhard DL, Whyte J, Sandel ME. Improved arousal and initiation following tricyclic antidepressant use in severe brain injury. *Arch Phys Med Rehabil*. 1996;77(1):80–83.

129. Arciniegas DB, Topkoff JL, Held K, et al. Psychosis due to neurologic conditions. *Curr Treat Options Neurol*. 2001;3(4):347–366.

130. Cowley A, Newton J, Sturmey P, et al. Psychiatric inpatient admissions of adults with intellectual disabilities: Predictive factors. *Am J Ment Retard*. 2005;110(3):216–225.

131. Michals ML, Crismon ML, Roberts S, et al. Clozapine response and adverse effects in nine brain-injured patients. *J Clin Psychopharmacol*. 1993;13(3):198–203.

132. Buzan RD, Dubovsky SL, Firestone D, et al. Use of clozapine in 10 mentally retarded adults. *J Neuropsychiatry Clin Neurosci.* 1998;10(1): 93–95.

133. Sajatovic M, Ramirez L. Clozapine therapy in patients with neurologic illness. *Int J Psychiatry Med.* 1995;25(4):331–344.

134. Shedlack KJ, Hennen J, Magee C, et al. Assessing the utility of atypical antipsychotic medication in adults with mild mental retardation and comorbid psychiatric disorders. *J Clin Psychiatry.* 2005;66(1):52–62.

135. Aman MG, Gharabawi GM. Treatment of behavior disorders in mental retardation: Report on transitioning to atypical antipsychotics, with an emphasis on risperidone. *J Clin Psychiatry.* 2004;65(9):1197–1210.

136. Janowsky DS, Barnhill LJ, Davis JM. Olanzapine for self-injurious, aggressive, and disruptive behaviors in intellectually disabled adults: A retrospective, open-label, naturalistic trial. *J Clin Psychiatry.* 2003;64(10):1258–1265.

137. Friedlander R, Lazar S, Klancnik J. Atypical antipsychotic use in treating adolescents and young adults with developmental disabilities. *Can J Psychiatry.* 2001;46(8):741–745.

138. Silver JM, Yudofsky SC. Aggressive disorders. In: Silver JM, Yudosfky SC, Hales RE, eds. *Neuropsychiatry of traumatic brain injury.* Washington, DC: American Psychiatric Press; 1994:313–353.

139. Pabis DJ, Stanislav SW. Pharmacotherapy of aggressive behavior. *Ann Pharmacother.* 1996; 30(3):278–287.

140. Fava M. Psychopharmacologic treatment of pathologic aggression. *Psychiatr Clin North Am.* 1997;20(2):427–451.

141. Mysiw WJ, Jackson RD, Corrigan JD. Amitriptyline for post-traumatic agitation. *Am J Phys Med Rehabil.* 1988;67(1):29–33.

142. Jackson RD, Corrigan JD, Arnett JA. Amitriptyline for agitation in head injury. *Arch Phys Med Rehabil.* 1985;66(3):180–181.

143. Szlabowicz JW, Stewart JT. Amitriptyline treatment of agitation associated with anoxic encephalopathy. *Arch Phys Med Rehabil.* 1990; 71(8):612–613.

144. Kant R, Smith-Seemiller L, Zeiler D. Treatment of aggression and irritability after head injury. *Brain Inj.* 1998;12(8):1–661.

145. Chatham-Showalter PE. Carbamazepine for combativeness in acute traumatic brain injury. *J Neuropsychiatry Clin Neurosci.* 1996;8(1):96–99.

146. Patterson JF. Carbamazepine for assaultive patients with organic brain disease. *Psychosomatics.* 1987;28(11):579–581.

147. Mattes JA. Comparative effectiveness of carbamazepine and propranolol for rage outbursts. *J Neuropsychiatry Clin Neurosci.* 1990; 2(2):159–164.

148. Geracioti TD Jr. Valproic acid treatment of episodic explosiveness related to brain injury. *J Clin Psychiatry.* 1994;55(9):416–417.

149. Giakas WJ, Seibyl JP, Mazure CM. Valproate in the treatment of temper outbursts. *J Clin Psychiatry.* 1990;51(12):525.

150. Mattes JA. Valproic acid for nonaffective aggression in the mentally retarded. *J Nerv Ment Dis.* 1992;180(9):601–602.

151. Horne M, Lindley SE. Divalproex sodium in the treatment of aggressive behavior and dysphoria in patients with organic brain syndromes. *J Clin Psychiatry.* 1995;56(9):430–431.

152. Wroblewski BA, Joseph AB, Kupfer J, et al. Effectiveness of valproic acid on destructive and aggressive behaviours in patients with acquired brain injury. *Brain Inj.* 1997;11(1):37–47.

153. Davanzo PA, King BH. Open trial lamotrigine in the treatment of self-injurious behavior in an adolescent with profound mental retardation. *J Child Adolesc Psychopharmacol.* 1996;6(4):273–279.

154. Bozikas V, Bascialla F, Yulis P, et al. Gabapentin for behavioral dyscontrol with mental retardation. *Am J Psychiatry.* 2001; 158(6):965–966.

155. Pachet A, Friesen S, Winkelaar D, et al. Beneficial behavioural effects of lamotrigine in traumatic brain injury. *Brain Inj.* 2003;17(8):715–722.

156. Childers MK, Holland D. Psychomotor agitation following gabapentin use in brain injury. *Brain Inj.* 1997;11(7):537–540.

157. Tallian KB, Nahata MC, Lo W, et al. Gabapentin associated with aggressive behavior in pediatric patients with seizures. *Epilepsia.* 1996;37(5):501–502.

158. Khurana DS, Riviello J, Helmers S, et al. Efficacy of gabapentin therapy in children with refractory partial seizures. *J Pediatr.* 1996;128(6):829–833.

159. Beran RG, Gibson RJ. Aggressive behaviour in intellectually challenged patients with epilepsy treated with lamotrigine. *Epilepsia.* 1998;39(3):280–282.

160. Hurtado B, Koepp MJ, Sander JW, et al. The impact of levetiracetam on challenging behavior. *Epilepsy Behav.* 2006;8(3):588–592.

161. Cohen SA, Underwood MT. The use of clozapine in a mentally retarded and aggressive population. *J Clin Psychiatry.* 1994;55(10):440–444.

162. Bellus SB, Stewart D, Vergo JG, et al. The use of lithium in the treatment of aggressive behaviours with two brain-injured individuals in a state psychiatric hospital. *Brain Inj.* 1996;10(11):849–860.

163. Glenn MB, Wroblewski B, Parziale J, et al. Lithium carbonate for aggressive behavior or affective instability in ten brain-injured patients. *Am J Phys Med Rehabil.* 1989;68(5):221–226.

164. Greendyke RM, Kanter DR, Schuster DB, et al. Propranolol treatment of assaultive patients with organic brain disease. A double-blind crossover, placebo-controlled study. *J Nerv Ment Dis.* 1986;174(5):290–294.

165. Silver JM, Yudofsky SC, Slater JA, et al. Propranolol treatment of chronically hospitalized aggressive inpatients. *J Neuropsychiatry Clin Neurosci.* 1999;11(3):328–335.

166. Brooke MM, Questad KA, Patterson DR, et al. Agitation and restlessness after closed head injury: A prospective study of 100 consecutive admissions. *Arch Phys Med Rehabil.* 1992;73(4): 320–323.

167. Alpert M, Allan ER, Citrome L, et al. A double-blind, placebo-controlled study of adjunctive nadolol in the management of violent psychiatric patients. *Psychopharmacol Bull.* 1990; 26(3):367–371.

168. Gualtieri CT. Buspirone: Neuropsychiatric effects. *J Head Trauma Rehabil.* 1991;6(1): 90–92.

169. Gualtieri CT. Buspirone for the behavior problems of patients with organic brain disorders. *J Clin Psychopharmacol.* 1991;11(4): 280–281.

170. Colella RF, Ratey JJ, Glaser AI. Paramenstrual aggression in mentally retarded adult ameliorated by buspirone. *Int J Psychiatry Med.* 1992; 22(4):351–356.

171. Ratey JJ, Leveroni CL, Miller AC, et al. Low-dose buspirone to treat agitation and maladaptive behavior in brain-injured patients: Two case reports. *J Clin Psychopharmacol.* 1992;12(5): 362–364.

172. Freinhar JP, Alvarez WA. Clonazepam treatment of organic brain syndromes in three elderly patients. *J Clin Psychiatry.* 1986;47(10): 525–526.

173. Mooney GF, Haas LJ. Effect of methylphenidate on brain injury-related anger. *Arch Phys Med Rehabil.* 1993;74(2):153–160.

174. Nickels JL, Schneider WN, Dombovy ML, et al. Clinical use of amantadine in brain injury rehabilitation. *Brain Inj.* 1994;8(8):709–718.

175. Chandler MC, Barnhill JL, Gualtieri CT. Amantadine for the agitated head-injury patient. *Brain Inj.* 1988;2(4):309–311.

176. Cutajar P, Wilson D. The use of ECT in intellectual disability. *J Intellect Disabil Res.* 1999; 43(Pt 5):421–427.

177. Thuppal M, Fink M. Electroconvulsive therapy and mental retardation. *J ECT.* 1999;15(2): 140–149.

178. Kant R, Bogyi AM, Carosella NW, et al. ECT as a therapeutic option in severe brain injury. *Convuls Ther.* 1995;11(1):45–50.

179. Kant R, Coffey CE, Bogyi AM. Safety and efficacy of ECT in patients with head injury: A case series. *J Neuropsychiatry Clin Neurosci.* 1999;11(1):32–37.

180. Ruedrich SL, Chu CC, Moore SL. ECT for major depression in a patient with acute brain trauma. *Am J Med Genet B Neuropsychiatr Genet.* 1983; 140(7):928–929.

181. Zwil AS, McAllister TW, Price TR. Safety and efficacy of ECT in depressed patients with organic brain disease: Review of a clinical experience. *Convuls Ther.* 1992;8(2):103–109.

182. Crow S, Meller W, Christenson G, et al. Use of ECT after brain injury. *Convuls Ther.* 1996; 12(2):113–116.

183. Clark AF, Davison K. Mania following head injury. A report of two cases and a review of the literature. *Br J Psychiatry Suppl.* 1987; 150(841):844.

184. Reinblatt SP, Rifkin A, Freeman J. The efficacy of ECT in adults with mental retardation experiencing psychiatric disorders. *J ECT.* 2004;20(4):208–212.

185. Little JD, McFarlane J, Ducharme HM. ECT use delayed in the presence of comorbid mental retardation: A review of clinical and ethical issues. *J ECT.* 2002;18(4):218–222.

186. Friedlander RI, Solomons K. ECT: Use in individuals with mental retardation. *J ECT.* 2002;18(1):38–42.

187. van Waarde JA, Stolker JJ, van der Mast RC. ECT in mental retardation: A review. *J ECT.* 2001;17(4):236–243.

188. Aziz M, Maixner DF, DeQuardo J, et al. ECT and mental retardation: A review and case reports. *J ECT.* 2001;17(2):149–152.

The Medically Ill or Pregnant Psychiatric Inpatient

JAMES J. AMOS, VICKI KIJEWSKI, AND ROGER KATHOL

T he goal of this chapter is to help general psychiatrists manage psychiatric inpatients who have active, severe general medical illnesses. The authors discuss delirium, a selected group of common medical illnesses, medical illness mimicry, bipolar disorder in pregnancy, and the medical psychiatry unit (MPU), which can be a valuable resource for addressing all of these issues.

Psychological Management of the Seriously Medically Ill Patient on the Psychiatric Unit

It is surprisingly easy for physicians to lose track of the psychological impact of severe general medical illness. For example, only recently was post-traumatic stress disorder recognized to be a common sequela of a stay in an intensive care unit.[1] Psychiatrists should assume, for each of their seriously ill patients on the psychiatric unit, that the general medical illness is a life crisis. Exactly how it is experienced of course varies from patient to patient. Factors influencing the impact include the patient's premorbid personality, the severity and nature of the patient's psychiatric illness, the patient's past experience of illness in general and personal or family experience of this sort of illness in particular, his or her knowledge and understanding of the current illness, the quality of the relationship with the doctor treating the illness, the acuity versus chronicity of the illness itself and its prognosis, the presence or absence of pain or other specific symptoms, and the nature of family and social support. Obviously in the case of pregnancy the "crisis" is of a somewhat different sort. Even with pregnancy, however, the "illness" is likely to cause major changes in the patient's life situation and to require psychological and family-system adaptation.

On the psychiatric unit, the psychiatrist should develop a formulation of the patient's experience and situation including these and other factors. In almost every case, the psychiatrist should devote a portion of each interview to discussing the patient's general medical illness and concerns, to allow the patient to bring these concerns into the conversation, and to improve the psychiatrist's understanding of the problems. "We're here to talk about your depression, Dr. Smith will be by later to talk about your cancer" is not an adequate approach to the care of the medically ill psychiatric inpatient. Work with the family and on the patient's discharge plan must include consideration of disability due to illness and the expected change in the patient's physical condition over time.

Nonpsychiatric physicians are likely to be involved with these patients during the psychiatric hospitalization, and finding ways to work with them collaboratively is another challenge for the psychiatric team. If possible, team meetings should at times include the nonpsychiatric physician (or other members of the medical treatment team), so that all members of the psychiatric team have the opportunity to familiarize themselves with the medical situation and to ask questions or make comments about it and so that the nonpsychiatric physician learns about the psychiatric situation. Nonetheless, often the psychiatrist has to explain general medical issues to nurses and nonmedical psychiatric staff and address their concerns about the illness and its management. The psychiatrist must be closely familiar with the treatment regimen, even if it is prescribed by others, to allow adequate monitoring for treatment-related side effects (including mental side effects) and drug interactions.

Delirium

Delirium is common in the medically ill.[2] It is a disturbance of consciousness that has an abrupt onset and is associated with fluctuating abnormalities in cognition, perception, emotions, and behavior. The disturbance often is not recognized by nonpsychiatric clinicians and sometimes missed by psychiatrists. Those suffering delirium are usually inpatients and, in this population, initial management goals are to control agitation and determine treatable medical causes.

Delirium is a sign of serious underlying systemic illness, and frequently, the afflicted patients need emergency treatment. It is often a harbinger of significant morbidity and mortality and frequently leads to increased in-hospital complications and length of stay.[3] Some patients with delirium have severe agitation that places them and those involved in their care at risk for physical injury.

Although the discussion focuses on the evaluation and management of delirium after it occurs, the reader should be aware of a growing trend to teach clinicians how to anticipate and prevent delirium. The Yale Delirium Prevention Trial was the first trial to show that delirium can be prevented.[4] The incidence of delirium was reduced from the expected 15% to just less than 10%. However, the severity and recurrence rate of delirium once it occurred were not affected. Interventions were targeted to specific risk factors, such as reality orientation for cognitive impairment, nonpharmacologic sleep enhancement for sleep deprivation, early mobilization for immobilization, vision and hearing aids, and volume repletion for dehydration.

Delirium most often has an acute onset, but some patients experience a prodrome of severe anxiety and autonomic instability. They may have poor short-term memory, display dependent behavior, or experience illusions; for example, an over-the-bed exercise bar may look like a gun. Later, they may become frankly disoriented and disorganized and have visual hallucinations. In most cases, the disorder lasts 1 to 2 weeks and resolves without residua. However, a few patients develop a chronic course or progress to dementia.

Fragmented sleep, sometimes with a complete reversal of the sleep–wake cycle, is common in delirium. Sundowning refers to deterioration of behavior marked by worsening agitation and disorientation late in the day, sometimes with frightening visual hallucinations and persecutory delusions. The affective, behavioral, and cognitive manifestations of delirium often mimic primary psychiatric disorders, including mood, psychotic, and anxiety syndromes. A major distinguishing feature of delirium is a fluctuating level of consciousness. Fluctuations in behavior often lead to conflicting reports by clinical staff about the status of the patient that, in themselves, are valuable clues to the diagnosis.

Disturbed psychomotor activity—increased or decreased—is also seen in delirium. Hyperactive or agitated patients quickly get the attention of clinicians because they climb out of bed, pull out their catheters and intravenous lines, and wander about the ward. Patients with hypoactive delirium often appear depressed because they are immobile and display a flat affect. However, when fully evaluated, they have the usual disorientation, inattentiveness, and perceptual disturbances diagnostic of delirium. Mortality seems to be higher in the hypoactive subtype relative to normal and hyperactive groups.[5]

Rating scales may aid in identifying delirium, of which in the authors' view the most promising is the Confusion Assessment Method (CAM).[6] Other rating scales can also be used as diagnostic aids and to assess response to pharmacologic treatment. The Delirium Rating Scale (DRS) and the Memorial Delirium Assessment Scale (MDAS) are examples.

There are many causes of delirium; often the disorder has multiple etiologies. Some causes of delirium are associated with irreversible central nervous system injury or death if they are not recognized and treated quickly. For example, Wernicke encephalopathy, the diagnosis of which commonly is missed, may lead to permanent memory impairment if not treated promptly with thiamine.[7] Patients with Wernicke encephalopathy are commonly slowed with flat affect and could be misdiagnosed as depressed if the clinician does not have a high index of suspicion, which should extend not just to alcoholics but to any patient who has had a substantially decreased nutritional intake.

The diagnostic workup of delirium includes the usual complete history and physical examination along with a mental status examination. The cognitive and physical examinations of the psychiatric inpatient are discussed in Chapters 4 and 5. A physical sign of particular importance is asterixis (or its inverse, multifocal myoclonus). As discussed in Chapter 5, finding this abnormality clinches the diagnosis of an organic mental state. A close review of the medication list is essential; prescribed medicines are the sole cause of delirium in as many as one third of cases, and they contribute to a multifactorial process in others.[8] Suggested laboratory and special test evaluation include electrolytes, urinalysis, brain imaging, and electroencephalogram (EEG). The EEG typically shows a pattern consistent with diffuse brain dysfunction, with slow wave activity except in nonalcohol withdrawal delirium. Faster β-wave activity is typical of alcohol withdrawal delirium. However, not every patient with delirium has an abnormal EEG, and it does not distinguish dementia from delirium.

According to a case–control study, delirium in psychiatric inpatients occurs significantly more frequently in those who are older, who have a history of cognitive impairment, and who are exposed to in-hospital lithium or anticholinergic medicines.[9] In this study, antipsychotic medicines were associated with delirium only at relatively high doses, and antidepressants and sedative hypnotics were not associated with delirium. These findings suggest that moderation in using anticholinergic and antipsychotic agents may help prevent delirium in psychiatric inpatients.

Because many psychiatric symptoms occur in delirium, it is generally unwise to diagnose a primary psychiatric disorder, such as major depression, when delirium is present. When the delirium resolves, these associated features may also disappear. Adding antidepressants or anxiolytics may further confuse the clinical picture by adding psychotropic side effects to an already overburdened brain.

Some specific considerations regarding delirium arise among psychiatric inpatients. Neuroleptic malignant syndrome (NMS) is caused by dopamine-blocking drugs (antipsychotic and antinausea agents) or the abrupt discontinuation of dopamine agonists. The syndrome features fever, extrapyramidal signs such as rigidity, and delirium. On the inpatient unit, any patient who becomes delirious while on an antipsychotic is a suspect for NMS. Stopping the neuroleptic and supportive measures—especially careful attention to hydration—are the mainstays of management. Antipsychotic agents should be held in patients who develop delirium while on them pending a diagnosis of the cause of the delirium. Unfortunately, measuring creatine kinase (CK) does not generally provide an answer to whether the delirium is due to NMS because the CK may rise in patients on neuroleptics who become febrile for other reasons.[10] Many clinicians use dopamine agonists, such as bromocriptine, and some use dantrolene, a muscle relaxant, in patients who do not respond to supportive measures and discontinuation of the dopamine blocker.[11] The utility of dantrolene is questionable. Electroconvulsive therapy (ECT) appears to be highly effective in the treatment of cases of NMS that do not respond to other measures.[12] NMS is discussed also in Chapter 4.

Serotonin syndrome is marked by tachycardia, fever, diarrhea and hyperactive bowel sounds, shivering, diaphoresis, myoclonus, hyperactive tendon jerks with clonus, and delirium, although not all of these phenomena are present in mild cases.[13] It is associated with increased serotonin levels and results from combinations of selective serotonin reuptake inhibitors (SSRIs) and monoamine oxidase inhibitors, other combinations of serotonergic agents, or the inhibition of hepatic enzymes degrading serotonergic drugs. The offending agents should be stopped, and supportive measures are the initial treatment; the use of the $5-HT_{2A}$ antagonist cyproheptadine can be considered.

The management of delirium begins with treatment of the underlying medical illness or removal of the offending toxin. Patients must be monitored closely to ensure safety. Protecting the patient may require restraints, although their use may increase agitation. However, improper use of restraints may lead to serious injuries, even death. Restraint is discussed more fully in Chapter 12.

In the authors' opinion and that of others,[2] the medicine of choice for the treatment of agitation in delirium is haloperidol. Numerous uncontrolled case studies show that it is effective in reducing the psychosis, disorganization, and psychomotor agitation. The choice of agent for agitation in general on the psychiatric unit is discussed further in Chapter 3. In general medical settings, intravenous haloperidol is often used, despite the lack of U.S. Food and Drug Administration (FDA) approval for this route of administration. Intravenous haloperidol is associated with cardiac side effects including hypotension, arrhythmias, and prolongation of the corrected QT (QTc) interval. Because it is most safely administered where telemetry is available, the use of intravenous haloperidol is generally inadvisable on the psychiatric unit.[14]

Dosing of haloperidol should be individualized based on the level of agitation. In general, a starting dose of 1 to 2 mg orally or intramuscularly every 2 to 4 hours is reasonable. Severely agitated patients may require much higher doses. Patients with cancer or acquired immunodeficiency syndrome (AIDS) may tolerate only lower doses combined with lorazepam. A starting dose of 3 mg of haloperidol followed by 0.5 to 1.0 mg of lorazepam has been recommended in these populations.[15]

Depression in the Cardiac Patient

Depression is the most common psychiatric disorder in patients with coronary artery disease. The point prevalence is estimated at approximately 15% to 20%, yet it is often undiagnosed and untreated. Patients with depression are about twice as likely to develop ischemic heart disease.[16] In those with preexisting coronary artery disease, the risk of death for patients with depression is three to four times higher than in those without depression. The association between depression and general medical illness is discussed further in Chapter 4.

The Sertraline Antidepressant Heart Attack Randomized Trial (SADHART), published in 2002, established the safety of sertraline and its efficacy in recurrent depression in patients with recent myocardial infarction (MI) or unstable angina when there are no other life-threatening medical conditions.[17] Other SSRIs are probably comparably efficacious, although they are likely all rarely cause bradycardia and presyncope as well. Some SSRIs, notably fluoxetine and fluvoxamine, can alter the effect of warfarin, as discussed further in subsequent text. Cognitive behavioral treatment of depression in this setting also is effective, although neither form of treatment can be counted on to reduce cardiac events or mortality.[18]

Although tricyclic antidepressants are not absolutely contraindicated in this population, they are often avoided. The Cardiac Arrhythmia Suppression Trial of the late 1980s and early 1990s demonstrated that antiarrhythmic drugs were unexpectedly linked to increased mortality rates in post-MI patients.[19] Tricyclic antidepressants are believed to be similar in effect to these antiarrhythmics because of their quinidine-like properties that have potential proarrhythmic effects. Ever since then, cautionary statements have been made against starting tricyclic antidepressants immediately in patients with ischemic heart disease. They also are associated with orthostatic hypotension and sinus tachycardia, which can increase myocardial oxygen demand.

The Patient with Hepatitis C

Hepatitis C virus infects >4 million Americans and is the leading cause of liver failure leading to transplantation. Patients with hepatitis C have high rates of psychiatric disorders even before treatment, including substance abuse, depression, and anxiety. Contrariwise, the rate of hepatitis C infection in the mentally ill, especially in injection drug abusers, is very high.[20] As discussed in Chapter 4, testing for hepatitis C should commonly be considered in psychiatric inpatients. The role of hepatitis C infection itself in causing cognitive and psychiatric symptoms is uncertain, but concurrent hepatitis C infection may be factor in aggravating the impairment in patients with AIDS.[21,22]

Currently, the only FDA-approved treatment for chronic hepatitis C infection is α-interferon, with or without ribavirin. This regimen is associated with a number of adverse neuropsychiatric side effects, especially depression, which affects roughly one third of those on interferon.[23] Other psychiatric side effects include cognitive impairment, personality changes, psychosis, delirium, and suicidality. Unstable mood and anxiety disorders are widely considered contraindications to interferon treatment.[24] Presumably this applies to most psychiatric inpatients, at least initially. Later, however, it appears to be possible to treat psychiatric patients with interferon without undue risk, as long as the patients receive appropriate concurrent psychiatric treatment. Probably psychiatric patients are substantially undertreated for this serious infectious disease, and part of the role of the psychiatrist is to ensure that hepatologists have the opportunity to provide the needed treatment.[20]

Depression due to interferon usually responds to standard doses of serotonergic agents.[23] A neurovegetative syndrome marked mainly by fatigue and anorexia may respond better to serotonin-norepinephrine reuptake inhibitors (SNRIs), bupropion, psychostimulants, or modafinil.[25]

End-Stage Renal Disease

More than 80,000 Americans develop end-stage renal disease (ESRD) each year; approximately half have diabetes mellitus. Depression and anxiety are common in this population, and depression has adverse effects on medical outcome.[26] Among the many issues relevant for inpatient psychiatrists treating these individuals is dosing of psychopharmacologic agents.

Most patients with ESRD tolerate ordinary doses of most psychotropic agents. However, the upper limit of the dosage range is often recommended to be two thirds of that for a patient without renal failure. Factors affecting drug metabolism in renal failure include abnormalities in hepatic metabolism, absorption, volume of distribution, and protein binding.[27,28] Even if drug levels are not abnormally high for pharmacokinetic reasons, patients are at risk of adverse mental side effects for pharmacodynamic reasons, that is, greater vulnerability to psychotoxicity. Dialysis almost completely removes hydrophilic medicines, such as lithium and gabapentin, but not lipophilic medicines, including most other psychotropic drugs.

Standard doses of most antidepressants are generally well tolerated. The doses of paroxetine and venlafaxine, however, should be lower by approximately half.[29] Because of the electrolyte imbalances that can occur in ESRD and because of its renally excreted active metabolites, bupropion is not a first-line choice in this population. In general, the dictum of "start low and go slow" should be followed.

Most patients on dialysis are on anticoagulants to maintain patency of shunts. As previously mentioned, SSRIs may alter metabolism of warfarin and its anticoagulant effect. Sertraline, citalopram, and escitalopram are relatively free of this risk. Information about the effect of antipsychotics on international normalized ratio (INR) is limited. Divalproex is strongly protein bound and displaces warfarin from protein binding, increasing the free fraction of warfarin and increasing the INR. Carbamazepine appears to increase metabolism of warfarin and has the opposite effect. In general, close monitoring of the INR when starting psychotropic drugs is advisable, starting with checking the INR 2 or 3 days after initiation.[30]

Lithium use in renal failure requires close communication with the patient's nephrologist. With reductions of the glomerular filtration rate, the dose of lithium must be reduced. Lithium is 100% dialyzed; patients on dialysis should get a single dose after each dialysis run. Because lithium is excreted completely through the renal route, the lack of renal clearance of the agent in the dialysis patient ensures that lithium serum levels remain constant. Starting low and making frequent check of serum levels during the initial week of treatment is recommended.[27,28]

Depression in the Cancer Patient

Depression often goes undetected and untreated by oncologists. The usual psychiatric concerns apply to the depressed cancer patient, including the need for suicide risk assessment.[31] Differentiating depressive hopelessness from a realistic understanding of the prognosis in advanced cancer requires considerable psychiatric skill. With experience, psychiatrists see that seriously and even terminally ill patients who lack a depressive cognitive bias often speak eagerly of what they are looking forward to in their lives. Although psychological treatment approaches are effective for depressive symptoms in cancer patients, evidence that either psychotherapy or pharmacotherapy is effective for syndromal depression is scant.[32,33] Combined approaches may be preferable.

Before instituting treatment for depression, the psychiatrist should consider whether the cancer patient is actually suffering from a hypoactive delirium, poorly controlled pain, fatigue, or the anorexia-cachexia syndrome.[34] The anorexia-cachexia syndrome is caused by gastrointestinal dysfunction, altered metabolism, cytokine production, hormone production by tumors, and anticancer treatments. Depression, eating disorder, and conditioned responses may contribute. Treatment includes parenteral or enteral hypercaloric feeding, cyproheptadine, ondansetron, megesetrol, melatonin, and dronabinol.

The SSRIs can be used for depression, including that associated with anorexia-cachexia syndrome.[31] Mirtazapine can be effective because of its propensity to combat anorexia, nausea, and weight loss. SSRIs and venlafaxine can both treat hot flashes associated with menopause after chemotherapy for breast cancer. Bupropion may not be an ideal choice because of its association with lowered seizure threshold, especially in those patients with brain cancers. Nortriptyline is the preferred tricyclic for treatment of comorbid depression and chronic pain caused by chemotherapy and surgery. The SNRI duloxetine is an alternative, although it is contraindicated in those with liver failure.

The psychostimulants, including methylphenidate, dextroamphetamine, and modafinil, may be effective for the more apathetic types of depression in late-stage cancer patients, although controlled-trial data are lacking.[35] They can promote energy, appetite, a sense of well-being, cognitive function often in a matter of hours or days—a definite boon for seriously or terminally ill patients.[31]

Management of Abnormal Illness Behavior (Medical Illness Mimicry)

Somatization was defined by Lipowski as "a tendency to experience and communicate somatic distress and symptoms unaccounted for by pathological findings, to attribute them to physical illness, and to seek medical help for them."[36] Somatization is associated with high economic costs due to medical tests and procedures, office visits, hospitalizations, and time lost from work or family.[37] Medically unexplained symptoms of bodily dysfunction and pain are common in primary care as well as in inpatient settings.[38] Patients with medically unexplained physical symptoms have high rates of depression and anxiety.[39] In some cases, anxiety and depression may be a reaction to bodily pain; in others, depression and anxiety may decrease the threshold for reporting pain and other bodily symptoms.

Treatment of somatization disorder, the most chronic and pervasive of the somatoform disorders, has been difficult, with limited clinical benefit from psychosocial or pharmacologic treatment. Cognitive behavioral therapy is associated with improvements in self-reported functioning and somatic symptoms and a decrease in health care costs in patients with somatization disorder.[40,41] The aims of cognitive behavioral therapy are to reduce physiologic arousal, enhance activity regulation, increase awareness of emotions, modify dysfunctional beliefs, enhance communication of thoughts and emotions, and reduce reinforcement of illness behavior. The inpatient psychiatrist should be aware that, once a diagnosis of somatization disorder is made on psychiatric grounds, simply recommending to primary care physicians that they examine patients with somatization disorder during regularly scheduled appointments while limiting additional diagnostic procedures and treatments is effective in reducing inappropriate medical care, with its attendant risks.[42]

Conversion disorder is another of the somatoform disorders. The essential feature is one or more symptoms that affect voluntary motor or sensory function and suggest a neurologic condition, but these symptoms are found not to be due to neurologic or musculoskeletal pathologies. Psychological factors are judged to be associated with the symptom because the symptom or deficit is exacerbated or initiated by conflicts or other stressors. Individuals with conversion disorder do not intentionally produce or feign their symptoms. Symptoms are often reinforced by social support from family and friends as well as by avoiding underlying emotional stress. The diagnosis of conversion disorder cannot be made until a thorough medical investigation has been performed to rule out a general medical condition or neurologic condition as the cause of the symptoms, but when properly made the diagnosis of conversion disorder is quite reliable.[43]

Once a diagnosis of conversion disorder is made, it is important to inform the patient that a full recovery is to be expected. Patients may believe that they have a particular medical or neurologic problem and often assume the "sick role" along with its privileged social status and rewards. A vicious cycle then develops as patients believe that they are sick and subsequently receive reinforcement of this belief through the attentions of others. A recent Cochrane Database Systematic Review could not uncover any evidence based on extant studies that psychosocial interventions alone are either beneficial or harmful.[44] That said, most practitioners believe that the plan of care should include either psychodynamic psychotherapy or cognitive behavioral therapy and in many cases physical therapy. Emphasis should be placed on the treatment of the symptoms and not the cause.

Ness (2007) described physical therapy management for conversion disorder in which unwanted behaviors such as paralysis, ataxia, or abnormal gait are ignored but not punished, and the desired behaviors such as normal gait or strength are rewarded. Part of the benefit of physical therapy is presumably that patients need to have a way to relinquish their symptoms without loss of self-esteem. Allowing the patient to experience the recovery as due to physical therapy and not requiring an acknowledgment of psychogenesis may be crucial to symptom reduction. The treatment team should remain positive and optimistic. Communication between team members and the patient's family members can help maintain reinforcement of normal movement behaviors.

Another group of patients with abnormal illness behavior patterns who may be admitted to psychiatric wards are those with factitious disorder. These patients show intentional production of either psychological or physical symptoms with the motivation of assuming the sick role, without prominent secondary gain for doing so. This last point makes the differentiation between factitious disorder and malingering, obviously a distinction that can at times be uncertain.

Gregory and Jindal suggested that the prevalence of this disorder among psychiatric inpatients may be higher than usually recognized.[45] In their case series, 6% of 100 psychiatric admissions merited a diagnosis of factitious disorder. Three of them alleged that they overdosed, but the accounts could not be confirmed. Most patients had other psychiatric disorders, notably depression and substance abuse along with borderline personality disorder. Although none of the patients had previously been given a diagnosis of factitious disorder, they had collected a variety of other diagnoses including schizoaffective disorder, bipolar disorder, and schizophrenia. Half of them had factitious physical symptoms as well.

Making a correct diagnosis of factitious disorder is the first step toward an effective intervention. Often the diagnosis is seen as pejorative and as impossible to prove beyond doubt; this attitude can delay identification of these patients and thereby expose them to iatrogenic harm. Inconsistencies between behavioral observations by ward staff and patient self-reports of medical and psychiatric symptoms can be helpful. For example, reports of hallucinations by a patient who does not seem to be responding to or particularly bothered by them can be a clue to lack of authenticity. Patients frequently are invested in a strictly biomedical treatment for their conditions and resist efforts at discharge.

Attempting to reframe the approach to patients with somatization and factitious disorders by emphasizing cognitive behavioral approaches over strictly biomedical treatments can be challenging, but in the long run will prevent harm from invasive procedures, avoid complicating things further with multiple medical specialist consultations, and reduce the obscuring of the underlying psychological issues. This reframing entails close communication amongst all members of the inpatient treatment team in order to avoid the splitting that the patients can engender.

Bipolar Disorder in the Pregnant Patient

The management of bipolar disorder during pregnancy is challenging.[46] Approximately half of women with bipolar disorder will relapse during pregnancy in the absence of continued pharmacotherapy. Relapse rates are higher after abrupt discontinuation of lithium, and postpartum recurrence of bipolar disorder is common. The prevalence of postpartum psychosis is 100-fold higher than the population rate of 0.05%. The high relapse rate and the evidence that maternal psychiatric illness is associated with increased risk for abnormal fetal development underline the need for effective clinical management of bipolar disorder during gestation. Updates on the complicated issues involved in medicating pregnant women and information for their own review can be found on the Internet, for example, at http://www.womensmentalhealth.org/.

Although lithium has been the mainstay of pharmacotherapy since the 1950s, it has been associated with a number of risks including Ebstein anomaly, a tricuspid valve malformation. Revised estimates of the risk have recently been published, indicating that it may be considerably lower than the 1 in 20,000 previously reported, perhaps 1 in 1,000.[27] Moreover, neurodevelopmental outcome data show a lack of adverse effects among prenatally exposed children compared with other mood stabilizers. Divalproex is known to be particularly teratogenic.[47] SSRIs also carry the risk of untoward fetal outcomes.[48] The risks of antipsychotics are incompletely known, but appear to be low.

However, numerous reports continue to surface about lithium use in late pregnancy, indicating neonatal complications such as cardiac dysfunction, low muscle tone, diabetes insipidus, hypothyroidism, hepatic abnormalities, and respiratory difficulties. A recent prospective study indicated that this may be related to lithium crossing the placenta and unrelated to maternal serum levels.[49] Guidelines for the use of lithium in late pregnancy based on these data include the following:

- Maintaining lithium concentrations at the minimum effective level for the patient
- Periodically monitoring of lithium levels during pregnancy, especially in late gestation
- Avoiding, if possible, treatments that tend to increase the risk for lithium toxicity, such as prescribing angiotensin-converting enzyme inhibitors, calcium channel blockers, nonsteroidal anti-inflammatory drugs, and diuretics as well as a sodium-restricted diet; and lowering the lithium dose and doing more frequent concentration monitoring if some conditions and treatments are not avoidable in for example, preeclampsia

- Suspending lithium administration 24 to 48 hours before scheduled caesarean section or induction, or at the onset of labor in spontaneous delivery
- Administering oral or intravenous fluids throughout labor and delivery, and checking maternal lithium concentration in the event of clinical evidence for toxicity
- Reinstituting lithium therapy as soon as the patient is medically stabilized after delivery

Medical Psychiatry Units for Patients with Serious Concurrent General Medical and Psychiatric Illnesses

One of the greatest challenges in treating patients with concurrent serious general medical and psychiatric illness is assuring that effective and coordinated intervention for both takes place from first day of hospitalization. For instance, many of the patients with psychiatric comorbidity associated with medical problems described in the foregoing sections become too complicated to manage on either psychiatric or general medical inpatient units. These patients, who account for 2% to 4% of admissions to general hospitals, consistently have worse clinical outcomes, longer lengths of stay, and discharges to more restrictive outpatient settings when treated using traditional sequential treatment techniques.[50] Some patients, such as those with delirium, even have documented higher mortality during hospitalization and postdischarge.

Traditional general hospital care forces these patients to be admitted to the "safest" clinical location, general medical or psychiatric. Medical units provide some psychosocial support but have little in the way of acute care psychiatric services. Psychiatry units can perform simple medical interventions, but are neither paid to complete medical evaluations by behavioral health payers nor accoutered to do so. Therefore, consultant physicians see patients with comorbid illness, make astute recommendations for clinical assessment and treatment, yet often fail to change patient outcomes because of barriers created by the referring unit's organization, geographic separation from needed discipline-specific capabilities, and lack of clinical expertise by nursing staff to follow through. As a result, psychotic or suicidal patients on medical units are restrained, observed through 24-hour shifts by nonpsychiatrically trained sitters, treated medically, and transferred to psychiatry when stable (sequential as opposed to concurrent, integrated care). Psychiatric patients needing acute general medical intervention remain at risk for adverse medical outcomes if they are placed on psychiatry units because of disruptive behavior since psychiatric nurses are not trained to intervene when potentially life-threatening health problems arise.

This is where MPUs could add value to outcomes for patients and reduce total cost for the health system. When correctly designed and accoutered, MPUs contain both medical and psychiatric safety features, are staffed by nursing personnel with combined general medical and psychiatric training and skills, use consolidated physical and mental health policies and procedures to assure safe and effective intervention, and are staffed by communicating and collaborating physicians from general medicine and psychiatry. These units are therefore able to provide psychiatric care to patients with significant general medical illness and vice versa.[50]

The MPUs that can bring the greatest value to patients are those capable of providing the highest level of general medical and psychiatric care, type IV units as they were previously called.[51] For instance, on the medical side, high-acuity capability may include use of central lines for parenteral nutrition, protective infectious isolation for tuberculosis, and peritoneal dialysis for renal failure. On the psychiatric side, it may include the ability to develop sophisticated behavior modification programs for patients with eating disorders, to administer intravenous haloperidol for delirium (see preceding text for caveats on the use of intravenous haloperidol), and to perform ECT. Because 5% of patients account for 50% of total health care costs[52] and most patients in MPUs are included among this population, the opportunity to maximize clinical outcomes and reduce cost of care is considerable. Traditional general medical and psychiatry units are unable to perform such cross-disciplinary functions, even when assisted by competent physician consultants. It is estimated that high-acuity MPUs in which patients with concurrent illness are proactively identified for admission and integrated care can shorten average lengths of stay by up to 4 days in complex patients and save an average of $6,000 per treated patient (unpublished data).

If the clinical capabilities of MPUs are as robust as described, one might ask why more are not in existence at the current time. Although many factors contribute, perhaps the most important and limiting one is that general medical and mental health/substance abuse services are reimbursed from segregated and competing physical health and mental health/substance abuse budgets. It takes careful attention to unit organization, bed licensure designation, clinical staff capabilities, and billing procedures to assure financial viability. Many hospitals have been unwilling to go to this trouble. The senior author of the present chapter, having received an increasing number of requests for assistance in setting up integrated inpatient programs, believes that only recently has there been an upsurge in the number of general hospitals interested in developing MPUs. The growth in interest stems from the recognition that hospitals are already spending far in excess of what it would cost to create an integrated unit in costs associated with constant observation and extended lengths of stay for complex comorbid patients hospitalized within a diagnosis-related group (DRG) system.

The severity of patients' medical illnesses affects their participation in psychiatric treatment. In order to support a psychiatric milieu and treatment program that includes group psychotherapy, occupational therapy, and activities therapy, the unit population needs to include patients appropriate for those interventions. Severely ill or bedridden patients may not be able to participate in all group activities offered, but a flexible group attitude can often adapt to patients' individual circumstances.[53] Coexisting medical illnesses often resolve or stabilize before accompanying psychiatric illnesses so that patients can participate in all group activities as their medical condition improves. This allows clinicians to provide comprehensive treatment, both medical and psychiatric, concurrently instead of sequentially. MPUs can help minimize transfers between services and interruptions in care.

Nursing staff need to be able to provide both medical and psychiatric interventions. Prioritizing care may be difficult from a nursing perspective. Psychiatric nursing interventions may be postponed, whereas tasks associated with medical care such as giving medications, bathing, toileting, and assessing patients' physical condition cannot be neglected. If there are many severely medically ill patients on the unit, patients who need primary psychiatric care may not receive their share of nursing time.

Careful planning is critical to establishing an MPU. What psychiatric treatment will be provided and by whom should be firmly established and agreed upon by all the stakeholders involved. Startup costs are high. Most units of this type have a small number of beds (usually ~12 to 14). The demand to fill them with demented and delirious patients can be an obstacle to developing self-sustained group psychotherapy treatment programs, as envisioned by some experts.[53] Efficient gatekeeping of admissions has been recommended to control this problem. However, having strict guidelines for admission gatekeeping by the medical director could be difficult to enforce in any hospital because of limited resources for management of violent, confused patients on open medical units or in the emergency room.

On the other hand, admitting a limited number of patients for brief lengths of stay with clearly defined preadmission goals for managing issues such as behavioral problems consequent to dementia and delirium can actually be a fiscally sound practice. Ensuring easy flow between the MPU and outpatient psychiatric treatment programs that span the continuum of care, including partial hospital programs and outpatient ECT, can also enhance the unit's viability.

Conclusions

The care of patients with concurrent serious general medical illness and psychiatric disorder is challenging. The problem is common, as discussed also in Chapter 4, and hospitals, psychiatrists, and psychiatric training programs should expect, plan for, and indeed welcome the opportunity to learn from and serve these complicated patients.

REFERENCES

1. Schelling G. Post-traumatic stress disorder in somatic disease: lessons from critically ill patients. *Prog Brain Res.* 2008;167:229–237.

2. Young J, Inouye SK. Delirium in older people. *Br Med J.* 2007;334(7598):842–846.

3. Siddiqi N, House AO, Holmes JD. Occurrence and outcome of delirium in medical in-patients:

A systematic literature review. *Age Ageing.* 2006;35(4):350–364.

4. Inouye SK, Bogardus ST Jr, Charpentier PA, et al. A multicomponent intervention to prevent delirium in hospitalized older patients. *N Engl J Med.* 1999;340(9):669–676.

5. Kiely DK, Jones RN, Bergmann MA, et al. Association between psychomotor activity delirium subtypes and mortality among newly admitted post-acute facility patients. *J Gerontol A Biol Sci Med Sci.* 2007;62(2):174–179.

6. Wei LA, Fearing MA, Sternberg EJ, et al. The confusion assessment method: A systematic review of current usage. *J Am Geriatr Soc.* 2008;56(5):823–830.

7. Sechi G, Serra A. Wernicke's encephalopathy: New clinical settings and recent advances in diagnosis and management. *Lancet Neurol.* 2007; 6(5):442–455.

8. Alagiakrishnan K, Wiens CA. An approach to drug induced delirium in the elderly. *Postgrad Med J.* 2004;80(945):388–393.

9. Patten SB, Williams JV, Petcu R, et al. Delirium in psychiatric inpatients: A case-control study. *Can J Psychiatry.* 2001;46(2):162–166.

10. O'Dwyer AM, Sheppard NP. The role of creatine kinase in the diagnosis of neuroleptic malignant syndrome. *Psychol Med.* 1993;23(2): 323–326.

11. Strawn JR, Keck PE Jr, Caroff SN. Neuroleptic malignant syndrome. *Am J Psychiatry.* 2007; 164(6):870–876.

12. Trollor JN, Sachdev PS. Electroconvulsive treatment of neuroleptic malignant syndrome: A review and report of cases. *Aust N Z J Psychiatry.* 1999;33(5):650–659.

13. Boyer EW, Shannon M. The serotonin syndrome. *N Engl J Med.* 2005;352(11):1112–1120.

14. Hassaballa HA, Balk RA. Torsade de pointes associated with the administration of intravenous haloperidol: A review of the literature and practical guidelines for use. *Expert Opin Drug Saf.* 2003;2(6):543–547.

15. Adams F, Fernandez F, Andersson BS. Emergency pharmacotherapy of delirium in the critically ill cancer patient. *Psychosomatics.* 1986; 27(Suppl 1):33–38.

16. Alspector SL, Shapiro PA. Heart disease. In: Levenson JL, ed. *Essentials of psychosomatic medicine,* 1st ed. Washington, DC: American Psychiatric Publishing; 2007:13–34.

17. Glassman AH, O'Connor CM, Califf RM, et al. Sertraline treatment of major depression in patients with acute MI or unstable angina. *JAMA.* 2002;288(6):701–709.

18. Writing Committee for the ENRICHD Investigators. Effects of treating depression and low perceived social support on clinical events after myocardial infarction: The Enhancing Recovery in Coronary Heart Disease Patients (ENRICHD)

randomized trial. *JAMA.* 2003;289(23): 3106–3116.

19. Roose SP, Glassman AH. Antidepressant choice in the patient with cardiac disease: Lessons from the Cardiac Arrhythmia Suppression Trial (CAST) studies. *J Clin Psychiatry.* 1994; 55(Suppl A):83–87; discussion 88–89, 98–100.

20. Loftis JM, Matthews AM, Hauser P. Psychiatric and substance use disorders in individuals with hepatitis C: Epidemiology and management. *Drugs.* 2006;66(2):155–174.

21. Reimer J, Backmund M, Haasen C. New psychiatric and psychological aspects of diagnosis and treatment of hepatitis C and relevance for opiate dependence. *Curr Opin Psychiatry.* 2005;18(6):678–683.

22. Hilsabeck RC, Castellon SA, Hinkin CH. Neuropsychological aspects of coinfection with HIV and hepatitis C virus. *Clin Infect Dis.* 2005; 41(s1):S38–S44.

23. Asnis GM, De La Garza R II. Interferon-induced depression in chronic hepatitis C: A review of its prevalence, risk factors, biology, and treatment approaches. *J Clin Gastroenterol.* 2006; 40(4):322–335.

24. Bini EJ. Singin' the blues: The downside of hepatitis C virus treatment. *Am J Gastroenterol.* 2007;102(11):2434–2436.

25. Raison CL, Demetrashvili M, Capuron L, et al. Neuropsychiatric adverse effects of interferon-alpha: Recognition and management. *CNS Drugs.* 2005;19(2):105–123.

26. Kimmel PL, Cukor D, Cohen SD, et al. Depression in end-stage renal disease patients: A critical review. *Adv Chronic Kidney Dis.* 2007; 14(4):328–334.

27. Cohen LM, Tessier EG, Germain MJ, et al. Update on psychotropic medication use in renal disease. *Psychosomatics.* 2004;45(1):34–48.

28. Wyszynski AA, Wyszynski B. The patient with kidney disease. In: Wyszynski AA, Wyszynski B, eds. *Manual of psychiatric care for the medically Ill,* 1st ed. Washington, DC: American Psychiatric Publishing; 2005:69–84.

29. Tossani E, Cassano P, Fava M. Depression and renal disease. *Semin Dial.* 2005;18(2):73–81.

30. Sayal KS, Duncan-McConnell DA, McConnell HW, et al. Psychotropic interactions with warfarin. *Acta Psychiatr Scand.* 2000;102(4): 250–255.

31. Miller K, Massie MJ. Depression and anxiety. *Cancer J.* 2006;12(5):388–397.

32. Akechi T, Okuyama T, Onishi J, et al. Psychotherapy for depression among incurable cancer patients. *Cochrane Database Syst Rev.* 2008;(2):CD005537.

33. Rodin G, Lloyd N, Katz M, et al. The treatment of depression in cancer patients: A systematic review. *Support Care Cancer.* 2007;15(2): 123–136.

34. Massie MJ, Greenberg DB. Oncology. In: Levenson JL, ed. *Essentials of psychosomatic medicine,* 1st ed. Washington, DC: American Psychiatric Publishing; 2007:109–132.

35. Orr K, Taylor D. Psychostimulants in the treatment of depression : A review of the evidence. *CNS Drugs.* 2007;21(3):239–257.

36. Lipowski ZJ. Somatization: The concept and its clinical application. *Am J Psychiatry.* 1988; 145(11):1358–1368.

37. Barsky AJ, Orav EJ, Bates DW. Somatization increases medical utilization and costs independent of psychiatric and medical comorbidity. *Arch Gen Psychiatry.* 2005;62(8):903–910.

38. Ovsiew F, Silver JM. Unexplained neuropsychiatric symptoms. In: Coffey CE, McAllister TW, Silver JM, eds. *Guide to neuropsychiatric therapeutics.* Philadelphia: Lippincott Williams & Wilkins; 2007:335–347.

39. Henningsen P, Zimmermann T, Sattel H. Medically unexplained physical symptoms, anxiety, and depression: A meta-analytic review. *Psychosom Med.* 2003;65(4):528–533.

40. Allen LA, Woolfolk RL, Escobar JI, et al. Cognitive-behavioral therapy for somatization disorder: A randomized controlled trial. *Arch Intern Med.* 2006;166(14):1512–1518.

41. Kroenke K, Swindle R. Cognitive-behavioral therapy for somatization and symptom syndromes: A critical review of controlled clinical trials. *Psychother Psychosom.* 2000;69(4):205–215.

42. Dickinson WP, Dickinson LM, deGruy FV, et al. A randomized clinical trial of a care recommendation letter intervention for somatization in primary care. *Ann Fam Med.* 2003;1(4):228–235.

43. Stone J, Smyth R, Carson A, et al. Systematic review of misdiagnosis of conversion symptoms and "hysteria". *Br Med J.* 2005;331(7523):989.

44. Ruddy R, House A. Psychosocial interventions for conversion disorder. *Cochrane Database Syst Rev.* 2005;(4):CD005331.

45. Gregory RJ, Jindal S. Factitious disorder on an inpatient psychiatry ward. *Am J Orthopsychiatry.* 2006;76(1):31–36.

46. Yonkers KA, Wisner KL, Stowe Z, et al. Management of bipolar disorder during pregnancy and the postpartum period. *Am J Psychiatry.* 2004;161(4):608–620.

47. Duncan S. Teratogenesis of sodium valproate. *Curr Opin Neurol.* 2007;20(2):175–180.

48. Oberlander TF, Warburton W, Misri S, et al. Neonatal outcomes after prenatal exposure to selective serotonin reuptake inhibitor antidepressants and maternal depression using population-based linked health data. *Arch Gen Psychiatry.* 2006;63(8):898–906.

49. Newport DJ, Viguera AC, Beach AJ, et al. Lithium placental passage and obstetrical outcome: Implications for clinical management during late pregnancy. *Am J Psychiatry.* 2005;162(11):2162–2170.

50. Kathol RG, Stoudemire A. Strategic integration of inpatient and outpatient medical-psychiatry services. In: Wise MG, Rundell JR, eds. *The American psychiatric publishing textbook of consultation-liaison psychiatry : psychiatry in the medically Ill,* 2nd ed. Washington, DC: American Psychiatric Publishing; 2002:871–887.

51. Kathol RG, Harsch HH, Hall RC, et al. Categorization of types of medical/psychiatry units based on level of acuity. *Psychosomatics.* 1992;33(4):376–386.

52. Kathol R, Saravay SM, Lobo A, et al. Epidemiologic trends and costs of fragmentation. *Med Clin North Am.* 2006;90(4):549–572.

53. Harsch HH, LeCann AF, Ciaccio S. Treatment in combined medical psychiatry units: An integrative model. *Psychosomatics.* 1989;30(3):312–317.

CHAPTER 19

Inpatient Treatment of Eating Disorders

WAYNE A. BOWERS, ARNOLD E. ANDERSEN, AND KAY EVANS

A lthough many patients with an eating disorder are successfully treated in an outpatient setting, hospital-based care by a skilled team remains the intervention of choice for those individuals who are very ill or who fail outpatient treatment. The literature has shown that inpatient care is an effective method to treat both the physical and psychological aspects of anorexia nervosa (AN).[1] The complex nature of eating disorders suggest a coordinated, interdisciplinary approach to treatment, focusing on the combined biological, social, behavioral, and psychological needs of the patient. A multidimensional perspective to the care of eating disorders[2-5] proposes that weight restoration achieved with a comprehensive treatment team is more enduring. Successful treatment has been described as a skillful blend of weight restoration, psychotherapy, psychoeducational interventions, medical management, and at times pharmacotherapy.[1,2,6]

However, inpatient treatment of eating disorders has dramatically changed in the last 15 years. The transformation of health care influenced by Health Maintenance Organization (HMO)s has moved treatment from "fee for service" to "managed care" with profound changes to inpatient treatment. Under pressure from managed care, the inpatient treatment of AN in the United States has "metamorphosed into management and stabilization of acute episodes."[7] The tight control of HMO on access to care has reduced cost and hospital length of stay (LOS). A review of a hospital program in the New York metropolitan area between 1984 and 1998 showed a dramatic decrease in the average LOS from approximately 150 to 24 days, as well as a decrease in patients' discharge weight from an average body mass index (BMI) of 19.3 to 17.7.[7] Bezold et al.[8] reported that the average LOS in a psychiatric hospital decreased 25% between 1988 and 1992. The pressure to reduce cost, the reduction in LOS for hospitalized patients and reduced insurance coverage affects the health of the patient, adversely influences long-term care and contributes to lower discharge weights and high remission rates.[9] In the 1970s patients stayed in the hospital longer, gained weight slower, and were less likely to be rehospitalized. Efforts to reduce time in hospital has also influenced an increased use of medications for the treatment of eating disorders especially among adolescents with AN even when no specific medication has been identified for the treatment of AN. An inpatient approach based on weight restoration, followed by diminishing intensity (partial hospital, then outpatient psychotherapy plus medication) when compared to limited intensity "usual treatment" resulted in a cost per year of life saved of $30,180. Efficient, cost-effective use of hospitalization is advocated as part of a successful treatment program for AN.[10]

The American Psychiatric Association (APA)[10] guidelines for the treatment of eating disorders offer specific and broad recommendations for evidence-based, current best practice treatment of eating disorders based on research studies and clinical consensus.[11] These guidelines detail the necessity of integrating nutritional rehabilitation, psychosocial treatments, medical procedures, and psychopharmacologic interventions along a treatment continuum. This continuum includes outpatient, intensive outpatient, partial hospitalization and full-day programming, residential, and inpatient care. The remainder of the chapter presents a prototype for inpatient hospitalization based on APA guidelines. Additionally, this chapter will focus on essential ingredients to good inpatient care as seen by patients and clinicians. Although the overall focus will be on inpatient care of eating disorders the ideas presented are basic to treatment of AN and bulimia nervosa.

The APA[11] guidelines suggest that each inpatient unit must determine how well they can meet these best practice standards. The APA recommends that inpatient units (practitioners in general) make a determination on initial level of care or change to a different level of care based on an overall assessment of the patient. This assessment needs to consider the patient's physical condition (particularly weight and cardiac status), psychology, behaviors, and social circumstances. Also the availability of the appropriate level of care (e.g., constraints of geography or insurance) must be considered. Determination for level of care must avoid basing the decision on a single or limited number of physical symptoms, such as weight alone. The guidelines also encourage hospitalization before a patient becomes medically unstable but to use the patient's general medical status to determine whether psychiatric or medical hospitalization is indicated.

Inpatient Treatment

The basic goals for the inpatient treatment of AN and bulimia nervosa are nutritional rehabilitation, psychosocial treatment, and if needed medical stabilization. Inpatient treatment is part of a continuum of care to restore healthy mental, physical, and social functioning. An inpatient program must achieve safe, prompt, and effective short-term improvement while preparing patients for transition to a less intense level of care. The conceptual model most appropriate for guiding the treatment of eating disorders emphasizes a multifactorial etiology. Because treatments logically grow out of assumptions of the nature of the disorder, the clearest possible description of known contributing factors is important for guiding effective treatment of eating disorders.

Admission to hospital for treatment of AN or bulimia nervosa remains a clinical decision based on multiple factors. Many of these factors interact with or potentiate each other. An initial goal of medical stabilization is intended to differentiate between symptoms produced by starvation or a chaotic binge and purge cycle, which will generally respond to simple nutritional rehabilitation versus those medical signs and symptoms that are either life threatening or atypical. For example, a very rapid weight loss of 25 lb may be medically more dangerous than a slower weight loss of 40 lb. Hypokalemia with an irregular but nonbradycardic heartbeat may be more medically serious than a gradually attained, very slow regular heart beat of 40. These distinctions require the clinician to thoroughly understand the adaptive responses of the body to an eating disorder. Many of the social behaviors and psychological symptoms attributed to the eating disorder may be due to the consequences of poor nutrition or chaotic eating and will normalize by restoration to a healthy body weight or a return to consistent adequate nutrition.

Medical indications for hospitalization among adult patients include an estimated healthy body weight below 85% of normal, a heart rate <40 bpm, blood pressure <90/60 mm Hg, glucose <60 mg per dL, potassium <3 mEq per L, and electrolyte imbalance. Consider hospitalization if an individual's temperature is <36.1°C (97.0°F), there is evidence of dehydration, hepatic, renal, or cardiovascular organ compromise requiring acute treatment. Also, consider hospitalization if there is poorly controlled diabetes. Along with the reasons mentioned in preceding text consider hospitalization for children and adolescents when weight <85% of estimated healthy body weight or acute weight decline with food refusal. Inpatient care needs to be initiated when the heart rate nears 40 bpm, there is orthostatic hypotension (with an increase in pulse of >20 bpm or a drop in blood pressure of >10 to 20 mm Hg per minute from supine to standing). Additional makers for hospitalization include blood pressure <80/50 mm Hg, hypokalemia, hypophosphatemia, or hypomagnesemia.

Other factors to assess when making a decision to hospitalize include a high level of suicide risk, suicidal intent, and suicide plan. Also, assess the individual's level of motivation to change. Hospitalization occurs when there is a need for supervision during and after all meals and in bathrooms; if there is uncontrolled vomiting or hemataemesis. Hospitalization needs to be considered if there is deterioration in any existing psychiatric disorder or severe co-occurring substance use disorder. Also, consider hospitalization if there are additional stressors interfering with the patient's ability to eat (e.g., significant psychosocial stressors or inadequate social supports). Additionally, an inpatient setting is important when the individuals weight is near that at which medical instability occurred in the past and/or there is severe disabling symptoms of bulimia that have not responded to outpatient treatment.

Hospitalization suggests that medical or psychological instability of the patient has occurred with an increased likelihood that outpatient or partial hospitalization has failed. The decision to hospitalize on a psychiatric versus a general medical or adolescent/pediatric unit depends on the patient's general medical status, the skills and abilities of local psychiatric and general medical staff, and the availability of suitable programs to care for the patient's general medical and psychiatric problems.[12] Even when admission has been primarily for medical stabilization, without changes in the psychological or environmental aspects of the disorder, there is a high probability those medical difficulties will return. The skilled management of inpatient care for patients with eating disorders is of paramount importance to the outcome of treatment. Because of the complex nature of treatment and consistency of goals and methods required to keep the focus of treatment, the best practice is inpatient care in a specialty eating disorder unit. A interdisciplinary team approach to treatment grows logically from a multifactorial concept of origin of the disorder. The interdisciplinary team provides patients with a consistent approach to a wide variety of their individual needs. The team focuses on the goal of changing illness behavior and thinking not only in the protected environment of the inpatient unit, but on an enduring basis after discharge. This interdisciplinary approach provides the patient with numerous opportunities to practice what they are learning and to receive consistent feedback in all parts of the therapeutic program. There is evidence to suggest that patients treated in specialized inpatient eating disorder units have better outcomes than patients treated in general inpatient settings where staff lacks expertise and experience in treating patients with eating disorders.[13]

The broad goals of inpatient care are weight restoration and initiation of treatment on the psychological and environmental factors that contribute to the maintenance of the disorder. Weight restoration (a vital but not exclusive goal), means restoration of a fully healthy body weight, with rebuilding of body and organ tissue as well as organ functioning. Restoration to a healthy body weight is a means, not an end, to comprehensive treatment. The conclusive work of treatment involves a fundamental and enduring change in overvalued ideas, dysfunctional family systems, and distorted beliefs concerning weight, shape, size, and appearance. Treatment is focused on decreasing the overinvestment in thinness as a means of dealing with crucial central issues in life, such as mood regulation, personal identity, or family stability.

Most patients and therapists agree that a healthy normal weight is an important condition for physical recovery. Clinicians place more importance on weight restoration and suggest it is important to psychological, emotional, and psychosocial well-being. Studies show that patients who do not attain a healthy normal weight are at a greater risk for relapse. There is no consensus on the question of what weight needs to be reached for recovery and clinicians have expressed different opinions on healthy normal, varying from a BMI of 18.5 to 19.5 or BMIs above 20. However, the establishment of a desired weight gain can be handled in different ways with the goal being a healthy normal weight. The three standards generally used are (a) the Metropolitan Life Tables[14] for patients aged 18 and older, (b) the nomograms devised by Frisch and McArthur[15] for achieving the weight necessary for return of periods in females and for adolescent girls, or (c) a BMI appropriate for age. A reasonable goal is the mid-range of the weight on the Metropolitan Life chart for a given height (with appropriate age correction and occasionally frame correction) or a BMI between 20 and 25. For female patients younger than age 18, with secondary amenorrhea, weights identified by Frisch and McArthur nomograms[15] for a 50% chance of return of menstrual cycles are suggested. It should be noted that the weight for return of periods is approximately 10 lb higher than the weight required to begin menstrual cycles during normal development. For patients younger than 14, 100% weight for height for age is used as the definition for 100% of expected weight in children and young adolescents, as available on the Internet at http://www.cdc.gov/growthcharts/.

Picking a number from a chart is not the whole answer, however. Some attention should be given to the weight at which the patient functioned well if she or he had a time of stable weight and height before the onset of illness. Establish a target weight and rates of weight gain at which normal menstruation and ovulation are restored or, in premenarchal girls, the weight at which normal physical and sexual development resumes. The average anorexic patient often begins dieting at 5% to 10% above the matched population ideal weight at the onset of dieting. There is a rationale for setting the goal weight of these patients at 5% to 15% above the "ideal" weight. Because many of these patients may, in fact, be biologically normal only when above the "ideal" in weight. However, few patients accept this reasoning and few clinicians practice individualization of weight goals within the normal range.

Where practical considerations dictate a short inpatient treatment period, moderate weight gain to 85% of normal may have to be accepted. In this case, close follow-up is required in a partial hospitalization program or the outpatient clinic. A goal weight range, rather than a single point, should be set so that patients can fluctuate comfortably within a 4 to 5 lb (1.4 kg) range. The weight goal is not firmly set when the patient comes into the hospital, but only after treatment has been under way for several weeks.

Nutritional Rehabilitation

Nutritional rehabilitation begins with the establishment of weight restoration goals. Along with restoration of weight is a goal to normalize eating patterns and to achieve normal perceptions of hunger and satiety. In the process of restoration the biological and psychological sequelae of malnutrition are diminished. The initial nutritional intake begins with 1,200 to 1,500 calories per day, according to the patient's admission weight, low in fat, salt, and lactose. Calories are increased by 500 every 4 to 5 days until a maximum of between 3,500 and 4,500 calories per day is achieved. The exact number will depend on the individual rate of weight gain, the height of the patient, and the presence of gastrointestinal discomfort. Once nutritional rehabilitation has been under way for several weeks, most calories can be prescribed in fairly dense form, including a moderate amount of fats and sweets. A safe continuing weight restoration averaging 3 lb a week in females, and 4 lb in males can be achieved without significant medical symptoms, except for occasional pedal edema, easily treated without diuretics by feet elevation, limitation of salt, and psychoeducation.

As restoration progresses it is important to help the patient cope with concerns about weight gain, body image changes, and to educate about the risks of eating disorders. Concurrent with restoration is helping the patient understand and cooperate with nutritional and physical rehabilitation, understanding and changing the behaviors and dysfunctional attitudes related to the eating disorder. Nutritional rehabilitation can improve interpersonal and social functioning, and lay the ground work to address comorbid psychopathology and psychological conflicts that reinforce or maintain eating disorder behaviors. During this phase of treatment, providing ongoing support to the family is critical.

The use of a treatment protocol that deals with all the specifics related to the management of the patient's weight restoration is vitally important. Members of the programs staff initially remain with patients for 24-hour support and supervision, until a normal eating pattern is established and comprehensive assessment of the patient's psychological and physical state has been obtained. Staff sits with patients at all meals and encourages them to eat. The emphasis is on psychological support and the use of the milieu for group encouragement. An empathic supervised weight restoration program using normal food in a milieu setting with group support, results in patients' beginning to eat three meals a day with only moderate anxiety within 24 hours. Food- and weight-related discussions are discouraged with an emphasis on self-understanding of the patient's feelings and thoughts.

During restoration help the patient limit physical activity and caloric expenditure according to food intake and fitness requirements. Monitor their vital signs, food and fluid intake/output, electrolytes, signs of fluid overload (e.g., presence of edema, rapid weight gain, congestive heart failure), or other evidence of a serious refeeding syndrome. Also, address gastrointestinal symptoms, particularly constipation, bloating, and abdominal pain. Provide cardiac monitoring, especially at night, for children and adolescents who are severely malnourished. Add vitamin and mineral supplements; for example, phosphorus supplementation may be particularly useful to prevent serum hypophosphatemia. Nasogastric feeding is a rare occurrence and is reserved for patients with extreme difficulty recognizing their illness, accepting the need for treatment, or tolerating guilt accompanying active eating even when done to sustain life.

Restoration encourages a wide variety of foods but diet foods are not allowed. On admission the dietitian takes a complete nutritional history from the patients and leads decisions about changes in dietary programs. Dietitians also play an essential role in relating to patients, families, and staff regarding restoration. However, they do not discuss treatment directly with the patient until weight is in the maintenance range. In conjunction with the dietitian a patient can name three specific foods to delete from their menu, but other than these three specific choices (i.e., artichoke, pork chops, scrambled eggs), they do not determine their foods. Vegetarianism is permitted only if part of an established religious or philosophical practice (for example, Seventh Day Adventist) preceding the eating disorder. Vegetarianism in eating disordered patients represents an early phase of their eating disorder. Direct or daily interaction between the dietitian and the patients is discouraged to reduce the potential for endless requests to change in menus.

With patients who binge and/or purge, healthy normal weight is determined and if needed restoration is begun to achieve and maintain healthy normal weight. Weights outside of healthy normal range may be a contributing factor to the bulimia nervosa. Additionally providing nutritional counseling can help the patient establish a pattern of eating regular, nonbinge meals, and increase the variety of foods eaten. A normal eating pattern can correct nutritional deficiencies, minimize food restriction, and encourage healthy exercise patterns.

Psychosocial Treatments

Although the initial emphasis of inpatient care is weight restoration and/or disrupting the chaotic binge-purge cycle, additional interventions especially psychoeducation and psychotherapy are provided once treatment has started. The goals of psychosocial interventions include reduction and, when possible, elimination of binge eating and purging, as well as understanding and cooperating with nutritional and physical rehabilitation. Treatment works to enhance motivation to cooperate in the restoration of healthy eating patterns and to participate in healthy nutrition. Psychotherapy of various theoretic models such as psychodynamic systems and cognitive behavioral therapies (CBTs) using individual, group, family, occupational, and recreational therapy formats can be implemented.[6] Also, an inpatient unit can be designed to support a specific theoretic perspective (i.e., cognitive therapy).

Beginning with and maintaining a psychotherapeutically informed relationship with the patient is critical. This includes being aware of the following: understanding deficits in sense of self, interpersonal and intrapsychic conflicts, cognitive and psychological development, as well as psychological defenses, and the complexity of family relationships. Therapy also focuses on the assessment and change in core dysfunctional thoughts, attitudes, motives, conflicts, and feelings related to the eating disorder. Additional goals are improvement of interpersonal and social functioning as well as, treating associated conditions, including deficits in mood, impulse regulation, self-esteem, and behavior. It is important to monitor how the patient reacts to and understands the therapy and if possible create a therapeutic plan that fits the patient's preferences. Complexity of family situation and relationships need to be assessed and if needed enlist family support and provide family counseling and therapy.

Increasing a patient's readiness and developing motivation to change is essential for a positive outcome. Developing a treatment to match the patient's motivation and readiness to change is critical. An empathic attitude on the part of the staff is highly valued by patients as a necessary condition for change in beliefs and behaviors related to an eating disorder. The growth process of patients is enhanced by skillful therapeutic use of the expression of empathy, creating and the understanding of psychological discrepancy, increasing individual self-efficacy, and meeting the patients where they are rather than battling with refusal to go along with treatment.

The APA guidelines[16] suggest the use of CBT to engage and create change in patients with an eating disorder. Because AN and bulimia nervosa share symptoms (overemphasis on body shape and weight as sources of self-esteem and identity, relentless drive for thinness, phobic fear of normal weight, rigid dietary habits), CBT seems well suited for the treatment of a heterogeneous mix of eating disorders during inpatient treatment when specifically directed at eating disorder symptoms, underlying maladaptive cognitions and working with relationship concerns.[17–20] CBT has been shown to be the most effective psychological method in the treatment of bulimia nervosa.[17] Although CBT can be effectively applied to treatment of AN, definitive demonstration of its effectiveness in AN has not yet been shown.[21]

A CBT conceptual model for eating disorders[22,23] proposes that an eating disorder is largely maintained by harmful beliefs that a patient holds about the self, the future, relationships, world, and the eating disorder. The self-destructive beliefs can take on a life of their own in which they develop a routine quality. The eating disorder symptoms act as precipitants and as responses to difficult life experiences, and the patient becomes consumed by negative beliefs about the self, the future, relationships, world, and the disorder. The model also posits that beliefs may be rigid and paralyzing, and prevent the patient from experimenting with different ways of thinking or behaving that could result in alternative ways of believing and interacting with the world. To change the belief system it must be tested through inquiry and experimentation. This can include looking at supporting and disconfirming evidence and setting up cognitive and behavioral experiments to determine whether anticipated outcomes will occur. The model and approach are especially important during inpatient treatment to overcome the difficulty in developing engagement with the patient during therapy.

A CBT individual therapy approach following Beck's model[24] with modifications specifically for an inpatient eating disorders unit is recommended.[19,25] Even patients who have difficulty with the more abstract concepts of cognitive therapy can benefit from the early behavioral components such as mood monitoring and problem solving. The cognitive model uses Socratic questioning and behavioral experiments to help patients understand that life does not occur in a vacuum. It focuses on the idea that interpersonal and intrapersonal factors contribute to the etiology and maintenance of the disorder. The cognitive model places a high value on developing alternate ways of seeing the world and coping with day-to-day events, as well as identifying and changing developmental templates, schemas, and core beliefs.[26–28]

A critical CBT intervention that helps patients engage in therapy and enhances motivation for change is Socratic questioning. Socratic questioning involves being empathic toward the experiences of the patient, as reflected in the acknowledgment of the possible function of the eating disorder symptoms and the recognition that changing behavior is a difficult task. Socratic questioning offers an encouraging framework so that patients can reach conclusions on their own concerning the origin of their symptoms or the pros and cons for change. The clinician's task consists of helping patients to find their own solutions and to make their own decisions to change. Clinicians can work to help patients to experience their changing behavior as fascinating and enjoyable. Statements (i.e., "just eat") imply that change is within the capacity of the patient and that failure to change signifies a deficiency for which they are being judged.

The core task of CBT is to create a therapeutic environment in which the patient is inspired to participate in this process of inquiry and experimentation. This cognitive model is highly adaptable and useful within an inpatient program. Therapists help patients understand and appreciate what has made change difficult by identifying factors that have prevented change from occurring. This may involve illustrating how the disorder is valued and serves many functions. Therapists provide the patient with the opportunity to see themselves through less critical eyes, which can cast the situation in a more acceptable light, and ultimately free them to experiment in a way that makes movement possible.[22,23]

A useful therapeutic approach is to encourage clients to engage in experimentation with feared situations and feelings. Repeated successful experimentation over time with opportunities to debrief and consolidate in a supportive environment can lead to increased self-acceptance, and confidence about being able to cope with difficult feelings in the future. The debriefing of experiments is extremely important and can help patients reformulate their beliefs simply by showing curiosity about whether the belief holds true when subjected to scrutiny and experimentation. The therapists' role is to use their experience and the patients' input to set up non-negotiable limits, and then assist the patient in making the best choices for themselves, given these constraints. Treatment non-negotiables (weight restoration, behavioral experiments) need to be clearly explained with a sound rationale in advance of their implementation and must be put into action respectfully and consistently. This emphasis on experimentation, Socratic questioning, and empathetic listening is the basic building block for CBT and all inpatient care.

Although this therapeutic model emphasizes changing beliefs it works to develop and places a high value on the articulate identification, expression, and understanding of emotions. Many times, "I feel fat" is the global and generic phrase for any dysphoria. Increased awareness, understanding, and expression of emotion are gradually achieved through the therapist's observation of inconsistencies, incongruities, and inappropriate emotional reactions from the patient's everyday events. Confirmation and reinforcement of emotions that are a genuine part of their past and present experience are essential. The patient is encouraged to express all emotions, especially "unacceptable" emotions. With the therapist serving as a model for expression of emotion, the patient can learn that open expression of emotions does not lead to rejection[29] or out-of-control behavior. There is a consistent emphasis on separating "I feel" from "I think" statements, for example, changing "I feel fat" to "When I experience being fat, I feel anxious and depressed and I see myself as out of control." Cognitive therapy helps the patient recognize and change the rigid standards employed to determine self-worth. The message communicated is that positive self-evaluation develops from success through mastery in small, step-wise increasingly challenging personal activities. Competence by way of reasonable standards (emphasizing adequacy, not perfection), as well as learning and accepting "in-betweens," are very important. Self-acceptance, despite personal shortcomings from unrealistic standards, is a fundamental goal for the psychotherapist working with a patient with an eating disorder. Individual therapy can also address the lack of trust in and the fear of feelings or expression of emotions.[29] This is accomplished by the therapist confirming genuine expressions of inner feelings, while assisting the patient to identify misconceptions or errors in their thinking. It is critical to progress slowly and let the patients learn to identify their affective states and in promoting acceptance of these feelings as there own.

Group psychotherapy based on cognitive-behavioral, interpersonal, psychodynamic, and/or supportive models can also influence beliefs and attitudes about restricting, bingeing, and purging and can help reduce the patient's sense of shame surrounding the disorder. Group therapy also provides effective peer-based feedback and support. As a basic approach, a blend of process orientation[30] and cognitive-behavioral principles[6,31] appear to be effective. Blending these two models gives the group latitude to deal with personal and interpersonal issues. Use of the curative factors of group[30] and cognitive therapy principles create a focus on cognitive and developmental aspects involved with eating disorders. The group can also influence the perceptions of the patients and permit the patients to assist in each other's recovery through confrontation of symptomatic behavior, self-disclosure of distorted ideas, and negative attitudes. Group work also helps patients understand how their cognitions influence their mood and consequent behaviors. Another healing factor is the ability of group members to easily identify in others the ramifications of their own eating disorder. As patients help each other identify and change negative cognitions, they also improve their own, often coming to resolution of their issues as reflected in others.

Family therapy is an important aspect of inpatient treatment. Family therapy is most effective with children and adolescents, particularly with illnesses lasting <3 years. Family therapy, especially with adolescents, has a primary focus on work with family communications and developmental issues.[32] Parents and siblings frequently exhibit a sense of hopelessness regarding the recovery of their family member, often intermixed with anger and anxiety. Families often have difficulty identifying feelings and expressing emotions and not infrequently there are family problems that are unspoken that impair open communication. Inpatient family therapy sessions are held on a regular basis with the patient, family members, and/or a significant other with content determined by the patient's concerns that have been pinpointed in the day-to-day treatment process. The focus of sessions is on the interactions between the patient and family and the resolution of the eating disorder. Additionally, families often need to be relieved of the belief that they could have prevented the illness, and that in fact this is an illness, not a personal or family failing.

A specific model for psychotherapeutic interventions with families for adolescent AN has recently been developed[33] incorporating elements of the Maudsley treatment program that have been found effective for adolescents patients with AN.[34] This protocol underscores the central role of parents as a resource in the treatment of adolescent patients with AN. Unlike more traditional family therapy models in which the patient is seen as having developed a problem in response to external or internal factors (e.g., genetic, physiologic, familial or sociocultural), the Maudsley approach focuses on how the family can effectively promote healthy eating behavior *per se*. This treatment emphasizes the parents' ability to help the adolescent overcome the "intrusion" of the AN in the adolescent's normal development. The main focus of treatment is the empowerment of the parents in order to succeed in restoring their starving child. It is only after the eating disorder has been successfully addressed that the parents will hand over the control of eating back to the adolescent. It is at this point that the family will begin to discuss other issues.

The theoretic underpinning of the Maudsley approach is the view that the adolescent is imbedded in the family, and that the parents are critical in the ultimate success in treatment. The eating disorder is seen to be interfering with regular adolescent development. Therefore, the parents should take an active role in their offspring's treatment while at the same time showing respect for the adolescent. This treatment pays close attention to adolescent development and guides the parents to assist their adolescent with developmental tasks once the eating disorders have been removed. In doing so, any meaningful work on other family conflicts or disagreements have to be deferred until the eating disorder is out of the way. In some cases, effective parental guidance may prevent the hospitalization of even very starved young adolescent patients.

Role of Medications in Treatment

ANOREXIA NERVOSA

Psychotropic medications are an adjunct to psychosocial interventions, not a sole or primary treatment for patients with AN. Antidepressants have been advocated for both AN and bulimia nervosa and may well have a role in treatment of comorbid depression in both.[35] Consider antidepressants to treat persistent depression or anxiety following weight restoration or if there is a documented preexisting depression. Selective serotonin reuptake inhibitors (SSRIs) have the most evidence for efficacy and the fewest difficulties with adverse effects. SSRIs may also be useful in patients with bulimic or obsessive compulsive symptoms. A suggested practice, however, has been to prescribe antidepressants only after patients' body weights are normal, their eating patterns are normal, and after they have had experience with intensive psychotherapy. After these three goals have been achieved, if the patient still meets criteria for major depressive illness, then antidepressants are prescribed. However, SSRIs are not seen to be effective in severely underweight patients.[36]

Bupropion should be avoided in patients with eating disorders because of increased risk of seizures. Tricyclic antidepressants (TCAs) and monoamine oxidase inhibitors (MAOIs) should be avoided in underweight patients due to their potential lethality and toxicity in overdose situations. Clinicians should attend to the black box warnings in the package inserts relating to antidepressants and discuss the potential benefits and risks of treatment with patients and families if such medications are to be prescribed. Whenever possible, defer making decisions about medications until after weight has been restored. Malnourished, depressed patients are more prone to side effects. Cardiovascular consultation may be helpful if there is concern about potential cardiovascular effects of a medication. The use of medicines to stimulate appetite is generally unhelpful and counterproductive.

Consider second-generation and low-potency antipsychotics for selected patients with severe symptoms. Evidence from controlled trials is limited. Clinical impression suggests that these agents may be useful for patients with severe unremitting resistance to gaining weight, severe obsessional thinking, and denial that approaches delusional proportions. If these agents are used, monitor for side effects, including laboratory abnormalities.

BULIMIA NERVOSA

Antidepressant medication has been shown to reduce the frequency of binge eating and vomiting, reduce associated symptoms (e.g., depression, anxiety, obsessions, impulsivity), and prevent relapse. The combination of psychotherapy and medication may be superior to either modality alone. Various antidepressants may have to be tried sequentially to achieve optimum effect. Clinicians should attend to the black box warnings in the package inserts relating to antidepressants and discuss the potential benefits and risks of treatment with patients and families if such medications are to be prescribed.

SSRIs have the most evidence for efficacy and the fewest difficulties with adverse effects. This class of medication can be helpful for the concurrent depression, anxiety, obsessions, and certain impulse disorder symptoms. Additionally, SSRIs can assist those patients with a suboptimal response to appropriate psychosocial therapy. Fluoxetine is the only medication currently approved by the U.S. Food and Drug Administration (FDA) for bulimia nervosa. Dosages may need to be higher than those used to treat depression (e.g., 60 to 80 mg per day of fluoxetine). Typical side effects include insomnia, nausea, asthenia, sexual side effects. TCAs and MAOIs should generally be avoided, due to potential lethality and toxicity in overdose situations and avoided for patients with chaotic binge eating and purging. Bupropion is contraindicated in patients with bulimia because of increased seizure risk. For patients who require a mood-stabilizing medication (e.g., for co-occurring bipolar disorder), choose an agent that is most compatible with the patient's preferences and disordered behaviors. Weight gain associated with lithium and valproic acid can distress patients with eating disorders and result in nonadherence. Levels of lithium carbonate can shift markedly with rapid volume changes that accompany bingeing and purging.

Inpatient Programming

Inpatient programs involve patients in some form of treatment throughout the day. A sample detailed weekly schedule is displayed in Table 19.1. Typical interventions conducted on an inpatient setting include a psychoeducational group where patients learn basic therapy principles, the effects of starvation, and principles of healthy social and psychological functioning. Patients participate in an activities therapy group with content focusing on building leisure time skills. Occupational therapy groups concentrate on meal preparation with one session focusing on meal planning and the purchase of food. The second session focuses on meal preparation and consumption of the prepared meal followed by a structured group discussion of attitudes and emotions after the meal. Group and individual psychotherapeutic interventions focus on various life experiences that create specific distorted ideas regarding the self, the world, and the future as well as are learned developmental experiences (schemas), which can create vulnerability to and maintain an eating disorder. Another important intervention is a body perception group that focuses on helping patients understand their body distortions and how these distortions influence their lives and maintain the eating disorder. Meals and snacks are provided in the groups with a structured discussion time following the snack. Daily meals are followed by a structured observation with the opportunity for discussion following the meal. Structured observation is set up on a continuum with the most intense level being 24-hour continuous observation by the unit staff. As a patient progresses through treatment, the amount of time under staff observation is reduced (see Table 19.2).

The nature of an inpatient setting creates an excellent opportunity for an interdisciplinary team to provide the patient with a comprehensive treatment program. This team establishes a clear understanding of the unique and shared treatment goals of each discipline. To function smoothly the team must work closely together. Team meetings must occur at least twice a week to provide the patients with the structure they need in treatment. The team goal is changing illness behavior and thinking, not only in the protected environment of the inpatient unit, but on an enduring basis after discharge. A basic treatment team consists of a psychiatrist, psychologist, Advance Registered Nurse Practitioner (ARNP), primary nurse, social worker, occupational therapist, dietitian, and an activities therapist. This team works with the patient to understand his or her individual life history, including the conceptualization behind the eating disorder. Working in collaboration with the patient the team addresses a multifaceted set of problems that include self-esteem, body image, possible sexual abuse, addictions, family issues, marital relationships, parent–child relationships, and interpersonal dynamics. There is also a focus on coping skills for stress management, compulsive exercise, leisure time activities, nutrition and cooking, assertiveness, relaxation, mood, and perfectionism.

A comprehensive psychiatric evaluation is obtained by a detailed psychiatric interview. This time-honored process is supplemented by a standardized written assessment tool, such as the Eating Disorders Evaluation or Eating Disorders Inventory.[37,38] These assessment tools are designed to assess broad clinical features of an eating disorder especially attitudes and behaviors related to the illness. The psychiatric conceptualization consists of all the features of the case, including the summary of pertinent features, diagnosis and differential diagnosis, etiologic factors, treatment plans, and prognosis. Often, treatment of comorbid conditions is equally challenging as the primary eating disorder itself. Personality functioning and the presence of Axis I comorbid disorders such as depression and anxiety disorders are important to assess. Affective disorders are the most commonly associated Axis I comorbidity, present in 50% to 80% of eating disorders with bulimic symptomology, and a substantial number of anorexic patients, with many having secondary but severe depressions. Intellectual functioning warrants assessment because many patients have expectations for academic or vocational performance beyond their ability. Evidence of actual level of intellectual functioning may be sympathetically used to change these expectations and therefore modify some of the cognitive distortions arising from such misperceptions. In addition, significant neuropsychological deficits are present in approximately 35% of starved patients.

The Discharge Process

Aftercare planning begins as close as possible to the time of admission. Eating disorders severe enough to require inpatient treatment will require experienced long-term follow-up, preferably partial hospital

TABLE 19.1 DAILY PATIENT SCHEDULE

Sunday	Monday	Tuesday	Wednesday	Thursday	Friday	Saturday
8:15–9:00 AM Breakfast	8:00–8:45 AM Breakfast	8:00–8:45 AM Breakfast	8:00–8:45 AM Breakfast	8:00–8:45 AM Breakfast	8:00–8:45 AM Breakfast	8:00–8:45 AM Breakfast
—	8:45–9:30 AM Psychoeducation group	8:45–9:30 AM Psychoeducation group	8:45–10:00 AM Individual therapy	8:45–10:00 AM Individual therapy	8:45–9:30 AM Psychoeducation group	
9:30–10:00 AM Religious service	9:30–10:00 AM Activity	9:30–10:00 AM Activity	9:30–10:00 AM Activity	9:30–10:00 AM Activity	9:30–10:00 AM Activity	
—	10:30–11:45 AM School	10:30–11:45 AM School	10:30–11:45 AM School	10:30–11:45 AM School	10:30–11:45 AM School	
	If needed	If needed	If needed	If needed	If needed	
	10:30–10:45 AM	10:30–11:45 AM	10:30–11:45 AM	10:30–10:45 AM	10:30–10:45 AM	
	Individual therapy	O.T. meal Preparation/shopping	O.T. meal Preparation/shopping	Individual therapy	Individual therapy	
11:45–12:30 PM Lunch	11:45–12:30 PM Lunch	11:45–12:30 PM Lunch	11:45–12:30 PM Lunch	11:45–12:30 PM Lunch	11:45–12:30 PM Lunch	11:45–12:30 PM Lunch
	12:30–1:00 PM	12:30–1:00 PM		12:30–1:00 PM		
	O.T. meal plan Preparation	O.T. coping Skills group		O.T. coping Skills group		
	2:00–3:00 PM	1:30–3:00 PM	2:00–3:00 PM	2:00–3:00 PM	2:00–3:00 PM	
	Body perception group	Cognitive therapy group	Body perception group	Cognitive therapy group	Body perception group	
2:30–3:00 PM Snack	2:30–3:00 PM Snack	2:30–3:00 PM Snack	2:30–3:00 PM Snack	2:30–3:00 PM Snack	2:30–3:00 PM Snack	2:30–3:00 PM Snack
	3:00–3:45 PM Activity	3:00–3:45 PM Activity	3:00–3:45 PM Activity	3:00–3:45 PM Activity	3:00–3:45 PM Activity	
5:00–5:45 PM	5:00–5:45 PM	5:00–5:45 PM	5:00–5:45 PM	5:00–5:45 PM	5:00–5:45 PM	5:00–5:45 PM
Supper	Supper	Supper	Supper	Supper	Supper	Supper
—	7:00–8:00 PM Activity	7:00–8:00 PM Activity	7:00–8:00 PM Activity	7:00–8:00 PM Activity	7:00–8:00 PM Activity	—
			8:30–9:30 PM Psychoeducation group	8:30–9:30 PM Psychoeducation group		
8:30–9:00 PM Snack	8:30–9:00 PM Snack	8:30–9:00 PM Snack	8:30–9:00 PM Snack	8:30–9:00 PM Snack	8:30–9:00 PM Snack	8:30–9:00 PM Snack
11:30 PM	11:30 PM	11:30 PM	11:30 PM	11:30 PM	11:30 PM	11:30 PM
Bedtime	Bedtime	Bedtime	Bedtime	Bedtime	Bedtime	Bedtime
Adolescents	Adolescents	Adolescents	Adolescents	Adolescents	Adolescents	Adolescents

TABLE 19.2 EATING DISORDER OBSERVATION LEVELS (EDO)

Inpatient EDO
24-h observation; patient is under continuous observation by staff with bathroom locked

Standard EDO on admission
Standard EDO is from 8 AM until 10 PM for at least 1 wk after admission; patients attend all unit activities provided their physical and mental health permit

EDO + 2
Patient is observed for 2 h after each meal by the unit staff

EDO + 1
Patient is observed for 1 h after each meal by the unit staff

EDO meals only
Patient has not been under observation after meals by unit staff

Indications for changing observation levels
Unexplained weight fluctuations
Strong impulse to behave inappropriately
Abnormal of increase in serum amylase

followed by experienced outpatient treatment usually from one to several years. The characteristics of satisfactory aftercare include predischarge decision making concerning step-down to partial hospitalization versus outpatient treatment alone. Involving the aftercare team in the discharge process, transmitting information about the course of treatment, sharing both the philosophy and practice of treatment is critical. Patients returning to rural areas or to areas without experienced professional may soon worsen in their symptomatology. This is particularly true in view of the increasingly frequent problem of managed care driven discharge of patients before a chance to establish adequate weight, healthy patterns of behavior (eating and exercise) and decreased cognitive distortions. Data do not support the frequently practiced discharge of patients at very low weight, immediately after medical danger or self-harm danger have passed, but while still far short of a healthy body weight.

Readmission to hospital for treatment of relapse will generally be more effective and shorter if it occurs sooner rather than later. Prompt readmission should occur when the patient falls below 85% of target weight but a higher threshold may be appropriate. Additionally, maintenance of body weight in the metastable weight range of 85% to 90% of target without improvement after 6 months may also warrant readmission. Other proven reasons for admission to a hospital include return of severe depressive illness or serious medical complications of the eating disorder. A subgroup of patients may require repeated admissions. There is a tendency to blame patients for return to illness as if the eating disorder was entirely voluntary and some health professionals or families take a negative or punitive view toward patients with eating disorder requiring readmission. For those patients, a minority who do have a chronic, severe, and relapsing eating disorder, readmission is necessary whenever indicated by clinical symptomatology and should not be a source of stigma or rejection.

Necessary Ingredients for Inpatient Care

Most specialized inpatient programs for eating disorders use an integrated approach including medical, psychological, nursing, and social interventions. Being able to create flexibility during inpatient care implies that a program asks and listens to the needs of the patient. Developing goals is a blend of sound clinical management (medical care, nutritional rehabilitation, psychosocial interventions) and addressing the needs of the patient. From the perspective of the patient it is important to understand their needs although those needs may not always be met. What a patient experiences from the treatment team or a specific team member can influence how well they adjust to treatment. This is important as most patients who have inpatient care are generally reluctant at best or involved in treatment under some form of duress.

With patients' needs as a background, here are some considerations that patients and caregivers find very significant. Of primary importance is consuming a normal amount of calories on a daily basis, no bingeing, moving away from "feeling fat," increasing a positive body image, and acceptance of one's appearance. Additionally, shared goals work to reduce obsessions with food, increase comfort in intimate relationships, expression of emotions (verbal and nonverbal) and expression of one's opinions. Equally important is not punishing oneself after eating a meal, reduction in perfectionism, and reducing fears about failure.[39] In addition to the above-mentioned goals, patients suggest having self-esteem not dependent on weight, a realistic body image, the ability to handle negative emotions, and a reduction in personal and interpersonal isolation as important goals during inpatient treatment.[40]

Another necessary condition for excellent inpatient care is meeting the patient with care and consideration during treatment. Often those behaviors that contribute to the need to use a hospital setting (reluctance to see a problem, reticent to engage in treatment) are observed as problems or resistance to treatment. Being able to see the person behind the disorder and the development of a supportive and understanding environment based on empathy and listening reduce the concerns about change while in treatment. Patients want to experience involvement in their treatment and desire less emphasis on interventions focusing on control of eating problems and more on creating comfort with food and meals. Additionally, assisting in meal planning at some point during their care is extremely important.

In the same context, it is essential for therapists to listen carefully to their patients' expectations when planning and providing treatment. Treatment can be jeopardized when the expectations of patients and therapist diverge. Patients want a focus on understanding the illness and having more opportunities to engage in therapy on the unit. When patients perceived that the staff viewed them as individuals with unique needs rather than "just another anorexic coming through on a conveyer belt" there was greater desire and interest with being involved in treatment.

Playing an active role in treatment and a collaborative atmosphere is highly important to a positive outcome for inpatient care. A program that is collaborative and rewarding of improvement increases desire to engage and comply with treatment.[40,41] The establishment of a therapeutic milieu is very important to promote readiness for change. One important aspect for the patient is being with others who understand the disorder ("been there done that"), which lends support for those individuals creating an "I'm not alone" environment. Another important feature is a setting that does not have a primary focus on weight restoration but rather an emphasis on psychotherapeutic interventions that focus on insight, reflection, and altering the patient's belief system. Placing more emphasis on psychological well-being is seen by patients as important for their long-term recovery.

Patients report feeling helped and, at times, punished by the structure and restrictions of a program. A patient is often expected to follow the structured treatment protocol (with a package of rather inflexible components) rather than participating in the development of their inpatient treatment. This can lead to tension (resistance) to the development of change. Balancing necessary restrictions with flexibility is fundamental; otherwise patients feel punished rather than helped, which will lessen the chances of successful recovery.[40,41] Keep in mind programs "that do not claim to use behavioral contingencies are usually dealing with subtler reinforcement: Most inpatient programs include some type of behavioral or contingency management, implicit or explicit."[6] Patients report that empathy and being listened to by staff are extremely important in facilitating psychological interventions and change.[40]

What are the ingredients that help the patient create new perspectives or insight regarding a problem? Patients use such words as safety, acceptance, empathy, trust. In order to speak freely, a patient must feel free of worries of being judged or of being punished for honest reflections or reactions. This is sometimes difficult during inpatient care especially when what the patient has to say conflicts or contradicts the perspective of the treatment team. The therapist's role is to be a supportive trustworthy person who provides ongoing reality-based feedback. The purpose of the therapeutic relationship is not to bring about immediate change, but rather to help patients make the best decisions for themselves, given the options with which they are faced. With the exception of an immediate health risk and treatment non-negotiables the less the therapist pushes the patient to change now, the more likely it is that the patient will be able to make a sustained change over time.

Conclusion

When deciding about inpatient care there is no data to guide the choice of treatment setting (inpatient, day hospital, outpatient). There is a dearth of information about the important aspects of inpatient care and even less understanding about what are the important ingredients for change during inpatient treatment. Randomized trials are needed to test theory-based psychosocial and medical treatments but are lacking due to consensus about what theories of interventions are most important. Sharp decreases in length of hospital stay for patients with AN, prompted by changes in economics of health care have demonstrated a concurrent dramatic increase in readmission rates. All these factors create difficulty and confusion as to the best practice during inpatient treatment although hospitalization is advocated as part of an efficient, cost-effective treatment program for AN.[10] The challenge for the clinician is to meet the demand of equitably allocating service resources, ensuring that patients receive evidence-based treatments that work not only in the controlled context of randomized trials but also in the context of daily clinical practice. Additionally, an inpatient program that provides the right mix of care within given resources is an important public health goal.[42]

The goal for the future of inpatient care will be the development of an individualized care-map algorithm based on quantitative assessment of individual risk factors and strengths.[6] However, clinicians have not approached this point in time although work is on to create individualized care-maps. Additionally, better outcomes may not always require hospitalization but might be achieved in outpatient settings with comprehensive case management.

REFERENCES

1. Andersen AE, Bowers WA, Evans KK. Inpatient treatment of anorexia nervosa. In: Garner DM, Garfinkel PE, eds. *Handbook of treatment for eating disorders*, 2nd ed. New York: Guilford Press; 1997:327–353.
2. Andersen AE, Morse C, Santmyer K. Inpatient treatment of anorexia nervosa. In: Garner DM, Garfinkel PE, eds. *Handbook of psychotherapy for anorexia nervosa and bulimia*. New York: Guilford Press; 1985:311–343.
3. Andersen AE. Inpatient and outpatient treatment of anorexia nervosa. In: Brownell KD, Foreyt JP, eds. *Handbook of eating disorders: physiology, psychology, and treatment of obesity, anorexia and bulimia*. New York: Basic Books; 1986.
4. Garner DM, Garfinkel PE, Irvine MJ. Integration and sequencing of treatment approaches for eating disorders. *Psychother Psychosom*. 1986; 46:67–75.
5. Vandereycken W. Inpatient treatment of anorexia nervoas: Some research-guided changes. *J Psychiatr Res*. 1985;19:413–422.
6. Bowers WA, Andersen AE. Inpatient treatment of anorexia nervosa: Review and recommendations. *Harv Rev Psychiatry*. 1994;2:193–203.
7. Wiseman CV, Sunday SR, Klapper F, et al. Changing patterns of hospitalization in eating disorder patients. *Int J Eat Disord*. 2001;30(69-74).
8. Bezold H, MacDowell M, Kunkel R. Predicting psychiatric length of stay. *Adm Policy Ment Health*. 1996;23:407–423.
9. Howard WT, Evans KK, Quintero-Howard CV, et al. Predictors of success or failure of transition to day hospital treatment for inpatients with anorexia nervosa. *Am J Psychiatry*. 1999;156(11): 1697–1702.
10. Crowe S, Nyman JA. The cost effectiveness of anorexia nervosa treatment. *Int J Eat Disord*. 2004;35:155–160.
11. APA. Practice guidelines for the treatment of patients with eating disorders (revision). *Am J Psychiatry*. 2002;157(1 Suppl).
12. Maxmen JS, Siberfarb PM, Ferrell RB: Anorexia nervosa: Practical initial management in a general hospital. *JAMA*. 1974;229(801-803).
13. Palmer RL, Treasure J. Providing specialized services for anorexia nervosa. *Br J Psychiatry*. 1999;175:306–309.
14. Metropolitan Life Insurance Company. *Metropolitan height and weight tables*. New York: Metropolitan Life Insurace Company; 1983.
15. Frisch RE, McArthur JW. Menstrual cycles: Fatness as a determinant of minimum weight for heigh necessary for their maintenance or onset. *Science*. 1974;1985(949-951).
16. American Psychiatric Association. Practice guideline for the treatment with eating disorders. *Am J Psychiatry*. 2000;157(Suppl):1–39.
17. Fairburn CG. Eating disorders. In: Clark DM, Fairburn CG, eds. *Science and practice of cognitive behavior therapy*. New York: Oxford Press; 1997.
18. Eckert ED, Mitchell JE: An overview of the treatment of anorexia nervosa. *Psychiatr Med*. 1989;7(293–315).
19. Bowers WA.Cognitive therapy for eating disorders. In: Wright JH, Thase ME, Beck AT, et al. eds. *Cognitive therapy with inpatients: developing a cognitive milieu*. New York: Guilford Press; 1993.
20. Garfinkel PE, Garner DM. *Anorexia nervosa: A multidimensional perspective*. New York: Brunner/Mazel; 1982.
21. Fairburn CG. Evidence-based treatment of anorexia nervosa. *Int J Eat Disord*. 2005;37(S1): S26–S30.
22. Bowers WA. Cognitive model of eating disorders. *J Cogn Psychother: An Int Q*. 2001;15(331-340).

23. Geller J. Mechanisms of action in the process of change: Helping eating disorder clients make meaningful shifts in their lives. *Clin Child Psychol Psychiatr.* 2006; 11(225–237).
24. Beck AT, Rush AG, Shaw BF, et al. *Cognitive therapy of depression.* New York: Guilford Press; 1979.
25. Garner DM. Psychoeducational principles in treatment. In: Garner DM, Garfinkel PE, eds. *Handbook of treatment for eating disorders*, 2nd ed. New York: Guilford Press; 1997.
26. Freeman A. A psychosocial approach to conceptualizing schematic development for cognitive therapy. In: Kuehlwein KT, Rosen H, eds. *Cognitive therapies in action.* New York: Jossey Bass; 1993:54–87.
27. Garner DM, Vitousek KM, Pike KM. Cognitive-behavioral therapy for anorexa nervosa. In: Garner DM, Garfinkel PE, eds. *Handbook of psychotherapy for anorexia nervosa and bulimia.* New York: Guilford Press; 1997.
28. Beck JS. *Cognitive therapy: basics and beyond.* New York: Guildford Press; 1995.
29. Garner DM. Individual psychotherapy for anorexia nervosa. *J Psychiatr Res.* 1985;19:423–433.
30. Yalom I. *The theory and practice of group therapy*, 4th ed. New York: Basic Books; 1995.
31. Bowers WA. Cognitive-behavioral group therapy for specific problems and populations. In: White JR, Freeman AS, ed. *Eating disorders.* Washington, DC: American Psychological Association; 2000.
32. Dare C, Eisler I. Family therapy for anorexia nervosa. In: Garner DM, Garfinkel PE, eds. *Handbook of treatment for eating disorders.* New York: Guilford Press; 1997.
33. Lock J, Le Grange D, Agras WS, et al. *Treatment manual for anorexia nervosa: a family-based approach.* New York: Guilford Press; 2001.
34. Lock J, Le Grange D. Family-based treatment of eating disorders. *Int J Eat Disord.* 2005;37(S1): S64–S67.
35. Kaye WH, Weltzin TE, Bulik CM. An open trial of fluoxetine in patients with anorexia nervosa. *J Clin Psychiatry.* 1991;52(464-471).
36. Walsh BT, Kaplan AS, Attia E, et al. Fluoxetine after weight restoration in anorexia nervosa. *JAMA.* 2006;295(2605-2611).
37. Garner DM, Olmstead MP. *Manual for the eating attitudes test (EDI).* Odessa: Psychological Assessment Resources; 1993.
38. Fairburn CG, Cooper PJ. Binge eating: Nature, assessment and treatment. In: Fairburn CG, Wilson GT, eds. *The eating disorders examination*, 12th ed. New York: Guilford Press; 1993.
39. Noordenbos G, Seubring A. Criteria for recovery from eating disorders according to patients and therapists. *Eat Disord.* 2006;14:41–54.
40. Colton A, Pistrang N. Adolescents' experiences of inpatient treatment for anorexia nervosa. *Euro Eating Disord Rev* 2004;12(307–316).
41. Clinton D, Bjorck C, Sohlberg S, et al. Patient satisfaction with treatment in eating disorders: Cause for complacency or concern? *Euro Eating Disord Rev.* 2004;12:240–246.
42. Streigel-Moore RH. Health services research in anorexia nervosa. *Int J Eat Disord.* 2005;37(S1): S31–S34.

CHAPTER 20

The Child or Adolescent Psychiatric Inpatient

FLYNN O'MALLEY AND NORMA V. L. CLARKE

T his chapter focuses on inpatient treatment for the child or adolescent patient. The authors view acute hospital care and more extended hospital or residential treatment as having commonalties, but also significant differences in regard to history, setting, goals, and current practice. They are treated in separate sections.

Geller and Beibel reported that psychiatric, behavioral, and substance use disorders are now the leading cause of hospital admission in the 5- to 19-year-old age-groups,[1] and self-injury is increasing among adolescents.[2] Yet child and adolescent psychiatry is currently in a dynamic state, with much new information to integrate into the development of treatment modalities. For example, for some children no diagnosis fits ("diagnostically homeless"), and the children are difficult to manage in any setting.[3] Determining whether a young patient has bipolar disorder or some other variant of mood dysregulation remains disputatious.[4] Very often, inpatient treatment provides the safest and most appropriate setting to evaluate the complexities of the interactions of biological, psychological, and social factors as they contribute to serious childhood and adolescent psychiatric illnesses.

The Biopsychosocial Model

Issues in acute care and extended treatment converge in the biopsychosocial model. A comprehensive model ensures that all essential areas of functioning are addressed.[5,6] The biological view recognizes that a youngster may be vulnerable to certain kinds of disorders because of inherited characteristics or physical trauma or illness. Common heritable features include difficult temperament, learning disabilities, attention deficit and hyperactivity, certain developmental delays and disorders, psychosis, mood disorders and emotional reactivity, and substance abuse. Patients who have a family history of mood disorder or substance abuse are not necessarily destined to manifest such disorders, but they may be more genetically predisposed than other youngsters to developing such problems under certain environmental circumstances. A patient with a schizoaffective disorder can be made aware of the potential for problems with thinking and affect management, begin to take responsibility for monitoring changes in thinking and moods, and develop plans for minimizing the effects of the illness. Similarly, patients with learning disabilities and developmental disorders, for example, Asperger syndrome, can be helped to understand and accept their vulnerabilities and limitations, and then develop coping and compensatory mechanisms for managing their problems. This approach allows patients to feel less guilt and shame and to acquire a greater sense of control over their lives. Another aspect of the biological view is a respect for the role of psychotropic medication in providing relief from the severity and frequency of many symptoms and allowing for greater accessibility to treatment. Child and adolescent patients are capable of learning that medications do not usually "cure" problems, but, rather, aid in helping patients manage their symptoms and vulnerabilities.

The psychological point of view recognizes that young people have a personal history and that some events and experiences may have affected them profoundly. Various forms of trauma including emotional, physical, and sexual abuse are common, and they vary in their intensity and the degree they have been repeated. Many youngsters have experienced developmental difficulties and academic failures. Others have become unhappy with their bodies and aspects of their personalities. Lack of peer acceptance and rejection in romantic relationships have an enormous impact on adolescents and are often the precipitants for self-destructive behavior. Divorce and the deaths of loved ones contribute to a young person's vulnerability to self-esteem problems and the development of attitudes of futility and despair. One's *interpretation* of experiences is also central to the development of psychiatric problems and also to their amelioration. How patients view themselves, the life events they have experienced, and their relationships with others are critical to a diagnostic understanding and treatment of the symptoms and problems they present.

Finally, the youngster's development occurs in a familial, cultural, and social context. This context may contribute resources and strengths along with challenges and difficulties. In addition, youngsters are likely to return to their environments, and even if they do not will certainly continue to be strongly influenced by their family and social origins. Achieving an understanding of the family system, including the extended family and multigenerational family patterns and events, is important in developing a sense of the context of the patient's problems. It is also crucial to engage the family members as participants in the diagnostic process and in accepting a sense of responsibility for successful outcome. A common challenge is how to create such a feeling of participation without stimulating an atmosphere of guilt and blame about past events and patterns of behavior. Creating defensiveness or self-hatred in parents invariably leads to self-protection rather than increased collaboration in problem solving.

The choice of level of care depends on the goals of intervention. Does the child or adolescent need the shorter intervention of acute care, which aims at immediate safety, or the longer intervention of residential care, which aims at solving long-standing problems that have resisted outpatient and brief hospital treatment?

Acute care inpatient units tend to be general units, with multiple diagnostic categories treated on one unit. Residential inpatient units are likely to be more specialized, with specific units for eating disorders, trauma, post-traumatic stress disorder (PTSD), obsessive compulsive disorder (OCD), and personality disorders. Residential care has a long and rich history with much written and clinical experience to guide the design of residential hospitals and other forms of residential care. The case is less clear with acute inpatient care. No extensive clinical literature provides a model of how acute care units are best designed for the patients they serve. The acute care unit as it now exists has evolved in response to rapidly decreasing third-party payments. Over the last decade lengths of stay have fallen from an average of 12 days to an average of 4 days.[7] The changes have been driven by financial realities and not by clinical knowledge or design. The section on acute care will focus on how the authors think such a unit should best be designed and run in order to attain maximum treatment benefit.

Acute Inpatient Treatment

What constitutes a clinically well-designed acute care unit for children and adolescents? What treatment modalities should be included? What staff training constitutes the minimal level of competence for nursing staff on an acute care unit? What clinical phenomena or psychiatric disorders are best treated in acute care settings? What is the acceptable milieu on an acute care unit? In answering these questions, consideration needs to be given to one of the primary difficulties of acute care units: patients with all diagnoses are admitted to acute care unit. A typical acute care unit may have at any one time suicidal patients, sexual offenders, trauma victims, substance abusers, people with personality disorders, those with eating disorders, psychotic patients, aggressive and assaultive children, or foster care children needing placement—all on a single 15-bed or 20-bed unit. That multiple diagnoses are served on one unit require particular attention to admission criteria, staff skills training, and unit design and milieu.

A well-designed acute inpatient program at minimum provides the following: patient safety; diagnostic understanding of a case; family intervention; sustained contact with outpatient providers if appropriate; medication management; and treatment modalities aimed toward helping patients understand, on a developmentally appropriate level, the various contributions to their admission. Equally important, the acute care unit provides discharge planning such that the patient moves smoothly from the unit to the next appropriate level of care.

The acute care admission is considered part of a continuum of care: a brief inpatient intervention can serve to diagnose a new-onset illness, clarify the diagnosis in a patient who has decompensated, redirect the course of a patient's care, or stabilize a patient to prepare the return to outpatient care or to move on to longer-term residential treatment. Ionescu and Ruedrich proposed such a model for adults.[8] The unit is likely to serve best those mental illnesses that respond to medication and brief psychosocial interventions. The acute care unit will be less effective in those illnesses that require extensive psychosocial or behavioral interventions, for example, eating disorders, personality disorders, OCDs, and substance use disorders.

TYPES OF ADMISSIONS AND FOCUS OF TREATMENT

Appropriate clinical circumstances for admission to the acute care unit include (a) new-onset mood or psychotic illness with no prior treatment, (b) decompensation during adequate outpatient treatment, (c) decompensation with no outpatient treatment, and (d) decompensation rooted in social and environmental chaos.

First-episode admissions with no outpatient treatment require the most extensive evaluations and perhaps the most energetic work on finding outpatient clinicians. Here both stabilization and treatment are the goals. Detailed assessment of symptoms, developmental issues, and community and family issues is necessary in order to arrive at the correct diagnosis and treatment and to begin planning for discharge.

Case Vignette

A 17-year-old boy was admitted 2 days after his return from a school trip to Germany. In Germany he had begun to behave oddly. He closed all the curtains in his room and talked of people who were persecuting him. He would neither sleep nor eat. His parents flew to Germany to bring the boy home. In 2 days at home he worsened. He began pacing, stopped sleeping, and became angry and irritable. His parents became frightened and arranged his admission. Urine drug screen was negative, as were electroencephalogram (EEG) and magnetic resonance imaging (MRI). Oral haloperidol was started and in 4 days the patient was significantly calmer, although still psychotic as manifested by his many paranoid statements and his acknowledgment that he was still hallucinating. The patient was discharged and readmitted several times in response to managed care demands. Finally, the patient was readmitted and remained for over 2 weeks. With the longer stay it was possible to make a diagnosis of schizophreniform disorder. During the longer stay, an atypical antipsychotic was substituted for haloperidol, and divalproex and lithium were discontinued. The patient gradually stabilized. He was discharged significantly less psychotic than on admission. He was subsequently managed in outpatient care and not readmitted.

Management of the decompensation of a patient receiving outpatient treatment entails substantial communication with the outpatient clinicians in order to clarify the nature of the patient's difficulties. Understanding the reason for the decompensation is the focus. Is the diagnosis accurate? Is there drug use or poor compliance? Is there previously unreported physical or sexual abuse? Is there an emerging personality disorder affecting the response to treatment? It is not always necessary to restart the diagnostic process, as is often done on the assumption that there has been some failure on the part of the outpatient clinician. Whenever possible, changes should be made with the involvement of the outpatient clinicians.

Case Vignette

A 16-year-old boy was admitted after a severe suicide attempt. He had been in outpatient treatment for depression for the past 6 months. He overdosed on his antidepressant medications and "everything else I could find" in his parents' medicine cabinet while his parents were away from home in the hope that he would not be found. He was transferred to acute psychiatric hospital care from the medical unit where he had been treated for his overdose. Evaluation revealed obsessive intrusive thoughts of a particularly distressing nature, which the boy tried to manage with a series of rituals that took up more and more of his time. He could manage and tolerate the hand washing and need for extra showers, but he "could not take one more day of having to deal with what goes on in my head." He had not told his outpatient clinician of his thoughts or, surprisingly, of his hand washing and showering. He gave the team permission to pass on this information. The outpatient clinician disclaimed expertise in managing OCD, which it was clear that the patient had. The outpatient clinician worked with the hospital team in trying to identify appropriate treaters. As none were found in the locality, the patient was transferred out-of-state to a hospital that specialized in OCD treatment.

Case Vignette

A 15-year-old girl had been in outpatient treatment with the same psychiatrist and therapist for the past 2 years. She had been diagnosed with a schizoaffective disorder and stabilized on a combination of risperidone and lithium. Over a period of 3 weeks she decompensated. She became suicidal with a plan to overdose on her medicines and drink alcohol "to make sure it works" and also became severely delusional. Voices told her that both her parents were demons and that her older brother had been poisoning her food. She secreted knives around the house against the possibility that she might need to defend herself against her demon parents and her brother, the poisoner. She was admitted for restabilization. Contact with her outpatient psychiatrist and therapist revealed that unknown to her treaters, the patient had discontinued both her medicines in the hope that this would make it easier for her to get a boyfriend. The inpatient team restarted the patient's medication and returned her to her treaters when she was stable (i.e., no longer suicidal or delusional.) Her outpatient therapist planned to work with the patient on how to navigate adolescence with a chronic and severe mental illness.

In cases of decompensation of a patient not receiving outpatient treatment, discharge planning becomes most important, and also determining the reasons for poor outpatient follow-up. If decompensation is medication related, then reasons for medication noncompliance are assessed.

Case Vignette

A 9-year-old boy was admitted for the second time in 8 weeks. Both admissions were for voicing intense suicidal ideation; but this time the boy had threatened to stab himself with a knife he had taken from the kitchen, and he had swallowed five pills he found in the medicine cabinet because he thought "they would make me die." After the first admission, the parents and the boy had been referred to outpatient treatment, but had not followed up. The parents were immigrants from Eastern Europe who spoke poor English. Neither parent believed in mental illness and interpreted the boy's previous admission as a shame to the family. Neither did they believe that a 9-year-old had the capacity to want to die, although both parents were frightened by the recent admission and voiced a willingness to get help for their son. The parents felt the therapist they had been referred to was annoyed with them for not speaking English, so they had not returned. When their son was stable enough for discharge, they were referred to a culturally sensitive therapist who worked in a center for immigrants.

Cases of social and environmental chaos are overrepresented in many acute care hospitals. Work with this group can be difficult as their issues are not illuminated by the medical model, and yet they are sometimes so angry and explosive as to be dangerous and unmanageable in less restrictive levels of care. Families of this group are sometimes difficult to engage in treatment. Contact with social services or foster care agencies is often needed. As much as possible, the acute care unit should avoid being used as respite care for social services.

Case Vignette

A 10-year-old boy returned for his fourth admission in the past year. He was the child of a single mother who was then living with one of her most recent ex-husbands, who was not the child's father. The boy's father, who was reported to be a substance abuser with a diagnosis of bipolar disorder, had no contact with the boy or his mother in the previous 5 years, but the boy was said to resemble him in looks and behavior. The boy was also diagnosed with bipolar disorder and prescribed thioridazine, lithium, and sertraline. The mother was not compliant in providing the boy with the medicine. She requested admission again because of the boy's assaultive and threatening behavior at home, destruction of property, lack of sleep, and screaming at night. However, the boy was well behaved during the admission and was observed unmedicated on the unit. For the next 5 days, no behavioral or psychiatric problems were noted; however, he complained about his circumstances. Throughout his hospital stay, it proved hard to get the mother in for family work or for visits with her son. He behaved badly when his mother came but did well after her departure. The patient was discharged with services recommended. The mother did not follow through in contacting the agencies. The mother made requests for readmission, but these were denied and the case referred to social services. The boy was ultimately placed outside the home.

Certain diagnostic categories are not best served in acute care settings. Eating disorders require specialized treatment with a structure focused on managing food and liquid intake and output. Acute care units do not easily lend themselves to an eating-disorder structure. OCD, which requires a combination of medication and cognitive behavioral therapy, should not be treated in acute care settings, which are typically not set up to provide the detailed behavioral interventions needed. Sexual offenders are often admitted to acute care units for want of anywhere else to send them. What constitutes effective treatment for sexual offenders remains controversial, but it seems clear that acute care units are not suited to their treatment.

THE INITIAL PSYCHIATRIC EVALUATION/ADMISSION PROCESS

There are two common models of physician management in acute care hospitals. One model uses physicians hired by the hospital to provide psychiatric care for the patients. In this model, rounds can be held at a set time each day, leaving the patients free for groups and other forms of treatment. The other model, common on units in general hospitals, is one where multiple private-practice physicians admit to one unit. This model is less supportive of the unit structure as the patient's care is directed by a physician who comes to rounds on a schedule fitting the physician's needs. The most predictable and efficient model, in the authors' opinion, is to have physicians hired by the hospital who work with a team of other mental health professionals.

Ideally the psychiatrist, social worker, and a nurse should be present for the initial admission interview. Obviously, if the patient has been admitted in the middle of the night, this will not be possible, but the next day, the treating team should meet with the patient and parents to go over the details of the history. The admission process should include the parents or guardians and should focus on obtaining the relevant information about which category the patient fits into (new-onset illness, decompensation, etc.). The team interview presents the beginning of teamwork to the patient and parents or guardians and lets them know that the observations of more than one person will matter. The psychiatrist should be careful to ask about previous and current treaters and should let the patient and parents know that contact with current treating clinicians is highly recommended. Evaluation of substance use and of a history of physical and sexual abuse is important, as these problems often underpin the failure of treatment. These evaluations often need to be done privately with the adolescent or child, as young patients may be less forthcoming in the presence of parents or guardians. A growing literature documents the effects of emerging personality disorders on treatment,[9] and the admission assessment should take into account the impact of Axis II diagnoses on presentation and acuity.

The psychiatrist should, at the end of the first evaluation, give parents or guardians some sense of what will happen from then on, when the psychiatrist will be in contact with the parents, and how medication, if necessary, will be handled. In other words, the psychiatrist should begin rudimentary treatment planning. The psychiatrist should confirm the goals of treatment with parents and adolescent: for example, reduction in suicidality, decrease in manic symptoms, ability to maintain safety, or completion of detoxification from an illicit substance. Parents should be told that the current admission is a part of treatment, not the complete treatment, and led to expect that treatment will continue in outpatient settings.

Particular care should be taken to assess for potential for assault and suicidality. Appropriate medicines should be given and proper safety plans made and these plans explained to patient and parents. It is best to do this before the milieu becomes disrupted. The seclusion room should be presented as being available and patients encouraged to use it voluntarily. Seclusion and restraint should not be relied upon as a management technique.

Inpatient stays need not be synonymous with medication changes. Instituting or changing multiple medicines at the same time is not recommended. This practice does not help to clarify which medicines are effective and which might be causing side effects. Medication management is one aspect of psychiatric care, and not always the most important. Medication changes need to be instituted in the context of careful and thoughtful consideration of each case. There are obvious cases, such as agitated psychotic or manic children or adolescents, where medication management is the primary and most effective modality. In such cases, careful and rapid medication stabilization is crucial to a good outcome. But medication management may not be the primary need in all cases. As noted in the introduction, the disturbed behavior of children and adolescents often arises from a complex mix of biological, psychological, and social difficulties. The domain of disruption should be an important factor in guiding medication management. Recent research suggests that dosing of medication might be more effective if based on diagnosis and knowledge of pharmacokinetics in children and adolescents. For example, children with pervasive developmental disorder (PDD) or conduct disorder may need lower doses of antipsychotics than children with mania or florid psychosis.[9,10] Most mood stabilizers, antipsychotics, antidepressants, and antianxiety agents are not approved by U.S. Food and Drug Administration (FDA) for use in children and adolescents, although community standards support their use. Since October 15, 2004 the FDA has added a "black box" warning about the increased risk of suicidal thoughts and behavior in children and adolescents being treated with antidepressant medication. This information should be passed on to parents whose children will need medication management.

Sedation and cognitive dulling can follow use of mood stabilizers. Atypical antipsychotics have seen a fivefold increase in use between 1993 and 2002.[10] Although these medicines are effective in the treatment of some childhood and adolescent disorders—mania, psychosis, aggression in PDD—their use is not without risk. Metabolic effects occur in children and adolescents as well as in adults, and appropriate monitoring of weight, blood glucose, and lipids needs to be a part of inpatient treatment and discharge planning.[11,12] Stimulants are among the few medicines with FDA approval for use in children and adolescents. The risk of diversion should be considered in children with comorbid conduct disorder, oppositional defiant disorder, and substance abuse. Long-acting forms which are less readily diverted, such as methylphenidate (Concerta) and possibly mixed amphetamine salts (Vyvanse), should be considered.

Good behavioral observations by well-trained staff can assist in making diagnostic assessments. Staff observations of interpersonal behavior provide important information. Throughout the admission, unit staff will be assessing the patient's behavior, response to medication, participation in groups and other unit activities, and behavior in family meetings in order to provide as comprehensive a picture as possible in a relatively short time.

MILIEU

Some clinicians more accustomed to outpatient or residential settings assume that acute care units are chaotic, dangerous, noisy places without form or structure. This need not be. The milieu of a child and adolescent acute care unit is as important as that of a child and adolescent long-term unit. The acute care unit has a different focus and a different purpose, but if the milieu is not attended to it will produce less favorable outcomes. Gunderson's five elements of containment, support, structure, involvement, and validation still hold.[13] In Chapter 2 of this volume Munich and Greene discuss the milieu in detail. What follows is a summary of details important to managing a child and adolescent milieu. Not surprisingly, many of the same points will hold for managing any psychiatric milieu whether it treats adults or children.

The unit must provide and encourage both internal and external containment of aggressive and destructive impulses without resorting to punitive means. There should be sufficient staff to provide support such as individual talks, helping with activities the patient may be temporarily unable to perform, and teaching patients effective ways to express emotion. Staff interactions should be therapeutic and not focused solely on giving orders or ensuring that the children follow the rules. More important, there should be enough staff to help patients feel safe and to manage whatever unit disruptions do arise. Uncontained aggression destroys the therapeutic function of the milieu. All staff should be trained in effective ways of managing out-of-control patients.

The rules and the daily program schedule are the most important scaffolding for the child and adolescent milieu. All patients, if they are not too agitated to cooperate, should be given the daily schedule and told the rules and behavioral expectations of the unit. Time spent providing a sense of security and safety will go a long way toward a more favorable outcome. Parents and guardians should be included in the explanation of unit rules and structure. Structure includes such features as morning meetings, set bedtimes and meal times, groups, and scheduled activities. The rules are best presented as part of the safety and treatment on the unit that allow all patients to progress, not as a punitive hammer that falls on the disobedient and disruptive.

Patient involvement in groups and activities should be encouraged, and as much as possible, treatment should be individualized. Patients who have suffered sexual trauma, for example, should not be in groups with sexual offenders or predators.

Care should be given to the rapid establishment of a therapeutic relationship with the patient. A therapeutic relationship does not require months for its establishment. Attention to language used, tone of voice, empathic statements, and nonjudgmental comments are all important. Terms such as *acting out* or *attention seeking* or *manipulating* are not often helpful to adolescent patients. Instead they feel misunderstood and accused of wrongdoing. It is far better to spend time helping the patient understand what a particular behavior is trying to communicate.

Treatment Modalities in the Milieu

Time is of the essence on an acute care unit. As much information as possible needs to be gathered as quickly as possible during a brief hospital stay. One of the best ways to collect and disseminate information regarding multiple aspects of the patient's treatment is to have daily team rounds. At its best the team would consist of psychiatrist, social worker, nurse, and mental health technician. The input of all team members is important to reviewing the patient's progress. Review of the admission, the issues which led to the admission, treatment goals for the admission, medication issues, and discharge planning should be discussed with the patient.

Regular daily meetings between the patient and the same clinician (psychiatrist, psychologist, or social worker) to talk about the admission and to explore the adolescent's ideas of what happened should be an expected part of treatment. The length of the meeting depends on the mental status of the patient, but these individual therapy sessions should be expected to last between 15 minutes and an hour.

The acute care setting lends itself best to groups that do not require consistency of membership for efficacy. Such groups are preferably educationally focused. Goals groups, groups on mindfulness, groups that teach self-regulation principles, medication teaching groups, and groups that help patients begin to see the effects of their environment on their lives are recommended. The overall focus of the groups should be affect and behavioral containment and rudimentary skills training. Groups should not be exploratory with the aim of uncovering traumatic memories or painful emotions. Acute care may not provide the length of stay or the type of milieu that can manage the profound emotional disruption that can accompany the revelation of trauma. School or tutors should be provided for a part of the day and should be an expectation of the milieu. Family therapy is essential but should be understood broadly to include guardians, caretakers, and other crucial members of the patient's intimate network. Activity therapy should be provided as a form of play and relaxation but also as a place to train assertiveness skills and social skills.

Staff Training and Support

The rapid rate of patient turnover on acute care units can lead to frustration and high burnout rates. Staff training and support are an important part of the unit design. Concepts such as transference and counter-transference need to be taught and utilized. Staffs need training in rapidly establishing therapeutic relationships, in effective interventions, and in how to talk with patients. Motivational interviewing provides a useful framework for staff–patient interactions. There needs to be training in behavioral methods of containing violence and aggression (some units focus too heavily on medications and the use of physical restraints). Training in managing suicidal patients and self-injury behaviors is available and should be provided for staff. Staff should be familiar with the rudiments of cognitive behavioral therapy (CBT) and other skills-training modalities. Work on an acute care unit requires a broad base of skills. Regular training helps to keep staff skills fresh and foster a sense of competence. Staff meetings should be held at least weekly to help staff deal with the intensity of the acute care unit by discussions of difficult cases, reactions to patients, or other issues affecting the smooth operation of the unit.

Family Work

Much research supports the inclusion of families in the treatment of patients.[14,15] Family meetings should be scheduled as soon as possible after the admission. Although there might not be sufficient time for a formal family-therapy process, focused family intervention is recommended. The goals might be to look at what was or was not working in the treatment before admission, look at triggers to the admission, suggest parenting classes, begin the exploration of family patterns, direct the family to the local chapter of National Alliance for the Mentally Ill (NAMI), recommend Alcoholic Anonymous (AA) or Narcotic Anonymous (NA) meetings, or provide whatever support the families need. It goes without saying that blaming of families should not occur and that everything should be done to support families and provide hope. Feedback from family meetings can be used in designing an appropriate discharge plan for the patient.

Discharge Planning

Social workers are usually in charge of this aspect of treatment and are usually the conduit to the family and the previous and current outpatient clinicians. Good follow-up can help prevent readmission. Patients should leave the hospital with appointments set up and a clearer sense of the direction of the treatment.

Extended Inpatient and Residential Psychiatric Treatment of Adolescents

Longer treatment courses of intensive inpatient and residential psychiatric treatment of adolescents are different from acute psychiatric hospitalization in a number of ways. Although the goals of acute care are to provide stabilization of psychiatric conditions and to plan outpatient care, the goal of more extended treatment is to understand and alter pathological, repetitive patterns of behavior, and functioning. Such treatment is usually recommended by community treaters when brief acute hospitalizations and outpatient treatment have been insufficient to produce lasting changes in symptom patterns, which may have become progressively more severe, refractory, and dangerous. Treatment in a contained setting is viewed as necessary to effect substantive changes.

Over time, the venues and processes for the provision of intensive, psychiatric treatment in 24-hour programs have gone through extensive changes. Before the 1980s residential treatment was largely based on developmental growth models.[16–18] These were long-term programs with lengths of stay of a year or more. The 1980s saw a growth spurt of various kinds of residential programs based on numerous models and often developed by proprietary organizations.[19] About the same time managed care companies emerged because of dramatic increases in overall health care costs, and one of their targets was the proliferation of residential treatment programs. The aggressive management of residential and extended inpatient treatment resulted in tighter control of authorization for payment for such treatment and drastic reductions in lengths of stay.

Presently, the environment for 24-hour psychiatric care involves stages and varieties of levels of care. A significantly reduced number of psychiatric hospitals provide intensive, individualized psychiatric treatment. A substantial, but reduced, number of residential treatment centers remain. Many offer treatment focused on specific problems, such as substance abuse and eating disorders. Others, such as wilderness programs, provide program-based, milieu experiences. A growing industry is in the area of therapeutic boarding schools, where live-in academic programs include strong therapeutic components.[20] Educational consultants, professionals who develop expertise in placement and knowledge of the variety of available programs, are now very much part of the scene in facilitating appropriate treatment.

Because of the cost of treatment in psychiatric hospitals and intensive residential treatment programs, and its aggressive management by third-party payers, lengths of stay of more than a few weeks or months are unusual. In order to have a successful therapeutic impact such programs must now quickly gain an understanding of the nature of the difficult-to-treat patient's refractory problems, focus treatment on specific objectives, and prepare such patients for transition to less intensive programs.

PATIENT CHARACTERISTICS AND ORIENTATION OF TREATMENT

Most patients referred for extended, intensive evaluation and treatment have had significant courses of previous treatment, including multiple brief hospitalizations, previous attempts at residential treatment, and outpatient treatment with numerous treaters.[21,22] Previous treatment has typically focused on repeated episodes of psychiatric and behavioral problems including self-endangering behaviors (suicide attempts, self-harm by cutting, eating disorders, problematic peer relationships, and drug and alcohol abuse), mood and anxiety disorders, conditions associated with the trauma of significant losses and sexual abuse, psychotic episodes, school failure, oppositional and defiant behavior, and serious family relational problems.

Treatment focuses on diagnostic understanding and treatment planning, the identification of core issues that have prevented progress or the maintenance of progress in other treatment settings, the establishment of a treatment alliance with both patient and family, the prioritization of problems and goals, careful review of psychiatric medication and aggressive medication trials where indicated, and systematic aftercare planning and collaboration with local treaters.

THE DIAGNOSTIC PROCESS: CORE ISSUES

Achieving a comprehensive diagnostic understanding of the patient's problems is crucial to creating a path for a functional life, as well as for treatment and aftercare. Patients with chronic, hard-to-treat problems are confused about what is wrong and what to do about it. The patients and their parents are seeking direction, a road map of sorts, which involves an understanding of the problems, clear options for treatment, and a long-range plan for managing the ups and downs of aftercare. Adolescents and their parents can tolerate struggles to the degree that chaos is not allowed to prevail; they need some guiding principles that enable them to feel more in control at times of crisis. Achieving a comprehensive diagnostic understanding of the patient's problems can be time-consuming and expensive. However, failing to focus attention on developing a careful understanding of the patient runs the risk of treatment failure because critical issues may not be understood and addressed.

Despite competent and thoughtful treatment these young patients have either failed to make significant progress or have been unable to sustain their gains. Rather than repeat treatment that has not been effective, a more focused approach is to ask questions about the problem of treatment. What are the factors that continue to drive the current pathology/or conflict? What has prevented previous treatment attempts from being successful? The work of trying to answer these questions leads to the identification of *core issues*, those problems or processes that are central to the refractory nature of the pathology.[23] The biopsychosocial model leads to a diagnostic process in which the core issues may be seen as reflective of biological issues, or having roots in psychological phenomena, or related to social or familial processes. Sometimes the core issues become readily identifiable. Often they have been previously hidden and elusive and require considerable exploration. Many times the core issues are multifaceted and appear to be combinations of several factors that have become interrelated.

A sample of commonly identified core issues includes the following:

Individual
- Multiple symptoms and confusion about primary problems and diagnosis
- Failure to respond to medication and the need for more systematic trials in a safe setting
- Unidentified and untreated subtle, but consequential, thought disorders or other cognitive deficits
- Separation and individuation issues that are masked by behavior problems
- Self-injurious behavior and the establishment of abusive relationships related to unidentified or unresolved trauma
- Distorted perceptions of self, for example, expectations that are inconsistent with abilities, patterns of self-loathing
- Vulnerability to emotional states and poor tolerance of emotions leading to impulsive behavior, for example, self-harm or externally focused outbursts

Family and Social
- Mismatch between the patient's abilities and parents' and patient's expectations of achievement
- Subtle expectations and messages in the family that prevent the expression of authentic thoughts and feelings
- Family myths and transgenerational expectations
- Unspoken issues, for example, trauma, relationship issues, "secrets" about family members
- Dysfunctional family patterns of handling conflict, emotions, dependence, and independence
- Failure to find acceptance in a peer group

The following vignettes are illustrative.

Case Vignette

Jane had suffered early, multiple losses. She grew up in foster care and institutions. She had a psychotic disorder, which was fairly well managed by medication. She hoped to eventually become more independent and move to a transitional program. However, her persistent self-injury by cutting prevented movement toward this goal. She acknowledged fear of failure and of being alone. Previous treatment had focused on the control and management of the self-harm, but this approach had not been successful. The focus of treatment was changed to helping Jane deal with separation and abandonment issues, along with learning more about the ongoing supports available in her current and transitional programs. This reduced Jane's view that "independence equals abandonment." Jane worked actively to stop her self-harming behaviors, and she was able to move forward.

Case Vignette

Kathy was admitted following suicide attempts and brief hospitalizations. These had been occasioned by the death by suicide of a close friend and Kathy having been raped by a male acquaintance. She continued to be depressed and vulnerable to self-harm. As she began to trust her treaters she acknowledged that she privately feared that her parents blamed her for and were humiliated by the rape despite their overtly supportive stance. Kathy assumed that her parents saw her as immoral and worthless. She felt responsible for the friend's death. She feared that she would never be able to please or separate from her parents. Treatment focused on helping Kathy distinguish between her own feelings and those of her parents, discuss her feelings openly with them, and work together to face gradual separation and growth.

Case Vignette

Chad, a 16-year-old boy from a very successful and affluent family, aspired to live up to and surpass his family's standards. In his senior year of high school he began to falter academically, developed severe anxiety about school performance, became depressed, and began to express suicidal ideation. Outpatient treatment for anxiety and depression was unsuccessful. Early in his intensive hospital treatment Chad acknowledged his puzzling symptoms but was very defensive about his abilities. Psychological testing revealed deficits in nonverbal cognitive functioning. Chad's supportive parents were quick to understand that the demands of his high achievement-oriented college preparatory school program were too much for him. Treatment focused on helping Chad accept his limitations, yet also see the successful future he could still have with appropriate academic planning.

The following case example highlights the problems involved in complicated core issues and the establishment of a treatment plan.

Case Vignette

Linda, a 15-year-old girl, had a history of potentially quite dangerous behaviors. She had long-standing depression, suicidal behavior, and a pattern of self-injury by inflicting cuts on herself. Most of the cutting was superficial, but she had literally dozens of scars on her arms and legs. At admission, Linda stated that her anxiety and depression got so unbearable at times that she felt hopeless, and this had frequently led to her cutting and suicidal behavior.

Linda's severe anxiety was persistent and particularly debilitating. It seemed related to multiple issues including inability to complete tasks and perform at school; extraordinary self-consciousness about her appearance, including her weight; and worry about her social acceptability to peers and often feeling unable to talk with them. Linda had developed a number of compulsive rituals that had increased over time and made her seem odd to others. A number of medicines for these problems had been tried with minimal success. In addition, on admission to the hospital Linda acknowledged a long history of bulimic symptoms, which she had never conveyed to her parents or other treaters. This array of problems, manifesting themselves prominently at varying times, had led to many diagnoses and treatment approaches at numerous facilities. Previous treatment had focused on the management of Linda's behavior and control of her mood states.

Despite efforts to establish an overall understanding of her problems, and how they each related to each other, Linda vacillated between symptom patterns. Linda demonstrated well above average intelligence, good long-term memory and executive function, and goal-directed behavior important for success in most activities. However, she had difficulties in short-term memory and auditory attention. Linda's distractibility revealed itself to be quite debilitating.

Linda acknowledged how hard and painful it was for her to try and articulate her difficulties concentrating, her volatile emotions, and other problems. She complained that she could not keep thoughts in her head, that she was distracted by both inner and outer stimuli, and that she just could not "think." She often became overwhelmed by the frustration of trying to put her thoughts into words when she was in the midst of mental confusion or emotional upset. Earlier in treatment she had been too embarrassed and felt "stupid," but she began to allow help and support in her communication with others. The entire treatment team focused on helping her to communicate in small and manageable doses. Linda began to trust this process, and her emotional tone brightened. Changes were made in Linda's medicines as she became able to communicate better about their effects on her. Over time, with the belief that she could make herself understood, Linda's other symptom patterns began to abate. Her management of emotions, including communicating about them, became the central focus of her treatment.

The focus on identifying core issues and establishing increasing clarity regarding the patient's diagnostic picture is essential to treatment progress. However, the diagnostic process is an ongoing aspect of treatment, and new information about the patient helps to clarify and refine this understanding. Each level of refinement, then, helps to inform the treatment plan, so that the diagnostic process and the provision of treatment are in continuous dialogue. The patient, the parents, and all members of the treatment team need to be encouraged to contribute actively to the identification of core issues and the refinement of diagnostic understanding and treatment planning.

THE TREATING MILIEU

The nature of the living milieu, including the relationships with treaters, unit staff, and fellow patients, constitutes the primary basis for the therapeutic encounter. Although the course of treatment may be a number of weeks rather than months, Winnicott's[24] concept of the treatment program as a *holding environment* may be even more important in the present environment than it was 40 years ago. In the intervening years the most significant change to the provision of extended inpatient and residential treatment for children and adolescents has been, of course, the drastic drop in length of stay and the need for more directly focused treatment. In addition, there have been numerous advances in specific treatment interventions for children and adolescents, which are reviewed and summarized in a number of works.[25,26] And, while the theoretic underpinnings of treatment have also undergone revision, the character and the essential elements of the day-to-day structure of the milieu[27-29] have remained more constant.

The development of a therapeutic alliance and the willingness to engage and share personal aspects of self are based in large part on the belief by the patient and family that the treating milieu is truly supportive of them as people and is a healthy environment. The milieu must be experienced as a safe place, both physically and emotionally, for patients to establish enough trust to address their personal issues. There should be well-established and clearly communicated expectations with consistent rules and structure. There is a balance between control of behavior on the one hand, and graded opportunities and practicing being more independent on the other. Staff members engage with patients in nonconflict and competence-building areas as well as in spheres of problems and conflict. Parents are valued as contributors to a positive outcome in addition to having issues of their own that require attention.

Individual work with patients and their families is a valued and necessary part of treatment, but the treatment takes place in the context of a treatment team and peer group who are aware of the patient's needs and goals, and who see themselves as having an active and specific responsibility for progress. The establishment of a connection between staff group, patient group, and individual patient is an essential element in creating a working alliance in focused treatment and is a goal that must be addressed upon admission. A collaborative treatment alliance is encouraged by careful attention to the presenting problems and shared identification of core issues, but also by engaging with the patient in the social activities of the unit and in supporting the patient's successes in the interpersonal world of the treatment milieu.

Ultimately, treatment is focused on the individual, not the group. However, the nature and functioning of the patient group is critical to individual progress. Most patients feel alone and isolated with their problems. Focus on group activities, shared experiences, and living together are accentuated and are nurtured for the purpose of developing a healthy context for the patient to feel a sense of belonging in a peer group where others are also struggling. A healthy, treatment-oriented peer group facilitates individual progress. A negative peer group that disparages treatment and reinforces negative behavior detracts from and hinders the individual patient's sense of emotional safety in addressing core issues.

THE TREATMENT TEAM

Historically, treatment teams in residential treatment functioned much like a therapeutic family, with the various members of the team taking on roles of consistent, parenting adults. Modern treatment that focuses on core issues requires the establishment of a *working team* in which there is greater delineation of function. Team members focus on various aspects of treatment based on their skills and expertise and identified areas of responsibility. Nurses and mental health counselors have a monitoring functioning related to safety and well-being. Chemical dependency counselors formulate and coordinate the aspects of treatment that pertain to substance abuse and addiction. Teachers attempt to help patients regain a sense of confidence and productivity at school. Social workers focus on interpersonal relatedness between the patient and family, strengths and dysfunctional aspects of family patterns, and the replication of such patterns in the treatment milieu. Individual and group psychotherapists work to help patients see their problems more clearly and to develop more functional perspective about their own roles in managing them. Various members of the team may be involved in the conducting of various program groups and activities that focus on the patients' targeted areas of need. The psychiatrist has medical and psychiatric responsibilities, especially in the establishment of diagnostic clarity and the direction and evaluation of medication strategies.

Although it is important to delineate specific roles and activities, such disparity of responsibilities can lead to isolation of the team members, and, therefore, fragmentation of the treatment. Team members share in common the importance of establishing trusting relationships with the patient and family. Team discussions may often focus on the contrasting experiences staff members have of the patients and families, and these differences of view are helpful in understanding the complexities and inconsistencies in the patients' and families' varying modes of conduct and relatedness. Ultimately, however, team members must have a shared vision of the treatment, especially with respect to the identified core issues and treatment goals.

Mental health colleagues who referred the patient for treatment or who are receiving the patient as part of the aftercare plan are also considered members of the treatment team. Reporting progress to them and seeking their consultation serve to protect a sense of continuity of care and secure their continued interest and participation, which are important to successful aftercare.

PSYCHOTHERAPIES AND PSYCHOEDUCATIONAL PROCESSES

Many programs focus on psychotherapy as the mainstay of treatment. Other treatment venues emphasize *the program*, generally referring to the focus on the patient group and the educational aspects of the program. Both points of view have advantages; however, there is a great deal of variability in the relative impact of various treatment experiences on individual patients. Individual, group, and family psychotherapy can open the doors to reflection, acceptance, and problem solving. These approaches are highly valued and emphasized as critical aspects of the treatment in many successful treatment programs. All provide venues for the establishment of relatedness between patients and treaters. Group therapy reduces experiences of isolation in the loneliness of one's problems and also offers a sense of a shared stake in problem solving with one's peers. Family therapy creates the potential for healing of long-standing resentments and the development of new, more effective ways of relating between family members.

However, some patients' functioning and development are hampered by their failure to develop certain skills or learn to cope with their limitations. Psychotherapy may be helpful in these situations, but other specialized training and education methods more specifically emphasize practical approaches and strategies for dealing with these problem areas. The specialized therapeutic school provides an opportunity for careful attention to the factors that have previously contributed to school failure; and individualized programs for learning can be put into place. Patients with a history of substance abuse require specific programs of individual and group approaches to address their addictive behaviors. Traumatized patients may benefit from problem-specific approaches such as eye movement desensitization and reprocessing (EMDR).[30] Patients with a history of inflicting injuries on themselves, such as cutting and burning, require specialized treatment depending on the function of the self-injurious behavior. Those with eating disorders also often benefit from groups that focus on body image, control, and one's relationship to food. A number of psychoeducational groups have been developed that focus on such areas as coping with trauma,[31] helping patients with psychotic disorders to think more clearly through neurocognitive training,[32] and management of anger and other emotions. Although dialectical behavior therapy[33] was originally formulated as an outpatient team treatment, variations of it are used in the hospital treatment phase of those patients who have significant borderline personality traits. These various approaches are determined based on assessment of the patient's core issues, assets, and limitations.

RECENT ADVANCES: AGENCY AND MENTALIZATION

The concept of the therapeutic alliance has a central place in the literature on psychological treatments of all kinds, from individual psychotherapy to hospital treatment. Treatments that are more behaviorally focused require the patient's cooperation, participation, and, ultimately, ownership of many aspects of the process. Collaboration and the therapeutic alliance have been specifically studied as part of the hospital and residential treatment of adolescents. O'Malley[34] focused on precursors to collaboration in the treatment of hospitalized adolescents. In that study collaboration was defined as "both the active use of treatment for constructive change, and the recognition of one's own contribution to problems and the taking of some responsibility for their resolution." In most cases adolescent patients do not actively collaborate as full partners in the process. Indeed, collaborative behavior is sometimes difficult to achieve with adolescents in residential or hospital care, who may have been coerced into treatment, do not trust adults, and rebel against their treaters as a way to hold on to some semblance of autonomy. Treaters need to look for and encourage "precursors" to collaboration. Examples include the patient's acceptance of containment, the communication of symptoms, working to meet developmental expectations (e.g., academic performance), the formation of attachments, and cooperation in solving problems related to conflict-free areas of the patient's functioning. Ideally, these processes lead to active collaboration regarding the patient's core problems. This last level of collaboration involves what has been characterized as the patient's acceptance of *agency* for the illness. Allen[35] described this attribute as making "active efforts to recover" and a feeling of being able to "do something" about one's problems. Ultimately, the presence of collaboration, or agency, is based on the nature of the relationship between the adolescent and the treatment team. Both sides have an investment in the outcome and share responsibility for the work involved.

Discussion of the nature of the relationship between adolescent and treater brings the authors to a more recently investigated concept—mentalization. According to Allen and Fonagy,[36] mentalizing is a capacity. Although it is related to such concepts as psychological mindedness, observing ego, empathy, and insight, it also involves additional properties that are central and essential to the mental activity of both the treating professional and the patient. Allen[37] describes mentalizing as treating others as persons rather than objects. Mentalizing involves the ability to think about another person—to formulate ideas about the person's mental life and also to empathize with and mirror back to the other person a sense of emotional attunement. Another way of putting it is that mentalizing involves the ability to entertain multiple perspectives about other people, their points of view, and the nature of one's own life experiences. From a developmental standpoint, the capacity to mentalize reflects the evolution of healthy and secure emotional attachments and is compromised by insecure attachments produced by maltreatment and emotional trauma.[38,39] Given such circumstances and experiences, many disturbed adolescent patients have great difficulty mentalizing. They have trouble examining their own inner worlds and in seeing things from another person's perspective. This capacity, essential for effective treatment and personal development, is facilitated by the actions of the therapist in psychotherapy and the entire team in hospital and residential treatment. So, as the therapist demonstrates the capacity and willingness to mentalize, to keep the patient's "mind in mind," the patient feels understood and valued, and, thereby, begins to develop the same capacity to examine oneself and develop an empathic attitude toward others. (See also, Chapter 14.)

Summary

Acute inpatient care is a necessary part of the continuum of care for children and adolescents. Well-designed acute care treatment concentrates on safety, diagnostic clarity, effective medication management, focused family intervention, and good discharge planning, The future will bring studies on what is effective in short-term care, leading to the design of even more effective acute care units.

Focused psychiatric hospital and residential treatment of adolescent patients with difficult-to-treat or refractory illnesses is driven and informed by a diagnostic understanding of the biopsychosocial elements that have affected and continue to affect the functioning of the patient. Identification of core issues that have compromised or prevented sustained progress is essential in order to effect successful treatment. Intensive treatment is multidimensional in nature, bringing to bear various complementary modes of therapy and education. The working team strives to operate as one unified force, with an eye on the core issues and attempting to engage the patient and family in working toward collaboration and problem solving. The power of positive relatedness in every aspect of the patient's treatment experience is critical to the development of a working relationship and the ability of the patient genuinely to explore those issues that may be most difficult, yet necessary to address.

REFERENCES

1. Geller JL, Beibel K. The premature demise of public child and adolescent inpatient beds. Part II: Challenges and implications. *Psychiatr Q.* 2006;77:273–291.
2. Walsh B. *Treating self injury: a practical guide.* New York: Guilford Press; 2005.
3. Weisbrot DM, Carlson GA. Diagnostically homeless. What to do if no diagnosis fits. *Curr Psychiatry.* 2005;4:25–42.
4. Liebenluft E, Charney DS, Towbin KE, et al. Defining clinical phenotypes of juvenile mania. *Am J Psychiatry.* 2003;160:430–437.
5. Munich RL. Efforts to preserve the mind in contemporary hospital treatment. *Bull Menninger Clin.* 2003;76:167–186.
6. O'Malley F. Contemporary issues in the psychiatric residential treatment of disturbed adolescents. *Child Adolesc Clin N Am.* 2004;13: 255–266.
7. Olfson M, Blanco C. National trends in the outpatient treatment of children and adolescents with anti psychotic drugs. *Arch Gen Psychiatry.* 2006;63:679–685.
8. Ionescu D, Ruedrich S. Inpatient treatment planning: Consider 6 pre-admission patterns. *Curr Psychiatry.* 2006;5(12):23–31.
9. Bleiberg E. *Treating personality disorders in children and adolescents.* New York: Guilford Press; 2001.
10. Kowatch RA, Fristad MA. Treatment guidelines for children and adolescents with bipolar disorder. *J Am Acad Child Adolesc Psychiatry.* 2005;44(3): 213–235.
11. Kowatch RA, Janicak PG. Are antipsychotics over prescribed in children? *Curr Psychiatry* 2006;5(9); [Online].
12. Cheng-Shannon J, McGough J. Second generation antipsychotic medications in children and adolescents. *J Child Adolesc Psychopharmacol.* 2004; 14(3):372–394.
13. Gunderson JG. Defining the therapeutic process in psychiatric milieus. *Psychiatry.* 1978;41(4): 337–335.
14. Bender K, Springer DW. Treatment effectiveness with dually diagnosed adolescents. *Brief treatment and crisis intervention.* 2006;6:177–205.
15. Werner-Wilson RJ. *Developmental systemic family therapy with adolescents.* Haworth Press; 2001.
16. Redl F. The concept of the therapeutic milieu. *Am J Orthopsychiatry.* 1950;29:721–736.
17. Bettleheim B. *Love is not enough.* Glencoe: Free Press; 1950.
18. Trieschman A, Whittaker J, Brendtro L. *The other 23 hours: child-care work with emotionally disturbed children in a therapeutic milieu.* New York: Aldine de Gruyter; 1969.
19. Wells K. Placement of emotionally disturbed children in residential treatment: A review of placement criteria. *Am J Orthopsychiatry.* 1991;61:339–347.
20. Santa J, Moss J. A brief history of the national association of therapeutic schools and programs. *J Therapeutic Schools Programs.* 2006;1:11–19.
21. Lyman R, Campbell N. *Treating children and adolescents.* Thousand Oaks: Sage Publications; 1996:25–30.
22. Khan A. *Short-term psychiatric hospitalization of adolescents.* Chicago: Year Book Medical Publishers; 1990:167–171.
23. O'Malley F. Critical issues in short-term residential treatment. *Res. Treat. Child. Youth.* 1996; 14(1):61–74.
24. Winnicott D. *The maturational processes and facilitating environment.* New York: International Universities Press; 1965.
25. Evans D, Foa E, Gur R, et al. *Treating and preventing adolescent mental health disorders: what we know and what we don't know.* Oxford: Oxford University Press; 2005.
26. Fonagy P, Target M, Cottrell D, et al. *What works for whom: a critical review of treatments for children and adolescents.* New York: Guildford Press; 2002.
27. Rinsley D. *Treatment of the disturbed adolescent.* New York: Aronson; 1980.
28. Masterson J. *Treatment of the borderline adolescent: a developmental approach.* New York: John Wiley & Sons; 1972.
29. Viner J. Milieu concepts for short-term hospital treatment of borderline patients. *Psychiatr Q.* 1985;57:127–133.
30. Shapiro F. *Eye movement desensitization and reprocessing: basic principles, protocols and procedures.* New York: Guilford Press; 1995.
31. Allen J. *Traumatic relationships and serious mental disorders.* New York: John Wiley & Sons; 2001.
32. Brenner H, Roder V, Hadel B, et al. Integrative psychological therapy for schizophrenic patients. Toronto: Hogrefe & Huber Publishers, 1994.
33. Linehan M. *Cognitive-behavioral treatment of borderline personality disorder.* New York: Guilford Press; 1993.
34. O'Malley F. Developing a therapeutic alliance in the hospital treatment of disturbed adolescents. In: Menninger W, Allen J, Leichtman M, et al. eds. *Hospitalization in the psychiatric treatment of children and adolescents.* Topeka, Kansas: The Menninger Foundation; 1990;13–24.
35. Allen J. Agency: How patients participate in their own recovery. *Menninger Perspect.* 2005;2:18–20.

36. Allen JG, Fonagy P. *Handbook of mentalization-based treatment.* New York: John Wiley & Sons; 2006.

37. Allen JG. Mentalizing. *Bull Menninger Clin.* 2003;67:87–108.

38. Bateman AW, Ryle A, Fonagy P, et al. Psychotherapy for borderline personality disorder: Mentalization based therapy and cognitive analytic therapy compared. *Int Rev Psychiatry.* 2007;19(1):51–62.

39. Fonagy P, Bateman AW. Mechanisms of change in mentalization-based treatment of BPD. *J Clin Psychol.* 2006;62(4):411–430.

Index